Colorectal Surgery
Third Edition

Take a look at the other great titles in the Companion Series...

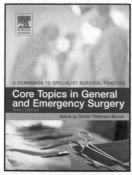

Paterson-Brown
Core Topics in
General and
Emergency Surgery
3rd Edition
0702027332

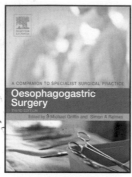

Griffin & Raimes
Oesophagogastric
Surgery
3rd Edition
0702027359

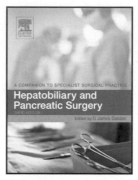

Garden
Hepatobiliary and
Pancreatic Surgery
3rd Edition
0702027367

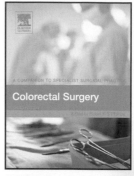

Phillips
Colorectal Surgery
3rd Edition
0702027324

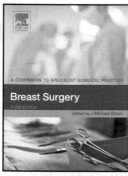

Dixon
Breast Surgery
3rd Edition
0702027383

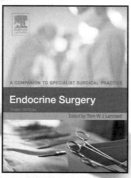

Lennard
Endocrine Surgery
3rd Edition
0702027391

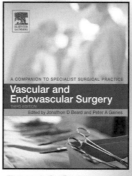

Beard & Gaines
Vascular and
Endovascular
Surgery
3rd Edition
0702027340

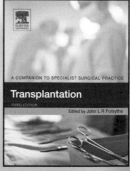

Forsythe
Transplantation
3rd Edition
0702027375

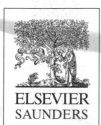

ELSEVIER
SAUNDERS

Order either through your local bookshop, direct from Elsevier
(call customer services on +44 (0)1865 474000) or log on to
http://www.elsevierhealth.com/surgery

A Companion to Specialist Surgical Practice
Third Edition

Series Editors
O. James Garden
Simon Paterson-Brown

Colorectal Surgery
Third Edition

Edited by
Robin K.S. Phillips
Professor of Colorectal Surgery
Imperial College London
and
Consultant Surgeon and Clinical Director
St Mark's Hospital
Harrow, Middlesex

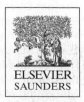

ELSEVIER
SAUNDERS

ELSEVIER
SAUNDERS

An imprint of Elsevier Limited

First edition 1997
Second edition 2001
Third edition 2005
Reprinted 2006
© 2005, Elsevier Limited. All rights reserved.

ISBN 0 7020 2732 4

British Library Cataloguing in Publication Data
A catalogue record for this book is available from the British Library

Library of Congress Cataloging in Publication Data
A catalog record for this book is available from the Library of Congress

Notice
Medical knowledge is constantly changing. Standard safety precautions must be followed, but as new research and clinical experience broaden our knowledge, changes in treatment and drug therapy may become necessary or appropriate. Readers are advised to check the most current product information provided by the manufacturer of each drug to be administered to verify the recommended dose, the method and duration of administration, and contraindications. It is the responsibility of the practitioner, relying on experience and knowledge of the patient, to determine dosages and the best treatment for each individual patient. Neither the Publisher nor the editor assumes any liability for any injury and/or damage to persons or property arising from this publication.
The Publisher

Printed in The Netherlands
Last digit is the print number: 9 8 7 6 5 4 3 2 1

Commissioning Editor: Michael Houston
Project Development Manager: Sheila Black
Editorial Assistants: Kathryn Mason, Liz Brown
Project Manager: Cheryl Brant
Design Manager: Jayne Jones
Illustration Manager: Mick Ruddy
Illustrator: Martin Woodward
Marketing Managers: Gaynor Jones (UK), Ethel Cathers (USA)

Contents

Contributors

David E. Beck MD FACS FASCRS
Chairman, Department of Colon and
Rectal Surgery
Ochsner Clinic Foundation
New Orleans, LA, USA

Sue Clark MD FRCS(Gen Surg)
Consultant Colorectal Surgeon
The Royal London Hospital
London, UK

**Sir Ara Darzi KBE MD FRCS FRCSI
FACS FRCPSG FMedSci**
Professor of Surgery and Head of
Division of Surgery, Anaesthetics and
Intensive Care
Imperial College London
London, UK

Paul Durdey MS FRCS
Consultant Surgeon
Bristol Royal Infirmary
Bristol, UK

Anton V. Emmanuel BSc MD FRCP
Senior Lecturer and Consultant in
Gastrointestinal Physiology
St Mark's Hospital
Harrow, Middlesex, UK

**Paul Hatfield BSc MB ChB MRCP
FRCR**
Specialist Registrar in Clinical
Oncology
Leeds Cancer Centre
Cookridge Hospital
Leeds, UK

**Alexander G. Heriot MA MD
FRCS(Gen Surg) FRCS(Ed)**
Consultant Colorectal Surgeon
St Mary's Hospital
London, UK

**Ming Hian Kam MB BS MRCS
MMed(Surg)**
Registrar, Department of Colorectal
Surgery
Singapore General Hospital
Singapore

**Zygmunt H. Krukowski MB ChB
PhD FRCS(Ed) Hon FRCS(Glasg)
FRCP**
Professor of Clinical Surgery
University of Aberdeen;
Consultant Surgeon
Aberdeen Royal Infirmary
Aberdeen, UK

**Peter J. Lunniss BSc MS
FRCS(Gen Surg)**
Senior Lecturer and Honorary
Consultant
Centre for Academic Surgery
Royal London and Homerton
Hospitals
London, UK

**Neil J.McC. Mortensen MB ChB
MD FRCS**
Professor of Colorectal Surgery
John Radcliffe Hospital
Oxford, UK

**R. John Nicholls MA BChir FRCS
FRCS(Glasg)**
Professor of Colorectal Surgery
Imperial College London;
Consultant Surgeon
St Mark's Hospital
Harrow, Middlesex, UK

Robin K.S. Phillips MB BS FRCS
Professor of Colorectal Surgery
Imperial College London;
Consultant Surgeon and Clinical
Director
St Mark's Hospital
Harrow, Middlesex, UK

**John H. Scholefield MB ChB MD
FRCS**
Professor of Surgery
Queen's Medical Centre
University Hospital
Nottingham, UK

**David Sebag-Montefiore FRCP
FRCR**
Consultant Clinical Oncologist
Leeds Cancer Centre
Cookridge Hospital
Leeds, UK

Asha Senapati PhD FRCS
Consultant Colorectal Surgeon
Queen Alexandra Hospital
Portsmouth, UK

**Francis Seow-Choen MB BS
FRCS(Ed) FAMS, FRES**
Senior Consultant Surgeon
Seow-Choen Colorectal Centre
Singapore

**Robert J.C. Steele MD FRCS(Ed)
FRCS FCSHK**
Professor of Surgery and Head of
Department of Surgery and Molecular
Oncology
University of Dundee Medical School
Ninewells Hospital
Dundee, UK

Paris P. Tekkis MD FRCS(Gen Surg)
Senior Lecturer
Imperial College London;
Consultant Colorectal Surgeon
St Mary's Hospital
London, UK

**Mark W. Thompson-Fawcett
MB ChB FRACS**
Senior Lecturer and Colorectal
Surgeon
University of Otago
Dunedin, New Zealand

**Jared Torkington MS
FRCS(Gen Surg)**
Consultant Surgeon
Llandough Hospital
Penarth, UK

**Charles B. Whitlow MD FACS
FASCRS**
Program Director, Colon and Rectal
Surgery Residency
and Staff Colorectal Surgeon
Ochsner Clinic Foundation
New Orleans, LA, USA

**Andrew B. Williams MS
FRCS(Gen Surg)**
Consultant Surgeon and
Director, Pelvic Floor Unit
St Thomas' Hospital
London, UK

**Alastair C.J. Windsor MD FRCS
FRCS(Ed)**
Consultant Colorectal Surgeon
St Mark's Hospital
Harrow, Middlesex, UK

Preface

The *Companion to Specialist Surgical Practice* series was designed to meet the needs of surgeons in higher training and practising consultants who wish up-to-date and evidence-based information on the subspecialist areas relevant to their surgical practice. In trying to meet this aim, we have recognised that the series will never be as all-encompassing as many of the larger reference surgical textbooks. However, by their very size, it is rare that the latter are completely up to date at the time of publication. The first edition of this series was published in 1997, with the second following in 2001. In this third edition, we have been able to bring up to date the relevant specialist information that we and the individual volume editors consider important for the practising subspecialist surgeon. Where possible, all contributors have attempted to identify evidence-based references to support key recommendations within each chapter. These should all be interpreted with the help of the guidance summary 'Evidence-based practice in surgery', which follows this preface.

We are extremely grateful to all volume editors and to their contributors to this third edition. It is thanks to their enthusiasm and hard work that the relatively short time frame between each of the editions has been maintained, thereby providing to the reader the most accurate and up-to-date information possible. We were all immensely saddened by the sudden and tragic death of Professor John Farndon, who edited the first and second editions of the volumes *Breast Surgery* and *Endocrine Surgery*. While recognising that he was a unique and talented individual, we are pleased to welcome the additional editorial skills of Mike Dixon and Tom Lennard for this third edition.

We are also grateful for the support and encouragement of Elsevier Ltd and hope that our aim – of providing up-to-date and affordable surgical texts – has been met and that all readers, whether in training or in consultant practice, will find this third edition a valuable resource.

Colorectal surgery has changed quite considerably in the last 4 years. Rectal cancer imaging has been transformed by thin-slice MRI, simplifying decision-making regarding adjuvant radiotherapy. A host of new approaches to haemorrhoidal disease are currently being explored. The previously undescribed recessive *MYH* polyposis explains a number of apparently *FAP*-gene-negative polyposis patients. The third edition reflects this, with an additional chapter on functional problems and their management along with completely rewritten chapters by a number of new, cutting-edge authors.

O. James Garden BSc, MB, ChB, MD, FRCS(Glasg), FRCS(Ed), FRCP(Ed)
Regius Professor of Clinical Surgery, Clinical and Surgical Sciences (Surgery), University of Edinburgh, and Honorary Consultant Surgeon, Royal Infirmary of Edinburgh

Simon Paterson-Brown MB, BS, MPhil, MS, FRCS(Ed), FRCS
Honorary Senior Lecturer, Clinical and Surgical Sciences (Surgery), University of Edinburgh, and Consultant General and Upper Gastrointestinal Surgeon, Royal Infirmary of Edinburgh

Robin K.S. Phillips MB, BS, FRCS
Professor of Colorectal Surgery, Imperial College London, and Consultant Surgeon and Clinical Director, St Mark's Hospital, Harrow, Middlesex

EVIDENCE-BASED PRACTICE IN SURGERY

The third edition of the *Companion to Specialist Surgical Practice* series has attempted to incorporate, where appropriate, **evidence-based practice in surgery**, which has been highlighted in the text and relevant references. A detailed chapter on evidence-based practice in surgery, written by Kathryn Rigby and Jonathan Michaels, has been included in the volume *Core Topics in General and Emergency Surgery*, to which the reader is referred for further information on assessing levels of evidence. We are grateful to them for providing this summary for each volume.

Critical appraisal for developing evidence-based practice can be obtained from a number of sources, the most reliable being randomised controlled clinical trials, systematic literature reviews, meta-analyses and observational studies. For practical purposes, three grades of evidence can be used, analogous to the levels of 'proof' required in a court of law:

1. **Beyond reasonable doubt** – such evidence is likely to have arisen from high-quality randomised controlled trials, systematic reviews, or high-quality synthesised evidence such as decision analysis, cost-effectiveness analysis or large observational data sets. The studies need to be directly applicable to the population of concern and have clear results. The grade is analogous to burden of proof within a crimimal court and may be thought of as corresponding to the usual standard of 'proof' within the medical literature (i.e. $P<0.05$).
2. **On the balance of probabilities** – in many cases a high-quality review of literature may fail to reach firm conclusions owing to conflicting or inconclusive results, trials of poor methodological quality or the lack of evidence in the population to which the guidelines apply. In such cases it may still be possible to make a statement as to the best treatment on the 'balance of probabilities'. This is analogous to the decision in a civil court where all the available evidence will be weighed up and the verdict will depend upon the balance of probabilities.
3. **Not proven** – insufficient evidence upon which to base a decision or contradictory evidence.

Depending on the information available, three grades of recommendation can be used:

a. strong recommendation, which should be followed unless there are compelling reasons to act otherwise;
b. a recommendaton based on evidence of effectiveness but where there may be other factors to take into account in decision-making, for example the user of the guidelines may be expected to take into account patient preferences, local facilities, local audit results or available resources;
c. a recommendation made where there is no adequate evidence regarding the most effective practice, although there may be reasons for making a recommendation in order to minimise cost or reduce the chance of error through a locally agreed protocol.

The text and references that are considered to be associated with reasonable evidence are highlighted in this volume with a 'scalpel code', leaving the reader to reach his or her own conclusion.

Acknowledgements

I should like to thank my personal assistant, Marie Gun, for all her hard work coordinating and marshalling the excellent group of contributors, and my wife, Janina, for her encouragement and support.

RKSP

CHAPTER
One
Anorectal investigation

Andrew B. Williams

INTRODUCTION

A wide range of tests is available to the clinician for investigating anorectal disorders. Each investigation will only provide part of a patient's assessment and results should be considered in conjunction with the other tests and the clinical picture as detailed by a careful history and physical examination.

Investigations provide information about structure alone, function alone, or both, and have been directed to five general areas of interest: faecal incontinence, constipation (including Hirschsprung's disease), anorectal sepsis, rectal prolapse (including solitary rectal ulcer syndrome) and anorectal malignancy.

ANATOMY AND PHYSIOLOGY OF THE ANAL CANAL

The anal canal in adults is approximately 4 cm long and begins as the rectum narrows, passing backwards between the levator ani muscles.[1] It has an upper limit at the pelvic floor and a lower limit at the anus.[2] The proximal canal is lined by simple columnar epithelium, which changes to stratified squamous epithelium lower in the canal via an intermediate transition zone just above the dentate line.[3] Beneath the mucosa is the subepithelial tissue, which is composed of connective tissue and smooth muscle.[1] This layer increases in thickness throughout life and forms the basis of the vascular cushions thought to be important in the maintenance of continence.[4,5]

Lateral to the subepithelial layer the caudal continuation of the circular smooth muscle of the rectum forms the internal anal sphincter,[3] which terminates caudally with a well-defined border, at a variable distance from the anal verge. Continuous with the outer layer of the rectum the longitudinal layer of the anal canal lies between the internal and external anal sphincters in the intersphincteric space. The longitudinal muscle comprises smooth muscle cells from the rectal wall, augmented with striated muscle from a variety of sources,[6] including the levator ani,[7] puborectalis[8] and pubococcygeus[9] muscles. Fibres from this layer traverse the external anal sphincter forming septa that insert into the skin of the lower anal canal and adjacent perineum as the corrugator cutis ani muscle.[6,8]

The striated muscle of the external sphincter surrounds the longitudinal muscle and forms the outer border of the intersphincteric space. The external sphincter is arranged as a tripartite structure, classically described by Holl and Thompson[10,11] and later adopted by Gorsch[12] and by Milligan and Morgan.[8] In this system the external sphincter is divided into deep, superficial and subcutaneous portions, with the deep and subcutaneous sphincter forming rings of muscle and, between them, the elliptical fibres of the superficial sphincter running anteriorly from the perineal body to the coccyx posteriorly.

Some authors consider the external sphincter to be a single muscle contiguous with the puborectalis muscle,[3] while others have adopted a two-part model.[13] This proposes a deep anal sphincter and a superficial anal sphincter, corresponding to the puborectalis and deep external anal sphincter combined and the fused superficial and subcutaneous sphincter of the tripartite model.

Anal endosonography (AES) and magnetic resonance imaging (MRI) have not resolved the dilemma, although most authors report a three-part sphincter where the puborectalis muscle is fused with the deep sphincter.[14,15] AES initially suggested that the anterior external anal sphincter is shorter than the posterior in women,[16,17] whereas in men the external sphincter forms a more cylindrical shape, in keeping with the description of the sphincters by Oh and Kark.[13] It is now thought that women simply have a shorter external sphincter per se which may not actually differ in configuration from men.[18]

The external anal sphincter is innervated by the pudendal nerve (S2–S4),[1,2] which leaves the pelvis via the lower part of the greater sciatic notch, where it passes under the lower border of the pyriformis muscle. It then crosses the ischial spine and sacrospinous ligament to enter the ischiorectal fossa through the lesser sciatic notch or foramen via the pudendal (or Alcock's) canal.

The pudendal nerve has two branches: the inferior rectal nerve, which supplies the external anal sphincter and sensation to the perianal skin; and the perineal nerve, which innervates the anterior perineal muscles together with the sphincter urethrae and forms the dorsal nerve of the clitoris (penis). There is a degree of cross-innervation between the two sides of the sphincter in monkeys,[19] although the degree of overlap in humans may be limited.[20] Although puborectalis receives its main innervation from a direct branch of the fourth sacral nerve root,[20] it may derive some innervation via the pudendal nerve.[21]

The autonomic supply to the anal canal and pelvic floor comes from two sources. The fifth lumbar nerve root sends sympathetic fibres to the superior and inferior hypogastric plexuses and the parasympathetic supply is from the second to fourth sacral nerve roots via the nervi erigentes.[1,22] Fibres of both systems pass obliquely across the lateral surface of the lower rectum to reach the region of the perineal body.

The internal anal sphincter has an intrinsic nerve supply from the myenteric plexus together with an additional supply from both the sympathetic and parasympathetic nervous systems. Sympathetic nervous activity is thought to enhance and parasympathetic activity to reduce internal sphincter activity.[23] Relaxation of the internal anal sphincter may be mediated via non-adrenergic, non-cholinergic nerve activity via the neural transmitter nitric oxide.[24,25]

Anorectal physiological studies alone cannot separate the different structures of the anal canal; instead they provide measurements of the resting and squeeze pressures along the canal. Between 60 and 85% of resting anal pressure can be attributed to the action of the internal anal sphincter.[18,26,27] The external anal sphincter and the puborectalis muscle generate maximal squeeze pressure. Symptoms of passive anal leakage (where the patient is unaware that episodes are happening) are attributed to internal sphincter dysfunction, whereas urge symptoms and frank incontinence of faeces are due to external sphincter problems.[28]

As the rectum distends there is reflex relaxation of the internal anal sphincter, called the rectoanal inhibitory reflex. Internal sphincter relaxation allows the rectal contents to enter the anal canal and to come in contact with the transition zone mucosa, allowing discrimination of solid from fluid and flatus, a process vital to the continence mechanism.[29,30] During this anorectal sampling there is reflex contraction of the external anal sphincter to prevent incontinence.[31]

Faecal continence is maintained by the complex interaction of many different variables. Stool must be delivered at a suitable rate from the colon into a compliant rectum of adequate volume. The consistency of this stool should be appropriate and accurately sensed by the sampling mechanism. Sphincters should be intact and able to contract adequately to produce pressures sufficient to prevent leakage of flatus, liquid and solid stool. For effective defecation there needs to be coordinated relaxation of the striated muscle components with an increase in intra-abdominal pressure to expel the rectal contents. The structure of the anorectal region should prevent herniation or prolapse of elements of the anal canal and rectum during defecation.

As a result of the complex interplay between the factors involved in continence and faecal evacuation, a wide range of investigations is needed for full assessment. A defect in any one element of the system in isolation is unlikely to have great functional significance and so in most clinical situations there is more than one contributing factor.

Rectoanal inhibitory reflex

Increasing rectal distension is associated with transient reflex relaxation of the internal anal sphincter and contraction of the external anal sphincter, known as the rectoanal inhibitory reflex (**Fig. 1.1**).[32] The exact neurological pathway for this reflex is unknown, although it may be mediated via the myenteric plexus[33] and stretch receptors in the pelvic floor.[20] It is absent in patients with Hirschsprung's disease,[33] progressive systemic sclerosis and Chagas' disease and initially absent after a coloanal anastomosis, although it rapidly recovers.[34] The rectoanal inhibitory reflex may enable rectal contents to be sampled by the tran-

sition zone mucosa to enable discrimination between solid, liquid and flatus.[30] The rate of recovery of sphincter tone after this relaxation differs for the proximal and distal canal, which may be important in maintaining continence.[31]

MANOMETRY

No standardisation exists for either the equipment or technique used for anal manometry. A variety of different catheter systems have been used, and it is important to note that measurements differ depending on the system employed. Available systems include microballoons filled with either air or water, microtransducers and water-perfused catheters. These systems may be hand-held or automated. Hand-held systems are withdrawn in a measured stepwise fashion with recordings made after each step (usually of 0.5–1.0 cm intervals); this is called a station pull-through. Automated withdrawal devices allow continuous data recording (vector manometry).

Water-perfused catheters use hydraulic capillary infusers to perfuse catheter channels, which are arranged either radially or obliquely staggered.

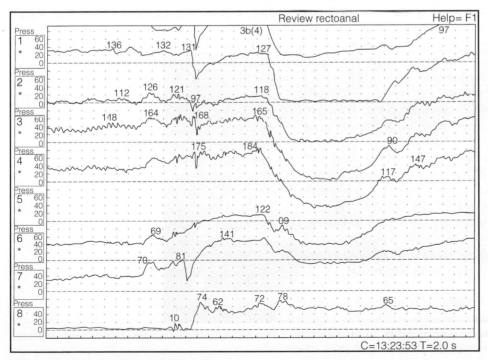

Figure 1.1 • Normal rectoanal inhibitory reflex.

Each catheter channel is then linked to a pressure transducer (**Fig. 1.2**). Infusion rates of perfusate (sterile water) vary between 0.25 and 0.5 mL/min per channel. Systems need to be free from air bubbles, which may lead to inaccurate recordings, and avoid leakage of perfusate onto the perianal skin, which may lead to falsely high resting pressures due to reflex external sphincter action. Perfusion rates should remain constant, because faster rates are associated with higher resting pressures,[35] while larger diameter catheters lead to greater recorded pressure.[36,37]

Balloon systems may be used to overcome some of these problems and may be more representative of pressure generated within a hollow viscus than recordings using a perfusion system. Furthermore, balloon systems are not subject to the same problems as a perfusion system when canal pressures are radially asymmetrical.[36] Balloons can be filled with either air[38,39] or water.[35,40] Over the range of balloon sizes used (diameter 2–10 mm), diameter appears to have less of an effect on the pressures recorded than it does with water-perfused catheter systems.

Microtransducers have been developed that can accurately measure canal pressure. However, these are expensive and fragile and more prone to inaccuracies when radial pressure asymmetry is present. They have been validated against water-filled balloon systems[30,41] and may be useful in the performance of ambulatory studies.[37]

Pressure changes in the anal canal can be measured in a number of ways and each method has been validated for its repeatability and reproducibility, although individual methods are not interchangeable. Although the correlation between measurements made using different systems and catheters is good, the absolute values are different and so when comparing the results of different studies it is essential to consider the method used to obtain the pressure measurements.

Significant variation exists in the results of anorectal manometry in normal asymptomatic subjects. Men have higher mean resting and squeeze pressures.[42,43] Pressures decline after the age of 60 years, changes most marked in women.[43,44] These facts must be considered when selecting appropriate control subjects for clinical studies.[45] Normal mean anal canal resting tone in healthy adults is 50–70 mmHg. Resting tone increases in a cranial to caudal direction along the canal such that the maximal resting pressure is found 1–2 cm from the anal verge.[18] The high-pressure zone (the part of the anal canal where the resting pressure is >50% of the maximum resting pressure) is longer in men than women (2.5–3.5 vs. 2.0–3.0 cm).[36,46] In a

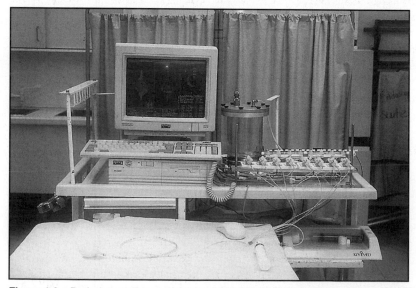

Figure 1.2 • Perfusion system used for anorectal manometry. Standard water perfusion set-up plus computer interface for anorectal manometry. The screen shows a vector volume profile.

normal individual the rise in pressure on maximal squeezing should be at least 50–100% of the resting pressure (usually 100–180 mmHg).[47] Reflex contraction of the external sphincter should occur when the rectum is distended, on coughing, or with any rise in intra-abdominal pressure.

Manometry has limited ability to discriminate between patients with faecal incontinence and normal age- and sex-matched controls. While both resting and maximal squeeze pressures are significantly lower in patients with incontinence than in matched controls,[48] there is considerable crossover between the pressures recorded in patients and controls. McHugh and Diamant found that in faecally incontinent patients, 39% of women and 44% of men had normal resting and squeeze pressures and 9% of asymptomatic normal individuals were unable to generate an appreciable pressure on maximal squeeze.[49] Whether manometry is better than a well-trained finger in assessing sphincter pressures has been disputed.[50]

Ambulatory manometry

The use of continuous ambulatory manometry to record rectal and anal canal pressures[51] has provided information on the functioning of the sphincter mechanism in a more physiological situation. The generation of giant waves of pressure in the rectum or neorectum may relate to episodes of incontinence in patients after restorative proctocolectomy.[52] Ambulatory manometry has also identified patients in whom episodes of internal sphincter relaxation are not accompanied by reflex external sphincter contraction,[53] a finding that may prove useful in selecting patients likely to benefit from biofeedback treatment.[54,55]

Vector volume manometry

This technique utilises a radially arranged eight-channel catheter that is automatically withdrawn from the anal canal during rest and squeeze and computer software that produces a three-dimensional reconstruction of the anal canal (**Fig. 1.3**).[56] This system is able to assess radial symmetry and produces a vector symmetry index (i.e. how far the radial symmetry of the anal canal differs from a perfect circle, which has a vector symmetry index

of 1). Sphincter defects are associated with symmetry indices of 0.6 or less.[57]

Vector volume manometry may differentiate between idiopathic and traumatic faecal incontinence by showing global external sphincter weakness rather than a localised area of scarred sphincter indicated by an asymmetrical vectogram.[56] However, there is poor correlation between vectogram and electromyographic or ultrasonic localisation of sphincter defects: the vectogram agrees with electromyographic localisation in only 13% and with ultrasonic localisation in 11%. Vector manometry also consistently records higher pressures than those obtained with conventional manometry.[58]

ANAL AND RECTAL SENSATION

The anal canal is rich in sensory receptors,[59] including those for pain, temperature and movement, with the somatic sensation of the anal transitional mucosa being more sensitive than that of the perianal skin. In contrast, the rectum is relatively insensitive to pain, although crude sensation may be transmitted via the nervi erigentes of the parasympathetic nervous system.[60]

A variety of methods have been used to measure anal sensation. Initial assessment of anal sensation used a stiff bristle to detect light touch in the anal canal and hot and cold metal rods to detect temperature sensation.[59] Thermal sensation has been assessed with water-perfused thermodes;[61] normal subjects can detect a change in temperature of 0.92°C.[61] The ability of the mucosa to detect a small electrical current can be assessed by the use of a double platinum electrode and a signal generator providing a square wave impulse at 5 Hz of 100 μs duration. The lowest recorded current of three readings at the point at which the subject feels a tingling or pricking sensation in the anal canal is noted as the sensation threshold. Normal electrical sensation for the most sensitive area of the anal canal (the transition zone) is 4 mA (2–7 mA).[62,63] Rectal mucosal electrical sensation may also be measured using the same technique as that used for anal mucosal electrical sensation measurement, with slight modification of the stimulus (500 μs duration at a frequency of 10 Hz)[60].

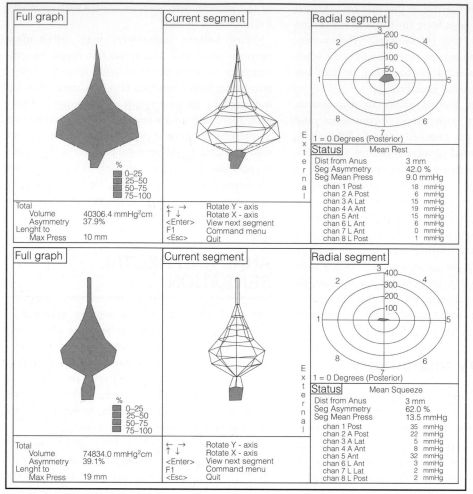

Figure 1.3 • Normal vector volume at squeeze and at rest. Note that asymmetry of the sphincter contour can be normal.

The sensation of rectal filling is measured by progressively inflating a balloon placed within the rectum or by intrarectal saline infusion.[60] Normal perception of rectal filling occurs after inflation of 10–20 mL, the sensation of the urge to defecate occurs after 60 mL, and normally up to 230 mL is tolerated in total before discomfort occurs.[60,64] The clinical use of these measurements may be limited due to the large inter- and intrasubject variation in values and the wide normal range, reducing the discriminatory value of this technique as a clinical investigation.[65]

Temperature sensation may be vital in the discrimination of solid stool from liquid and flatus[61] and is reduced in patients with faecal incontinence. It is thought that this sensation is important in the sampling reflex, although this is brought into

question by the fact that the sensitivity of the anal mucosa to temperature change is not great enough to detect the very slight temperature gradient between the rectum and anal canal.[66]

Anal mucosal electrical sensation threshold increases with age and thickness of the subepithelial layer of the anal canal.[62] Anal canal electrical sensation is reduced in idiopathic faecal incontinence,[63] diabetic neuropathy,[67] descending perineum syndrome[68] and haemorrhoids.[63] There are differing reports on whether there is any correlation between electrical sensation and measurement of motor function of the sphincters (pudendal terminal motor latency and single-fibre electromyography).[62,69]

The sampling mechanism and maintenance of faecal continence are complex multifactorial processes, as seen by the fact that the application of local anaesthetic to the sensitive anal mucosa does not lead to incontinence and in some individuals actually improves continence.[70]

RECTAL COMPLIANCE

The relation between changes in rectal volume and the associated pressure changes is termed compliance, which is calculated by dividing the change in volume by the change in pressure. Compliance is measured by inflating a rectal balloon with saline or air[64] or by directly infusing saline at physiological temperature into the rectum.[71] In the former method, the filling of the rectal balloon can be either incremental or continuous.[72] When continuous inflation of the rectal balloon is used, the rate of inflation should be 70–240 mL/min.[65] Mean rectal compliance is about 4–14 mL/cmH$_2$O, with pressures of 18–90 cmH$_2$O at the maximum tolerated volume.[73] Reports on the reproducibility of the measurement of rectal compliance are varied and many have found great variation within the same subject;[65,73] the most reproducible measurement is usually the maximum tolerated volume.

The compliance of the rectum does not differ between men and women up to the age of 60 years, but after this age women have more compliant rectums. It is reduced in Behçet's disease and Crohn's disease and after radiotherapy in a dose-related fashion.[74,75] The association between changes in rectal compliance and faecal incontinence is less clear. Some state that compliance is normal in incontinence[76] whereas others have found a reduction in compliance associated with faecal incontinence,[77,78] although changes in compliance may be secondary to the incontinence and not causative.[77] Altered compliance may play a role in soiling and constipation associated with megarectum.[42]

PELVIC FLOOR DESCENT

Parks et al.[79] first described the association between excessive descent of the perineum and anorectal dysfunction, and subsequently it has been described in a number of conditions: faecal incontinence, severe constipation, solitary rectal ulcer syndrome and anterior mucosal and full-thickness rectal prolapse.[76,80,81] The presumption in all these conditions is that abnormal perineal descent, especially during straining, causes traction and damage to the pudendal and pelvic floor nerves leading to progressive neuropathy and muscular atrophy.[80] Irreversible pudendal nerve damage occurs after a stretch of 12% of its length, and often the descent of the perineum in these patients is of the order of 2 cm, which is estimated to cause pudendal nerve stretching of 20%.[82]

Descent of the perineum was initially measured using the St Marks' perineometer. The perineometer is placed on the ischial tuberosities and a moveable latex cylinder is positioned on the perineal skin. The distance between the level of the perineum and the ischial tuberosities is measured at rest and during straining.[83] Negative readings indicate that the plane of the perineum is above the tuberosities and a positive value indicates descent below this level. In normal asymptomatic adults the plane of the perineum at rest should be –2.5 ± 0.6 cm, descending to +0.9 ± 1.0 cm on straining. When measured using dynamic proctography, similar measurements of pelvic floor descent are obtained. The anorectal angle normally lies on a line drawn between the coccyx and the most anterior part of the pubis and descends by 2 ± 0.3 cm on straining.[76] More recently dynamic MRI has been used to assess the pelvic floor at rest and during straining;[84] this technique has the advantage of being able to demonstrate prolapse and enteroceles as they occur.

Excessive perineal descent is found in 75% of subjects who chronically strain during defecation. The degree of descent correlates with age and is greater in women.[76,85] Although increased perineal descent on straining has been shown to be associated with features of neuropathy, namely decreased anal mucosal electrical sensitivity and increased pudendal nerve terminal motor latency, not all patients with abnormal descent have abnormal neurology.[81,86] Perineal descent is also associated with faecal incontinence, although the degree of incontinence and the results of anorectal manometry do not correlate with the extent of pelvic floor laxity.[76,87]

ELECTROPHYSIOLOGY

Neurophysiological assessment of the anorectum includes assessment of the conduction of the pudendal and spinal nerves and electromyography (EMG) of the sphincter.

Electromyography

Electromyographic traces can be recorded from the separate components of the sphincter complex both at rest and during active contraction of the striated components. Initially, EMG was used to map sphincter defects prior to consideration for surgery but AES is now so superior in its ability to map defects and is so much better tolerated by patients[88,89] that EMG has largely become a research tool. Broadly, two techniques of EMG are used: concentric needle studies and single-fibre studies.

Concentric needle EMG records the activity of up to 30 muscle fibres from around the area of the needle both at rest and during voluntary squeeze. The amplitude of the signal recorded correlates with the maximal squeeze pressure,[90] polyphasic long-duration action potentials indicating reinnervation subsequent to denervation injury. The main use of this technique has been in the confirmation and mapping of sphincter defects. Examination of puborectalis EMG may be more sensitive than cinedefecography in the detection of paradoxical puborectalis contraction in obstructed defecation,[91] although paradoxical puborectalis contraction is also present in normal subjects.[92]

The use of an anal plug or sponge can record global electrical activity from the anal sphincters,[90,93] EMG amplitudes recorded in this way correlating with voluntary squeeze pressure. In the future, sponge electrode EMG may have a role in directing biofeedback retraining for anismus.[94]

When EMG is performed using a needle with a smaller recording area (25 μm diameter) the action potential from individual motor units is recorded. Denervated muscle fibres can regain innervation from branching of adjacent axons, leading to an increase in the number of muscle fibres supplied by a single axon. With multiple readings (an average of 20) using this small-diameter needle the mean fibre density (MFD) for an area of sphincter can be calculated (i.e. the mean number of muscle action potentials per unit area or axon). Denervation and subsequent reinnervation are also indicated by neuromuscular 'jitter', which are caused by variation in the timing of triggering and non-triggering potentials.[95] An increase in sphincter MFD is often found in cases of idiopathic incontinence[96] and is associated with recognised histological changes in sphincter structure.[97] Atrophic sphincter muscle shows a loss of the characteristic mosaic pattern of distribution of type 1 and type 2 muscle fibres.[98] There is also selective muscle fibre hypertrophy together with fibro-fatty fibre degeneration. These changes predominantly affect the external anal sphincter but the puborectalis and levators are also affected to a lesser extent.[98]

MFD correlates inversely with squeeze pressure[99] and is increased in patients with excessive perineal descent.[78] The correlation with direct assessment of the integrity of sphincter innervation (pudendal nerve terminal motor latency) is less clear.

Electromyographic examination of the internal sphincter is also possible by inserting a bipolar electrode (under ultrasound guidance) and recording the resting electrical activity.[100] Ambulatory studies have shown sustained hypertonia of the internal sphincter in patients with non-healing anal fissures.[101]

Pudendal nerve terminal motor latency

Pudendal nerve conduction can be assessed by stimulating it as it enters the ischio-rectal fossa at the ischial spines. The mass production of self-adhesive disposable electrodes, which can easily be mounted on a gloved finger, has enabled this assessment to become routine in most centres.[102] The nerve latency is measured from the stimulus spike to the beginning of the motor response; standard tracings are shown in **Fig 1.4**. This investigation only examines the fastest conducting fibres of the pudendal nerve and so can still be normal even in the presence of abnormal sphincter innervation.[103] The normal value for pudendal nerve terminal motor latency (PNTML) is 2.0 ± 0.5 ms.[104]

Prolongation of PNTML is associated with idiopathic faecal incontinence, rectal prolapse, solitary rectal ulcer syndrome, severe constipation and sphincter defects.[81,105] Nerve latency is delayed with increasing age[96,106] and is prolonged in 24% of all faecally incontinent patients and 31% of those presenting with constipation.[107] The association of PNTML with manometry is less clear, with an inverse correlation between PNTML and squeeze

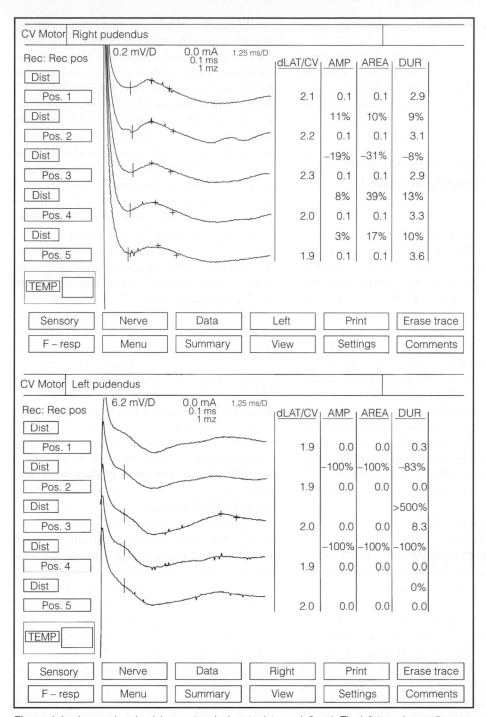

Figure 1.4 • A normal pudendal nerve terminal motor latency (<2 ms). The left trace is usually represented as a downward deflection.

pressure only in incontinent patients with intact anal sphincters.[106]

A prolonged PNTML may be a negative prognostic factor in the results from anterior sphincter repair.[41,108] Nerve latencies are known to deteriorate with time, partly explaining deterioration of incontinent patients with increasing age.[105]

Spinal motor latency and somatosensory evoked potentials

Transcutaneous stimulation of the sacral motor nerve roots provides further information on the innervation of the pelvic floor. The motor response from stimulation at the level of the first and fourth lumbar vertebrae can be recorded using standard EMG needles inserted into the puborectalis and external sphincter. By comparing the latency times between the two levels, the latency of the motor component of the cauda equina can be assessed. Up to 23% of patients with idiopathic faecal incontinence will have cauda equina delay.[109]

The sphincters can also be stimulated transcranially using magnetic impulses to investigate patients with spinal and central neurological conditions,[110] although at present these techniques have not reached the clinical arena.

DEFECOGRAPHY/ EVACUATION PROCTOGRAPHY

Defecography or evacuation proctography involves video fluoroscopy of the patient evacuating barium paste of stool consistency. Barium-soaked gauze may also be inserted into the vagina in women and barium paste applied to the perineum to aid in assessing the anorectal angle and perineal descent.[111,112] Opacification of the small bowel with an orally ingested contrast medium or injection of contrast into the peritoneum (peritoneography) will reveal enteroceles in 18% of patients with pelvic floor weakness,[113] with only half filling with bowel.[114] Defecography is a dynamic examination; it not only provides information on anorectal structural changes during defecation but it also assesses function. While anatomical changes during evacuation (namely rectocele, enterocele, rectoanal intussusception, rectal prolapse and changes in anorectal angle) may be evident, the extent and duration of emptying is of more clinical significance.[115]

Interobserver agreement is good for the reporting of rectocele and internal prolapse.[116] However, these findings often occur in normal asymptomatic indicividuals[117] such that anatomical abnormalities demonstrated on proctography are of poor discriminatory value in determining patients from controls.[118] Furthermore, defecation patterns do not appear to be consistently related to symptomatology, manometric assessment or duration of the complaint.[119] The only measurements that can discriminate between normal subjects and those with severe constipation are the time taken to evacuate and the completeness of evacuation.[120]

During normal evacuation the anorectal angle increases because of relaxation of puborectalis. The maintenance of an acute anorectal angle during evacuation may be due to obstructed defecation or anismus[121] (where the puborectalis and external anal sphincter contract paradoxically during attempted evacuation). Normal evacuation should be 90% complete (and 60% complete with a pouch). Rectoceles are significant if they are greater than 3 cm or require digitation to empty.[122]

SCINTIGRAPHY

Scintigraphy using technetium-labelled sulphur colloid mixed with dilute veegum powder may also be used for defecography.[123] The advantages of this technique are that a quantitative result is obtained and a lower dose of radiation is used. However, the study is not dynamic and does not correlate with patient symptoms or manometric assessment. Radioisotope testing may also be used to assess colonic transit time to diagnose idiopathic slow transit constipation.[124] Colonic transit time is measured more easily by tracking the progress of ingested sets of radio-opaque markers with plain abdominal radiography. Standard protocol takes a single plain abdominal radiograph 5 days after commencing ingestion of the markers (usually different-shaped markers are taken daily over the first 3 days).

IMAGING THE RECTUM AND ANAL SPHINCTERS

The indications for anorectal imaging may be divided into three broad clinical areas: sepsis and fistula disease, malignancy, and faecal incontinence. The available techniques include surface scanning techniques, namely computed tomography (CT) and body coil MRI, and endoanal imaging, namely AES, with or without subsequent multiplanar (three-dimensional) reconstruction, and endocoil MRI.

Anal endosonography/endorectal ultrasound

Endoluminal ultrasound of the rectum utilises a transducer that rotates through 360° within a water-filled balloon in order to provide acoustic coupling. The ultrasonic anatomy has been described in detail as a result of scanning dissected specimens and comprises alternating bands of reflection created by the interfaces between the different anatomical structures present.[125] An alternating bright and dark pattern of rings is seen corresponding to the layers of the rectal wall.

To enable examination of the anal sphincters, endorectal ultrasound (EUS) has been adapted by replacing the water-filled balloon with a water-filled plastic cone and by using a 10-MHz transducer (Fig 1.5a).[126] The anatomy of the anal canal has been described using dissection and, more recently, by comparison with MRI.[127–129] The anal canal mucosa is generally not seen on AES. The sub-epithelial tissue is highly reflective and surrounded by the low reflection from the internal anal sphincter. The width of the internal sphincter increases with age: the normal width for a patient aged 55 years or younger is 2.4–2.7 mm, whereas in an older patient the normal range is 2.8–3.4 mm. As the width of the sphincter increases it becomes progressively more reflective and more indistinct, which may be due to a relative increase in the fibroelastic content of this muscle as a consequence of ageing.[130] Both the external anal sphincter and the longitudinal muscle are of moderate reflectivity. The intersphincteric space often returns a bright reflection (Fig 1.5b).

Endocoil receiver MRI

MRI provides images with excellent tissue differentiation, although spatial resolution of the anal sphincters using a body coil receiver is poor. When an endoanal receiver coil is used, spatial resolution is vastly improved locally around the coil (within about 4 cm), enabling the acquisition of images of the anal sphincters with both excellent tissue differentiation and spatial resolution. Endocoils have

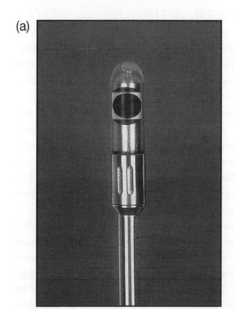

(a)

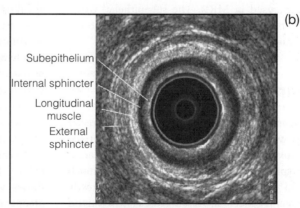

(b)

Subepithelium
Internal sphincter
Longitudinal muscle
External sphincter

Figure 1.5 • (a) Bruel-Kjaer 7·5-MHz endoanal ultrasound probe. **(b)** The layers of the sphincter are depicted by the endoanal ultrasound probe.

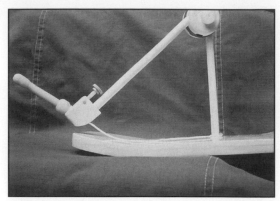

Figure 1.6 • Endoanal magnetic resonance coil with stand.

either rectangular or saddle geometry and measure 6–10 cm in length and 7–12 mm in diameter. This increases to 17–19 mm after encasement in an acetal homopolymer (Delrin) former. The coil is inserted in the left lateral position and then secured with sandbags or with a purpose-built holder to avoid movement artefact (**Fig 1.6**).[14,131]

Much has been learnt about the anatomy of this region using endoanal MRI with anatomical correlation from dissected specimens.[15,132,133] On T2-weighted images, the external sphincter and longitudinal muscle return a relatively low signal. The internal sphincter returns a relatively high signal and enhances with gadolinium (an intravenous contrast agent used in MRI). The subepithelial tissue has a signal intensity value between that of the internal and external sphincters (**Fig 1.7**).

Imaging in rectal cancer

CT has an accuracy of 89% in assessing rectal tumours with extensive spread beyond the serosal layer; however, when only cases of moderate tumour spread are assessed, the accuracy is much lower (55%).[134] EUS by comparison can correctly T-stage rectal cancers in 75% of cases, with a trend to overstage in 22%,[135] and is considered by many as the first-choice investigation for the local staging of rectal cancer.[136,137] Perirectal lymph nodes involved with tumour are seen on EUS as well-defined areas of low reflectivity, although malignant nodal status has also been associated with a degree

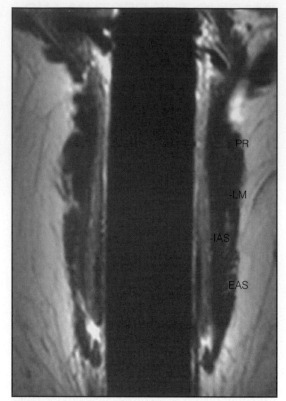

Figure 1.7 • A mid-coronal image of the anal canal using endocoil MRI. EAS, external anal sphincter; IAS, internal anal sphincter; LM, longitudinal muscle; PR, puborectalis.

of inhomogeneity on EUS. EUS is superior to CT and has a positive predictive value for tumour invasion beyond the muscularis propria of 98%. If a lymph node measures greater than 5 mm in diameter on EUS, there is a 45–70% chance that it is involved with tumour.[138]

Body coil MRI has been used to assess the stage of rectal tumours and it would appear to give comparable results to EUS.[139] When assessing nodal involvement, MRI may be slightly inferior to EUS.[140] Recent work using thin-section MRI has shown very accurate T-staging of rectal tumours preoperatively.[141]

Body coil MRI has the advantage over EUS in that it can be performed even in the presence of stenotic tumours, which the ultrasound probe may not be able to traverse. Furthermore, after radiotherapy EUS will tend to overstage tumours, leading to a marked reduction in its diagnostic accuracy, especially in the differentiation between T2 and T3 tumours.[142] The other area where MRI is superior to EUS is in the assessment of recurrent tumours. The appearances of fibrosis after surgery and recurrent tumour in the pelvis are very similar using either EUS or CT, which makes assessment for recurrent disease very difficult. On MRI the signals from these two tissue types (especially on T2-weighted images) are quite different, allowing greater tissue differentiation.[143]

Imaging in anal sepsis and anal fistulas

Both surface imaging and endoanal imaging have been employed in the assessment of perianal sepsis. CT is unsatisfactory for the assessment of fistulas because of the poor definition of tracks, which is largely due to volume averaging.[144] AES is used to assess anal fistulas and has been shown to be accurate for the definition of the anatomy of anal sepsis, especially horseshoe collections and the anatomy of complex fistulas.[145] Endosonography is also able to detect and assess sphincter damage caused by chronic sepsis.[146]

Endosonography is less accurate in the assessment of suprasphincteric sepsis and it is often difficult to differentiate between supra-levator and infra-levator collections, leading to inaccuracy in up to 20% of cases.[147] Furthermore, AES is poor at defining the internal opening of a fistula because of the lack of definition of the mucosa (penetration of the internal anal sphincter by the track acts as a surrogate for the opening) and is of limited value close to the anal margin.[145] Whether the diagnostic accuracy of AES will increase with the use of hydrogen peroxide injected into fistulous tracks to act as a contrast medium remains to be seen.

MRI has the most to offer in the assessment of perianal sepsis. Anal sepsis appears on MRI as areas of very high signal, which enhance with the administration of the intravenous contrast agent gadolinium. Definition is further increased with the use of STIR (short τ inversion recovery) sequences to suppress the signal returned by fat (**Fig 1.8**). Excellent correlation has been shown between the findings during examination under anaesthesia (EUA) and the appearances shown by MRI for the anatomy of fistulous tracks.[148,149] MRI is at least as accurate, if not more so, than digital examination for the assessment of anal fistulas.[150] The use of dynamic contrast-enhanced MRI has been reported to provide better delineation of fistulas than that found during EUA,[151] and MRI may be better at predicting outcome than the findings at surgery.[152]

Imaging in faecal incontinence

AES has revealed that many patients who were thought to have idiopathic faecal incontinence in fact have a surgically remediable sphincter defect.[153] It has also been shown that a much higher proportion of women sustain sphincter damage during childbirth than is suspected by clinical assessment alone.[154,155] While the true incidence of sphincter tears may be lower than initially thought,[156] many women have important morphological changes to the sphincter following delivery.[157]

The ability of AES to diagnose and correctly assess the extent of external sphincter damage has been validated by comparison with EMG studies and findings at surgery.[158,159] AES is superior in the differentiation between those patients with idiopathic faecal incontinence and those with a sphincter defect when compared with either simple manometric assessment or vector volume studies.[160]

More recently, MRI has been used to assess patients with faecal incontinence. The diagnosis of sphincter defects using endocoil MRI has been validated with surgical confirmation of defect presence and extent.[161,162] Endocoil MRI may be superior to AES in the detection and assessment of external sphincter defects as a result of better sphincter definition using MRI,[162] although it is more important that the clinician is familiar with the imaging technique used.[163]

MRI has multiplanar capability (i.e. axial, sagittal and coronal images can be acquired), whereas standard AES provides only axially oriented images. The acquisition of volume ultrasound data has overcome this problem,[164] and using three-dimensional AES has led to a better understanding of sphincter injury. A direct correlation exists between the length of a defect and the arc of displacement of the two ends of the sphincter.[165]

(a)

(b)

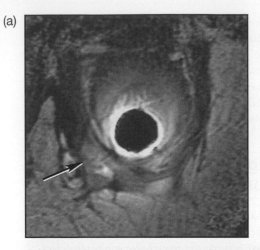

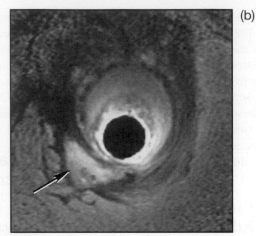

(c)

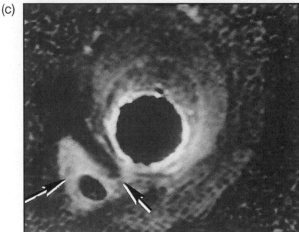

Figure 1.8 • Examples of complex perirectal sepsis as shown by the endoanal magnetic resonance probe. **(a, b)** T1-weighted images of an intersphincteric collection prior to and following gadolinium-DTPA contrast (arrow). **(c)** STIR image of the abscess cavity showing a central gas-containing cavity (long arrow) and a fistula at the 7 o'clock position (short arrow).

The use of endocoil MRI has shown that incontinence in the absence of a sphincter defect may be due to atrophy, where the sphincter has been replaced by fat and fibrous tissue.[131,166] The presence of external anal sphincter atrophy on endocoil MRI has been associated with poor results from anterior sphincteroplasty.[167]

SUMMARY

A wide variety of physiological and morphological tests are available for the assessment of the anus and rectum. Although there is no clear correlation between manometric/neurophysiological testing and clinical symptomatology in patients with idiopathic faecal incontinence, there is considerable value in performing these tests before surgery in order to predict long-term outcome. Furthermore, anorectal investigation has revealed a large group of parous women who have occult sphincter trauma which may have a clinical impact as the women get older.

Anorectal physiological assessment is essential as an objective measure in patients with faecal incontinence and for the diagnosis of Hirschsprung's disease, and may help select those patients who will have acceptable function after colo-anal anastomosis or an ileo-anal pouch.

Endoanal imaging is becoming the gold standard in the preoperative determination of sphincter integrity and defines those patients most likely to benefit from surgical intervention. Endorectal imaging of rectal tumours correlates well with histological assessment of tumour depth and is accurate for the diagnosis of recurrent tumour after anterior resection (especially when using MRI).

In patients with primary evacuatory disorders, neurophysiological testing and defecography assist in the demonstration of unsuspected rectoanal intussusception or rectocele who may benefit from surgery and those who may be suitable candidates for biofeedback therapy.

Anorectal investigation continues to have a major role in clinical research and has helped outline the anatomy of the component parts of the sphincter complex as well as to define the physiology of both defecation and anal continence. The understanding of these processes is vital to the correct management of patients with anorectal disorders.

• Key points

- Normal pelvic floor function relies on a complex interplay between various mechanisms.
- Sphincter function may be assessed using anal manometry and electrophysiology.
- Sphincter anatomy may be assessed using AES and MRI, the former being the standard for the diagnosis of sphincter trauma.
- Evacuation proctography is useful in the assessment of patients with evacuatory disorders.
- Pelvic MRI is the best imaging modality for anorectal sepsis and can predict recurrence of anal fistulas after surgery.
- Preoperative staging of rectal cancer is most accurate using MRI for moderately to advanced tumours and endorectal ultrasound for early lesions.

REFERENCES

1. Walls EW. Anatomy of the anal canal. Ann R Coll Surg Engl 1983; Symposium on Sir Alan Parks 1920–1982, Surgeon and Scientist: 1–3.

2. Lawson JON. Pelvic anatomy. II. Anal canal and associated sphincters. Ann R Coll Surg Engl 1974; 54:287–300.

3. Goligher JC, Leacock AG, Brossy JJ. The surgical anatomy of the anal canal. Br J Surg 1955; 43:51–61.

4. Parks AG. The surgical treatment of haemorrhoids. Br J Surg 1956; 43:337–51.

5. Haas PA, Fox TA. Age-related changes and scar formations of perianal connective tissue. Dis Colon Rectum 1990; 23:160–9.

6. Lunniss PJ, Phillips RKS. Anatomy and function of the anal longitudinal muscle. Br J Surg 1992; 79:882–4.

7. Courtney H. Anatomy of the pelvic diaphragm and anorectal musculature as related to sphincter preservation in anorectal surgery. Am J Surg 1950; 79:155–73.

8. Milligan ETC, Morgan CN. Surgical anatomy of the anal canal with special reference to anorectal fistulae. Lancet 1934; ii:1150–6, 1213–14.

9. Shafik AA. Concept of the anatomy of the anal sphincter mechanism and the physiology of defecation. Dis Colon Rectum 1987; 30:970–82.

10. Thompson P. The myology of the pelvic floor. In: Newton J. (ed.) A contribution to human comparative anatomy. London: McCorquodale & Co., 1899.

11. Holl K. Bardeleben's Handbuch der Anatomie des Menschen. Fischer, 1897.

12. Gorsch RV. Proctologic anatomy. Baltimore: Williams and Wilkins, 1955.

13. Oh C, Kark AE. Anatomy of the external anal sphincter. Br J Surg 1972; 59:717–23.

14. deSouza NM, Kmiot WA, Puni R et al. High resolution magnetic resonance imaging of the anal sphincter using an internal coil. Gut 1995; 37:284–7.

15. Hussain SM, Stoker J, Lameris JS. Anal sphincter complex: endoanal MR imaging of normal anatomy. Radiology 1995; 197:671–7.

16. Nielsen MB, Pedersen JF, Hauge C, Rasmussen OO, Christiansen J. Endosonography of the anal sphincter: findings in healthy volunteers. Am J Roentgenol 1991; 157:1199–202.

17. Sultan AH, Kamm MA, Hudson CN, Nicholls JR, Bartram CI. Endosonography of the anal sphincters: normal anatomy and comparison with manometry. Clin Radiol 1994; 49:368–74.

18. Williams AB, Cheetham MJ, Bartram CI, Halligan S, Kmiot WA, Nicholls RJ. Gender differences in the longitudinal pressure profile of the anal canal related to anatomical structure as demonstrated on three-dimensional anal endosonography. Br J Surg 2000; 87:1674–9.

19. Wunderlich M, Swash M. The overlapping innervation of the two sides of the external anal sphincter by the pudendal nerves. J Neurol Sci 1983; 59:97–109.

20. Percy JP. Anatomy and innervation of the pelvic floor. Ann R Coll Surg Engl 1983; Symposium on Sir Alan Parks 1920–1982, Surgeon and Scientist: 5–16.

21. Uher EM, Swash M. Sacral reflexes, physiology and clinical application. Dis Colon Rectum 1998; 41:1165–77.

22. Lawson JON. Pelvic anatomy. I. Pelvic floor muscles. Ann R Coll Surg Engl 1974; 54:244–52.

23. Sangwan YP, Solla JA. Internal anal sphincter, advances and insights. Dis Colon Rectum 1998; 41:1297–311.

24. Chakder S, Rattan S. Release of nitric oxide by activation of nonadrenergic noncholinergic neurons of the internal anal sphincter. Am J Physiol 1993; 264:G7–G12.

25. O'Kelly TJ, Davies JR, Brading AF, Mortensen NJ. Distribution of nitric oxide synthase containing neurons in the rectal myenteric plexus and anal canal. Morphologic evidence that nitric oxide mediates the rectoanal inhibitory reflex. Dis Colon Rectum 1994; 37:350–7.

26. Duthie HL, Watts JM. Contribution of the external anal sphincter to the pressure zone in the anal canal. Gut 1965; 6:64–8.

27. Lestar B, Penninckx F, Kerremans R. The composition of anal basal pressure. An in vivo and in vitro study in man. Int J Colorectal Dis 1989, 4:118–22.

28. Engel AF, Kamm MA, Bartram CI, Nicholls RJ. Relationship of symptoms in faecal incontinence to specific sphincter abnormalities. Int J Colorectal Dis 1995; 10:152–5.

29. Lubowski DZ, Nicholls RJ, Swash M, Jordan MJ. Neural control of internal anal sphincter function. Br J Surg 1987; 74:668–70.

30. Miller R, Bartolo DC, Cervero F, Mortensen NJ. Anorectal sampling: a comparison of normal and incontinent patients. Br J Surg 1988; 75:44–7.

31. Goes RN, Simons AJ, Masri L, Beart RW Jr. Gradient of pressure and time between proximal anal canal and high-pressure zone during internal anal sphincter relaxation. Its role in the fecal continence mechanism. Dis Colon Rectum 1995; 38:1043–6.

32. Gowers WR. The automatic action of the sphincter ani. Proc R Soc Lond 1877; 26:77–84.

33. Lawson J, Nixon HH. Anal canal pressures in the diagnosis of Hirschsprung's disease. J Pediatr Surg 1967; 2:544–52.

34. Lewis WG, Williamson MER, Miller AS, Sagar PM, Holdsworth PJ, Johnston D. Preservation of complete anal sphincteric proprioception in restorative proctocolectomy: the inhibitory reflex and fine

control of continence need not be impaired. Gut 1995; 36:902–6.

35. Hancock BD. Measurement of anal pressure and motility. Gut 1976; 17:645–51.

36. Taylor BM, Beart RW, Phillips SF. Longitudinal and radial variations of pressure in the human anal sphincter. Gastroenterology 1984; 86:693–7.

37. Johnson GP, Pemberton JH, Ness J, Samson M, Zinsmeister AR. Transducer manometry and the effects of body position on anal canal pressures. Dis Colon Rectum 1990; 33:469–75.

38. Miller R, Bartolo DCC, James D, Mortensen NJM. Air-filled microballoon manometry for use in anorectal physiology. Br J Surg 1989; 76:72–5.

39. Orrom WJ, Williams JG, Rothenberger DA, Wong WD. Portable anorectal manometry. Br J Surg 1990; 77:876–7.

40. Gibbons CP, Bannister JJ, Trowbridge EA, Read NW. An analysis of anal sphincter pressure and anal compliance in normal subjects. Int J Colorectal Dis 1986; 1:231–7.

41. Varma JS, Smith AN. Anorectal profilometry with the microtransducer. Br J Surg 1984; 71:867–9.

42. Loening-Baucke V, Anwar M. Effects of age and sex on anorectal manometry. Am J Gastroenterol 1985; 80:50–3.

43. Enck P, Kuhlbusch R, Lubke H, Frieling T, Erckenbrecht JF. Age and sex and anorectal manometry in incontinence. Dis Colon Rectum 1989; 32:1026–30.

44. Laurberg S, Swash M, Henry MM. Delayed external sphincter repair for obstetric tear. Br J Surg 1988; 75:786–8.

45. Read NW, Abouzekry L, Read MG, Howell P, Ottewell D, Donnelly TC. Anorectal function in elderly patients with faecal impaction. Gastroenterology 1985; 89:959–66.

46. Sun WM, Read NW. Anorectal function in normal subjects: effect of gender. Int J Colorectal Dis 1989; 4:188–96.

47. Jorge JM, Wexner SD. Anorectal manometry: techniques and clinical applications. South Med J 1993; 86:924–31.

48. Hiltunen KM. Anal manometric findings in patients with anal incontinence. Dis Colon Rectum 1985; 28:925–8.

49. McHugh SM, Diamant NE. Effect of age, gender, and parity on anal canal pressures. Contribution of impaired anal sphincter function to fecal incontinence. Dig Dis Sci 1987; 32:726–36.

50. Hallan RI, Marzouk DEMM, Waldron DJ, Womack NR, Williams NS. Comparison of digital and manometric assessment of anal sphincter function. Br J Surg 1989; 76:973–5.

51. Kumar D, Waldron D, Williams NS, Browning C, Hutton MRE, Wingate DL. Prolonged anorectal manometry and external anal sphincter electromyography in ambulant human subjects. Dig Dis Sci 1990; 35:641–8.

52. Holdsworth PJ, Sagar PM, Lewis WG, Williamson M, Johnston D. Internal anal sphincter activity after restorative proctocolectomy for ulcerative colitis: a study using continuous ambulatory manometry. Dis Colon Rectum 1994; 37:32–6.

53. Sun WM, Read N, Miner PB, Kerrigan DD, Donnelly TC. The role of transient internal anal sphincter relaxation in faecal incontinence. Int J Colorectal Dis 1990; 5:31–6.

54. Enck P. Biofeedback training in disordered defecation. A critical review. Dig Dis Sci 1993; 38:1953–60.

55. Sangwan YP, Coller JA, Barrett RC, Roberts PL, Murray JJ, Schoetz DJ Jr. Can manometric parameters predict response to biofeedback therapy in fecal incontinence? Dis Colon Rectum 1995; 38:1021–5.

56. Braun JC, Treutner KH, Dreuw B, Klimaszewski M, Schumpelick V. Vectormanometry for differential diagnosis of fecal incontinence. Dis Colon Rectum 1994; 37:989–96.

57. Perry RE, Blatchford GJ, Christensen MA, Thorson AG, Attwood SEA. Manometric diagnosis of sphincter injuries. Am J Surg 1990; 159:112–16.

58. Yang YK, Wexner SD. Anal pressure vectography is of no apparent benefit for sphincter evaluation. Int J Colorectal Dis 1994; 9:92–5.

59. Duthie HL, Gairns FW. Sensory nerve-endings and sensation in the anal region of man. Br J Surg 1960; 47:585–95.

60. Kamm MA, Lennard-Jones JE. Rectal mucosal electrosensory testing: evidence for a rectal sensory neuropathy in idiopathic constipation. Dis Colon Rectum 1990; 33:419–23.

61. Miller R, Bartolo DCC, Cervero F, Mortensen NJM. Anorectal temperature sensation: a comparison of normal and incontinence patients. Br J Surg 1987; 74:511–15.

62. Felt BR, Poen AC, Cuesta MA, Meuwissen SG. Anal sensitivity test: what does it measure and do we need it? Cause or derivative of anorectal complaints. Dis Colon Rectum 1997; 40:811–16.

63. Roe AM, Bartolo DC, Mortensen NJ. New method for assessment of anal sensation in various anorectal disorders. Br J Surg 1986; 73:310–12.

64. Ihre T. Studies on anal function in continent and incontinent patients. Scand J Gastroenterol 1974; 9:1–64.

65. Kendall GPN, Thompson DG, Day SJ, Lennard-Jones JE. Inter- and intraindividual variation in pressure–volume relations of the rectum in normal subjects and patients with irritable bowel syndrome. Gut 1990; 31:1062–8.

66. Rogers J, Hayward MP, Henry MM, Misiewicz JJ. Temperature gradient between the rectum and the anal canal: evidence against the role of temperature sensation as a sensory modality in the anal canal of normal subjects. Br J Surg 1988; 75:1083–5.

67. Rogers J, Levy DM, Henry MM, Misiewicz J. Pelvic floor neuropathy: a comparative study of diabetes mellitus and idiopathic faecal incontinence. Gut 1988; 29:756–61.

68. Miller R, Bartolo DC, Cervero F, Mortensen NJ. Differences in anal sensation in continent and incontinent patients with abnormal perineal descent. Int J Colorectal Dis 1989; 76:607–9.

69. Rogers J, Henry MM, Misiewicz JJ. Combined sensory and motor deficit in primary neuropathic faecal incontinence. Gut 1988; 29:5–9.

70. Read MG, Read NW, Haynes WG, Donnelly TC, Johnson AG. A prospective study of the effect of haemorrhoidectomy on sphincter function and faecal continence. Br J Surg 1982; 69:396–8.

71. Read NW, Harford WV, Schmulen AC, Read MG, Santa Ana C, Fordtran JS. A clinical study of patients with fecal incontinence and diarrhoea. Gastroenterology 1979; 76:747–56.

72. Allen ML, Orr WC, Robinson MG. Anorectal functioning in fecal incontinence. Dig Dis Sci 1988; 33:36–40.

73. Sorensen M, Rasmussen OO, Tetzschner T, Christiansen J. Physiological variation in rectal compliance. Br J Surg 1992; 79:1106–8.

74. Broens P, Van Limbergen E, Penninckx F, Kerremans R. Clinical and manometric effects of combined external beam irradiation and brachytherapy for anal cancer. Int J Colorectal Dis 1998; 13:68–72.

75. Buchmann P, Mogg GAG, Alexander Williams J, Allan RN, Keighley MRB. Relationship of proctitis and rectal capacity in Crohn's disease. Gut 1980; 21:137–40.

76. Bartolo DCC, Read NW, Jarrat JA, Read MG, Donnelly TC, Johnson AG. Differences in anal sphincter function and clinical presentation in patients with pelvic floor descent. Gastroenterology 1983; 85:68–75.

77. Rasmussen O, Christiansen B, Sorensen M, Tetzschner T, Christiansen J. Rectal compliance in the assessment of patients with faecal incontinence. Dis Colon Rectum 1990; 33:650–3.

78. Womack NR, Morrison JFB, Williams NS. The role of pelvic floor denervatoin in the aetiology of idiopathic faecal incontinence. Br J Surg 1986; 73:404–7.

79. Parks AG, Porter NH, Hardcastle JD. The syndrome of the descending perineum. Proc R Soc Lond 1966; 59:477–82.

80. Swash M, Snooks SJ, Henry MM. Unifying concept of pelvic floor disorders and incontinence. J R Soc Med 1985; 78:906–11.

81. Jones PN, Lubowski DZ, Swash M, Henry MM. Relation between perineal descent and pudendal nerve damage in idiopathic faecal incontinence. Int J Colorectal Dis 1987; 2:93–5.

82. Henry MM. The descending perineum syndrome. Ann R Coll Surg Engl 1983; Symposium on Sir Alan Parks 1920–1982, Surgeon and Scientist: 24–5.

83. Lubowski DZ, Swash M, Nicholls RJ, Henry MM. Increase in pudendal nerve terminal motor latency with defaecation straining. Br J Surg 1988; 75:1095–7.

84. Healy JC, Halligan S, Reznek RH et al. Dynamic MR imaging compared with evacuation proctography when evaluating anorectal configuration and pelvic floor movement. Am J Roentgenol 1997; 169:775–9.

85. Ho YH, Goh HS. The neurophysiological significance of perineal descent. Int J Colorectal Dis 1995; 10:107–11.

86. Engel AF, Kamm MA. The acute effect of straining on pelvic floor neurological function. Int J Colorectal Dis 1994; 9:8–12.

87. Read NW, Bartolo DC, Read MG, Hall J, Haynes WG, Johnson AG. Differences in anorectal manometry between patients with haemorrhoids and patients with descending perineum syndrome: implications for management. Br J Surg 1983; 70:656–9.

88. Enck P, von Giesen HJ, Schafer A et al. Comparison of anal sonography with conventional needle electromyography in the evaluation of anal sphincter defects. Am J Gastroenterol 1996; 91:2539–43.

89. Law PJ, Kamm MA, Bartram CI. A comparison between electromyography and anal endosonography in mapping external anal sphincter defects. Dis Colon Rectum 1990; 33:370–3.

90. Sorensen M, Tetzschner T, Rasmussen OO, Christiansen J. Relation between electromyography and anal manometry of the external anal sphincter. Gut 1991; 32:1031–4.

91. Karlbom U, Edebol Eeg-Olofsson K, Graf W, Nilsson S, Pahlman L. Paradoxical puborectalis contraction is associated with impaired rectal evacuation. Int J Colorectal Dis 1998; 13:141–7.

92. Voderholzer WA, Neuhaus DA, Klauser AG, Tzavella K, Muller-Lissner SA, Schindlbeck NE. Paradoxical sphincter contraction is rarely indicative of anismus. Gut 1997; 41:258–62.

93. Pinho M, Hosie K, Bielecki K, Keighley MRB. Assessment of noninvasive intra-anal electromyography to evaluate sphincter function. Dis Colon Rectum 1991; 34:69–71.

94. Wexner SD, Cheape JD, Jorge JM, Heymen S, Jagelman DG. Prospective assessment of biofeedback for the treatment of paradoxical puborectalis contraction. Dis Colon Rectum 1992; 35:145–50.

95. Wexner SD, Marchetti F, Salanga VD, Corredor C, Jagelman DG. Neurophysiologic assessment of the anal sphincters. Dis Colon Rectum 1991; 34:606–12.

96. Roig JV, Villoslada C, Lledo S et al. Prevalence of pudendal neuropathy in fecal incontinence. Results of a prospective study. Dis Colon Rectum 1995; 38:952–8.

97. Swash M. Pathophysiology of idiopathic (neurogenic) faecal incontinence. Ann R Coll Surg Engl 1983; Symposium on Sir Alan Parks 1920–1982, Surgeon and Scientist:22–4.

98. Beersiek F. The pelvic floor: pathophysiology. Ann R Coll Surg Engl 1983; Symposium on Sir Alan Parks 1920–1982, Surgeon and Scientist:17–19.

99. Fink RL, Roberts LJ, Scott M. The role of manometry, electromyography and radiology in the assessment of faecal incontinence. Aust N Z J Surg 1992; 62:951–8.

100. Sorensen M, Nielsen MB, Pedersen JF, Christiansen J. Electromyography of the internal anal sphincter performed under endosonographic guidance. Description of a new method. Dis Colon Rectum 1994; 37:138–43.

101. Farouk R, Duthie GS, MacGregor AB, Bartolo DC. Sustained internal sphincter hypertonia in patients with chronic anal fissure. Dis Colon Rectum 1994; 37:424–9.

102. Rogers J, Henry MM, Misiewicz JJ. Disposable pudendal nerve stimulator: evaluation of the standard instrument and new device. Gut 1988; 29:1131–3.

103. Sangwan YP, Coller JA, Barrett RC, Murray JJ, Roberts PL, Schoetz DJ Jr. Prospective comparative study of abnormal distal rectoanal excitatory reflex, pudendal nerve terminal motor latency, and single fiber density as markers of pudendal neuropathy. Dis Colon Rectum 1996; 39:794–8.

104. Kiff ES, Swash M. Slowed conduction in the pudendal nerve in idiopathic (neurogenic) faecal incontinence. Br J Surg 1984; 71:614–16.

105. Hill J, Mumtaz A, Kiff ES. Pudendal neuropathy in patients with idiopathic faecal incontinence progresses with time. Br J Surg 1994; 81:1494–5.

106. Vernava AM, Longo WE, Daniel GL. Pudendal neuropathy and the importance of EMG evaluation of faecal incontinence. Dis Colon Rectum 1993; 36:23–7.

107. Vaccaro CA, Cheong DM, Wexner SD et al. Pudendal neuropathy in evacuatory disorders. Dis Colon Rectum 1995; 38:166–71.

108. Wexner SD, Marchetti F, Jagelman DG. The role of sphincteroplasty for fecal incontinence reevaluated: a prospective physiologic and functional review. Dis Colon Rectum 1991; 34:22–30.

109. Snooks SJ, Swash M, Henry MM. Abnormalities in central and peripheral nerve conduction in patients with anorectal incontinence. J R Soc Med 1985; 78:294–300.

110. Speakman CT, Kamm MA, Swash M. Cerebral evoked potentials: are they of value in anorectal disease? Gut 1990; 31:A1173.

111. Delemarre JB, Kruyt RH, Doornbos J et al. Anterior rectocele: assessment with radiographic defecography, dynamic magnetic resonance imaging, and physical examination. Dis Colon Rectum 1994; 37:249–59.

112. Mahieu P, Pringot J, Bodart P. Defecography: I. Description of a new procedure and results in normal patients. Gastrointest Radiol 1984; 9:247–51.

113. Kelvin FM, Maglinte DD, Benson JT. Evacuation proctography (defecography): an aid to the investigation of pelvic floor disorders. Obstet Gynecol 1994; 83:307–14.

114. Halligan S, Bartram CI. Evacuation proctography combined with positive contrast peritoneography to demonstrate pelvic floor hernias. Abdom Imaging 1995; 20:442–5.

115. Halligan S, Bartram CI. Is barium trapping in rectoceles significant? Dis Colon Rectum 1995; 38:764–8.

116. Klauser AG, Ting KH, Mangel E, Eibl-Eibesfeldt B, Muller-Lissner SA. Interobserver agreement in defecography. Dis Colon Rectum 1994; 37:1310–16.

117. Agachan F, Pfeifer J, Wexner SD. Defecography and proctography. Results of 744 patients. Dis Colon Rectum 1996; 39:899–905.

118. Hiltunen KM, Kolehmainen H, Matikainen M. Does defecography help in diagnosis and clinical decision-making in defecation disorders? Abdom Imaging 1994; 19:355–8.

119. Wald A, Jafri F, Rehder J, Holeva K. Scintigraphic studies of rectal emptying in patients with constipation and defecatory difficulty. Dig Dis Sci 1993; 38:353–8.

120. Turnbull GK, Bartram CI, Lennard-Jones JE. Radiologic studies of rectal evacuation in adults with idiopathic constipation. Dis Colon Rectum 1988; 31:190–7.

121. Halligan S, Bartram CI, Park HJ, Kamm MA. Proctographic features of anismus. Radiology 1995; 197:679–82.

122. Halligan S, Bartram CI. The radiological investigation of constipation. Clin Radiol 1995; 50:429–35.

123. McLean RG, King DW, Talley NA, Tait AD, Freiman J. The utilization of colon transit scintigraphy in the diagnostic algorithm for patients with chronic constipation. Dig Dis Sci 1999; 44:41–7.

124. Gattuso JM, Kamm MA, Morris G, Britton KE. Gastrointestinal transit in patients with idiopathic megarectum. Dis Colon Rectum 1996; 39:1044–50.

125. Beynon J, Foy DMA, Temple LN, Channer JL, Virjee J, Mortensen NJMcC. The endosonic appearances of normal colon and rectum. Dis Colon Rectum 1986; 29:810–13.

126. Bartram CI, Sultan AH. Anal endosonography in faecal incontinence. Gut 1995; 37:4–6.

127. Sultan AH, Nicholls RJ, Kamm MA, Hudson CN, Beynon J, Bartram CI. Anal endosonography and correlation with in vitro and in vivo anatomy. Br J Surg 1993; 80:508–11.

128. Williams AB, Bartram CI, Halligan S, Marshall MM, Nicholls RJ, Kmiot WA. Endosonographic anatomy of the normal anal canal compared to endocoil magnetic resonance imaging. Dis Colon Rectum 2002; 45:176–83.

129. Tjandra JJ, Milsom JW, Stolfi VM et al. Endoluminal ultrasound defines anatomy of the anal canal and pelvic floor. Dis Colon Rectum 1992; 35:465–70.

130. Burnett SJ, Bartram CI. Endosonographic variations in the normal internal anal sphincter. Int J Colorectal Dis 1991; 6:2–4.

131. Stoker J, Rociu E, Zwamborn AW, Schouten WR, Lameris JS. Endoluminal MR imaging of the rectum and anus: technique, applications and pitfalls. Radiographics 1999; 19:398.

132. deSouza NM, Puni R, Zbar A, Gilderdale DJ, Coutts GA, Krausz T. MR imaging of the anal sphincter in multiparous women using an endoanal coil: correlation with in vitro anatomy and appearances in fecal incontinence. Am J Roentgenol 1996; 167:1465–71.

133. Tan IL, Stoker J, Zwamborn AW, Entius CA, Calame J, Lameris JS. Female pelvic floor: endovaginal MR imaging of normal anatomy. Radiology 1998; 206:777–83.

134. Nicholls RJ, York Mason A, Morson BC, Dixon AK, Kelsey Fry I. The clinical staging of rectal cancer. Br J Surg 1982; 69:404–9.

135. Orrom WJ, Wong WD, Rothenberger DA, Jensen LL, Goldberg SM. Endorectal ultrasound in the preoperative staging of rectal tumours. Dis Colon Rectum 1990; 33:654–9.

136. Romano G, de Rosa P, Vallone G, Rotondo A, Grassi R, Santangelo ML. Intrarectal ultrasound and computed tomography in the pre- and post-operative assessment of patients with rectal cancer. Br J Surg 1985; 9(suppl.): S117–S119.

137. Kramann B, Hildebrandt U. Computed tomography versus endosonography in the staging of rectal carcinoma: a comparative study. Int J Colorectal Dis 1986; 1:216–18.

138. Beynon J, Mortensen NJ, Foy DM, Channer JL, Rigby H, Virjee J. Preoperative assessment of mesorectal lymph node involvement in rectal cancer. Br J Surg 1989; 76:276–9.

139. McNicholas MM, Joyce WP, Dolan J, Gibney RG, MacErlaine DP, Hyland J. Magnetic resonance imaging of rectal carcinoma: a prospective study. Br J Surg 1994; 81:911–14.

140. Thaler W, Watzka S, Martin F et al. Preoperative staging of rectal cancer by endoluminal ultrasound vs. magnetic resonance imaging. Preliminary results of a prospective, comparative study. Dis Colon Rectum 1994; 37:1189–93.

141. Brown G, Richards CJ, Newcombe RG et al. Rectal carcinoma: thin-section MR imaging for staging in 28 patients. Radiology 1999; 211:215–22.

142. Napoleon B, Pujol B, Valette PJ, Gerard JP, Souquet JC. Accuracy of endosonography in the staging of rectal cancer treated by radiotherapy. Br J Surg 1991; 78:785–8.

143. Krestin GP, Steinbrich W, Friedmann G. Recurrent rectal cancer: diagnosis with MR imaging versus CT. Radiology 1988; 168:307–11.

144. Schratter-Shen AU, Lochs H, Vogelsang H, Schurawitzki H, Herold C, Schratter M. Comparison of transrectal ultrasonography and computed tomography in the diagnosis of peri-anorectal fistulae in patients with Crohn's disease. Gastroenterology 1992; 102:A691.

145. Deen KI, Williams JG, Hutchinson R, Keighley MR, Kumar D. Fistulas in ano: endoanal ultrasonographic assessment assists decision making for surgery. Gut 1994; 35:391–4.

146. Law PJ, Talbot RW, Bartram CI, Northover JM. Anal endosonography in the evaluation of perianal sepsis and fistula in ano. Br J Surg 1989; 76:752–5.

147. Choen S, Burnett S, Bartram CI, Nicholls RJ. Comparison between anal endosonography and digital examination in the evaluation of anal fistulae. Br J Surg 1991; 78:445–7.

148. Lunniss PJ, Barker PG, Sultan AH et al. Magnetic resonance imaging of fistula-in-ano. Dis Colon Rectum 1994; 37:708–18.

149. Buchanan GN, Halligan S, Williams AB et al. Magnetic resonance imaging for primary fistula in ano. Br J Surg 2003; 90:877–81.

150. Van Beers B, Grandin C, Kartheuser A. MRI of complicated anal fistulae: comparison with digital examination. J Comput Assist Tomogr 1994; 18:87–90.

151. Spencer JA, Ward J, Ambrose NS. Pictorial review: dynamic contrast-enhanced MR imaging of perianal fistulae. Clin Radiol 1998, 53:96–104.

152. Spencer JA, Chapple K, Wilson D, Ward J, Windsor ACJ, Ambrose NS. Outcome after surgery for perianal fistula: predictive value or MR imaging. Am J Roentgenol 1998; 171:403–6.

153. Law PJ, Kamm MA, Bartram CI. Anal endosonography in the investigation of faecal incontinence. Br J Surg 1991; 78:312–14.

154. Burnett SJD, Spence-Jones C, Speakman CT, Kamm M, Hudson CN, Bartram CI. Unsuspected sphincter damage following childbirth revealed by anal endosonography. Br J Radiol 1991; 64:225–7.

155. Donnelly V, Fynes M, Campbell D, Johnson H, O'Connell PRO'H. Obstetric events leading to anal sphincter damage. Obstet Gynecol 1998; 92:955–61.

156. Williams AB, Bartram CI, Halligan S, Spencer JA, Nicholls RJ, Kmiot WA. Sphincter damage after vaginal delivery: a prospective study. Obstet Gynecol 2000; 97:770–5.

157. Williams AB, Bartram CI, Halligan S et al. Alteration of anal sphincter morphology following vaginal delivery revealed by multiplanar anal endosonography. Br J Obstet Gynaecol 2002; 109:942–6.

158. Tjandra JJ, Milsom JW, Schroeder T, Fazio VW. Endoluminal ultrasound is preferable to electro-myography in mapping anal sphincteric defects. Dis Colon Rectum 1993; 36:689–92.

159. Sultan AH, Kamm MA, Talbot IC, Nicholls RJ, Bartram CI. Anal endosonography for identifying external sphincter defects confirmed histologically. Br J Surg 1994; 81:463–5.

160. Sentovich SM, Blatchford GJ, Rivela LJ, Lin K, Thorson AG, Christensen MA. Diagnosing anal sphincter injury with transanal ultrasound and manometry. Dis Colon Rectum 1997; 40:1430–4.

161. deSouza NM, Hall AS, Puni R, Gilderdale DJ, Young IR, Kmiot WA. High resolution magnetic resonance imaging of the anal sphincter using a dedicated endoanal coil. Comparison of magnetic resonance imaging with surgical findings. Dis Colon Rectum 1996; 39:926–34.

162. Stoker J, Hussain SM, Lameris JS. Endoanal magnetic resonance imaging versus endosonography. Radiol Med (Torino) 1996; 92:738–41.

163. Malouf AJ, Williams AB, Halligan S, Bartram CI, Dhillon S, Kamm MA. Prospective assessment of accuracy of endoanal MR imaging and

endosonography in patients with fecal incontinence. Am J Roentgenol 2000; 175:741–5.

164. Williams AB, Bartram CI, Halligan S. Review of three-dimensional anal endosonography. RAD 1999; 25:47–8.

165. Gold DM, Bartram CI, Halligan S, Humphries KN, Kamm MA, Kmiot WA. Three-dimensional endoanal sonography in assessing anal canal injury. Br J Surg 1999; 86:365–70.

166. Williams AB, Bartram CI, Modhwadia D et al. Endocoil magnetic resonance imaging quantification of external anal sphincter atrophy. Br J Surg 2001; 88:853–9.

167. Briel JW, Stoker J, Rociu E, Lameris JS, Hop WC, Schouten WR. External anal sphincter atrophy on endoanal magnetic resonance imaging adversely affects continence after sphincteroplasty. Br J Surg 1999; 86:1322–7.

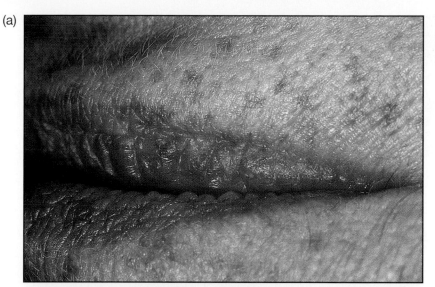

(a)

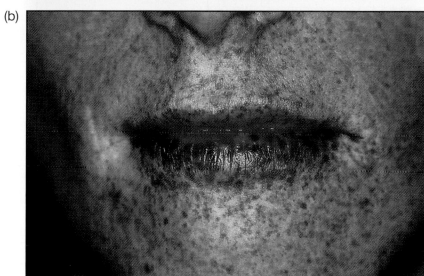

(b)

Plate 1 • Comparison of common perioral freckling **(a)** with Peutz–Jeghers pigmentation **(b)**.

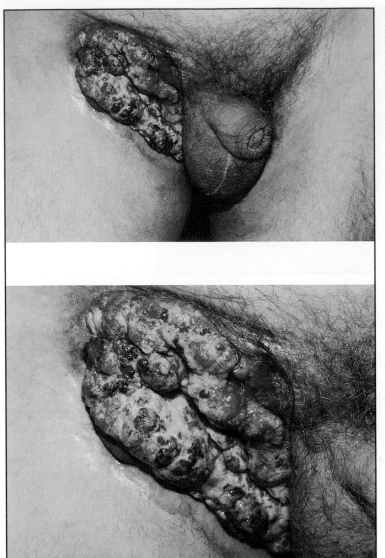

Plate 2 • Locally advanced anal cancer involving the anal canal, perianal skin, perineal skin and base of scrotum. Treatment with chemo-irradiation failed to control the disease and the patient underwent a salvage abdominoperineal excision.

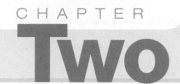

CHAPTER

Two

Inherited bowel cancer

Sue Clark

INTRODUCTION

Individuals develop colorectal cancer as a result of interactions between their genotype and the environment to which they, and their large bowel, are exposed. The lifetime risk of colorectal cancer in the UK population is about 5%. As it is a common cancer, many people are quite likely by chance alone to have at least one affected relative;[1] as the number of affected relatives increases, so does the risk of developing the disease.[2] As far as the genetic factors are concerned, there is a spectrum of risk, at one end of which are those who have no particular genetic predisposition, and at the other end those who will almost inevitably develop bowel cancer. In between the two extremes lie those whose genetic constitution plays a variable role. While to some extent an oversimplification, it is possible to divide the population's risk for colorectal cancer into three broad categories: low risk, moderate risk and high risk.

In the high-risk group, the contribution of inheritance or genotype is overwhelming, though environmental influences may modify disease severity (phenotype). It is this minority (amounting to less than 5% of the total large bowel cancer load) that is traditionally described as being at risk of 'inherited bowel cancer'.

In the low- and moderate-risk groups, genotype may still contribute to risk, but in a less marked fashion, and is thought to play a part in about 30% of colorectal cancers.[3] This may be due to modifying genes that influence responses to carcinogen exposure and to protective dietary nutrients.

This chapter deals predominantly with those in the high-risk group, where inheritance of the risk of developing bowel cancer is very strong. Although these individuals make up only a minority of those at risk overall, there is now sufficient knowledge about the specific syndromes that fall within this category to provide important opportunities for cancer prevention.

ASSESSMENT OF RISK

The crucial step in allocating individuals to one of the three risk categories is the documentation of an accurate family history which, in the absence of a diagnosis of familial adenomatous polyposis (FAP) or hereditary non-polyposis colorectal cancer (HNPCC), allows an empirical assessment of risk.[2] It should focus on the site and age at diagnosis of all cancers in family members, as well as the presence of related features such as colorectal adenomas. This can be a time-consuming task, especially when the information needs to be verified. Few surgeons are able to devote the necessary time or skill to do this satisfactorily, and it is here that family cancer clinics or family cancer registries for inherited bowel cancer have an important role to play (grade 2 evidence).[4]

A full personal history should also be taken, with particular attention to the following.

- presence of symptoms (e.g. rectal bleeding, change in bowel habit), which should be investigated as usual;
- previous large bowel polyps;
- previous large bowel cancers;
- cancers at other sites;
- Other risk factors for colorectal cancer (inflammatory bowel disease, ureterosigmoidostomy, acromegaly); these conditions are not discussed further in this chapter, but may warrant surveillance of the large bowel.

The family history has many limitations, particularly in small families. Other difficulties arise because of incorrect information, lack of contact between family members, early death of individuals before they develop cancers, and non-paternity. A vast range of complex pedigrees arise, and rather than try to devise equally complex guidelines to cover all of them, common sense is needed. If a family seems to fall between risk groups (e.g. one first-degree relative aged 55 years and a second-degree relative aged 50 years on the same side of the family, both with bowel cancer), it would be safest to manage the family as if in the higher risk group. Despite this, some families will appear to be at high risk simply because of chance clustering of truly sporadic cancer while some, particularly small families with HNPCC, will be assigned to the low- or moderate-risk groups. In addition, even in families affected with an autosomal dominant condition, 50% of family members will not have inherited the causative mutated gene and will therefore not be at any increased risk of developing bowel cancer.

It should also be borne in mind that family histories evolve, so that the allocation of an individual to a particular risk group may change if further family members develop tumours. It is important that patients are informed of this, particularly if they are in the low- or moderate-risk

groups and are therefore not undergoing regular surveillance.

Low-risk group

This group encompasses the majority of the population. Individuals have:

1. no personal history of bowel cancer; no confirmed family history of bowel cancer; or
2. no first-degree relative (i.e. parent, sibling or child) with bowel cancer; or
3. one first-degree relative with bowel cancer diagnosed at age 45 years or older.

Moderate-risk group

Individuals are allocated to this category if there is:

1. one first-degree relative with bowel cancer diagnosed before the age of 45 years (without the high-risk features outlined below); or
2. two first-degree relatives with bowel cancer diagnosed at any age (without the high-risk features outlined below).

High-risk group

This category encompasses HNPCC and the various polyposis syndromes. Criteria for inclusion include:

1. member of a family with known (FAP) or other polyposis syndrome; or
2. member of a family with known HNPCC; or
3. pedigree suggestive of autosomal dominantly inherited colorectal (or other HNPCC-associated) cancer; various different criteria are used, for example
   (a) three or more first- or second-degree (grandparent, uncle/aunt, niece/nephew) relatives with bowel cancer on the same side of the family;
   (b) two or more first- or second-degree relatives with bowel cancer on the same side of the family with bowel cancer and one or more of the following high-risk features:
   (i) multiple bowel cancers in an individual;
   (ii) diagnosis before age 45 years; and
   (iii) a relative with endometrial or another HNPCC-associated cancer.

Diagnosis of the polyposis syndromes is comparatively straightforward as there is a recognisable phenotype in each. HNPCC is much more difficult as there is no recognisable phenotype, other than the occurrence of cancers.

MANAGEMENT

Low-risk group

The risk of bowel cancer even in these individuals may be up to twice the average risk,[2] although this tends to be expressed after the sixth decade of life. There is no evidence to support invasive surveillance in this group.[5] It is important to explain to these individuals that they are at average or only marginally above average risk of developing colorectal cancer, but that this risk is not sufficient to outweigh the disadvantages of colonoscopy. They should be aware of the symptoms of colorectal cancer, and the importance of reporting if further members of the family develop tumours. In addition, population screening, in the form of either faecal occult blood testing or flexible sigmoidoscopy, is likely to be introduced in the UK in the foreseeable future, and individuals in this risk category should be encouraged to take part.

Moderate-risk group

There is a threefold to sixfold relative risk for individuals in this category,[2] but probably only a marginal benefit from surveillance.

Part of the reason for this is that the incidence of colorectal cancer is very low in the young but rises markedly in the elderly. Thus even those aged 50 who have a sixfold relative risk by virtue of their family history are less likely to develop colorectal cancer in the following 10 years than are 60 year olds at average risk.[6]

Current recommendations[5] are that individuals in this risk group should be offered colonoscopy at 35–40 years of age (or at presentation if they are older), and again at the age of 55 years. If polyps are found, follow-up is modified accordingly. Flexible sigmoidoscopy is not sufficient, as neoplasms in individuals with a strong family history are often proximal; if the caecum is not reached, barium enema or CT colography should be performed.

Again, these individuals should be informed of the symptoms of colorectal cancer, the importance of reporting changes in family history and that they should take part in population screening when it is introduced.

High-risk group

There is up to a 1 in 2 chance of inheriting a high risk of developing bowel cancer in this group, and referral to a clinical genetic service is essential. The polyposis syndromes are usually diagnosed from the phenotype, which can be supplemented by genetic testing. Diagnostic confusion can arise, particularly in cases where there are adenomatous polyps insufficient to be diagnostic for FAP. This may occur in FAP with an attenuated phenotype, or in HNPCC. A careful search for extracolonic features, mistach repair immunohistochemistry and microsatellite instability assessment of tumour tissue, and germline mutation detection can sometimes help. Despite this, the diagnosis in some families remains in doubt. In these circumstances the family members should be offered thorough surveillance.

HEREDITARY NON-POLYPOSIS COLORECTAL CANCER

HNPCC is responsible for about 2% of colorectal cancers and is the commonest of the two main inherited bowel cancer syndromes. HNPCC was previously known as Lynch syndrome and is inherited in an autosomal dominant fashion. Labelled first as the 'cancer family syndrome', the name was changed to HNPCC to distinguish it from the polyposis syndromes and to highlight the absence of the high numbers of colorectal adenomas found in FAP. However, adenomatous polyps are a feature of HNPCC. The terms Lynch syndrome I and II were proposed in 1984 to describe those with predominantly colorectal cancer at a young age (Lynch I) and those with both colorectal and extracolonic cancers (Lynch II).[7]

Clinical features

HNPCC is characterised by early onset of colorectal tumours, the average age at diagnosis being 45 years compared with approximately 65 years in the general population. These tumours have certain distinguishing pathological features. There is a predilection for the proximal colon, and tumours are also frequently multiple (synchronous and metachronous). They tend to be mucinous, poorly differentiated and of 'signet-ring' appearance, with marked infiltration by lymphocytes and lymphoid aggregation at their margins. The associated cancers and their frequencies are detailed in **Table 2.1**.[8] The prognosis of all these cancers tends to be better than in the same tumours arising sporadically.

Genetics

HNPCC is due to germline mutations in mismatch repair (MMR) genes, whose role is to correct errors in base-pair matching during replication of DNA or to initiate apoptosis when DNA damage is beyond repair. The following MMR genes have been identified and mutations in them may be associated with HNPCC: *hMLH1*, *hMSH2*, *hMSH6*, *hPMS1*, *hPMS2* and *hMSH3*. The MMR genes are tumour-suppressor genes: patients with HNPCC inherit a defective copy from one parent and tumorigenesis is triggered when the solitary normal gene in a cell becomes mutated or lost due to environmental factors, so that DNA mismatches are no longer repaired in that cell. Defective MMR results in the accumulation of mutations in a host of other genes, leading to tumour formation.

Defective MMR also results in microsatellite instability (MSI), a hallmark of tumours in HNPCC.[9] Microsatellites are regions where a short DNA sequence (up to five nucleotides) is repeated. There are large numbers of such sequences in the human genome, the majority in non-coding DNA. Base-pair mismatches occurring during DNA replication are normally repaired by the MMR proteins. In tumours with a deficiency of these proteins this mechanism fails and microsatellites become mutated, resulting in a change in the number of sequence repeats and hence the length of the microsatellite (microsatellite instability). Typically in such a tumour over half of all microsatellites will exhibit this phenomenon.

About 25% of colorectal cancers show MSI. Some of these are from individuals with HNPCC, and are due to inherited MMR mutation. The majority, however, occur in older patients and are thought to be due to inactivation of MMR genes by methylation over time, a change that takes place in the colonic epithelial cells with ageing but which is not inherited.

Although predominantly a disorder based on MMR mutations, there is evidence to suggest that other influences affect expression in HNPCC populations. Thus, a comparative study between Korean and Dutch families with *hMLH1* mutations found that there were more gastric and pancreatic cancers and fewer endometrial cancers in the Koreans than in the Dutch.[10] This implies either that these Korean families were affected by a modifying gene or genes also prevalent in the general population (which has a high risk for gastric cancer), or that environmental influences exist to which the Korean population are exposed and which interact with the mutations responsible for HNPCC-related cancers.

Diagnosis

PEDIGREE

Over the years a confusing range of 'criteria' have emerged. The International Collaborative Group on HNPCC (ICG-HNPCC), established in 1989, proposed the Amsterdam criteria in 1990 (**Box 2.1**). These were not intended as a diagnostic definition but rather as a means to identify families very likely to be harbouring HNPCC. The aim of this was to allow genetic research to be targeted on a well-defined group that was likely to yield positive results. While families fulfilling these criteria very likely have HNPCC, many affected families will not meet the stringent conditions.[11] The Amsterdam criteria were modified by the ICG-HNPCC in 1999

Table 2.1 • Cancers associated with HNPCC

Site	Frequency (%)
Large bowel	80
Endometrium	40 (of women)
Stomach	15
Ovary	12
Urothelium (renal pelvis, ureter, bladder)	5
Other (small bowel, pancreas, brain)	<5

Box 2.1 • HNPCC: Amsterdam criteria I

- At least three relatives with colorectal cancer, one of whom should be a first-degree relative of the other two
- At least two successive generations should be affected
- At least one colorectal cancer should be diagnosed before age 50 years
- FAP should be excluded
- Tumours should be verified by pathological examination

(**Box 2.2**) to include HNPCC-associated cancers other than colorectal cancer (Amsterdam II criteria), so that a diagnosis of HNPCC might be made using either set of criteria.[12] However, some HNPCC-affected families will still fail to meet them.

Genetic testing is expensive and time-consuming. The circumstances under which it is offered vary from centre to centre, but generally an affected individual (i.e. with an HNPCC-related cancer) from a family fulfilling the Amsterdam I or II criteria would be offered testing. In families in whom the risk of HNPCC is not obviously high but where clinical suspicion remains, analysis of tumour tissue can provide further useful information.

ANALYSIS OF TUMOUR TISSUE

A reference panel of five microsatellite markers is used to detect MSI; if two of the markers show

Box 2.2 • HNPCC: Amsterdam criteria II

- At least three relatives with an HNPCC-associated cancer (colorectal, endometrial, small bowel, ureter, renal pelvis), one of whom should be a first-degree relative of the other two
- At least two successive generations should be affected
- At least one colorectal cancer should be diagnosed before age 50 years
- FAP should be excluded
- Tumours should be verified by pathological examination

From Vasen HFA, Watson P, Mecklin J-P et al. New clinical criteria for hereditary nonpolyposis colorectal cancer (HNPCC, Lynch syndrome) proposed by the International Collaborative Group on HNPCC. Gastroenterology 1999; 116:1453–6, with permission from the American Gastroenterological Association.

instability, the tumour is designated 'MSI-high'. About 25% of colorectal cancers are MSI-high, but only a minority of these will be from patients with HNPCC. The value of MSI testing stems from the fact that HNPCC is due to MMR mutation and therefore virtually all tumours arising as a result of HNPCC will be MSI-high. The Bethesda guidelines[13] (**Box 2.3**) have been suggested for determining whether the tumour tissue from an individual should be tested for MSI. The aim was to provide a sensitive set of guidelines that would encompass nearly all HNPCC-associated colorectal cancers but also many 'sporadic cancers', and to use MSI testing to exclude those individuals lacking MSI-high, whose cancers are therefore extremely unlikely to be caused by HNPCC. Those designated MSI-high can then be further investigated using immunohistochemistry and genetic testing. Using this approach, approximately 95% of individuals with colorectal cancer due to HNPCC can be identified.

MSI testing is expensive, requiring DNA extraction and 'relatively inaccessible'[14] technology. A simpler approach, which could be performed routinely on all colorectal cancer specimens, is to use standard immunohistochemical techniques to identify MMR proteins.[9,15] The results of immunohistochemistry, if reported on the standard histopathology form,

Box 2.3 • Bethesda criteria for determining whether the tumour tissue from an individual with colorectal cancer should be tested for microsatellite instability

- Individuals with colorectal cancer diagnosed at age 50 years
- Individuals with multiple colorectal or other HNPCC-associated tumours, either at the same time (synchronous) or occurring over a period of time (metachronous)
- Individuals diagnosed with colorectal cancer at < 60 years, in whom the tumour has microscopic characteristics indicative of microsatellite instability
- Individuals with colorectal cancer who have one or more first-degree relatives diagnosed with an HNPCC-related tumour at age 50 years or younger
- Individuals with colorectal cancer who have two or more first- or second-degree relatives diagnosed with an HNPCC-related tumour at any age

will also serve to remind the surgeon on each occasion of the possibility of HNPCC and of the relevance of genetic testing. Care is needed in interpreting the results, as abnormal MMR protein, which stains normally but does not function, can be present in HNPCC.

GENETIC TESTING

The decision whether to perform germline genetic testing on a blood sample from an at-risk or affected person takes the features of the patient, family and tumour into account. This cautious approach is currently justified on the grounds of cost, since genetic testing for MMR genes in the first member of the family (mutation detection) currently costs around £1000. Logistic models for estimating the likelihood of an MMR gene mutation, based on the Amsterdam I criteria, the average age of diagnosis of colorectal cancer in the family and the presence of endometrial cancer, have been derived to produce a strategy for molecular analysis. Where the probability of mutation detection is greater than 20%, germline testing is recommended; where less than 20%, MSI analysis is suggested, on the basis of cost-effectiveness.[16] Once a mutation has been detected in a family, testing other at-risk family members to determine whether they too carry the abnormal gene (predictive testing) is much more straightforward, and allows those without the mutation to be discharged from further surveillance.

As with the other syndromes described in this chapter, testing should be undertaken only after the patient has been counselled appropriately and given informed consent. The consent process should include an offer to provide written information, including a frank discussion of the benefits and risks (e.g. to employment, insurance) of genetic testing. A multidisciplinary clinic where counselling is available is ideal.[7,17] However, not every individual will accept an offer of genetic testing. Significant predictors of test uptake by individuals include an increased perception of risk, greater confidence in the ability to cope with unfavourable genetic news, more frequent thoughts of cancer and having had at least one colonoscopy.[18]

Germline gene testing may have several outcomes (**Box 2.4**) and the results should be relayed via the multidisciplinary clinic, where counselling is available.[19]

Box 2.4 • Outcomes of genetic testing in HNPCC

Mutation detected

Test at-risk family members (predictive testing): if positive, surveillance and/or other management (e.g. surgery); if negative, no surveillance required

Mutation not detected

Keep all at-risk members under surveillance (current tests have a sensitivity of approximately 80%)

There are also complexities of interpretation of results that mandate this (missense mutations, genetic heterogeneity, limited availability of validated assays).[20]

Unregulated genetic testing for cancer risk has led to errors and adverse events for individuals,[21] lending further support to the need for thoughtful organisation of the system involved in gene testing for cancer susceptibility. Failure to detect a mutation may be due to a variety of factors: some cases may be due to mutation in regulatory genes rather than the MMR genes themselves; there may be other genes involved that have not yet been identified; there may be a technical failure to identify a mutation which is present; or the family history may be a cluster of sporadic tumours. When this happens, the at-risk family members should continue to be screened.

Surveillance

There is good evidence that regular colonoscopy significantly reduces the 80% risk of colorectal cancer in HNPCC patients.[22]

Colonoscopy must be meticulous, because tiny cancers may be present.[23] Thus, for individuals with HNPCC, colonoscopy every 2 years from age 25 years (or 5 years younger than the youngest affected relative, whichever is the earlier) is recommended for at-risk individuals. Surveillance should continue until 75 years or until the causative mutation in that family has been excluded.[5]

The risk for extracolonic cancers appears to depend on which MMR gene is mutated, being

Box 2.5 • Extracolonic surveillance in HNPCC

- Annual transvaginal ultrasound ± colour flow Doppler imaging ± endometrial sampling
- Annual CA125 level and clinical examination (pelvic and abdominal)
- Upper gastrointestinal endoscopy every 2 years
- Annual urinalysis/cytology
- Annual abdominal ultrasound/renal tracts, pelvis, pancreas
- Annual liver function tests, CA19-9, CEA

nearly 50% for carriers of the *hMSH2* mutation compared with approximately 10% for carriers of the *hMLH1* mutation.[7] Screening for extracolonic cancers is available, but there is currently little evidence of benefit. Recommendations vary from centre to centre, but surveillance is generally advised where there is a family history of cancers at a particular site. **Box 2.5** shows the options for extracolonic surveillance.

Intervention

SURGERY
Prophylactic
The option of prophylactic colectomy rather than colonoscopic surveillance should be discussed with mutation carriers, because of the high risk of colorectal cancer. A similar situation pertains to prophylactic hysterectomy and bilateral salpingo-oophorectomy at the time of colectomy in women who have completed their families.

Colectomy might be subtotal, with an ileorectal anastomosis, or might take the form of a restorative proctocolectomy. The risk of metachronous cancer in the retained rectum after ileorectal anastomosis has been estimated to be about 12% at 12 years.[24] Regardless of the operation performed, regular endoscopy via the anus should be carried out post-operatively, at intervals no greater than 12 months, depending on findings. Use of a decision analysis model indicates large gains in life expectancy for carriers of an HNPCC mutation when offered some intervention. Benefits were quantified as 13.5 years from surveillance, 15.6 years from proctocolectomy and 15.3 years from subtotal colectomy compared

with no intervention.[25] Adjusting for quality of life showed that surveillance led to the greatest quality-adjusted life expectancy benefit. This study provides a mathematically based indication of benefit only: individual circumstances need to be incorporated into the decision-making process when making recommendations.

Treatment

There is a risk of metachronous bowel tumours of 45% (grade 2 evidence).[26]

For those with colonic tumours, colectomy with ileorectal anastomosis has a prophylactic element in that the entire colon is removed, but without the additional morbidity of proctectomy. Procto-colectomy (with or without ileo-anal pouch reconstruction, which depends on the height of the tumour, the age and general fitness of the patient, and the quality of the anal sphincter) is the option of choice in patients who present with rectal cancer.

MEDICAL
Studies of in vitro colorectal cancer using cells deficient in MMR genes has shown that MSI is reduced in cells exposed to non-steroidal anti-inflammatory drugs (NSAIDs).[27] This provides some theoretical support for the CAPP2 (Colorectal Adenoma/Carcinoma Prevention Programme 2) study, currently underway in HNPCC patients, using aspirin and resistant starch as chemopreventive agents. As yet, however, there is no evidence to support the use of any medical therapy in HNPCC.

The benefit of cytotoxic chemotherapy for cancers in the setting of HNPCC has been questioned, but the evidence to date is contradictory. Some agents (notably 5-fluorouracil) act by damaging DNA, which results in apoptosis. MMR proteins are thought to play a part in signalling the presence of irreversible DNA damage and initiating apoptosis, a pathway absent in these tumours.

Future developments

Screening, surveillance and treatment may be more individualised in future, as more is understood about genotype–phenotype interactions.[28] Gene therapy for HNPCC (as in other inherited bowel cancer syndromes) remains a focus of research. HNPCC may yet undergo another change in nomenclature, with the suggestion that it be replaced by 'hereditary mismatch repair deficiency syndrome' (HMRDS).[29] Unless colorectal surgeons and others are acquainted with the molecular basis for diagnosis, HMRDS will not be an easily understood or clinically meaningful acronym. If one fails to understand this condition, and this applies to inherited bowel cancer in general, then one also runs the risk of prejudicing the survival of patients. This now carries with it a risk of medicolegal action.[30]

FAMILIAL ADENOMATOUS POLYPOSIS

Less common than HNPCC, the risk of colorectal cancer in patients with FAP is nearly 100%. FAP is usually characterised by:

- hundreds of colorectal adenomatous polyps at a young age (second or third decade of life);
- duodenal adenomatous polyps;
- multiple extraintestinal manifestations (**Box 2.6**);

Box 2.6 • Extracolonic manifestations in FAP

Ectodermal origin
• Epidermoid cysts
• Pilomatrixoma
• Tumours of central nervous system
• Congenital hypertrophy of the retinal pigment epithelium
Mesodermal origin
• Connective tissue: desmoid tumours, excessive adhesions
• Bone: osteoma, exostosis, sclerosis
• Dental: dentigerous cyst, odontoma, supernumerary teeth, unerupted teeth
Endodermal origin
• Adenomas and carcinomas of duodenum, stomach, small intestine, biliary tract, thyroid, adrenal cortex
• Fundic gland polyps
• Hepatoblastoma

- mutation in the tumour-suppressor adenomatous polyposis coli (*APC*) gene on chromosome 5q;
- autosomal dominant inheritance (offspring of affected individuals have a 1 in 2 chance of inheriting FAP).

Diagnosis

FAP was originally defined by the presence of over 100 colorectal adenomas. This clinical definition is still useful, as a mutation in the *APC* gene can only be identified in up to 80% of affected individuals. The majority of new cases come from families with a known history of the disease, but confusion can arise as approximately 20% are due to a new mutation.[31] In these circumstances there will be no family history of colorectal cancers at a young age or of multiple polyps. A further potential source of confusion is the well-documented existence of a milder form of the condition, known as attenuated FAP.[32]

Inadequate colonoscopy may lead to a false diagnosis of attenuation, an error that can be avoided by the use of dye-spray.[33] In this technique, either indigo-carmine or diluted writing ink is sprayed down a catheter in the biopsy channel of the colonoscope, adding a contrast to the transparent mucosal surface and thereby accentuating the profile of diminutive polyps that might otherwise be missed. A further point that needs to be borne in mind is that some individuals with HNPCC have a number of adenomatous polyps. Where the diagnosis requires confirmation, the use of dye-spray and random biopsies looking for microadenomas (a hallmark of FAP, but which are not seen in HNPCC) are helpful, as are testing for MSI and immunohistochemistry of tumours.

Genetic testing

The issue of genetic testing is a useful paradigm highlighting the fundamental role played by registries. Identification of at-risk family members who might be offered gene testing is critical and is usually made possible by the comprehensive collation of family pedigrees that such registries are uniquely positioned to obtain and update.[34] Once tested, results need to be given to the individual. An uncontrolled approach to testing and the release of results leads to inadequate counselling and the provision of incorrect information to patients.[35]

An affected family member should be tested first. The mutation can be located in approximately 80% of affected individuals. Once the mutation has been identified, at-risk members of the family can be offered testing. Should the known family mutation not be found in the at-risk individual, that person can be discharged from continued surveillance[36] but should be informed that he or she remains at the same risk of sporadic colorectal cancer as any member of the general population. Such an approach eliminates unnecessary colonic examination and costs less than conventional clinical screening.[37]

GENOTYPE–PHENOTYPE CORRELATION

The site of the mutation in the *APC* gene can influence the expression of FAP.[38]

This genotype–phenotype correlation is seen in the association between certain mutations and severe FAP (dense colorectal polyposis with relatively early colorectal cancer development), and between other mutations and less severe FAP ('attenuated' polyposis).[39] However, individuals with identical mutations can display differences in phenotypic expression, suggesting that other modifying genes and the environment play a role in disease severity and expression.[40]

Nevertheless, there is molecular support for the existence of the attenuated FAP variant, based on the finding that the gene product in attenuated FAP interferes only weakly with *APC* gene expression when compared with the gene product associated with a mutation in the area associated with severe FAP (codon 1309).[41] Some of the multiple extra-colonic manifestations of FAP (see **Box 2.6**),[42] such as desmoid disease, also show some correlation with the mutation site; others, notably duodenal polyposis and malignancy, do not.

These genotype–phenotype correlations have led to suggestions that the findings of molecular analysis might guide both surveillance and treatment regimen.[39,43,44] At present, however, it is important to emphasise that prophylactic colectomy or procto-colectomy (almost always with a pouch) remains the management option of choice for all patients with proven FAP (grade 2 evidence).

Surveillance

If the family mutation is known, at-risk family members are usually offered predictive genetic testing in their early teens. If this is not possible, then clinical surveillance is required. It is very unusual for colorectal polyps to develop before the teenage years and while cancers have been described in this age group, they are exceptionally rare. If an individual has symptoms attributable to the large bowel (anaemia, rectal bleeding or change in bowel habit), then of course colonoscopy should be performed. Otherwise annual flexible sigmoidoscopy starting at 13–15 years of age is recommended. If no polyps are detected, colonoscopy should be started at the age of about 20 years, alternating with flexible sigmoidoscopy, so that one or other examination is performed annually.

Colorectal polyps

SURGERY
Prophylactic

Once the diagnosis has been made, either by predictive genetic testing or by the detection of adenomatous polyposis during surveillance of an at-risk family member, the aim is to offer prophylactic surgery before a cancer develops. If the diagnosis has been made on the basis of flexible sigmoidoscopy, colonoscopy should be performed to assess the severity of the polyps throughout the colon. If the individual is symptomatic or the polyps are dense or large, surgery should be undertaken as soon as is practical. In other cases it is usual to defer surgery until a time when its social and educational impact will be minimised, usually a long summer vacation or 'gap' after leaving school.

As the surgical options have increased, so has the controversy surrounding the choice between them. Increasingly, laparoscopically assisted surgery is becoming available and has great attractions in this group where a good cosmetic result makes surgery more acceptable. The available operations are:

- colectomy and ileorectal anastomosis (IRA);
- restorative proctocolectomy (RPC) with an ileal pouch–anal anastomosis;
- total proctocolectomy and end ileostomy (almost exclusively for those with low rectal cancer).

Most young people facing prophylactic colectomy will want to avoid a permanent ileostomy, so the choice really lies between the first two options. The biggest attraction of RPC is that the entire large bowel is removed, so that there is no risk of polyps and cancers developing in a retained rectum. However, this is not entirely true, as a cuff of rectal mucosa is retained when the operation is performed using a stapled anastomosis, and cancers at this site have been reported.[45] At operation, a mucosectomy can be performed to remove this area and a hand-sewn pouch anal anastomosis created, but this is a more technically demanding technique, which probably also results in marginally poorer functional outcome. Furthermore, follow-up studies are beginning to show adenoma formation within ileo-anal pouches, so there is concern that over time these may develop into invasive cancers.[46]

The advantages of IRA are that it is a one-stage procedure (whereas RPC often involves a temporary defunctioning ileostomy) with lower morbidity and mortality. The functional results in terms of stool frequency and leakage are generally slightly better than after RPC, although it is difficult to know how much impact these small differences make.

Sexual and reproductive function can both be compromised by proctectomy. There is a small but definite risk of erectile and ejaculatory dysfunction in men undergoing proctectomy, and recent studies have shown that RPC for both FAP[47] and ulcerative colitis affects fertility in women. These potential complications are particularly difficult to accept for essentially healthy young people undergoing surgery for prophylaxis rather than treatment.

It is known that some groups are at particular risk of developing rectal cancer after IRA. These are individuals with numerous rectal polyps, carriers of certain mutations and those presenting over the age of 25–30 years. Historical data show a cumulative rectal cancer risk of up to 30% by 60 years of age and a subsequent proctectomy rate of up to 30%, but at the time many of these patients underwent IRA, RPC was not available. IRA was the only option to avoid a permanent ileostomy, and thus was done in circumstances when it would not now be recommended.

In selected cases the risk of rectal cancer is low and IRA is a reasonable option.[48]

Many patients will have experience of one or both operations from other family members who have undergone them, which may affect their choice. Ultimately, they need to be informed about the advantages and disadvantages of both procedures, as well as the implications of their genotype (if identified) so that their decision can be as informed as possible.

Treatment

In the presence of a colonic cancer, the surgical decision-making is essentially the same as in prophylactic surgery. In individuals with severe rectal polyposis, in those carrying a mutation at codon 1309 of the *APC* gene or in those aged over 25–30 years, the risk of subsequent uncontrollable rectal polyposis requiring completion proctectomy, or of rectal cancer itself, are high and outweigh the disadvantages of RPC. In younger patients, those with few rectal polyps (or mutations at other sites) and older patients with a genuine attenuated phenotype, IRA may represent a better option. Ultimately, it remains for the informed patient to make a choice.

When rectal cancer is present, the choice is between RPC and proctocolectomy and ileostomy. As in any case of rectal cancer, a very low tumour precludes reconstruction. A further factor that needs to be taken into account is that pelvic radiotherapy given before or after formation of an ileo-anal pouch results in either anal or pouch dysfunction, so it should be avoided if oncologically possible. Careful local staging and multidisciplinary management are crucial in these cases.

SURVEILLANCE AFTER SURGERY

Follow-up is required after all procedures. After IRA or RPC, peranal digital and flexible endoscopic examination are mandatory at intervals of up to 12 months, depending on findings. The NSAID sulindac has been used to control rectal adenomas[49] and pouch adenomas.[50]

A recent trial using the selective cyclooxygenase (COX)-2 inhibitor celecoxib has shown a moderate reduction in large bowel polyps in treated patients,[51] but must be used with caution in view of earlier reports of cancer despite chemoprevention (with sulindac) and surveillance in this setting.

Following colectomy, the major causes of mortality and morbidity are duodenal cancers, desmoid tumours and, in those who have an IRA, rectal cancers. This knowledge guides postoperative management.[34]

Upper gastrointestinal tract polyps

Non-adenomatous gastric polyps (fundic gland polyps) occur in approximately 50% of patients with FAP. Their malignant potential is extremely low but not non-existent.[52]

 Duodenal adenomas occur in nearly all patients with FAP but are severe in only 10%, with malignant change occurring in 5%.[53]

SURVEILLANCE OF THE UPPER GASTROINTESTINAL TRACT

Surveillance usually begins in the third decade of life (in the asymptomatic patient), with endoscopies at intervals of between 6 months and 3 years depending on the severity of duodenal polyposis.[54] A staging system for duodenal polyposis has been developed (**Table 2.2**) to allow surveillance to be tailored to disease severity and to identify individuals at high risk of developing malignant

Table 2.2 • Spigelman staging of severity of duodenal polyposis in FAP

	Points allocated		
	1	2	3
Number of polyps	1–4	5–20	>20
Polyp size (mm)	1–4	5–10	>10
Histological type	Tubular	Tubulovillous	Villous
Degree of dysplasia	Mild	Moderate	Severe
Total points			
0	Stage 0		
1–4	Stage I		
5–6	Stage II		
7–8	Stage III		
9–12	Stage IV		

change.[55] Upper gastroduodenal endoscopy leads to a moderate gain in life expectancy.[56] The periampullary area must be examined, being at particularly high risk, so a side-viewing as well as end-viewing scope should be used in the examination.[57]

MANAGEMENT OF DUODENAL POLYPOSIS

 Management of severe duodenal polyposis is difficult. Chemopreventive options have some benefit.[58,59]

Interventions such as endoscopic removal or open duodenotomy are associated with high recurrence rates.[60] The risk of endoscopic-induced duodenal perforation may be obviated by using argon plasma coagulation.[61] Advanced endoscopic techniques, often under general anaesthesia, are currently being investigated in patients with Spigelman stage III disease.

 While prophylactic pancreatico-duodenectomy or pylorus-preserving pancreatico-duodenectomy has been described with good outcomes,[53,60] associated morbidity and mortality are substantial. However, the poor prognosis once invasive disease is present and the high rate of progression to cancer of advanced polyposis (36% in one series) means that this aggressive approach can be justified in some cases with Spigelman stage IV disease. Cancer risk and hence the need for intervention is minimal in patients with stage 0–II disease.

Desmoid tumours

Desmoid tumours are fibromatous lesions consisting of clonal proliferations of myofibroblasts.[62] They occur in approximately 15% of individuals with FAP, with a mortality rate of about 10%.[63,64] However, the majority exhibit cycles of growth and resolution and, while causing discomfort and being unsightly, may not cause significant problems. Most desmoids associated with FAP arise either intra-abdominally (usually within the small bowel mesentery) or on the abdominal wall, although they can appear in the extremities and trunk. They are histologically benign, but within the abdomen can cause small bowel and ureteric obstruction, intestinal ischaemia or perforation, all of which can be fatal. A model of desmoid tumour development, based on the appearance of a precursor plaque-like lesion, has been proposed, offering a possibility for prevention.[65]

The aetiology of desmoid tumours is multi-factorial, with contributions from trauma (e.g. operative), oestrogens, specific *APC* gene mutations and modifier genes. Currently, it is thought that both alleles of the *APC* gene must be mutated or lost, one mutation/loss being 3′ of codon 1444. Families where such a 3′ mutation is inherited in the germline have a high rate of desmoid disease.

MANAGEMENT

The challenge in the management of these bizarre tumours is to identify the minority which are rapidly and relentlessly progressive and to avoid harming patients with unnecessarily aggressive attempts to treat the rest. Ureteric obstruction is not infrequent, and as the consequences can be obviated by ureteric stenting it is wise to perform regular renal tract imaging in patients otherwise being managed non-operatively.

CT provides the best imaging with respect to size and relationship to surrounding structures, but T2-weighted MRI sequences may provide useful information about cellularity and progressive potential. Ultrasound can be used to monitor the state of the kidneys.

Treatment options include NSAIDs, antioestrogens, surgical excision and cytotoxic chemotherapy. Anecdotal successes with a variety of NSAIDs and antioestrogens abound (e.g. sulindac 150–200 mg twice daily alone or in combination with tamoxifen 80–120 mg daily), although evidence for efficacy based on prospective studies on large numbers of patients is lacking. Evaluation of these treatments is further hampered by the natural history of desmoids, which have been documented to regress spontaneously and exhibit relentless growth in only a small minority of patients.

Grade 2 evidence[63] supports the use of surgery as first-line treatment for abdominal and body wall desmoids, although the recurrence rate is high. There is no evidence to support the concern that this might be increased by the use of prosthetic materials to repair any resulting defect. Surgery should usually be avoided where possible for intra-abdominal desmoids, being associated with a high mortality rate, high recurrence rate and high morbidity rate requiring long-term parenteral nutrition. However, perforation with peritonitis, complete intestinal obstruction or erosion through the body wall to ulcerate on the surface may force the surgeon's hand.

PEUTZ–JEGHERS SYNDROME

Peutz–Jeghers syndrome is an autosomal dominant condition that was first described by Peutz in 1921 in a Dutch family, a report supplemented by the description of ten additional cases by Jeghers in 1942. The condition is characterised by mucocutaneous pigmentation (**Fig. 2.1**; see also Plate 1, facing p. 22) together with multiple gastrointestinal hamartomatous polyps. The gene responsible in some patients is the *STK11* (*LKB1*) gene on chromosome 19p13, although there is evidence of genetic heterogeneity as mutation at this site has been excluded in some families.

A 78-year follow-up of the original family described by Peutz is instructive.[66] Survival of affected family members was found to be reduced as a result of bowel obstruction and the development of a range of cancers.

Bowel obstruction

The commonest polyp-related complication is bowel obstruction, often caused by intussusception with a polyp at the apex. Repeated episodes result in increasingly difficult laparotomies and loss of bowel length. The incidence of subsequent bowel obstruction can be reduced by adequate intra-operative small bowel enteroscopy, allowing identification and removal of all polyps at the time of initial laparotomy.[67]

Cancer risk

Individuals with Peutz–Jeghers syndrome are at increased risk particularly of gastrointestinal malignancy, with a lifetime risk of colorectal cancer of about 20% and of gastric cancer of about 5%. Other areas at increased risk include the breasts (female), ovaries, cervix, pancreas and testes.[68]

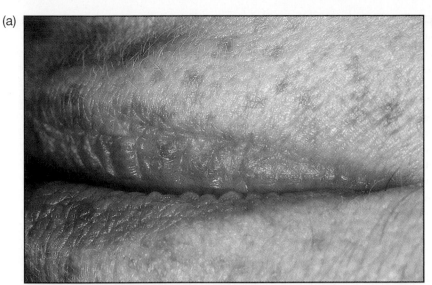

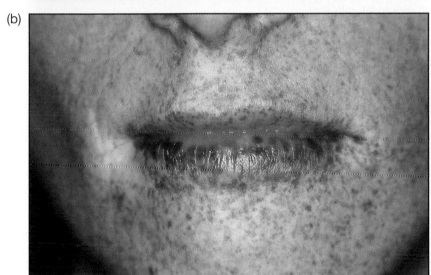

Figure 2.1 • Comparison of common perioral freckling **(a)** with Peutz–Jeghers pigmentation **(b)**.

Surveillance and management

Up-to-date surveillance protocols are best obtained from local registries. Most involve annual review with physical examination and measurement of haemoglobin. Upper and lower gastrointestinal endoscopies (with polypectomy) and barium follow-through examinations or capsule endoscopy of the small bowel are performed every 2–3 years to detect premalignant polyps or early cancers. If large polyps are seen in the small bowel or symptoms suggesting intermittent small bowel obstruction occur, or if there are small bowel polyps with anaemia, a laparotomy with on-table enteroscopy and polypectomy is recommended to clear the small bowel of polyps and prevent frank obstruction.

As far as malignancy at other sites is concerned, where surveillance programmes have been shown to be useful in the general population they should be used. Breast and testicular self-examination can be advised, and it is important to stress that females should remain up to date with cervical smears and standard breast screening. However, ovarian and pancreatic ultrasound are much more controversial as benefit is not likely.

JUVENILE POLYPOSIS

Not to be confused with the finding of an isolated juvenile polyp (which has very low, if any, malignant potential), juvenile polyposis is an autosomal dominant condition where multiple characteristic hamartomatous juvenile polyps occur, mostly in the colon but also in the upper gastrointestinal tract and small bowel. Other features sometimes associated are macrocephaly and congenital heart disease. Some affected individuals harbour germline mutations in the SMAD4 gene,[69] while others have germline mutations in the BMPR1A gene.

There is a risk of gastrointestinal cancer in excess of 50%, warranting regular endoscopic screening.[70] Regular oesophago-gastroduodenoscopy and colonoscopy, with polypectomy for large polyps, is mandatory; there may be an occasional role for prophylactic colectomy.

COWDEN DISEASE

The PTEN gene on chromosome 10q22 is associated with this syndrome, which consists of gastrointestinal hamartomas and cancers, plus a high risk of cancer of the female breast, thyroid, uterus and cervix, benign fibrocystic breast disease, non-toxic goitre and varied benign mucocutaneous lesions, particularly trichilemmomas. Targeted screening seems sensible, but there is little evidence to support it.

OTHER INHERITED COLORECTAL CANCER SYNDROMES

Multiple hyperplastic polyps that have adenomatous features (mixed polyposis syndromes) are associated with a high risk for colorectal cancer,[71] as is giant hyperplastic polyposis. Both conditions can be inherited. Endoscopy and even timely colectomy may be necessary.

A variant mutation of the APC gene on chromosome 5q (E1317Q) has been associated with an increased risk of colorectal cancer without any of the syndromes described above, particularly in the Ashkenazi Jewish population.[72] Research into the same population has provided evidence for the existence of another colorectal cancer susceptibility gene on chromosome 15q.[73] Caution should therefore be exercised in discharging Ashkenazi Jewish kindred on the basis of a negative HNPCC gene test, as mutations in the other colorectal cancer genes found in this population may be present.[74]

More recently, biallelic mutation of the MYH gene has been associated with multiple colorectal adenomas,[75] in some cases numbering over 100. Thus for the first time autosomal recessive inheritance has been described in the context of inherited bowel cancer, although individuals who are heterozygotes do not appear to be at increased risk.

SUMMARY

The emerging complexity of inherited bowel cancer, coupled with rapid advances in knowledge,[66–70] reinforce the need for the availability of experienced, informed and up-to-date opinion in the areas of diagnosis and management. Individual surgeons will rarely be able to meet all of these needs. Patients and their families are best served by the existence of good working relationships between managing clinicians, family cancer clinics and registries.

• Key points

- Genetic factors make a significant contribution to colorectal cancer.
- High-risk families should be referred to special-interest registries or genetics units.
- HNPCC and FAP are the main autosomal dominant conditions involved.
- An understanding of these conditions is required to recognise and diagnose them.
- Individuals with these conditions are at risk of a range of extracolonic tumours, so need specialised follow-up.

REFERENCES

1. Fuchs CS, Giovannucci EL, Colditz GA et al. A prospective study of family history and the risk of colorectal cancer. N Engl J Med 1994; 331:1669–74.

2. Houlston RS, Murday V, Harocopos C et al. Screening and genetic counselling for relatives of patients with colorectal cancer in a family cancer clinic. Br Med J 1990; 301:366–8.

3. Lichtenstein P, Holm NV, Verkasalo PK et al. Environmental and heritable factors in the causation of cancer: analyses of cohorts of twins from Sweden, Denmark and Finland. N Engl J Med 2000; 343:78–85.

4. Lips CJM. Registers for patients with familial tumours: from controversial areas to common guidelines. Br J Surg 1998; 85:1316–18.

5. Dunlop MG. Guidance on large bowel surveillance for people with two first degree relatives with colorectal cancer or one first degree relative diagnosed with colorectal cancer under 45 years. Gut 2002; 51(suppl. V):17–20.

6. Dunlop MG, Campbell H. Screening for people with a family history of colorectal cancer. Br Med J 1997; 314:1779–80.

7. Thorson AG, Knezetic JA, Lynch HT. A century of progress in hereditary nonpolyposis colorectal cancer (Lynch syndrome). Dis Colon Rectum 1999; 42:1–9.

8. Aarnio M, Sankila R, Pukkala E et al. Cancer risk in mutation carriers of DNA-mismatch repair genes. Int J Cancer 1999; 81:214–18.

9. Frayling IM. Microsatellite instability. Gut 1999; 45:1–4.

10. Park JG, Park YJ, Wijnen JT, Vasen HF. Gene–environment interaction in hereditary nonpolyposis colorectal cancer with implications for diagnosis and genetic testing. Int J Cancer 1999; 82:516–19.

11. Simmang CL et al. and the Standards Committee of the American Society of Colon and Rectal Surgeons. Practice parameters for detection of colorectal neoplasms. Dis Colon Rectum 1999; 42:1123–9.

12. Vasen HFA, Watson P, Mecklin J-P et al. New clinical criteria for hereditary nonpolyposis colorectal cancer (HNPCC, Lynch syndrome) proposed by the International Collaborative Group on HNPCC. Gastroenterology 1999; 116:1453–6.

13. Umar A, Boland CR, Terdiman JP et al. Revised Bethesda Guidelines for hereditary nonpolyposis colorectal cancer (Lynch syndrome) and microsatellite instability. J Natl Cancer Inst 2004; 96:261–8.

14. Talbot IC. Mismatch repair deficit: a gain for diagnostic histopathology. Gut 1999; 45:324–6.

15. Cawkwell L, Gray S, Murgatroyd H et al. Choice of management strategy for colorectal cancer based on a diagnostic immunohistochemical test for defective mismatch repair. Gut 1999; 45:409–15.

16. Wijnen JT, Vasen HFA, Khan PM et al. Clinical findings with implications for genetic testing in families with clustering of colorectal cancer. N Engl J Med 1998; 339:511–18.

17. Scholefield JH, Johnson AG, Shorthouse AJ. Current surgical practice in screening for colorectal cancer based on family history criteria. Br J Surg 1998; 85:1543–6.

18. Esplen MJ, Madlensky L, Butler K et al. Motivations and psychosocial impact of genetic testing for HNPCC. Am J Med Genet 2001; 103:9–15.

19. Burke W, Petersen G, Lynch P et al. Recommendations for follow-up care of individuals with an inherited predisposition to cancer: I. Hereditary nonpolyposis colon cancer. JAMA 1997; 277:915–19.

20. Syngal S, Fox EA, Li C et al. Interpretation of genetic test results for hereditary nonpolyposis colorectal cancer: implications for clinical predisposition testing. JAMA 1999; 282:247–53.

21. Neergaard L. Unregulated gene tests can cause life altering errors. Associated Press, 20 September 1999. Available at http://www.nandotimes.com

22. Jarvinen HJ, Aarnio M, Mustonen H et al. Controlled 15-year trial on screening for colorectal cancer in families with hereditary nonpolyposis colorectal cancer. Gastroenterology 2000; 118:829–34.

23. Church J. Hereditary colon cancers can be tiny: a cautionary case report of the results of colonoscopic surveillance. Am J Gastroenterol 1998; 93:2289–90.

24. Rodriguez-Bigas MA, Vasen HF, Mecklin J-P et al. Rectal cancer risk in hereditary nonpolyposis colorectal cancer after abdominal colectomy. Ann Surg 1997; 225:202–7.

25. Syngal S, Weeks JC, Schrag D et al. Benefits of colonoscopic surveillance and prophylactic colectomy in patients with hereditary nonpolyposis colorectal cancer mutations. Ann Intern Med 1998; 129:787–96.

26. Fitzsimmon RJ Jr, Lynch HT, Stanislav GV et al. Recognition and treatment of patients with hereditary nonpolyposis colorectal cancer (Lynch syndromes I and II). Ann Surg 1987; 206:289–94.

27. Ruschoff J, Wallinger S, Dietmaier W et al. Aspirin suppresses the mutator phenotype associated with hereditary nonpolyposis colorectal cancer by genetic selection. Proc Natl Acad Sci USA 1998; 95:11301–6.

28. Bell J. The human genome. In: Marinker M, Peckham M (eds) Clinical futures. London: BMJ Books, 1998; pp. 20–42.

29. Jass JR. Diagnosis of hereditary non-polyposis colorectal cancer. Histopathology 1998; 32:491–7.

30. Lynch HT. Cancer family history and genetic testing: are malpractice adjudications waiting to happen? Am J Gastroenterol 2000; 97:518–20.

31. Bisgaard ML, Fenger K, Bulow S et al. Familial adenomatous polyposis (FAP): frequency, penetrance and mutation rate. Hum Mutat 1994; 3:121–5.

32. Hernegger GS, Moore HG, Guillem JG. Attenuated familial adenomatous polyposis: an evolving and poorly understood entity. Dis Colon Rectum 2002; 45:127–34.

33. Wallace MH, Frayling IM, Clark SK et al. Attenuated adenomatous polyposis coli: the role of ascertainment bias through failure to dye-spray at colonoscopy. Dis Colon Rectum 1999; 42:1078–80.

34. Vasen HFA, Bülow S and the Leeds Castle Polyposis Group. Guidelines for the surveillance and management of familial adenomatous polyposis (FAP): a world wide survey among 41 registries. Colorectal Dis 1999; 1:214–21.

35. Giardiello FM, Brensinger JD, Petersen GM et al. The use and interpretation of commercial APC gene testing for familial adenomatous polyposis. N Engl J Med 1997; 336:823–7.

36. Berk T, Cohen Z, Bapat B, Gallinger S. Negative genetic test results in familial adenomatous polyposis: clinical screening implications. Dis Colon Rectum 1999; 42:307–10.

37. Bapat B, Noorani H, Cohen Z et al. Cost comparison of predictive genetic testing versus conventional clinical screening for familial adenomatous polyposis. Gut 1999; 44:698–703.

38. Wu JS, Paul P, McGannon EA, Church JM. APC genotype, polyp number, and surgical options in familial adenomatous polyposis. Ann Surg 1998; 227:57–62.

39. Vasen HFA, van der Luijt RB, Slors JFM et al. Molecular genetic tests as a guide to surgical management of familial adenomatous polyposis. Lancet 1996; 348:433–5.

40. Crabtree MD, Tomlinson IPM, Hodgson SV et al. Explaining variation in familial adenomatous polyposis: relationship between genotype and phenotype and evidence for modifier genes. Gut 2002; 51:420–3.

41. Dihlmann S, Gebert J, Siermann A et al. Dominant negative effect of the APC 1309 mutation: a possible explanation for genotype–phenotype correlations in familial adenomatous polyposis. Cancer Res 1999; 59:1857–60.

42. Brett MCA, Hershman MJ, Glazer G. Other manifestations of familial adenomatous polyposis. In: Phillips RKS, Spigelman AD, Thomson JPS (eds) Familial adenomatous polyposis and other poly- posis syndromes. London: Edward Arnold, 1994; pp.142–58.

43. Soravia C, Berk T, Madlensky L et al. Genotype– phenotype correlations in attenuated adenomatous polyposis coli. Am J Hum Genet 1998; 62:1290–301.

44. Bertario L, Russo A, Radice P et al. Genotype and phenotype factors as determinants for rectal stump cancer in patients with familial adenomatous polyposis. Ann Surg 2000; 231:538–43.

45. Van Duijvendijk P, Vasen HA, Bertario L et al. Cumulative risk of developing polyps or malig- nancy at the ileal pouch–anal anastomosis in patients with familial adenomatous polyposis. J Gastrointest Surg 1999; 3:325–30.

46. Parc YR, Olschwang S, Desaint B et al. Familial adenomatous polyposis: prevalence of adenomas in the ileal pouch after restorative proctocolectomy. Ann Surg 2001; 233:360–4.

47. Olsen KO, Juul S, Bulow S et al. Female fecundity before and after operation for familial adenomatous polyposis. Br J Surg 2003; 90:227–31.

48. Church J, Burke C, McGannon E et al. Risk of rectal cancer after colectomy and ileorectal anastomosis for familial adenomatous polyposis: a function of available options. Dis Colon Rectum 2003; 46:1175–81.

49. Giardiello FM, Offerhaus JA, Tersmette AC et al. Sulindac induced regression of colorectal adenomas in familial adenomatous polyposis: evaluation of predictive factors. Gut 1996; 38:578–81.

50. Ho JWC, Yuen ST, Chung LP, So HC, Kwan KYM. The role of sulindac in familial adenomatous polyposis patients with ileal pouch polyposis. Aust N Z J Surg 1999; 69:756–8.

51. Steinbach LT, Lynch P, Phillips RKS et al. The effect of celecoxib, a cyclo-oxygenase inhibitor, in familial adenomatous polyposis. N Engl J Med 2000; 342:1946–58.

52. Hofgartner WT, Thorp M, Ramus MC et al. Gastric adenocarcinoma associated with fundic gland polyps in a patient with attenuated familial adenomatous polyposis. Am J Gastroenterol 1999; 94:2275–81.

53. Groves CJ, Saunders BP, Spigelman AD, Phillips RKS. Duodenal cancer in patients with familial adenomatous polyposis (FAP): results of a 10 year prospective study. Gut 2002; 50:636–41.

54. Burke CA, Beck GJ, Church JM, van Stolk RU. The natural history of untreated duodenal and ampullary adenomas in patients with familial adenomatous polyposis followed in an endoscopic surveillance program. Gastrointest Endosc 1999; 49:358–64.

55. Spigelman AD, Williams CB, Talbot IC et al. Upper gastrointestinal cancer in patients with familial adenomatous polyposis. Lancet 1989; ii:783–5.

56. Vasen HFA, Bülow S, Nyrhøj T et al. Decision analysis in the management of duodenal adenomatosis in familial adenomatous polyposis. Gut 1997; 40:716–19.

57. Wallace MH, Phillips RKS. Upper gastrointestinal disease in patients with familial adenomatous polyposis. Br J Surg 1998; 85:742–50.

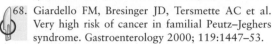

58. Phillips RKS, Wallace MH, Lynch PM et al. A randomised, double blind, placebo controlled study of celecoxib, a selective cyclooxygenase 2 inhibitor, on duodenal polyposis in familial adenomatous polyposis. Gut 2002; 50:857–60.

59. Seow-Choen F, Vijayan V, Keng V. Prospective randomized study of sulindac versus calcium and calciferol for upper gastrointestinal polyps in familial adenomatous polyposis. Br J Surg 1996; 83:1763–6.

60. Penna C, Bataille N, Balladur P, Tiret E, Parc R. Surgical treatment of severe duodenal polyposis in familial adenomatous polyposis. Br J Surg 1998; 85:665–8.

61. Grund KE, Storek D, Farin G. Endoscopic argon plasma coagulation (APC). First clinical experiences in flexible endoscopy. Endosc Surg Allied Technol 1994; 2:42–6.

62. Middleton SB, Frayling IM, Phillips RK. Desmoids in familial adenomatous polyposis are monoclonal proliferations. Br J Cancer 2000; 82:827–32.

63. Clark SK, Neale KF, Landgrebe JC, Phillips RKS. Desmoid tumours complicating familial adenomatous polyposis. Br J Surg 1999; 86:1185–9.

64. Church JM, McGannon E, Ozuner G. The clinical course of intra-abdominal desmoid tumours in patients with familial adenomatous polyposis. Colorectal Dis 1999; 1:168–73.

65. Clark SK, Smith TG, Katz DE et al. Identification and progression of a desmoid precursor lesion in patients with familial adenomatous polyposis. Br J Surg 1998; 85:970–3.

66. Westerman AM, Entius MM, de Baar E et al. Peutz–Jeghers syndrome: 78-year follow-up of the original family. Lancet 1999; 353:1211–15.

67. Edwards DP, Khosraviani K, Stafferton R, Phillips RKS. Long-term results of polyp clearance by intraoperative enteroscopy in the Peutz–Jeghers syndrome. Dis Colon Rectum 2003; 46:48–50.

68. Giardello FM, Bresinger JD, Tersmette AC et al. Very high risk of cancer in familial Peutz–Jeghers syndrome. Gastroenterology 2000; 119:1447–53.

69. Friedl W, Kruse R, Uhlhaas S et al. Frequent 4-bp deletion in exon 9 of the SMAD4/MADH4 gene in familial juvenile polyposis patients. Genes Chrom Cancer 1999; 25:403–6.

70. Howe JR, Mitros FA, Summers RW. The risk of gastrointestinal carcinoma in familial juvenile polyposis. Ann Surg Oncol 1998; 5:751–6.

71. Ilyas M, Straub J, Tomlinson IPM, Bodmer WF. Genetic pathways in colorectal and other cancers. Eur J Cancer 1999; 35:335–51.

72. Lamlum H, Al Tassan N, Jaeger E et al. Germline APC variants in patients with multiple colorectal adenomas, with evidence for the particular importance of E1317Q. Hum Mol Genet 2000; 9:2215–21.

73. Tomlinson I, Rahman N, Frayling I et al. Inherited susceptibility to colorectal adenomas and carcinomas: evidence for a new predisposition gene on 15q14–q22. Gastroenterology 1999; 116:789–95.

74. Yuan ZQ, Wong N, Foulkes WD, Alpert L, Manganaro F. A missense mutation in both hMSH2 and APC in an Ashkenazi Jewish HNPCC kindred: implications for clinical screening. J Med Genet 1999; 36:793–4.

75. Sieber OM, Lipton L, Crabtree M et al. Multiple colorectal adenomas, classic adenomatous polyposis and germ-line mutations in MYH. N Engl J Med 2003; 348:791–9.

Three

Colonic cancer

Robert J.C. Steele

INTRODUCTION

Colorectal cancer is a major health problem in the Western world. In the UK, it is the second most common cause of cancer death, accounting for some 16 000 deaths in 2003. In 1999 there were approximately 35 000 new cases, of which about 13 000 were rectal and 22 000 colonic.[1] Although the overall numbers in men and women are similar, the incidence of rectal cancer is higher in men, while the incidence of colonic cancer is higher in women. The 5-year relative survival rate is currently in the region of 45%, and has improved slightly over the last 30 years from around 30% in 1971–75.[2]

Perhaps surprisingly, there is no precise definition of colonic cancer. Although the colon comprises all the large bowel proximal to the rectum, the definition of the rectum is unclear. Anatomical texts describe the top of the rectum as the point where the sigmoid mesocolon ends or that part of the large bowel level with the third sacral vertebra.[3] Surgeons, on the other hand, prefer to think of the rectum as the segment of large bowel lying within the true pelvis.[4] As far as rectal cancer is concerned, in 1989 the United Kingdom Coordinating Committee on Cancer Research (UKCCCR) defined this as a tumour within 15 cm of the anal verge on rigid sigmoidoscopy,[4] whereas authorities in the USA have preferrred 11 or 12 cm.[5] Perhaps the simplest definition is the intraoperative identification of the

fusion of the two antemesenteric taenia into an amorphous area where the true rectum begins.

These distinctions are important for two practical reasons. First, adjuvant radiotherapy is not appropriate for colonic tumours and, secondly, comparisons between outcomes for colorectal cancer surgery in different series are impossible unless clear and uniform definitions are adopted. This is an important problem that has yet to be addressed by international consensus.

NATURAL HISTORY

Within the colon, about 50% of cancers arise in the left side and 25% in the right (**Fig. 3.1**); in 4–5% of cases there are synchronous lesions.[6,7] It is now widely accepted that the majority of colonic cancers arise from pre-existing adenomatous polyps, the supporting evidence being as follows.

1. The prevalence of adenomas correlates well with that of carcinomas, the average age of patients with adenomas being around 5 years younger than patients with carcinomas.[8,9]
2. Adenomatous tissue often accompanies cancer, and it is unusual to find small cancers with no contiguous adenomatous tissue.[10]
3. Sporadic adenomas are identical histologically to the adenomas of familial adenomatous

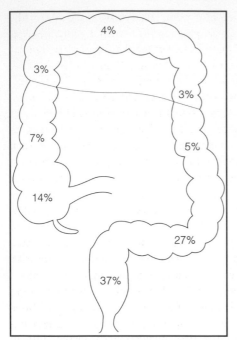

Figure 3.1 • Frequency of anatomical locations of colorectal cancer. Based on data from the Royal College of Surgeons audit in Trent Region and Wales.

polyposis (FAP), and this condition is unequivocally premalignant.[11]

4. Large adenomas are more likely to display cellular atypia and genetic abnormalities than small lesions.[8,12]

5. The distribution of adenomas throughout the colon is similar to that for carcinomas.[13]

6. Adenomas are found in up to one-third of all surgical specimens resected for colorectal cancer.[14,15]

7. The incidence of colorectal cancer has been shown to fall with a long-term screening programme involving colonoscopy and polypectomy.[16]

It should be recognised that although the majority of adenomas diagnosed in the West are polypoid or exophytic, the flat adenoma (defined as an adenoma where the depth of the dysplastic tissue is no more than twice that of the mucosa) is now a recognised entity.[17] There is good evidence that these lesions are premalignant, and may indeed have a greater tendency towards malignant transformation than polypoid adenomas. They are difficult to find, but may account for up to 40% of all adenomas.[17] Reliable diagnosis requires a skilful experienced colonoscopist and the use of dye sprayed onto the colonic mucosa to highlight the contours of the abnormal tissue.

When invasion has taken place, colonic cancer can spread directly and via the lymphatic, blood and transcoelomic routes.

Direct spread

Direct spread occurs longitudinally, transversely and radially, but as adequate proximal and distal clearance is technically feasible in the majority of colonic cancers, it is radial spread which is of most importance. In a retroperitoneal colonic cancer, radial spread may involve the ureter, duodenum and muscles of the posterior abdominal wall; the intraperitoneal tumour may involve small intestine, stomach, pelvic organs or the anterior abdominal wall.

Lymphatic spread

In general, the lymphatic spread of colonic cancer progresses from the paracolic nodes along the main colonic vessels to the nodes associated with either cephalad or caudal vessels, eventually reaching the para-aortic glands in advanced disease. This orderly process does not always occur, however, and in about 30% of cases nodal involvement can skip a tier of glands.[18] In contrast to rectal disease, it is rare for a colonic cancer that has not breached the muscle wall to exhibit lymph node metastases[18] (overall, about 15% of cases confined to the bowel wall will be found to have lymph node metastases).

Blood-borne spread

The most common site for blood-borne spread of colorectal cancer is the liver, presumably arriving by the portal venous system. Up to 37% of patients may have detectable liver metastases at the time of operation, and around 50% of patients may be expected to develop overt disease at some time.[19] The lung is the next most common site, with around 10% of patients developing lung metastases at some stage; other reported sites include ovary, adrenal, bone, brain and kidney.

Transcoelomic spread

Colonic cancer may spread throughout the peritoneum, either via the subperitoneal lymphatics or by virtue of viable cells being shed from the serosal surface of a tumour, giving rise to malignant ascites, which is relatively rare.[20]

AETIOLOGY

Knowledge of molecular genetics in sporadic colorectal cancer has increased rapidly in recent years, but the stimuli which lead to these carcinogenic changes are still obscure. In this section, a brief consideration of the genetic basis of colorectal cancer is followed by discussion of aetiological factors.

Genetic factors

The genetic changes associated with colorectal cancer have been widely studied, and the molecular background to inherited colorectal cancer is dealt with in Chapter 2. However, the genetic events that take place in the development of sporadic colorectal

cancer are also being elucidated. Mutations of the adenomatous polyposis coli (APC) gene, which is probably involved in cell–cell adhesion, are thought to occur early as they are found in 60% of all adenomas and carcinomas.[21] K-ras mutations, which probably stimulate cell growth by activating growth factor signal transduction, similarly occur in both adenomas and carcinomas. However, as they are more common in large adenomas than small adenomas they are thought to represent a later event.[12,22] The deleted in colorectal cancer (DCC) gene is a tumour-suppressor gene that may be responsible for cell–cell or cell–matrix interactions,[23] and its deletion may be important in further progression towards the malignant state. Mutation of the p53 gene is common in invasive colonic cancers but rare in adenomas and is therefore deemed to be a late event which accompanies the development of the invasive phenotype.[24] This is thought to be important as the p53 protein has roles in the repair of DNA and the induction of programmed cell death.[25,26]

The sequence of events described above is depicted in **Fig. 3.2**, but it must be stressed that this merely illustrates one possible multistep process; indeed,

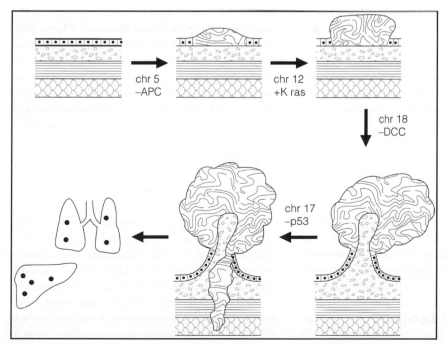

Figure 3.2 • A possible sequence of genetic changes in the development of colorectal polyps and invasive cancer.

there is now good evidence that K-*ras* and *p53* mutations very rarely occur in the same tumour, suggesting alternative pathways to carcinogensis.[27] Many other genetic events have been observed in sporadic colorectal cancer, and no single event has been seen in all cancers. Thus the range of mutations, inactivations and deletions is wide, and it is likely that no single pattern will be applicable to every tumour. Nevertheless, knowledge of specific genetic events that take place in colorectal carcinogenesis may well have implications for diagnosis, prognosis and ultimately for gene therapy. For example, there is now evidence that K-*ras* mutations are not only associated with advanced stage at presentation but also with poor prognosis in node-negative disease.[28] This information is now being used in some centres to select patients with apparently early disease for adjuvant chemotherapy.

Diet

It is widely held that lack of fibre in the diet is an important factor in the high incidence of colorectal cancer in the West. Burkitt[29] first suggested that, by reducing intestinal transit time and by acting as a diluent, dietary fibre could reduce the exposure of the large intestinal mucosa to potential carcinogens. This hypothesis gained support from epidemiological studies[30] and the effect of wheat fibre on mucosal cell turnover,[31] and two recently published major dietary questionnaire studies have indicated strong associations between dietary fibre intake and decreased risk of colorectal cancer or adenoma.[32,33]

Another dietary influence is animal fat. It has been suggested that a diet rich in animal fats not only causes increased excretion of bile salts in the faeces but also promotes the growth of bacteria that can degrade bile salts to carcinogens.[30] It is also well established that a diet lacking in vegetables is associated with colorectal cancer,[29,34] and there is good evidence that isothiocyanates in cruciferous vegetables (e.g. broccoli) may be protective by enhancing the expression of carcinogen metabolising enzymes and inducing apoptosis in neoplastic cells.[35]

Other lifestyle factors

Other lifestyle factors that have been associated with colon cancer include physical activity, smoking and alcohol intake. There is a consistent inverse relationship between exercise and colon cancer risk in all studies, although the effect seems to be greater in men than in women;[36] avoidance of weight gain also appears to be important. Although earlier studies did not uncover a clear association between smoking and colon cancer, more recent work has shown that long-term smokers are at elevated risk, with relative risks between 1.5 and 3.0.[37] Finally, alcohol consumption may have an assocation with the disease but the evidence is conflicting, and no definitive statement can be made as yet.[38]

Bile acids

There is good evidence that bile acids may act as carcinogens,[39,40] and this may be related to calcium in the diet. Calcium binds bile acids, and it has been shown that calcium supplementation can bring about a reduction in the risk of recurrent colonic adenomas.[41] It is also of note that secondary bile acid secretion is increased after cholecystectomy, and there is some evidence that this operation may increase the risk of colorectal cancer.[42]

Bacteria

Until recently, the role of the colonic flora in the aetiology of cancer has attracted little interest. However, a recent study found that intraepithelial *Escherichia coli* were present in the colonic mucosa of the majority of patients with adenomas or carcinomas but rarely in individuals with normal colons.[43] This interesting finding has opened up a new area of research that has yet to be exploited.

Predisposing conditions

Long-standing inflammatory bowel disease, both ulcerative colitis and Crohn's disease, increases the risk of colorectal cancer, and this is discussed in Chapters 8 and 9. Previous gastric surgery has also been implicated,[44,45] and although the association is controversial, the risk may be about twofold. Altered bile acid metabolism may play a role in this process, both after gastrectomy[44] and after vagotomy.[46] The risk after uretero-sigmoidostomy is well established, although this operation has now been largely superseded by the use of an isolated ileal conduit for urinary diversion.

PRESENTATION

Colon cancer can present as an emergency or with chronic symptoms that are well recognised.[47] Right-sided cancer typically presents with anaemia, as the liquid nature of the faeces and the wider diameter of the colon make obvious tumour-related symptoms unusual. When the tumour is situated in the descending or sigmoid colon, change of bowel habit, colicky abdominal pain and blood in the stool are the commonest symptoms. Occasionally, the patient may notice the primary tumour as a mass and even more rarely as symptoms of fistulation. A sigmoid cancer may cause pneumaturia and urinary infection by fistulation into the bladder, and a gastrocolic fistula may cause faecal vomiting or severe diarrhoea and weight loss.

Unfortunately, many of the symptoms of colon cancer are common and non-specific, and there has been a good deal of recent work attempting to refine the indications for investigation. Guidelines have been developed to classify those at high risk warranting urgent investigation based on change in bowel habit, rectal bleeding in the absence of anal symptoms, palpable abdominal or rectal masses, and anaemia (**Box 3.1**).[48] These guidelines are not particularly discriminatory, however, and weighted scoring systems may be more accurate.[49]

INVESTIGATION

When the decision to investigate a patient for colorectal cancer has been made, the choice lies between the combination of barium enema and sigmoidoscopy, colonoscopy or computed tomography (CT) colography.

A barium enema usually demonstrates a colonic cancer as an irregular polypoid lesion or as an 'apple-core' stricture with destruction of the mucosal pattern; benign polyps may also be seen as typical filling defects. It must be stressed, however, that false-positive and false-negative results may occur in up to 1% and 7% of cases respectively, and errors usually occur in the sigmoid colon and caecum.[50] These errors can be divided into:

1. perceptive errors, where the original films did indeed show the lesion but the radiologist failed to spot it;

Box 3.1 • UK Department of Health criteria for high and low risk of colorectal cancer

Higher risk

- Rectal bleeding with a change in bowel habit to looser stools or increased frequency of defecation persisting for 6 weeks (all ages)
- Change in bowel habit as above without rectal bleeding and persisting for 6 weeks (>60 years)
- Persistent rectal bleeding without anal symptoms* (>60 years)
- Palpable right-sided abdominal mass (all ages)
- Palpable rectal mass (not pelvic) (all ages)
- Unexplained iron deficiency anaemia (all ages)

Low risk
Patients with no iron deficiency anaemia, no palpable rectal or abdominal mass and

- Rectal bleeding with anal symptoms and no persistent change in bowel habit (all ages)
- Rectal bleeding with an obvious external cause, e.g. anal fissure (all ages)
- Change in bowel habit without rectal bleeding (<60 years)
- Transient changes in bowel habit, particularly to harder or decreased frequency of defecation (all ages)
- Abdominal pain as a single symptom without signs and symptoms of intestinal obstruction (all ages)

*Soreness, discomfort, itching, lumps, prolapse or pain. From Thompson MR, Heath I, Ellis BG et al. Identifying and managing patients at low risk of bowel cancer in general practice. Br Med J 2003; 327:263–5, with permission.

2. technical errors, such as too few films, lack of air contrast and overfilling with barium;
3. limitations of barium radiology itself, particularly in demonstrating small lesions, usually in the caecum, sigmoid colon (especially in the presence of diverticular disease) and rectum, and most particularly when bowel preparation has been poor.

Although rigid sigmoidoscopy can often provide satisfactory views of the rectum, flexible sigmoidoscopy after a cleansing enema is preferred by many. It will provide useful supplementary information, and neoplasia may be detected in the sigmoid colon in 25% of cases with 'normal' barium enemas, especially if there is coexisting diverticular disease.[51,52] It may therefore be argued that colonoscopy should be the investigation of choice, but there is little doubt that it carries a risk of perforation (much greater than barium enema), and even in good hands failure to achieve a total colonic examination can be expected in 10% of cases.[53] In addition, the precise position of a tumour seen at colonoscopy can be very difficult to determine as the only reliable landmarks are the anus and the terminal ileum.[54]

In the UK, the choice between barium enema and colonoscopy usually depends on local availability and expertise, but if radiology is to be used the rectum must be visualised endoscopically as it is not seen well on radiographs.[55] If a barium enema is normal in the face of continuing suspicious symptoms, then flexible sigmoidoscopy or colonoscopy as appropriate is mandatory. Likewise, if a primary colonoscopy fails to achieve total colonic visualisation, a completion barium enema should be carried out. Given equal access to either technique, then colonoscopy would be the method of choice when the presenting complaint suggested mucosal pathology (e.g. bleeding or a family history of polyps/cancer) whereas barium radiology would be indicated when there were functional symptoms of altered bowel habit, and especially fistulation or a suspicion of megabowel or sigmoid volvulus.

Preoperative histological confirmation of colonic cancer is ideal, but this can be achieved only by performing endoscopy in every case. If a barium enema demonstrates an unequivocal carcinoma, then biopsy may be deemed unnecessary, but where there is any doubt regarding the nature of a stricture or other lesion, then endoscopic visualisation and biopsy are mandatory.

Occasionally, both barium enema and colonoscopy will be unsatisfactory, either because of poor bowel preparation or through inability to retain contrast or air, especially in elderly patients. In such instances, careful spiral CT of the abdomen may be useful.[56] CT is also attracting interest as, with appropriate software, it is now possible to carry out CT colography or 'virtual colonoscopy', which is effective in detecting polypoid lesions down to 6 mm in diameter.[57] Although not yet widely available in the UK, this technology is fast becoming a standard investigation and will almost certainly replace barium enema as the radiological investigation of choice.

Many surgeons think it sensible to screen for liver and lung metastases. A fit patient with liver metastases may be suitable for active treatment, whereas an elderly patient with a relatively asymptomatic primary and evidence of widespread dissemination may escape resection. For pulmonary lesions, a chest radiograph is adequate; for hepatic involvement, preoperative ultrasonography, although widely used, does not always achieve an 85% accuracy.[58,59] For this reason the use of intraoperative ultrasonography has gained ground in recent years, and several studies now indicate its superiority over preoperative examination and intraoperative clinical assessment.[60]

CT is generally regarded as superior to preoperative ultrasonography[59] and is accurate in the detection of liver metastases over 1.5 cm in diameter.[61] It may also provide information on local extension and possible ureteric involvement. Until recently, magnetic resonance imaging (MRI) was considered to be less useful because the long image acquisition time resulted in movement artefact. With ultrafast scanning, however, MRI may yet prove the investigation of choice for both distant and local disease.[62]

A routine preoperative intravenous urogram, particularly for tumours of the left colon, was once regarded as important,[63] but opinion has changed and few now perform it as a routine.[64,65] Under certain circumstances, however, particularly where there is evidence of ureteric obstruction on CT or ultrasound, an intravenous urogram may still be needed.

SCREENING

Colon cancer would seem to be a very suitable candidate for screening. Prognosis after treatment is much better in early-stage disease and the polyp–carcinoma sequence (see above) offers an opportunity to prevent cancer by treating premalignant disease. The ideal screening test should detect the majority of tumours without a large number of false positives, i.e. it should have high sensitivity and specificity. In addition, it must be safe and acceptable to the population offered screening.

In colorectal cancer, the most widely studied test is Haemoccult, a guaiac-based test that detects the peroxidase-like activity of haematin in faeces. Because this activity is diminished as haemoglobin travels through the gastrointestinal tract,[66] upper gastrointestinal bleeding is less likely to be detected than colonic bleeding. On the other hand, false-positive results may be produced by ingestion of animal haemoglobin or vegetables containing peroxidase, and dietary restriction is necessary to confirm marginally positive results.[67] In addition, because of the intermittent nature of bleeding from tumours, the sensitivity of Haemoccult is only about 50–70%.[68]

Screen-detected tumours are much more likely to be at an early stage than symptomatic disease, but this does not prove that screening is beneficial. Even improved survival in patients whose tumours are detected by screening is not conclusive because of the biases inherent in screening. These biases are threefold, and comprise selection bias, length bias and lead-time bias.

Selection bias arises from the tendency of people who accept screening to be particularly health conscious and therefore atypical of the population as a whole. Length bias indicates the tendency for screening to detect a disproportionate number of cancers that are slow-growing, and which thereby have a good prognosis. Lead-time bias results from the time between the date of detection of a cancer by screening and the date when it would have been diagnosed had the subject not been screened. As survival is measured from the time of diagnosis, screening advances the date at which diagnosis is made, thus lengthening the survival time without necessarily altering the date of death.

Because of these biases, effectiveness can be assessed only by comparing disease-specific mortality in a population offered screening with that in an identical population not offered screening. This has to be done in the context of a well-designed randomised controlled trial, and for colorectal cancer three trials using faecal occult blood (FOB) have reported mortality data.[69–71]

The first of these was carried out in Minnesota[69] and showed a significant 33% reduction in colorectal cancer-specific mortality with annual FOB testing and a significant 21% reduction in a group offered biennial screening. However, this study was carried out on volunteers so that it was not a true population study. In addition, the test used rehydrated Haemoccult, which was not very specific and resulted in a large proportion of subjects undergoing negative colonoscopies.

In Nottingham, a strictly population-based randomised study of 150 251 subjects aged 45–74 years has been carried out, with recruitment between 1981 and 1991.[70] At the first round, tests were sent to 75 253 individuals, of whom 53.4% accepted. The test was positive in 906 (2.1%) and, of these, 104 (11%) were found to have carcinoma (46% stage A). Those who completed the tests were offered further screening at 2-year intervals, and an extra 132 cancers (37% stage A) were found. In total, 893 cancers were diagnosed in the study group, of which 26% were detected by screening, 28% presented as interval cancers and 46% arose in patients who had refused the test. At a median follow-up of 7.8 years, 360 individuals had died of colorectal cancer in the study group compared with 420 in the control group. This represents a significant 15% reduction in cumulative mortality (odds ratio 0.85, 95% confidence interval 0.74–0.98). An almost identical study carried out in Funen, Denmark, has obtained very similar results, showing an 18% reduction in mortality.[71]

There seems little doubt that FOB screening can reduce mortality from colorectal cancer, albeit modestly when applied to unselected populations, and the challenges for the future are to increase compliance and to improve the sensitivity and specificity of the screening test.

As 70% of cancers and large adenomas are found in the distal 60 cm of the large bowel,[72] flexible sigmoidoscopy has been proposed as a screening test and there is good evidence that it is more sensitive than FOB testing.[73] The Imperial Cancer Research Fund (now Cancer Research UK) has investigated the role of once-only flexible sigmoidoscopy as a screening modality in a multicentre randomised study,[74] but the effect on mortality is not yet known. Another approach for improving the test is to examine stool for DNA mutations that are known to occur in colorectal cancer. This would be highly specific, but for it to be sensitive such a test would have to be capable of detecting mutations in a number of genes, as there is no uniform pattern of genetic mutation common to all cancers. However, researchers have been successful in picking up mutations in the APC,[75] K-ras[76] and p53[77] genes in stool samples from patients with colorectal cancer, and the prospect of a stool test that would scan for a panel of appropriate genetic mutations is not far away.

SURVEILLANCE OF HIGH-RISK GROUPS

Individuals at high risk of colon cancer are not suitable for the population screening strategies described above, as the tests employed are not sufficiently sensitive. Surveillance of patients with inflammatory bowel disease is dealt with in Chapters 8 and 9, and of individuals with a family history of colon cancer in Chapter 2. However, another important group comprises those with adenomatous polyps and, particularly where screening is available, these individuals pose a significant challenge in terms of the use of colonoscopy resources. For this reason, guidelines have been developed that classify patients as being at low, intermediate or high risk of adenoma recurrence.[78] In the low-risk category (those with one or two adenomas <1 cm in diameter), either no follow-up or a repeat colonoscopy at 5 years is recommended. In the intermediate-risk category (those with three to four adenomas or at least one adenoma >1 cm in diameter), colonoscopy at 3 years is recommended. In the high-risk category (those with five or more small adenomas or three or more where at least one is >1 cm in diameter), patients should have another colonoscopy at 1 year. While the evidence upon which these guidelines is based is not very strong, they represent a very sensible approach, and one that has been adopted widely in the UK.

ELECTIVE SURGERY

Given that a patient is fit for surgery and does not have advanced disseminated disease, resection of colonic cancer is the only advisable primary treatment. It is important to stress that surgery offers a realistic hope of cure in this disease, as two-thirds of patients will survive 5 years after potentially curative resection[79] and recurrence is very rare after 4 years of disease-free survival.[80] In colon cancer,

there is now evidence that adjuvant chemotherapy may also be of value; this is dealt with in Chapter 5.

Preparation for surgery

The first priority is to obtain informed consent, and the surgeon must be prepared to discuss the risks of death, complications such as anastomotic dehiscence, venous thromboembolism and wound infection, and disease recurrence. The patient must also be assessed for fitness for operation. This implies obtaining a full history and examination, full blood count, urea and electrolytes, and ECG where indicated. In addition, investigations for disseminated disease should be performed as outlined above.

Blood transfusion

The patient must have blood taken for crossmatch, but the amount of blood requested will depend on the individual procedure. Group and save alone will be suitable for most right hemicolectomies, whereas for other types of colectomy and depending on the operating technique it is prudent to have at least two units of blood available.[81]

There is still some debate as to the effects of blood transfusion on prognosis in colorectal cancer. Since the report by Burrows and Tartter[82] that blood transfusion may be associated with an increased likelihood of recurrence, there have been many reports, some making allowance for case mix, that have reached conflicting conclusions.[83]

 Recently, however, a randomised trial comparing the use of predeposited autologous and allogeneic blood in patients undergoing resection for colorectal cancer showed no difference in prognosis.[84] For this reason, the observed effects of blood transfusion on recurrence must be treated with caution.

Bowel preparation

Immediately before surgery, most surgeons require the patient to undergo some form of mechanical bowel preparation. A wide variety of washouts, enemas and purgatives have been used, and one of the most popular regimens uses Picolax. This combines a senna compound (10 mg sodium

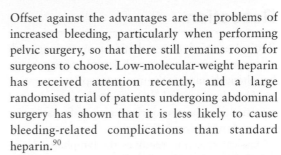
picosulphate), which is activated by colonic bacteria and causes vigorous mass contraction, with magnesium citrate, which reduces water and sodium reabsorption so that a large hyperosmolar fluid load reaches the caecum. This is usually given in the morning and the afternoon of the day before operation; however, although it is easy to take, it often causes abdominal discomfort and may cause dehydration unless extra fluids are taken either by mouth or intravenously.[85]

A popular alternative is polyethylene glycol salt solution, which can achieve preparation within 3 hours, and this appears to be preferred by patients to more conventional approaches.[86] However, it does necessitate 4–5 L of oral intake, and some elderly patients find this difficult. Nasogastric whole-gut irrigation with an electrolyte solution obtains excellent results, but patients find it very unpleasant.[87]

Whatever approach is taken, care must be taken not to attempt preoperative preparation in the presence of obstruction. If a patient experiences excessive pain or abdominal distension during preparation, it should be stopped. In such cases, the use of intraoperative preparation should be considered (see below).

Finally, it is by no means certain that bowel preparation is essential to prevent anastomotic leakage[88] or its consequences. Most anastomotic leaks are caused by technical error (such as poor knotting/suturing or too much tension) or biological failure (usually from ischaemia), neither of which will be influenced by bowel preparation. The effects of an early leak (usually due to poor technique) would probably be obviated by bowel preparation, but most leaks occur late after the patient has recommenced oral feeding so that any value of preoperative bowel preparation will have been lost.

Thromboembolism prophylaxis

Although there have been no studies confined to patients with colorectal cancer, a meta-analysis of appropriate randomised trials has shown that rates of deep vein thrombosis, pulmonary embolism and death from pulmonary embolism can all be significantly reduced by the use of subcutaneous heparin in general surgical patients.[89]

Offset against the advantages are the problems of increased bleeding, particularly when performing pelvic surgery, so that there still remains room for surgeons to choose. Low-molecular-weight heparin has received attention recently, and a large randomised trial of patients undergoing abdominal surgery has shown that it is less likely to cause bleeding-related complications than standard heparin.[90]

Other measures include graduated compression stockings, intravenous dextran and intermittent pneumatic calf compression. Stockings alone are less effective than other methods and dextran is not as effective as heparin, but there is at least one trial indicating that intermittent compression is equivalent to heparin in reducing the incidence of deep vein thrombosis.[91]

Antibiotic prophylaxis

All patients should receive antibiotic prophylaxis, as there is good evidence from several randomised trials that systemic antibiotics reduce the risk of sepsis after colorectal surgery.[92]

The choice of antibiotic and the route of administration are still open to debate, but in the UK the intravenous use of metronidazole for *Bacteroides fragilis* combined with broad-spectrum cover against gut anaerobes is favoured.[92]

A single dose of cephalosporin plus metronidazole is just as effective as a three-dose regimen in preventing wound infection.[93]

If there is significant contamination at the time of surgery, then prolonging antibiotic therapy for 3–5 days may be appropriate. Whatever regimen is used, it is important that the antibiotics are given immediately before the inoculation of bacteria into the wound, and the ideal timing is immediately after induction of anaesthesia.

Bladder catheterisation

This is usually done after the patient has been anaesthetised in order to monitor urine output peroperatively and postoperatively. The urethral route is most commonly used, although there is evidence that suprapubic catheterisation may be preferable.[94]

Resection

Radical excision of a colonic tumour along with the appropriate vascular pedicle and accompanying lymphatic drainage is the most appropriate operation to obtain local control.[95] Occasionally, a very limited resection may be appropriate in an unfit patient or one with widespread disease.

Classical resection removes the lymphatic drainage that lies along the arterial blood supply, thereby rendering the associated colon ischaemic; thus right hemicolectomy removes the ileocolic and right colic arteries, transverse colectomy removes the middle colic artery and left hemicolectomy removes the left colic artery. However, transverse colectomy has fallen out of favour owing to a perception that anastomotic leakage is unacceptably high,[96] and the distinction between left hemicolectomy and sigmoid colectomy is irrelevant if the principle of radical excision of the vascular pedicle is accepted. Thus, many surgeons would now hold that the decision as to type of operation lies between right hemicolectomy and left hemicolectomy, with the extent of bowel resection dependent on site of tumour.

A standard right hemicolectomy involves division of the ileocolic and right colic arteries at their origins from the superior mesenteric artery (**Fig. 3.3**). The marginal artery or the right branch of the middle colic artery will also need division to complete vascular isolation. For tumours of the descending colon and sigmoid colon, a formal left hemicolectomy involves division of the inferior mesenteric artery at its origin from the aorta (**Fig. 3.4**).

Splenic flexure carcinoma

The main controversy arises with tumours in the region of the splenic flexure, and here there are two options. One is to regard the tumour as left sided and to carry out a left hemicolectomy, dividing the inferior mesenteric artery at its origin and dividing the left branch of the middle colic artery. A more conservative approach to this operation is to preserve the inferior mesenteric trunk, but this is essentially a segmental resection. The other approach is to carry out an extended right hemicolectomy, dividing the middle colic artery and the ascending branch of the left colic artery.

Expert opinion is divided as to which approach to take, but left hemicolectomy will necessitate

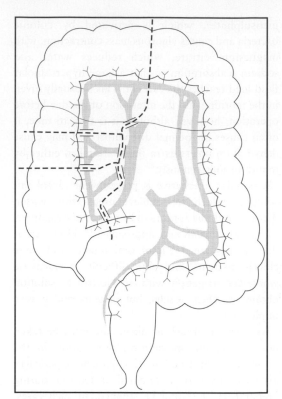

Figure 3.3 • Alternative sites of vascular division in right hemicolectomy.

anastomosis between right colon and rectum, which may be difficult to achieve without tension in some patients. Furthermore, the blood supply of the colon is inconstant. In 6% of cases there is no left colic artery and the blood supply of the splenic flexure is from the middle colic artery. In 22% of cases the middle colic artery is absent and the blood supply of the splenic flexure comes from both the left and right colic arteries. A cancer operation involves removing the tumour with its associated lymphatic drainage, and as the lymphatic drainage follows the arterial blood supply, it would seem sensible to ligate the right colic, middle colic and left colic arteries, making extended right hemicolectomy necessary.[97]

For these reasons, I prefer extended right hemicolectomy, with an anastomosis between sigmoid colon and mobile well-vascularised ileum. It must be stressed, however, that the ideal operation will be dictated by individual anatomy, the most important criteria being lack of tension and good blood supply as evidenced by brisk bleeding and good colour at the cut bowel ends.

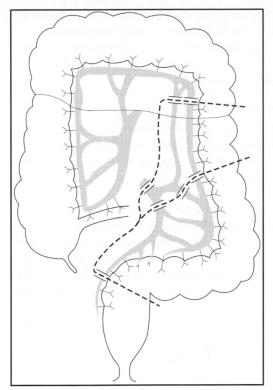

Figure 3.4 • Alternative sites of vascular division in left hemicolectomy.

The Large Bowel Cancer Project found a high local recurrence rate and poor survival for patients with splenic flexure carcinoma, regardless of stage and presentation, which may reflect surgical inadequacy of primary treatment.[98]

Advanced tumours

When a tumour is locally advanced, it may still be possible to achieve a curative resection if the surgeon is prepared to resect adjacent involved organs, such as ureter, duodenum, stomach, spleen, small bowel, bladder and uterus (Rupert Turnbull at the Cleveland Clinic classified tumours that involved other organs as Dukes' D, for which he achieved a number of cures). In addition, about 5% of women will have macroscopic ovarian metastases[99] and a further 2% will have microscopic disease.[100] For this reason, a few surgeons carry out routine oophorectomy in all women with colorectal cancer.

In a patient with a truly inoperable tumour of the colon an ileocolonic bypass may be appropriate

for lesions of the right side, whereas for tumours of the distal colon a defunctioning colostomy may be preferable. With multiple colonic tumours, a subtotal or total colectomy should be considered.

Operative technique

RIGHT HEMICOLECTOMY

I prefer midline incisions for all colonic resections, as there is no muscle damage and access is gained to all parts of the abdomen and pelvis. For a right hemicolectomy it is useful to have two-thirds of the incision above the umbilicus to facilitate mobilisation of the hepatic flexure.

With the surgeon standing on the patient's left, the right colon is retracted towards the midline, and the peritoneum in the right paracolic gutter is divided. This extends from the caecal pole to the hepatic flexure, and distal to this point the lesser sac is entered and the greater omentum divided below the gastroepiploic arcade up to the point of intended division of the transverse colon. The right colon is then retracted firmly towards the midline, and the plane between the colonic mesentery and the posterior abdominal wall is carefully developed with diathermy or scissors, taking care not to damage the duodenum. If this is done, the ureter and gonadal vessels will fall away safely.

It then remains to divide the appropriate colonic vessels as described above, which can be facilitated by transillumination of the mesentery. Once done, the bowel wall is cleared at the sites of transection and single crushing clamps are applied. Soft clamps may be applied on proximal small bowel and distal large bowel, and the bowel is divided on the crushing clamps, leaving them on the specimen.

LEFT HEMICOLECTOMY

For all left-sided colonic resections, it is advisable to place the patient in the Lloyd-Davies position, as standing between the legs is an advantageous position for an assistant, and it also allows the operator excellent access to the splenic flexure. (Editor's note: at St Mark's Hospital even patients for right colon operations are placed in the lithotomy–Trendelenburg position, not only for distribution of surgeon, assistants and scrub nurse around the operating table but also because at times right-sided tumours or Crohn's disease will be found to involve the rectum.) A long midline incision is employed, extending from above the umbilicus to the pubis. The operator stands on the patient's left side, and one assistant retracts the sigmoid colon medially while the other retracts the lower left abdominal wall.

The peritoneum lateral to the sigmoid and descending colon is divided close to the 'white line' of fusion using diathermy or a knife. It should then be possible to see the plane between the mesentery and the retroperitoneal structures, which can be further developed using a combination of firm medial traction of the bowel by the assistant and countertraction applied by the operator on the retroperitoneum using a swab or forceps.

This manoeuvre will ensure that ureter and gonadal vessels are swept away. Care must be taken to identify the hypogastric nerves, and these should be separated from the mesentery or they may be damaged as the upper rectum is prepared for anastomosis. The splenic flexure should then be mobilised, and this is best done by dissecting the greater omentum off the transverse colon and continuing laterally towards the flexure. However, if the tumour is in the region of the splenic flexure, it is advisable to divide the gastrocolic ligament and take the omentum with the specimen. In either event, the spleen is at risk from tears caused by traction on its peritoneal attachments, and despite extreme care splenectomy is sometimes necessary. For minor tears, however, application of a haemostatic agent such as oxycellulose is sufficient.

Once the left colon has been mobilised, the origin of the inferior mesenteric artery is identified by dividing the peritoneum over the aorta close to the fourth part of the duodenum, ligated and divided. To obtain full mobility it is then necessary to divide the inferior mesenteric vein just below the inferior border of the pancreas. The colon is then divided as described for right hemicolectomy at a convenient point in the transverse colon and at the rectosigmoid junction.

'NO-TOUCH' TECHNIQUE

It has been argued that early vascular ligation before mobilisation of the tumour, sometimes even supported by the use of proximal and distal occluding tapes around the bowel, prevents embolisation of tumour cells and improves survival.

The technique was popularised by Rupert Turnbull at the Cleveland Clinic,[101] but a recent randomised controlled clinical trial in the Netherlands has shown no survival advantage to this otherwise elegant variation.[102]

ANASTOMOSIS

For anastomosis after resection of a colonic cancer, I prefer to use hand suturing, although it is appreciated that stapling may produce excellent results.

Appositional serosubmucosal anastomosis

This method, initially described by Matheson et al.,[103] utilises a single layer of interrupted 3/0 braided polyamide. For mobile anastomoses (usually ileocolic) the first step is to ensure that the ends to be anastomosed are roughly equal in circumference. This is usually achieved by making an incision on the antemesenteric aspect of the small bowel, although some surgeons prefer to use an end-to-side technique. One side of the anastomosis is performed on the serosal aspect of the bowel between the mesenteric and antemesenteric borders, placing the sutures 4 mm apart and 4 mm deep, ensuring that the muscle layer and the submucosa but not the mucosa have been included (Fig. 3.5). The sutures are left untied until they have all been inserted (Fig. 3.6), and each knot is then tied by hand to ensure a snug but non-constrictive result. The half-completed anastomosis is then turned over and the process repeated. Mesenteric defects are not closed.

For colorectal or ileorectal anastomoses, the posterior row of sutures is inserted first, holding each suture with a specially designed suture clamp or individual artery forceps. If artery forceps are used, they should be threaded on to a forceps holder to avoid tangling. Again, the sutures are tied by hand after insertion of the whole row, the knots being tied on the luminal side of the anastomosis

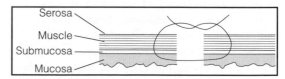

Figure 3.5 • Placement of the appositional serosubmucosal suture.

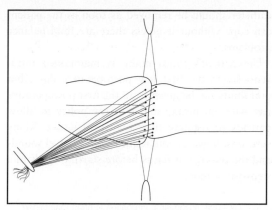

Figure 3.6 • Ileocolic anastomosis. The sutures are left untied until they have all been inserted.

after the proximal bowel has been 'parachuted' down the sutures to the upper rectum (**Fig. 3.7**). The knot tails are then cut so that they are covered by the cut edges of the undisturbed mucosal layers. On completion of the posterior aspect of the anastomosis, the anterior part is performed in a similar fashion but with the knots tied on the extraluminal side. This type of anastomosis is greatly facilitated by the use of curved 'Heaney' needle holders, with the needle mounted facing out from the convex side of the tip.

Stapled anastomoses

After right hemicolecomy the most widely employed stapled anastomosis is the 'functional end-to-end'.

Here, the ends of the colon and ileum are stapled closed at the time of specimen excision, and two small enterotomies are made to permit insertion of the limbs of a linear cutting stapler. The anastomosis is then performed by firing the stapler, taking care not to include mesentery (**Fig. 3.8**), and after checking the staple line for bleeding the remaining defect is closed with a linear stapler. After left hemicolectomy, a true end-to-end anastomosis can be performed using a circular anastomosing stapler introduced per anum (**Fig. 3.9**), although in some male patients the intact rectum can be difficult to negotiate.

Results of anastomotic techniques

The interrupted serosubmucosal technique is recommended for its adaptability to any anastomosis involving the colon, but it is also associated with the best results in the literature, being associated with leak rates of 0.5–3% in sizeable series.[104,105]

Stapling has been compared with hand suturing in several randomised trials.[106–110] Although the results vary, there seems to be no consistent difference in colonic anastomotic dehiscence between the two approaches.

In one trial there was evidence that tumour recurrence was less in the stapled group, but no

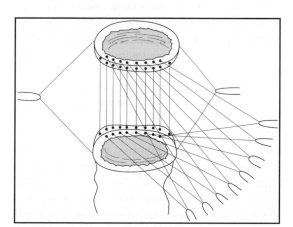

Figure 3.7 • Colorectal anastomosis. The sutures are held in individual forceps, and the colon slid down to the rectum before tying.

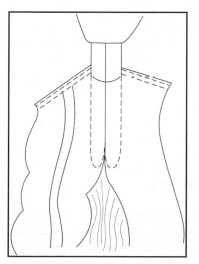

Figure 3.8 • 'Functional end-to-end' ileocolonic stapled anastomosis.

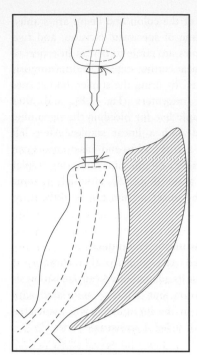

Figure 3.9 • End-to-end colorectal anastomosis using a circular stapling device.

distinction between rectal and colonic resections was made.[111]

DRAINS

After the anastomosis is complete, many surgeons will leave a drain in the peritoneal cavity either to minimise the consequences of an anastomotic leak or to prevent the accumulation of fluid that might be infected.

However, there is no evidence to support this practice and three randomised trials have shown there to be no advantage associated with drainage of colonic or colorectal anastomoses.[112–114]

Postoperative care/ complications

After colectomy, postoperative care is similar to that of any patient undergoing major abdominal surgery. Opiate analgesia is best administered by a patient-driven system, and is usually required for the first two or three postoperative days. Early mobilisation is encouraged, and the urethral catheter should be removed as soon as the patient can cope without it unless there are fluid balance problems.

The patient's fluid intake is maintained intravenously in the first few postoperative days, but oral fluids can be given from the first postoperative day without mishap and it is my policy to allow patients to regulate their own oral intake. Many surgeons, however, still require active bowel sounds and the passage of flatus before starting fluids in a stepwise fashion.

Likewise, nasogastric intubation is often maintained until there is evidence of intestinal activity, although there is good evidence from a randomised trial that it confers no benefit in elective colorectal surgery.[115]

It is my policy to avoid routine nasogastric intubation after colectomy.

Anastomotic dehiscence

Although patients undergoing colectomy may suffer any of the complications associated with major abdominal surgery, it is anastomotic breakdown that is the major source of morbidity specific to this type of operation. Subclinical leaks occur more frequently than clinically obvious leaks,[116] but after resection of a colonic tumour the overall significant leak rate is currently in the region of 4%.[6]

A leak may present in a variety of ways and the onset of symptoms may be quite insidious. Warning signs are pyrexia, increasing pulse rate and abdominal distension due to paralytic ileus. The patient may then develop localised or generalised peritonitis, or a faecal fistula, usually through the wound. Occasionally a patient will develop sudden generalised peritonitis and septicaemic shock as a result of rapid faecal contamination of the peritoneal cavity.

Because of the heterogeneous nature of the symptoms, a leak should be suspected in any patient with an anastomosis who is not progressing as well as expected, including those with apparent cardiac events. Investigations that may prove useful in a doubtful case include a full blood count, abdominal and chest radiography, water-soluble contrast enema and CT. The white cell count is usually raised, but not inevitably. Plain radiographs will frequently demonstrate distended loops of bowel and gas may be seen under the diaphragm, although both may be seen after any laparotomy in the absence of a leak. Surgeons often consider the most useful investigation to be a water-soluble contrast enema but many radiologists now favour CT.

The treatment of an anastomotic dehiscence depends on the specific mode of presentation. The patient with general peritonitis requires laparotomy after appropriate resuscitation. The anastomosis should be taken down and the two ends exteriorised if possible; primary repair of the anastomotic dehiscence is doomed to failure and should not be attempted. After dealing with the anastomosis, careful peritoneal toilet must be performed using copious quantities of warm saline with or without antibiotic, and the patient will require at least 5 days of intravenous antibiotic therapy.

In the patient with localised peritonitis who remains otherwise well a conservative approach with systemic antibiotics may be appropriate, although laparotomy should not be delayed if there is any deterioration. A faecal fistula can also be treated in this way but care must be taken with the surrounding skin, and nutritional support may be required if drainage is prolonged.

Laparoscopic surgery

Laparoscopic surgery for colonic cancer has excited a great deal of interest in recent years, but there are serious concerns regarding this type of surgery.[117] First, it is technically difficult. As in open surgery, the important principles of traction and precise dissection in the correct plane must be observed for colonic mobilisation, and it can be difficult to obtain adequate vision and the correct angles for this to be done. Intracorporeal anastomosis is likewise awkward, and most surgeons will use an extracorporeal technique where possible. To facilitate complex laparoscopic surgery the concept of hand assistance has arisen; this utilises a special sealing device that allows the introduction of the surgeon's hand into the peritoneal cavity via a small incision.[118] Although this overcomes some of the problems outlined above, it sacrifices some of the advantages of minimal access in colonic surgery.[119]

The second problem is that of specimen retrieval, and for colonic cancers a relatively large incision

has to be made. This negates a lot of the benefit in terms of postoperative pain, and the duration of hospital stay after laparoscopic colorectal surgery is currently little different from that achieved by open surgery.[117]

Port-site tumour recurrence has also been a major concern; although its incidence varies from 1.5 to 21% depending on the series,[117] it is unlikely to be much more than the 1% abdominal wall recurrence rate reported after conventional surgery.[120] Crucial to the future of laparoscopic surgery are long-term data indicating the survival and rates of distant or local recurrence that can be expected after laparoscopic colonic cancer resection. For this reason, randomised trials are being carried out, and in the UK the results of a trial sponsored by the Medical Research Council are awaited.[121] Recently, a Spanish group has reported follow-up of 3–9 years in a randomised trial that has shown a significant benefit for laparoscopic surgery in terms of cancer-related survival.[122] If these findings are replicated by other studies, laparoscopic surgery for colorectal cancer will have come of age, and the onus will be on coloproctologists to embrace this technique.

EMERGENCY MANAGEMENT

In the UK, about 20% of patients with colonic cancer will present as an emergency while 16% will present with obstruction.[5] Bleeding and perforation are less common modes of emergency presentation; when perforation occurs, it is often in the caecum as a result of distal obstruction in the face of a competent ileocaecal valve. Obstruction is thus the most likely reason for emergency or urgent operation.

Investigation

The patient with obstruction will usually present with colicky abdominal pain and abdominal distension, with a variable degree of vomiting and change in bowel habit. Paradoxically, the obstructed patient may complain of diarrhoea rather than constipation owing to overflow. The first specific investigation in this case will be a plain abdominal radiograph, which will demonstrate the typical features of large or, in the case of an obstructing caecal cancer, small bowel obstruction.

Particular attention should be paid to the size of the caecum on the radiograph, and whether gas is present in small bowel loops. If the caecum is 12 cm or more in diameter and there is no evidence of decompression into the small bowel, then there is significant risk of caecal perforation and urgent intervention is required, particularly if there is local tenderness.

However, before committing the patient to laparotomy, it is important to identify the site of obstruction, as colonic pseudo-obstruction can mimic the clinical and radiological signs of mechanical obstruction. Thus, every patient should have rigid sigmoidoscopy at least to exclude rectal pathology, followed by a water-soluble contrast enema.[123] Barium should not be used as it can become inspissated in the segment of colon distal to the obstruction, and if there is a perforation barium can enter the peritoneal cavity with disastrous consequences.

Management of obstruction

Once mechanical obstruction is diagnosed and the patient resuscitated, laparotomy should proceed with experienced surgical and anaesthetic staff in attendance, preferably during daylight hours. The first task at laparotomy is usually to decompress the gaseous distension of the large bowel, and this can be achieved by inserting a 19G (white) needle attached to suction into the lumen through a convenient taenia. If a larger tube is required to evacuate large amounts of liquid faeces, this should be inserted into the caecum via an enterotomy in the terminal ileum.

When the bowel can be safely handled, a decision must be made as to the type of operation required. If the obstruction is due to a right-sided lesion, it is usually easy and safe to carry out a standard right hemicolectomy. If, however, the cancer is on the left side, several options are available. Traditionally, obstructing left-sided cancers were treated by a three-stage approach, starting with a defunctioning loop colostomy followed by resection and anastomosis, and then by closure of the defunctioning stoma. This gradually gave way to a two-stage procedure, with primary resection of the tumour in the form of a Hartmann's operation where the proximal colon is brought out as an end colostomy and the distal

segment either closed off or brought out as a mucous fistula.[124]

Recently, however, there has been a move towards one-stage procedures, and here the choice lies between subtotal colectomy with ileocolic or ileorectal anastomosis and left hemicolectomy after on-table colonic irrigation.[125] For tumours in the region of the splenic flexure, the former approach is often sensible, especially if there is doubt about the viability of the caecum.

There is also an argument for subtotal colectomy for tumours in the more distal colon, but a recent randomised trial comparing both strategies found that patients treated by left hemicolectomy had more acceptable postoperative bowel function.[126]

If a decision is made to perform a left hemicolectomy, then the colon proximal to the site of obstruction should be irrigated using the technique originally described by Dudley et al.[127] to produce ideal conditions for the anastomosis. A colostomy is made just proximal to the lesion, taking care not to spill bowel contents, and anaesthetic scavenging tubing is inserted and secured with heavy silk around the bowel wall. The end of this tubing is tied into a large plastic bag which is placed into a bucket on the floor. A large Foley catheter is then inserted into the caecum by means of an enterotomy in the appendix or the terminal ileum, and the balloon inflated (**Fig. 3.10**). About 3–4 L of warm saline are then infused into the caecum and massaged around the colon to the anaesthetic tubing, pieces of solid faeces being broken up within the lumen by gentle manipulation. This should continue until the effluent is clear. A standard resection and anastomosis can then be safely performed.

Clearly, the choice of operation will depend on individual circumstances, and few surgeons would attempt an anastomosis in the presence of severe intra-abdominal sepsis or in a severely ill patient. In these cases, a Hartmann's resection is perfectly acceptable, and in some situations a defunctioning stoma may be the best option. Increasingly, expanding metal (wall) stents are being used in obstructing left-sided colonic tumours. Although most experience has been palliative in intent, more lesions are now being treated in this way to allow

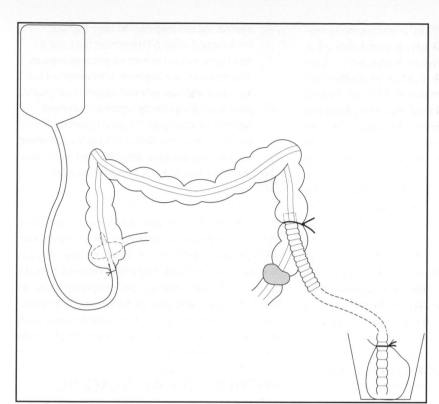

Figure 3.10 • On-table colonic irrigation.

decompression followed by bowel preparation and elective resection of the tumour.[128]

Management of perforation

In the patient who is found to have a perforated caecum as a result of an obstructing distal cancer, an extended right hemicolectomy or subtotal colectomy is the treatment of choice. Whether an anastomosis is fashioned will depend on the degree of peritoneal contamination. For the cancer which has perforated primarily, it is important to resect the lesion itself to eliminate not only the malignancy but also the source of sepsis. This can be technically demanding, and for left-sided lesions will almost always necessitate a Hartmann's procedure.

MANAGEMENT OF ADVANCED DISEASE

The surgical management of the advanced primary tumour is covered in the section on elective surgery. In colonic cancer, local recurrence usually occurs at the suture line and, in the absence of disseminated disease, re-resection should be attempted, although palliative bypass may be all that can be achieved. The patient with distant metastases poses different challenges.

Operable metastases

Hepatic resection for colorectal cancer metastases is now widely practised, but there is still debate as to its value. It has never been tested in a randomised trial, and all comparative studies have used retrospective data from historical controls.[129]

Nevertheless, with careful patient selection, hepatectomy for colorectal metastases can be associated with a 5-year survival of around 30%.[130] Although the most widely accepted criterion for resection is one to three resectable metastases in one lobe of the liver, many surgeons are now extending their indications.

Perhaps the most persuasive argument in favour of hepatectomy comes from the Registry of Hepatic

Metastases in the USA.[131] In a multicentre long-term follow-up study, this group found that after resection of colorectal hepatic metastases, recurrence was very rare after 3 years of disease-free survival, suggesting that about 30% of treated patients were effectively cured. Recently, however, this observation has been challenged by the prospective Gastrointestinal Tumour Study Group trial, which shows a continuing attrition rate up to 5 years after surgery.[132]

The timing of liver resection is also debatable. Although some surgeons advocate immediate operation, especially when the metastases are found synchronously with the primary tumour, leading authorities suggest that a delay of 3–4 months with intensive restaging investigations at the end of this time is appropriate.[133] In this way patients with rapidly progressive disease that is unlikely to benefit from resection will be spared fruitless major surgery. In a proportion of patients with liver disease that is not amenable to resection, in situ ablation using cryotherapy or radiofrequency energy may be employed.[134] This may prolong survival, but as yet must be regarded as palliative.

Pulmonary metastases may also be amenable to resection, but as only 10% of patients develop such metastases and only 10% of these have disease confined to the lung, very few patients will be suitable. Nonetheless, segmental resection of the lung may be associated with 5-year survival rates of 20–40%.[135]

Inoperable disseminated disease

In the patient with widespread disease, chemotherapy containing 5-fluorouracil (5-FU) is the only established therapeutic option, but this can only be regarded as palliative. Few studies have compared chemotherapy with supportive treatment only, and the survival benefits, though significant, are not great.

Nevertheless, 5-FU and folinic acid (FUFA) are now regarded as standard palliative therapy, and this can be given in bolus form (Mayo regimen), as an intermittent infusion (de Gramont regimen) or as a continuous infusion (Lokich regimen). Trials have indicated that the infusional techniques are more

effective and less toxic than the Mayo regimen.[136] For patients in whom 5-FU treatment has failed, the new topoisomerase I inhibitor irinotecan provides an effective second-line treatment. In a randomised trial comparing irinotecan with best supportive care, such patients had a significantly improved survival and quality of life when given the active treatment.[137] First-line combination therapy with FUFA and irinotecan has also been compared with FUFA alone and shown to improve survival, but at the cost of increased toxicity.[138,139]

In patients with disease confined to the liver, regional perfusion chemotherapy offers the delivery of high concentrations of drug to the disease-bearing organ with relatively low systemic toxicity. However, despite evidence that response rates are higher than with systemic chemotherapy,[140] improvements in survival are modest, and the advantages of intra-arterial hepatic chemotherapy tend to be offset by technical difficulties.

PATHOLOGICAL STAGING

Accurate, detailed and consistent pathology reporting for colorectal cancer is important for estimating prognosis and planning further treatment in terms of adjuvant therapy (see Chapter 5). Both macroscopic and histological appearances must be described in some detail, and the following information should be available.

Macroscopic description
1. Size of the tumour (greatest dimension).
2. Site of the tumour in relation to the resection margins.
3. Any abnormalities of the background bowel.

Microscopic description
1. Histological type.
2. Differentiation of the tumour, based on the predominant grade within the tumour.[141]
3. Maximum extent of invasion into/through the bowel wall (submucosa, muscularis propria, extramural).
4. Serosal involvement by tumour, if present.[142]
5. A statement on the completeness of excision at the cut ends (including the 'doughnuts' from stapling devices).

6. Number of lymph nodes examined, the number containing metastases, and whether the apical node is involved.
7. Extramural vascular invasion if present.[143]
8. Pathological staging of the tumour according to Dukes' classification.[144]

Dukes' staging is simple, reproducible and widely recognised, and it should always be used. TNM staging may also be used and the two systems are described in **Box 3.2**. Some pathologists use the Jass classification,[145] although its usefulness may be limited by observer variation in the degree of lymphocytic infiltration at the advancing margin of the tumour (one of the four parameters that contribute to the classification) and the fact that its prognostic value appears to be confined to rectal tumours.

After curative resection, cancer registry data indicate that age-adjusted 5-year survival for Dukes' stage A colonic cancer is 85%, for stage B 67% and for stage C 37%. These results can be improved as evidenced by individual series,[146] and the 'Will Rogers' effect (stage migration owing to variable quality of pathology reporting) may play a role in this respect.

RECOMMENDATIONS FOR BEST PRACTICE

The recommendations given here represent a summary of the evidence-based guidelines from the Association of Coloproctology and the Scottish Intercollegiate Guidelines Network for the management of colorectal cancer as they apply to colonic tumours.[147,148]

Investigation

1. Patients with suspicious symptoms or a proven colorectal cancer should be investigated with either endoscopic visualisation of the whole rectum plus a high-quality double-contrast barium enema or a total colonoscopy. Supplementary flexible endoscopy should be carried out where it is impossible, with any certainty, to exclude neoplasia on barium enema.
2. All patients should have preoperative full blood count and urea and electrolyte estimations, and, unless it cannot alter management, screening

---

Box 3.2 • Clinicopathological staging of colorectal cancer

Dukes' staging (based on histological examination of the resection specimen)

A   Invasive carcinoma not breaching the muscularis propria
B   Invasive carcinoma breaching the muscularis propria, but not involving regional lymph nodes
C1 Invasive carcinoma involving the regional lymph nodes (apical node negative)
C2 Invasive carcinoma involving the regional lymph nodes (apical node positive)

Note: Dukes' stage D has come to mean the presence of distant metastases.

TNM staging

T – primary tumour

TX Primary tumour cannot be assessed
T0 No evidence of primary tumour
Tis Carcinoma *in situ*
T1 Tumour invades submucosa
T2 Tumour invades muscularis propria
T3 Tumour invades through muscularis propria into subserosa or into non-peritonealised pericolic or perirectal tissues
T4 Tumour perforates the visceral peritoneum or directly invades other organs or structures

Note: direct invasion in T4 includes invasion of other segments of the colorectum by way of the serosa, e.g. invasion of the sigmoid colon by a carcinoma of the caecum

N – regional lymph nodes

NX Regional lymph nodes cannot be assessed
N0 No regional lymph node metastasis
N1 Metastasis in 1 to 3 pericolic or perirectal lymph nodes
N2 Metastasis in 4 or more pericolic or perirectal lymph nodes
N3 Metastasis in any lymph node along the course of a named vascular trunk

M – distant metastasis

M0 No distant metastases
M1 Distant metastases

---

for lung and liver metastases should be carried out by means of chest radiography and CT or ultrasound.

Preparation for surgery

1. All patients undergoing surgery for colorectal cancer should give informed consent. This

implies being given information about the likely benefits and risks of the proposed treatment and details of any alternatives.

2. Blood should not be withheld if there is a clinical indication to give it, and preparations for blood transfusion should be made in all patients undergoing surgery for colorectal cancer except where an individual patient refuses.

3. Mechanical bowel preparation prior to surgery is recommended.

4. Subcutaneous heparin or intermittent compression should be employed as thromboembolism prophylaxis in surgery for colorectal cancer unless there is a specific contraindication.

5. All patients undergoing surgery for colorectal cancer should have antibiotic prophylaxis. It is impossible to be dogmatic as regards the precise regimen, but a single dose of appropriate intravenous antibiotics appears to be effective.

Elective surgical treatment

1. Any tumour with a distal margin at 15 cm or less from the anal verge using a rigid sigmoidoscope should be classified as rectal.

2. Although no definite recommendations can be made regarding anastomotic technique, the interrupted serosubmucosal method is adaptable to all colonic anastomoses and has the lowest reported leak rate in the literature.

3. Laparoscopic surgery for colorectal cancer should be performed only by experienced laparoscopic surgeons who have been properly trained in colorectal surgery, and who are prepared to audit their results very carefully.

Emergency treatment

1. Emergency surgery should be carried out during daytime hours as far as possible, by experienced surgeons and anaesthetists.

2. In patients presenting with obstruction, steps should be taken to exclude pseudo-obstruction before operation.

3. Stoma formation should be carried out in the patient's interests only and not as a result of lack of experienced surgical staff.

4. The overall mortality for emergency/urgent surgery should be 20% or less.

Adjuvant therapy

Patients with stage C colonic cancer who are medically and psychosocially fit should be offered fluorouracil-containing adjuvant chemotherapy.

Treatment of advanced disease

1. It is recommended that effective palliation with optimal quality of remaining life should be the main aim of therapy in advanced disease.

2. Consideration should be given to palliative chemotherapy in patients with local advanced and metastatic disease. Thus, patients with advanced disease who remain in good general condition should have the opportunity to discuss the possible benefits of palliative therapy with an oncologist.

3. Consideration should also be given to surgical treatment in selected patients with locally advanced and metastatic disease. In particular, the patient with limited hepatic involvement should be considered for partial hepatectomy by an experienced liver surgeon.

Outcomes

Surgeons should carefully audit the outcome of their colorectal cancer surgery.

1. They should expect to achieve an operative mortality of less than 20% for emergency surgery and 5% for elective surgery for colorectal cancer.

2. Wound infection rates after surgery for colorectal cancer should be less than 10%.

3. Surgeons should expect to achieve an overall leak rate below 4% for colonic resection.

4. Surgeons should carefully examine their practice with a view to meeting or improving targets set by national long-term mortality statistics.

Pathology

All resected colorectal tumours should be submitted for histological examination. For this to be useful, the report should reach an acceptable standard, providing information that will be useful in assessing prognosis, planning treatment and carrying out audit.

• **Key points**

- It is now accepted that most if not all colon cancers arise from pre-existing adenomatous polyps. However, it has to be recognised that the flat adenoma which can be difficult to detect endoscopically may be a significant precursor lesion.
- While genetic background is clearly important in the aetiology of colorectal cancer, it is now recognised that lifestyle factors are also important. Diet contributes to colorectal cancer in that red meat appears to be a risk factor and both green vegetables and fibre are protective. There is also evidence that exercise and avoidance of weight gain are important protective factors.
- Colonoscopy is the gold standard investigative procedure but there is increasing evidence that CT colography will have an important role to play in the future.
- It is now established that faecal occult blood test screening can reduce colon cancer mortality. The evidence to support flexible sigmoidoscopy screening is awaited.
- Surgery is the only definitive curative treatment for the majority of colon cancers and technique is important to ensure a good outcome. The evidence for laparoscopic surgery for colon cancer is accumulating rapidly and this may be an important therapeutic modality in the future.
- The majority of colon cancers that present as an emergency do so because of intestinal obstruction. It is important that these patients are dealt with by specialist teams and the role of radiological stenting is rapidly expanding.

REFERENCES

1. Cancer Research UK. Statistics on colorectal cancer. Available at http://www.cancerresearchuk.org/aboutcancer/statistics/statstables/colorectalcancer
2. ISD Scotland. Key health topics. Colorectal cancer. Available at http://www.show.scot.nhs.uk/isd/cancer/facts_figures/types/colorectal.htm
3. Williams PL, Warwick R. Gray's anatomy. Edinburgh: Churchill Livingstone, 1980; p. 1356.
4. United Kingdom Coordinating Committee on Cancer Research (UKCCCR). Handbook for the clinicopathological assessment and staging of colorectal cancer. London: UKCCCR, 1989.
5. Bass BL, Enker WE, Lightdale CJ. Advances in colorectal carcinoma surgery. New York: World Medical Press, 1993; p. 37.
6. Mella J, Biffin A, Radcliffe AG, Stamatakis JD, Steele RJC. Population-based audit of colorectal cancer management in two UK health regions. Br J Surg 1997; 84:1731–6.
7. Wessex Audit of Colorectal Cancer Management (Thompson M, personal communication, 2000).
8. Muto T, Bussey HJ, Morson BC. The evolution of cancer of the colon and rectum. Cancer 1975; 36:2251–70.
9. Winawer SJ, Zauber A, Diaz B. Temporal sequence of evolving colorectal cancer from the normal colon (abstract). Gastrointest Endosc 1987; 33:167.
10. Morson BC. Factors influencing the prognosis of early cancer of the rectum. Proc R Soc Med 1966; 59:607–8.
11. Bussey HJ. Familial polyposis coli. Baltimore: Johns Hopkins University Press, 1975.

12. Vogelstein B, Fearon ER, Hamilton SR et al. Genetic alterations during colorectal-tumour development. N Engl J Med 1988; 319:525–32.

    This seminal paper established the concept of colorectal cancer developing as a result of a stepwise accumulation of genetic mutations, phenotypically expressed as the adenoma–carcinoma sequence.

13. Granqvist S. Distribution of polyps in the large bowel in relation to age. A colonoscopic study. Scand J Gastroenterol 1981; 16:1025–31.
14. Chu DZ, Glacco G, Martin RG, Guinee VF. The significance of synchronous carcinoma and polyps in the colon and rectum. Cancer 1986; 57:445–50.
15. Eide TJ. Prevalence and morphological features of adenomas of the large intestine with and without colorectal carcinoma. J Histopathol 1986; 10:111–18.
16. Mandel JS, Church TR, Bond JH et al. The effect of fecal occult-blood screening on the incidence of colorectal cancer. N Engl J Med 2000; 343:1603–7.
17. Rembacken BJ, Fujii T, Cairns A et al. Flat and depressed colonic neoplasms: a prospective study of 1000 colonoscopies in the UK. Lancet 2000; 355:1211–14.
18. Jinnai D. Incidence and pathology of carcinoma of the colon and rectum. In: Goligher JC (ed.) Surgery of the anus, rectum and colon, 4th edn. London: Baillière Tindall, 1982; p. 447.
19. Cedermark BJ, Shultz SS, Bakshi S et al. The value of liver scan in the follow-up study of patients with

adenocarcinoma of the colon and rectum. Surg Gynecol Obstet 1977; 144:745–8.

20. Moore GE, Sako K, Kondo T et al. Assessment of the exfoliation of tumour cells into the body cavities. Surg Gynecol Obstet 1961; 112:469.

21. Powell SM, Zilz N, Beazer-Barclay Y et al. APC mutations occur early during colorectal tumorigenesis. Nature 1992; 359:235–7.

22. Scott N, Bell SM, Sagar P, Blair GE, Dixon MF, Quirke P. p53 expression and K-ras mutation in colorectal adenomas. Gut 1993; 34:621–4.

23. Fearon ER, Cho KR, Nigro JM et al. Identification of a chromosome 18q gene that is altered in colorectal cancers. Science 1990; 247:49–56.

24. Kikuchi-Yanoshita R, Konishi M, Ito S et al. Genetic changes of both p53 alleles associated with the conversion from colorectal adenoma to early carcinoma in familial adenomatous polyposis and non-familial adenomatous polyposis patients. Cancer Res 1992; 52:3965–71.

25. Kastan MB, Onyekwere O, Sidransky D et al. Participation of p53 protein in the cellular response to DNA damage. Cancer Res 1991; 51:6304–11.

26. Shaw P, Bovey R, Tardy S, Sahli R, Sordat B, Costa J. Induction of apoptosis by wild-type p53 in a human colon tumour-derived cell line. Proc Natl Acad Sci USA 1992; 89:4495–9.

27. Smith G, Carey FA, Beattie J et al. Mutations in APC, Kirsten-ras, and p53: alternative genetic pathways to colorectal cancer. Proc Natl Acad Sci USA 2002; 99:9433–8.

28. Font A, Abad A, Monzo M et al. Prognostic value of K-ras mutations and allelic imbalance on chromosome 18q in patients with resected colorectal cancer. Dis Colon Rectum 2001; 44:549–57.

29. Burkitt DP. Epidemiology of cancer of the colon and rectum. Cancer 1971; 28:3–13.

30. Modan B, Barell V, Lubin F et al. Low fibre intake as an aetiological factor in cancer of the colon. J Natl Cancer Inst 1975; 55:15–18.

31. Rooney PS, Hunt L, Clarke PA. Wheat fibre, lactulose and rectal mucosal proliferation in individuals with a family history of colorectal cancer. Br J Surg 1994; 81:1792–4.

32. Bingham SA, Day NE, Luben R et al. Dietary fibre in food and protection against colorectal cancer. The European Prospective Investigation into Cancer and Nutrition (EPIC): an observational study. Lancet 2003; 361:1496–501.

33. Peters U, Sinha R, Chatterjee N et al. Dietary fibre and colorectal adenoma in a colorectal cancer detection programme. Lancet 2003; 361:1491–5.

34. Bjelke E. Epidemiologic studies of cancer of the stomach, colon and rectum with special emphasis on the role of diets, vols I–IV. Thesis, University of Minnesota, 1973.

35. Thornalley P. More good things in vegetables than you ever imagined. Biochemist 1999; 21:19–23.

This review sets out current concepts of the biochemistry underlying the protective effect of vegetables in colorectal cancer.

36. IARC Working Group on the Evaluation of Cancer Preventive Agents. Weight control and physical activity. Lyon: International Agency for Research on Cancer, 2002.

37. Giovannucci E. An updated review of the epidemiological evidence that cigarette smoking increases risk of colorectal cancer. Cancer Epidemiol Biomarkers Prev 2001; 10:725–31.

38. Corrao G, Bagnardi V, Zambon A, Arico S. Exploring the dose–response relationship between alcohol consumption and the risk of several alcohol-related conditions: a meta-analysis. Addiction 1999; 94:1551–73.

39. Rainey JB, Maeda M, Williams C, Williamson RCN. The co-carcinogenic effect of intrarectal deoxycholate in rats is reduced by oral metronidazole. Br J Cancer 1984; 49:631–6.

40. Imray CHE, Radley S, Davis A et al. Biliary bile acid profiles in patients with colorectal cancer or polyps. Gut 1992; 33:1239–45.

41. Baron JA, Beach M, Mandel JS et al. Calcium supplements for the prevention of colorectal adenomas. N Engl J Med 1999; 340:101–7.

42. Schottenfeld D, Winawer SJ. Cholecystectomy and colo-rectal cancer (editorial). Gastroenterology 1983; 85:966–70.

43. Swidsinski A, Khilkin M, Kerjaschki D et al. Association between intraepithelial Escherichia coli and colorectal cancer. Gastroenterology 1998; 115:281–6.

44. Bundred NJ, Whitfield BCS, Stanton E, Prescott RJ, Davies GC, Kingsnorth AN. Gastric surgery and the risk of subsequent colorectal cancer. Br J Surg 1985; 72:618–19.

45. Caygill CPJ, Hill MJ, Hall CN, Kirkham JS, Northfield TC. Increased risk of cancer at multiple sites after gastric surgery for peptic ulcer. Gut 1987; 28:924–8.

46. Mullan FJ, Wilson HK, Majury CW. Bile acids and the increased risk of colorectal tumours after truncal vagotomy. Br J Surg 1990; 77:1085–90.

47. Keddie N, Hargreaves A. Symptoms of carcinoma of the colon and rectum. Lancet 1968; ii:749–50.

48. Thompson MR, Heath I, Ellis BG, Swarbrick ET, Wood LF, Atkin WS. Identifying and managing patients at low risk of bowel cancer in general practice. Br Med J 2003; 327:263–5.

49. Selvachandran SN, Hodder RJ, Ballal MS, Jones P, Cade D. Prediction of colorectal cancer by a patient consultation questionnaire and scoring system: a prospective study. Lancet 2002; 360:278–83.

50. Anderson N, Cook HB, Coates R. Colonoscopically detected colorectal cancer missed on barium enema. Gastrointest Radiol 1991; 16:123–7.

51. Farrands PA, Vellacott JD, Amar SS, Balfour TW, Hardcastle JD. Flexible fibreoptic sigmoidoscopy and double contrast barium enema examination in the identification of adenomas and carcinoma of the colon. Dis Colon Rectum 1983; 26:725–7.

52. Boulos PB, Karamanolis DG, Salmon PR, Clarke CG. Is colonoscopy necessary in diverticular disease? Lancet 1984; i:95–6.

53. Williams CB. Colonoscopy. Curr Opin Gastroenterol 1985; 1:54–9.

54. Cotton PB, Williams CB. Practical gastrointestinal endoscopy, 3rd edn. Oxford: Blackwell Scientific Publications, 1990.

55. Reeders JWAJ, Bakker AJ, Rosenbusch G. Contemporary radiological examination of the lower gastrointestinal tract. Baillières Clin Gastroenterol 1995; 9:701–28.

56. Amin Z, Boulos PB, Lees WR. Spiral CT pneumocolon for suspected colonic neoplasm. Clin Radiol 1996; 51:56–61.

57. Kuwayama H, Imiuro M, Kitazumi Y, Luk G. Virtual endoscopy: current perspectives. J Gastroenterol 2002; 37(suppl. 13):100–5.

58. Lamb G, Taylor I. An assessment of ultrasound scanning in the recognition of colorectal liver metastases. Ann R Coll Surg Engl 1982; 64:391–3.

59. Williams NS, Durdey P, Quirk P. Pre-operative staging of rectal neoplasm and its impact on clinical management. Br J Surg 1985; 72:868–74.

60. Stone MD, Kane R, Bothe A et al. Intraoperative ultrasound imaging of the liver at the time of colorectal cancer resection. Arch Surg 1994; 129:431–5.

61. Levitt RG, Dagel SS, Stanley RJ, Jost RG. Accuracy of computed tomography of the liver and biliary tract. Radiology 1977; 124:123–8.

62. DeLange EE. Cross-sectional imaging of the liver. Baillières Clin Gastroenterol 1995; 9:97–120.

63. Cameron A. Left colon resection. Br J Hosp Med 1977; 17:281–9.

64. Phillips R, Hittinger R, Saunder V et al. Pre-operative urography in large bowel cancer: a useless investigation. Br J Surg 1983; 70:425–7.

65. Kettlewell MGW. Neoplasm: present surgical treatment. Curr Opin Gastroenterol 1988; 4:19–27.

66. Burton RM, Landreth KS, Barrows GH et al. Appearance, properties and origin of altered human haemoglobin in faeces. Lab Invest 1976; 35:111–15.

67. Robinson MHE, Thomas WM, Pye G et al. Is dietary restriction always necessary in Haemoccult screening for colorectal neoplasia? Eur J Surg Oncol 1993; 19:539–42.

68. Bennett DH, Hardcastle JD. Early diagnosis and screening. In: Williams NS (ed.) Colorectal cancer. Clinical surgery international, vol. 20. Edinburgh: Churchill Livingstone, 1996; pp. 21–37.

69. Mandel JS, Church TR, Ederer F, Bond JH. Colorectal cancer mortality: effectiveness of biennial screening for fecal occult blood. J Natl Cancer Inst 1999; 91:434–7.

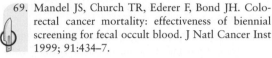

70. Hardcastle JD, Robinson MHE, Moss SM et al. Randomised controlled trial of faecal occult blood screening for colorectal cancer. Lancet 1996; 348:1472–7.

71. Kronborg O, Fenger C, Olsen J et al. A randomized study of screening for colorectal cancer with fecal occult blood test at Funen in Denmark. Lancet 1996; 348:1467–71.

These three randomised trials (69–71) provide evidence that disease-specific mortality can be reduced by faecal occult blood screening for colorectal cancer, and form the basis for current debates regarding the introduction of national screening programmes in several countries.

72. Kronborg O, Fenger C, Olsen J et al. Repeated screening for colorectal cancer with faecal occult blood test. Scand J Gastroenterol 1989; 24:599–606.

73. Wherry DC, Thomas WM. The yield of flexible fibreoptic sigmoidoscopy for the detection of asymptomatic colorectal neoplasia. Surg Endosc 1994; 8:393–5.

74. UK Flexible Sigmoidoscopy Screening Trial Investigators. Single flexible sigmoidoscopy screening to prevent colorectal cancer: baseline findings of a UK multicentre randomised trial. Lancet 2002; 359:1291–300.

75. Deuter R, Muller O. Detection of APC mutations in stool DNA of patients with colorectal cancer by HD-PCR. Hum Mutat 1998; 11:84–9.

76. Villa E, Dugani A, Rebecchi AM et al. Identification of subjects at risk for colorectal carcinoma through a test based on K-ras determination in the stool. Gastroenterology 1996; 110:1346–53.

77. Eguchi S, Kohara N, Komuta K, Kanematsu T. Mutations of the p53 gene in the stool of patients with resectable colorectal cancer. Cancer 1996; 77:1707–10.

78. Atkin WS, Saunders BP. Surveillance guidelines after removal of colorectal adenomatous polyps. Gut 2002; 51(suppl. v):v6–v9.

79. Gordon NML, Dawson AA, Bennett B et al. Outcome in colorectal adenocarcinoma: two seven-year studies of a population. Br Med J 1993; 307:707–10.

80. Berge T, Ekelund C, Mellner BP. Carcinoma of the colon and rectum in a defined population: an epi-

demiological, clinical and post-mortem investigation of colorectal cancer and co-existing benign polyps in Malmo. Acta Chir Scand 1973; 438:1–86.

81. Harrison S, Steele RJC, Johnston AK, Jones JA, Morris DL, Hardcastle JD. Predeposit autologous blood transfusion in patients with colorectal cancer: a feasibility study. Br J Surg 1992; 79:355–7.

82. Burrows L, Tartter P. Effect of blood transfusions on colonic malignancy recurrence rate. Lancet 1982; ii:662.

83. Bentzen SM, Balsev I, Pedersen M et al. Blood transfusion and prognosis in Dukes' B and C colorectal cancer. Eur J Cancer 1990; 26:457–63.

84. Busch ORC, Hop WCJ, Hoynck van Papendrecht MAW, Marquet RL, Jeekel J. Blood transfusions and prognosis in colorectal cancer. N Engl J Med 1993; 328:1372–6.

85. Takada H, Ambrose NS, Galbraith K et al. Quantitative appraisal of Picolax (sodium picosulphate/magnesium citrate) in the preparation of the large bowel for elective surgery. Dis Colon Rectum 1989; 33:679–83.

86. Ambrose NS, Hohnson M, Burdon DW, Keighley MRB. A physiological appraisal of polyethylene glycol and a balanced electrolyte solution as a bowel preparation. Br J Surg 1983; 70:428–30.

87. Downing R, Dorricott NJ, Keighley MRB et al. Whole gut irrigation: a survey of patient opinion. Br J Surg 1979; 66:201–2.

88. Irving AD, Scrimgeour D. Mechanical bowel preparation for colonic resection and anastomosis. Br J Surg 1987; 74:580–1.

89. Collins R, Scrimgeour A, Yusuf S, Peto R. Reduction in fatal pulmonary embolism and venous thrombosis by perioperative administration of subcutaneous heparin. N Engl J Med 1988; 318:1162–73.

This important meta-analysis established the use of low-dose subcutaneous heparin as a prophylactic measure in abdominal surgery.

90. Kakkar VV, Cohen AT, Edmonson RA et al. Low molecular weight versus standard heparin for prevention of venous thromboembolism after major abdominal surgery. Lancet 1993; 341:259–65.

91. Persson AV, Davis RJ, Villavicencio JL. Deep venous thrombosis and pulmonary embolism. Surg Clin North Am 1991; 71:1195–9.

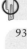

92. Keighley MRB. Sepsis and the use of antibiotic cover in colorectal surgery. In: Keighley MRB, Williams NS (eds) Surgery of the anus, rectum and colon. Philadelphia: WB Saunders, 1993; pp. 66–101.

93. Rowe-Jones DC, Peel ALG, Kingston RD, Shaw JFL, Teasdale C, Cole DS. Single dose cefotaxime plus metronidazole versus three dose cefotaxime plus metronidazole as prophylaxis against wound infection in colorectal surgery: multicentre prospective randomised study. Br Med J 1990; 300:18–22.

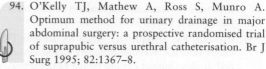

As a result of several trials, the place of prophylactic antibiotics in colorectal surgery is now firmly established, and the second of the above two publications (92, 93) provides important evidence that a single dose is as effective as multiple doses.

94. O'Kelly TJ, Mathew A, Ross S, Munro A. Optimum method for urinary drainage in major abdominal surgery: a prospective randomised trial of suprapubic versus urethral catheterisation. Br J Surg 1995; 82:1367–8.

95. Enker WE. Extent of operations for large bowel cancer. In: DeCosse JJ (ed.) Large bowel cancer. Clinical surgery international, vol. 1. Edinburgh: Churchill Livingstone, 1981; pp. 78–93.

96. Bouwman DL, Weaver DW. Colon cancer: surgical therapy. Gastroenterol Clin North Am 1988; 17:859–72.

97. Griffiths JD. Surgical anatomy of the blood supply of the distal colon. Ann R Coll Surg Engl 1956; 19:241–56.

98. Aldridge MC, Phillips RKS, Hittinger R, Fry JS, Fielding LP. Influence of tumour site on presentation, management and subsequent outcome in large bowel cancer. Br J Surg 1986; 73:663–70.

99. Blamey S, McDermott F, Pihl E et al. Ovarian involvement in adenocarcinoma of the colon and rectum. Surg Gynecol Obstet 1981; 153:42.

100. MacKeigan JM, Ferguson IA. Prophylactic oophorectomy and colorectal cancer in pre-menopausal patients. Dis Colon Rectum 1979; 22:401.

101. Turnbull RB, Kyle K, Watson FR, Spratt J. Cancer of the colon: the influence of the no-touch technique on survival rates. Ann Surg 1967; 166:420–7.

102. Wiggers T, Jeebel J, Arends JW et al. No-touch isolation technique in colon cancer: a controlled prospective trial. Br J Surg 1988; 75:409–15.

103. Matheson NA, McIntosh CA, Krukowski ZH. Continuing experience with single layer appositional anastomosis in the large bowel. Br J Surg 1985; 72:S104–S106.

These results have yet to be bettered, and form a persuasive argument for the use of the serosubmucosal anastomotic technique.

104. Carty NJ, Keating J, Campbell J, Karanjia N, Heald RJ. Prospective audit of an extramucosal technique for intestinal anastomosis. Br J Surg 1991; 78:1439–41.

105. Leslie A, Steele RJC. The interrupted serosubmucosal anastomosis: still the gold standard. Colorectal Dis 2003; 5:362–6.

106. Beart RW, Kelly KA. Randomised prospective evaluation of the EEA stapler for colorectal anastomoses. Am J Surg 1981; 141:143–7.

107. Brennan SS, Pickford IR, Evans M, Pollok AV. Staples or sutures for colonic anastomoses: a controlled clinical trial. Br J Surg 1982; 69:722–4.

108. Everett WG, Friend PJ, Forty J. Comparison of stapling and hand suture for left-sided large bowel anastomosis. Br J Surg 1986; 73:345–8.

109. McGinn FP, Gartell PC, Clifford PC, Brunton FJ. Staples or sutures for low colorectal anastomoses: a prospective randomised trial. Br J Surg 1985; 72:603–5.

110. West of Scotland and Highland Anastomosis Study Group. Stapling or suturing in gastrointestinal surgery: a prospective randomised study. Br J Surg 1991; 78:337–41.

111. Docherty JG, McGregor JR, Akyol AM et al. Comparison of manually constructed and stapled anastomoses in colorectal surgery. Ann Surg 1995; 221:176–84.

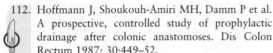
112. Hoffmann J, Shoukouh-Amiri MH, Damm P et al. A prospective, controlled study of prophylactic drainage after colonic anastomoses. Dis Colon Rectum 1987; 30:449–52.

113. Johnson CD, Lamont PM, Orr N, Lennox M. Is a drain necessary after colonic anastomosis? J R Soc Med 1989; 82:661–4.

114. Sagar PM, Couse N, Kerin M et al. Randomised trial of drainage of colorectal anastomosis. Br J Surg 1993; 80:769–71.

115. Olesen KL, Birth M, Bardram L, Burcharth F. Value of nasogastric tube after colo-rectal surgery. Acta Chir Scand 1984; 150:251–3.

116. Goligher JC, Graham NG, De Dombal FT et al. Anastomotic dihiscence after anterior resection or rectum and colon. Br J Surg 1970; 57:109–18.

117. Teoh TA, Wexner SD. Laparoscopic surgery in colorectal cancer. In: Williams NS (ed.) Colorectal cancer. Clinical surgery international, vol. 20. Edinburgh: Churchill Livingstone, 1996; pp. 103–21.

118. Southern Surgeons' Study Group. Handoscopic surgery: a prospective multicentre trial of a minimal invasive technique for complex abdominal surgery. Arch Surg 1999; 134:477–85.

119. Psaila J, Bulley SH, Ewings P et al. Outcome following laparoscopic resection for colorectal cancer. Br J Surg 1998; 85:662–4.

120. Hughes SE, McDermott FT, Proligase AI, Johnson WR. Tumour recurrence in abdominal wall scar after large bowel cancer surgery. Dis Colon Rectum 1983; 26:571–2.

121. Guillou PJ. Laparoscopic surgery for diseases of the colon and rectum: quo vadis? Surg Endosc 1994; 8:669–71.

The results of the MRC trial of laparoscopic surgery for colorectal cancer may have an important effect on attitudes to this approach.

122. Lacy AM, Garcia-Valdecasas JC, Delgado S et al. Laparoscopy-assisted colectomy versus open colectomy for treatment of non-metastatic colon cancer: a randomised trial. Lancet 2002; 359:2224–9.

123. Koruth NM, Koruth A, Matheson NA. The place of contrast enema in the management of large bowel obstruction. J R Coll Surg Edinb 1985; 30:258–60.

124. Rothenberger DA, Mayoral J, Deen K. Obstruction and perforation. In: Williams NS (ed.) Colorectal cancer. Clinical surgery international, vol. 20. Edinburgh: Churchill Livingstone, 1996; pp. 123–33.

125. Koruth NM, Krukowski ZH, Youngson GG et al. Intra-operative colonic irrigation in the management of left-sided large bowel emergencies. Br J Surg 1985; 72:708–11.

126. SCOTIA Study Group. Single-state treatment for malignant left-sided colonic obstruction: a prospective randomised trial comparing subtotal colectomy with segmental resection following intraoperative irrigation. Br J Surg 1996; 82:1622–7.

One of the few randomised trials of surgical technique in emergency colonic surgery, this study indicates that segmental resection of obstructed colon cancer provides better long-term results than subtotal colectomy.

127. Dudley HAF, Radcliffe AG, McGeehan D. Intra-operative irrigation of the colon to permit primary anastomosis. Br J Surg 1980; 67:80.

128. Mainar A, De Gregorio Ariza MA, Tejero E et al. Acute colorectal obstruction: treatment with self-expandable metallic stents before scheduled surgery. Results of a multicenter study. Radiology 1999; 10:65–9.

129. Barr LC, Skene AI, Meirion Thomas J. Metastasectomy. Br J Surg 1992; 79:1268–74.

130. Geoghegan JG, Scheele J. Treatment of liver metastases. Br J Surg 1999; 86:158–69.

This article provides a state-of-the-art review of optimum treatment of liver metastases and examines developments in neoadjuvant therapy.

131. Hughes KS for the Registry of Hepatic Metastases. Resection of the liver for colorectal cancer metastases: a multi-institutional study of indications for resection. Surgery 1988; 103:278–88.

132. Babineau TJ, Steele G. Treatment of colorectal liver metastases. In: Williams NS (ed.) Colorectal cancer. Clinical surgery international, vol. 20. Edinburgh: Churchill Livingstone, 1996; pp.173–83.

133. Bismuth H, Castaing D, Traynor O. Surgery for synchronous hepatic metastases of colorectal cancer. Scand J Gastroenterol Suppl 1988; 149:144–9.

134. Yoon SS, Tanabe KK. Surgical treatment and other regional treatments for colorectal cancer liver metastases. Oncologist 1999; 4:197–208.

135. Pahlman L. Surveillance and recurrence. In: Williams NS (ed.) Colorectal cancer. Clinical surgery international, vol. 20. Edinburgh: Churchill Livingstone, 1996; pp. 159–72.

136. Meta-analysis group in cancer. Efficacy of intravenous infusion of fluorouracil compared with bolus administration in advanced colorectal cancer. J Clin Oncol 1998; 16:301–8.

137. Cunningham D, Pyrhonen S, James RD et al. Randomised trial of irinotecan and supportive care after fluorouracil failure for patients with metastatic colorectal cancer. Lancet 1998; 352:1413–18.

This trial provides evidence for the effectiveness of a new chemotherapeutic agent in colorectal cancer.

138. Salz LB, Cox JV, Blanke C et al. Irinotecan plus fluorouracil and leucovorin for metastatic colorectal cancer. Irinotecan Study Group. N Engl J Med 2000; 343:905–14.

139. Doullard JY, Cunningham D, Roth AD et al. Irinotecan combined with fluorouracil compared with fluorouracil alone as first-line treatment for metastatic colorectal cancer: a multicentre randomised trial. Lancet 2000; 355:1041–7.

140. Hamantas A, Rotstein LE, Langer B. Regional versus systemic chemotherapy in the treatment of colorectal carcinoma metastatic to the liver. Is there a survival difference? Meta-analysis of the published literature. Cancer 1996; 78:1639–45.

141. Halvorsen TB, Seim E. Degree of differentiation in colorectal adenocarcinomas: a multivariate analysis of the influence on survival. J Clin Pathol 1988; 41:532–7.

142. Shepherd NA, Baxter KJ, Love SB. Influence of local peritoneal involvement on pelvic recurrence and prognosis in rectal cancer. J Clin Pathol 1995; 48:849–55.

143. Talbot IC, Ritchie S, Leighton M, Hughes AO, Bussey HJR, Morson BC. Invasion of veins by carcinoma of the rectum: method of detection, histological features and significance. Histopathology 1981; 5:141–63.

144. Dukes CE, Bussey HJR. The spread of rectal cancer and its effect on prognosis. Br J Cancer 1958; 12:309–20.

145. Jass JR, Love SB, Northover JMA. A new prognostic classification of rectal cancer. Lancet 1987; i:1303–6.

146. Hawley PR. Treatment of carcinoma of the colon. In: Goligher JC (ed.) Surgery of the anus, rectum and colon, 4th edn. London: Baillière Tindall, 1984; p. 549.

147. Association of Coloproctology of Great Britain and Ireland. Guidelines for the management of colorectal cancer. London: ACPGBI, 2001.

148. Scottish Intercollegiate Guidelines Network. Guidelines for the management of colorectal cancer. Edinburgh: SIGN, 2003.

Four
Rectal cancer

Robin K.S. Phillips

INTRODUCTION

From a surgeon's perspective, the rectum begins where the two antemesenteric taenia on the sigmoid colon fuse together. This is roughly at the level of the sacral promontory and may be some 15 cm from the anus.

Rectal cancer at presentation is either truly local (or locoregional) or has spread elsewhere, usually to the liver. Preoperative scanning and intraoperative palpation may not always demonstrate small occult metastases within the liver substance but, if present, they will be responsible for death over the next 5 years.[1]

ROLE OF PATHOLOGY

Histopathological examination of the resected specimen simply allows an estimate of any occult hepatic metastases already present in the liver at the time of apparently curative resection, the chance increasing with depth of primary tumour penetration, grade and lymph node status.

The depth of primary tumour penetration can be gauged very accurately by endoanal ultrasound,[2] but intra- and interobserver variation[3] and variation within the tumour[4] make estimation of grade inexact. Thus a preoperative biopsy may reveal a rectal cancer that is not obviously poorly differ-entiated and yet examination of the subsequently resected whole specimen may show unsuspected areas of poor differentiation within the tumour.

It is not possible to combine the information on depth of primary tumour penetration and on grade and thereby make the information on lymph node status redundant. This is important, as depth and grade (subject to the caveat raised above) can be assessed preoperatively much more accurately than lymph node status. Nevertheless, lymph node status remains central to all rectal cancer staging systems (TNM,[5] Dukes,[6] Jass[7]).

OBJECTIVES OF RECTAL CANCER SURGERY

A tumour that is truly local will be cured by adequate locoregional therapy; inadequate loco-regional therapy will lead to local recurrence. A tumour that has already spread to the liver will be incurable by surgical means alone. It does not matter whether abdominoperineal excision of the rectum is performed, or indeed an anterior resection, the occult hepatic metastases will still kill the patient. Similarly, in the presence of occult hepatic metastases, it does not matter whether preoperative or postoperative radiotherapy is used, or no radio-therapy, the patient will still die.

From time to time it is stated that preoperative radiotherapy can 'downstage' the primary tumour, but one must be very careful in interpreting this downstaging. The original histology provides an estimate of the likelihood of occult hepatic metastases already present in the liver at the time of resection; the application of radiotherapy makes no difference to this original estimate, even if it makes the primary tumour smaller (or makes it go away completely) and lymph nodes disappear. Thus one must be very cautious about estimating likely outcome based on the histopathological examination of a resected pre-irradiated rectal cancer. This is because there is no useful yardstick by which to measure the likelihood of occult hepatic metastases based on the pathology of irradiated rectal cancer specimens.

From the above discussion, it can be seen that longer term survival is in many ways outside the control of the rectal cancer surgeon, being dependent on the presence or absence of occult hepatic metastases at the time of presentation. However, the surgeon can control (i) death in hospital, (ii) local recurrence and (iii) quality of life.

DEATH IN HOSPITAL

Death in hospital involves patient factors, tumour factors and surgeon-related factors. Clearly, in an elderly patient with an obstructing tumour the risks of death are much higher than in a younger patient undergoing elective surgery. Elective surgery under the age of 80 years has an overall in-hospital mortality of 8% compared with a 16% mortality in those over the age of 80. An elderly patient over the age of 80 years with malignant large bowel obstruction has a 1 in 3 chance of in-hospital mortality.[8] Similarly, the in-hospital mortality in the presence of an anastomotic leak is much higher than when there has been no leak.[9]

There is thus enormous scope for a skilled surgeon to make a very great difference to in-hospital outcome in patients with rectal cancer. Anastomotic leak rate is a surgeon-related variable. The organisation of a dedicated daytime operating list for the treatment of urgent cases by a senior team has now largely been achieved. From time to time the decision to adopt a local approach, for example local excision, transanal endoscopic microsurgery (TEM) or even local radiotherapy, will be influenced

by knowledge of the likely cost benefit of the alternative (local excision of a tumour confined to the rectal wall has an approximately 15% chance of leaving involved lymph nodes behind compared with an approximate 16% mortality for radical surgery in those aged over 80).

LOCAL RECURRENCE

Local recurrence arises for one of the following reasons.

1. The primary tumour was disrupted in some way at the time of the original operation.
2. Local excision was inadequate.
3. Viable exfoliated cells have implanted into the wound/tumour bed/port site/anastomosis.

Tumour disruption

Clearly, cutting into a primary tumour while mobilising it will run a very high risk of spilling viable cancer cells. The occasions when this may happen in rectal cancer surgery include the following.

1. When an adherent loop of intestine is thought to be stuck onto the tumour by 'inflammatory' adhesions. The loop should be resected en bloc with the primary tumour rather than pinched off.[10]
2. Through fragmentation of the envelope of the mesorectum. Heald has done more than anyone else to popularise the importance of maintaining the integrity of the mesorectal envelope.[11,12] It has been claimed that rough traction, blunt dissection and less-than-total mesorectal excision contribute to disruption of the mesorectal envelope, which on removal will look ragged and shredded. Precise surgery using sharp or diathermy dissection under vision will avoid this problem.
3. Injudicious exploration of the anterior plane in a man with an anterior encroaching tumour.

ANTERIOR ENCROACHING TUMOUR IN THE MALE

Rectal cancer rarely penetrates through Denonvillier's fascia to involve the seminal vesicles, prostate or base of bladder. However, all surgeons have experience of cases where this has proved to be the case. The problem does not really arise in women, as the vagina acts as a barrier to involvement of the bladder, and surgeons are used to performing en-bloc hysterectomy when the uterus/back of the vagina is involved.

 Specialised imaging using magnetic resonance (MRI) has transformed the preoperative evaluation of rectal cancer in the UK.

In the best hands,[13,14] exquisite images can be obtained that clearly show the mesorectal envelope and which allow assessment of the circumferential resection margin (**Fig. 4.1**). Whereas endoanal ultrasound permits local evaluation of depth and may help predict cases suited to local excision, MRI examines the margin and helps the clinician choose those most likely to benefit from preoperative chemo-irradiation or those males with anterior encroachment sufficient to warrant primary exenteration. In the past, surgeons largely encountered the problem of anterior encroachment unexpectedly during the operation. Given surgeons' natural reluctance to embark unnecessarily on synchronous en-bloc removal of the bladder with construction of an ileal conduit, the fairly modest results of such extensive surgery[15] and the lack of confidence of many surgeons in their own skills in this area, the natural response was to remain in the normal anterior dissection plane, hoping that the tumour and the seminal vesicles could be shaved off the back of the prostate/bladder.

This situation should no longer arise if a standard preoperative work-up (**Box 4.1**) for all cases of rectal cancer includes first-class MRI. For the now hopefully rare occasion when a surgeon is confronted by such a conundrum, it would be wise to pause and take stock. Would it be better to back out, give a course of radiotherapy and then return

Box 4.1 • Standard preoperative work-up for rectal cancer

- Full blood count, electrolytes, liver function tests
- Serum carcinoembryonic antigen (optional)
- Group and save serum
- Colonoscopy
- MRI
- Transrectal ultrasound (if considering local therapy)
- Chest radiography
- Liver ultrasound
- Preoperative discussion at multidisciplinary team meeting

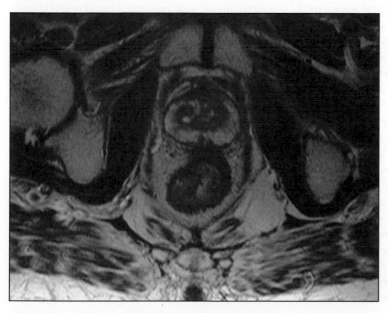

Figure 4.1 • An anterior tumour invading into the prostate can clearly be seen.

at a later date, when hopefully tumour shrinkage may allow an uninvolved plane to be found? (In these circumstances, a wait of 3 months would be advised; see below.) Is the patient young enough and fit enough to be considered for pelvic exenteration? Such an operation should be preceded in all cases by chemoradiotherapy and performed by a joint colorectal surgical and urological surgical team.

Inadequate local excision

How radical does the pelvic clearance need to be in a standard case of rectal cancer? The issues to be addressed here are total mesorectal excision, extended pelvic lymphadenectomy[16,17] and high vs. low vascular ligation (with or without a pre-aortic strip).[18,19] In addition, the role of local excision needs to be considered.

TOTAL MESORECTAL EXCISION

The history of gastric cancer surgery included a vigorous debate on whether total excision of the stomach should always be done or whether it should be undertaken only when it was essential.[20] The debate was summarised as total *gastrectomie de principale* vs. total *gastrectomie de necessitaire*. The debate on total mesorectal excision is identical in its content, the two views being (i) total mesorectal excision should be used but only in certain circumstances and (ii) total mesorectal excision should always be used in all cases of rectal cancer. Few surgeons would now doubt the advisability of performing total mesorectal excision when operating on a case of low or mid-rectal cancer. The debate is focused on upper rectal cancer.

First, there is a lack of clear cancer-related evidence when dealing with upper rectal cancer. Heald has shown that in some cases satellite deposits of cancer, not always in lymph nodes, may be present in the mesorectum distal to the lower palpable margin of the tumour.[11] Does this apply to cases of cancer of the upper rectum? How often? And how far below the lower palpable border of the tumour can some of these deposits be found? The answers to these questions are not very clear from reading the literature. One recent study suggests that extension in the mesorectum may be as much as 3 cm

below the distal margin of the tumour,[21] whereas Heald described them extending as far as 4 cm below.[11] Extrapolating from these figures, it would seem reasonable in oncological terms to perform a mesorectal clearance 5 cm below the tumour, which in an upper rectal cancer would not always involve total mesorectal excision.

It might be argued that the good results of total mesorectal excision make these questions redundant but, in practice, function in the absence of a small colonic pouch (see below) or a short rectal remnant[22] is inferior when total mesorectal excision is performed, and complications are high,[23] making a temporary stoma advisable in all cases.

Thus, given this background, there are many surgeons who, when confronted with an upper rectal cancer, would perform a less-than-total mesorectal excision. Nevertheless, they would all perform quite an extensive distal clearance of mesentery, of the order of at least 5 cm, thereby making their anastomosis effectively somewhere in the region of the junction of the mid and lower thirds of the rectum.

EXTENDED PELVIC LYMPHADENECTOMY

There seems little doubt, at least in the Japanese literature, that lymph nodes are involved in cases of rectal cancer along the internal iliac vessels. These involved lymph nodes lie outside the boundaries of a conventional total mesorectal excision and should, on the face of it, be responsible for local recurrence in cases where they have not been removed.

As an example, one Japanese paper has shown these lymph nodes to be involved in 18% of cases overall and in 36% of Dukes' C cases. In addition, in 6% of cases lateral pelvic side-wall lymph nodes were the only lymph nodes involved. That is to say, if an extended pelvic side-wall lymphadenectomy had not been performed, these cases would have been considered Dukes' A or B.[17] Based on this evidence, the biological rate of local recurrence for total mesorectal excision should be around 18%, not the 3–5% claimed by its protagonists. What are the possible explanations for these discrepancies?

First, the Japanese literature does not make it clear whether the majority of these involved lymph nodes are along the main trunk of the internal iliac vessels (where they would indeed be left behind by total mesorectal excision) or whether they are in fact in the vicinity of the lateral ligaments, where conceivably they would be removed as part of a total mesorectal excision anyway.

Second, post-mortem studies have clearly identified instances of local recurrence in terminal cases not identified in life as they caused no clinical problem.[24] Thus a patient dying with disseminated disease may have undetected recurrence in the pelvic side-wall lymph nodes: the clinical rate of local recurrence will inevitably be quite a lot smaller than the biological rate. Perhaps where the tumour burden is excessive and the patient is doomed anyway, pelvic side-wall lymph nodes may be involved, but their removal in these circumstances will add nothing to the patient's cancer-related outcome.

Third, there is the charge of selection. Perhaps the cases operated upon by those with a low local recurrence rate are not representative of those seen by the rest of us. My own view is to reject this as anything but a most marginal explanation. There is growing evidence that surgeons who have adopted total mesorectal excision have significantly reduced their local recurrence rates; and independent review of Heald's cases does not support selection as a reasonable explanation for his very good results.[12]

Extended pelvic lymphadenectomy is unlikely to become popular in the West, largely because of the poor functional result and because of the perceived success of total mesorectal excision. Half the cases reported in one series had the operation performed unnecessarily, as they did not have any lymph nodes involved at all. Operating times were lengthy, averaging 5.5 hours, and blood loss was excessive (average 1.5 L). All patients had sexual and urinary disturbance, 10% needing a permanent urinary catheter.[17]

Nerve-sparing operations are being developed that combine the potential advantages of an extended lymph node dissection with less collateral nerve damage.[25] Nevertheless, the excellent results of total mesorectal excision make it unlikely that they will ever become popular.

HIGH VS. LOW VASCULAR LIGATION

The inferior mesenteric artery can be divided either flush on the aorta (high ligation) or at the level of the sacral promontory, in effect preserving the left colic artery (low ligation). There have been quite a number of studies that have compared these two approaches in terms of cancer survival and have found no benefit to high ligation.[18,26]

About 20% of cases with apical lymph node involvement will be cured. Presumably, had they had a ligation that left the involved apical lymph node behind, they would all have died. A possible explanation for a lack of benefit in studies of high ligation is that the operation was not simultaneously extended in a lateral direction, i.e. lateral pelvic side-wall lymphadenectomy was not also performed at the same time. Presumably, cases with extensive lymph node involvement in one plane will also have extensive lymph node involvement in another, so leaving one set of lymph nodes untreated while solely concentrating on the treatment of the other is unlikely to show benefit.

When performing an anastomosis to the anus it has generally been the view that the descending colon should be used in preference to the sigmoid colon. Not only does the sigmoid colon generate fairly high pressures, which could therefore lead to relatively poor function, but more importantly the marginal artery is absent in the sigmoid colon, which is thus prone to ischaemia if it is used for anastomosis. However, the descending colon will not reach the anus unless the splenic flexure is mobilised in all cases, and there is a flush tie of the inferior mesenteric artery on the aorta. This is because the left colic artery is too short and will not permit the descending colon to reach the anus if a low ligation that preserves the left colic artery is performed. Hence a low anastomosis will always need a high ligation, but for technical rather than cancer-specific reasons. A high anastomosis can be achieved quite easily with either a high or a low ligation.

An international randomised controlled trial comparing colonic pouches with straight coloanal anastomoses employed the sigmoid colon in 42% of cases and these showed no functional or complication disadvantage.[27] It would seem that the earlier favouring of descending colon for anastomosis can now be tempered by issues of practicality: where the splenic flexure is easy to mobilise, then it would still seem appropriate to do so and use descending colon; but with a high and difficult splenic flexure, sigmoid colon might be the best choice, avoiding a difficult mobilisation.

BLOOD SUPPLY AT THE SPLENIC FLEXURE

There is one other point of importance when preparing the left colon for anastomosis, and that is to do with the precariousness of the marginal artery blood supply in the region of the splenic flexure (Griffiths' point).[28] Between the terminal two branches of the left colic artery the marginal artery can be quite thin (**Fig. 4.2**). It is important when mobilising the blood supply at the splenic flexure to preserve these two branches to act as a support for the marginal artery at this point.

ROLE OF LOCAL EXCISION

A tumour confined to the bowel wall has an approximately 15–20% chance of lymph node involvement,[29,30] whereas a tumour penetrating through the full thickness of the bowel wall has an approximately 40% chance. In addition, a well-differentiated tumour has about a 25% chance of having lymph node involvement, whereas a poorly differentiated tumour has a greater than 50% chance. Thus a well-differentiated tumour, confined to the bowel wall, would have a reasonably low prospect of lymph node involvement.

An analysis of 151 malignant polyps showed that pedunculated polyps had no risk of lymph node involvement when the degree of spread was limited to the head, neck or stalk of the polyp, but was 27% when invasion reached the base of the polyp (however, numbers were small, 3 of 11 having lymph node involvement). Patients with sessile polyps had a 10% chance of lymph node invasion.[31]

A small (say <3 cm in diameter) low rectal cancer, which on biopsy was well differentiated, would be a potential candidate for local excision, whether by TEM or by a conventional transanal approach. As

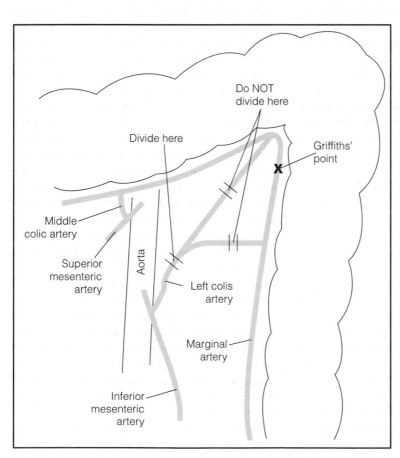

Figure 4.2 • When mobilising the vascular supply to the splenic flexure, it is important not to divide the two terminal branches of the left colic artery, but rather to leave them supporting the marginal artery at the splenic flexure, where it can be deficient, and instead divide the main trunk of the left colic artery as indicated. Frequently, the inferior mesenteric vein also needs to be divided again at the inferior border of the pancreas to gain further length.

mentioned earlier, the preoperative biopsy may not be truly representative of the histology of the whole tumour once it has been excised, but this has to be accepted.

Assessment of depth of primary tumour penetration with the examining finger is notoriously unreliable. Rectal endosonography is extremely accurate[2] but not all surgeons have ready access to the technique. The alternative is simply to treat the excised specimen as a large biopsy and allow the pathologist to report on the depth of primary tumour penetration and the completeness of excision, as well as commenting finally on the tumour grade. Using this approach, the surgeon can then decide, based on the full histology report, either to continue with a policy of local excision or to advise the patient that further more radical surgery is advisable.

The updated results of local excision from St Mark's Hospital have been reported. Of 152 patients with tumours confined to the bowel wall, 11% died of cancer.[32] Against this background, it would be hard to advise a young and fit patient to have local excision. However, in the elderly and less fit there does still seem to be a place for this technique. Furthermore, local excision does not require a pelvic dissection, with all its attendant risks to erection, ejaculation and bladder function. Bowel function is also significantly better afterwards than with a straight coloanal anastomosis. For these reasons there will still be some younger patients who, while adequately informed, may nevertheless prefer to avoid conventional surgery and opt for local excision, however performed. This issue has recently been addressed using decision analysis, paying particular attention to comparison between abdominoperineal excision and local excision.[33] As expert colorectal surgeons are more likely than general surgeons to have a choice between sphincter-preserving local excision and sphincter-preserving radical surgery,[34] the conclusion in favour of local excision for early low rectal cancer may not be so applicable to them.

Local excision as practised in the UK has not usually been followed by the application of postoperative radiotherapy, unlike in France[35] and the USA,[36] or sometimes chemoradiotherapy.[37] This is because surgeons have been concerned that any metastases in lymph nodes are unlikely to be eradicated by radiotherapy and because function in an irradiated rectum may become suboptimal, thereby obviating one of the specific advantages of a local approach. Finally, detection of recurrence in an irradiated pelvis may be more difficult than in the absence of postoperative radiotherapy, making the potential for salvage in the presence of recurrence less likely. Nevertheless, although radiotherapy in general will certainly make function worse,[38] it does reduce failure.[36] Its role may apply particularly to the higher risk surgical patient.[39]

Implantation of viable tumour cells

The role of implantation remains controversial. On the one hand, there is clear experimental evidence that colorectal cancer cells are shed into the lumen of the bowel, that they are viable and that they represent clones of cells capable of transplanting.[40] On the other hand, most North American surgeons ignore the risk when operating conventionally, and all surgeons ignore the risk (in fact, they cannot avoid it) when performing any form of transanal local excision, whether conventionally or by TEM.

Not only are viable colorectal cancer cells present in the lumen of the bowel, where presumably they may give rise to anastomotic recurrence if left untreated, but they are also able to cross an otherwise watertight anastomosis, where they potentially might result in the much more common locoregional recurrence.[41,42] In the test tube, colorectal cancer cells are effectively killed by povidone iodine, mercuric perchloride and chlorhexidine/cetrimide. Other agents such as water are not effective.[43] However, blood makes povidone iodine and chlorhexidine/cetrimide much less efficient at killing colorectal cancer cells.[44]

Most British surgeons would strongly recommend steps to prevent implantation. The use of tapes both proximally and distally, as advocated by Cole,[45] is no longer advised, but a right-angled clamp should be placed across the bowel just distal to the tumour and the bowel then washed out below the clamp. This means that unprotected cross-stapling below a low rectal cancer is considered inadvisable in the UK. Instead, a right-angled clamp should be introduced first and cross-stapling should be done beyond the clamp, after a cytocidal washout.

However, there are circumstances where it is simply not possible to place a right-angled clamp distal to a rectal cancer and then to manage to place a cross-stapling instrument below that. What should the surgeon then do? There are also some circumstances where a tongue of tumour extends down towards the dentate line, when transanal division of the bowel and internal sphincter at this level would permit an otherwise impossible restorative operation to be done (**Fig. 4.3**), but only if a clamp is not used below the tumour.

Some surgeons would argue that a restorative operation should not be attempted in these circumstances, and argue in favour of abdominoperineal excision. Others would argue that, in the first example, a right-angled clamp should be applied and the anus washed out below the clamp, before the gut tube is then divided either from above or from below and an endoanal coloanal anastomosis constructed.

However, there are occasions when a restorative operation is technically possible but the application of a distal clamp and washout below this clamp would not be possible. In these circumstances, I (and others[46]) think it reasonable to continue with a restorative operation, although cytocidal agents should be instilled after specimen removal and before anastomosis. Thus the use of a distal clamp with washout below it is in my view relative and not absolute. In support of the relative rather than absolute nature of this choice is the very obvious advantage of a restorative operation as against a permanent stoma, the fact that there are many surgeons, particularly in the USA, who think the risk of implantation metastases has been exaggerated, and the fact that British surgeons, who have vehemently argued in favour of protecting the anastomotic line from exposure to viable tumour cells, have still been prepared in certain circumstances to entertain local excision, where all these potential risks apply.

QUALITY OF LIFE

In rectal cancer surgery quality of life issues include preservation of continence, preservation of reasonable bowel frequency and avoidance, as far as possible, of permanent sexual and urinary disturbance.

Preservation of continence

The reasons for abdominoperineal excision include the following.

1. Cancer involves the sphincter or is so near to it that attempts to preserve it are unjustified.

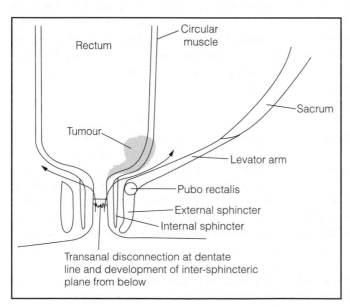

Figure 4.3 • A fairly small, well-differentiated tumour close to the anus may have a superficial extension into the upper anal canal. Transanal full-thickness division of the anus and underlying internal sphincter at the level of the dentate line permits entry to the intersphincteric space and may assist completion of an ultra-low attempt at restorative surgery. However, in these circumstances it is impossible both to gain the necessary anal access and to use a right-angled clamp below the tumour with a cytocidal washout below that.

2. The functional result of restorative surgery is likely to be so poor that a colostomy would be an advantage.

3. The potential complications of attempts to restore intestinal continuity are not worth risking, particularly in the frail and elderly.

DISTAL CLEARANCE MARGIN

It is not always clear from an examination of the literature what is meant by the distal margin. A distance of 5 cm at rigid sigmoidoscopy in the living may expand to 8 cm after rectal mobilisation, then shrink to 3 cm after specimen removal, simply because of contraction of the longitudinal muscle. If an attempt is then made to pin out the specimen, a margin of 4.5 cm may be achieved after fixation, but without pinning out the final margin may measure only 2 cm.[47]

Against this background, it is very uncommon for rectal cancer to spread more than 1.5 cm below the distal palpable margin of the tumour, and then only when the tumour is poorly differentiated, when distances as far as 4.5 cm have rarely been reported.[48] Of course, the preoperative biopsy may not accurately represent the final tumour histology, but given this caveat it is usually advised that a 5 cm distal clearance margin should still be considered for a poorly differentiated tumour, whereas a 2 cm margin should suffice otherwise.

In practice, the distal margin is now largely irrelevant for most rectal cancer, as the amount of bowel removed is determined more by a policy of performing total mesorectal excision than it is by considering the distal clearance margin. Nevertheless, the issue does apply when considering cancer in the lower third of the rectum, where it has been argued that, given a tumour that is not poorly differentiated, being able to apply a right-angled clamp below the lower margin of the tumour is clearance enough.[49]

From time to time, the histology report will describe the tumour abutting the distal margin (i.e. being within 1 cm or less of the margin) but not involving it. Studies of resected specimens have shown that so long as the margin itself is uninvolved then the risk of recurrence is not increased,[49,50] provided that adequate lateral clearance has been achieved. There is a tendency for the inexperienced surgeon to cone in on the distal clearance margin, thereby leaving some of the mesorectum behind on the pelvic side walls. This practice is considered likely to increase the chance of local recurrence and should therefore be avoided.[51]

TUMOUR HEIGHT

It has been commonplace to advise measuring the height of the lower border of the tumour from the anal verge. I have always been puzzled by this advice, as the anal verge is often a variable point, for example being much further from the dentate line (in my view the critical point) in patients with a funnel anus.

In fact the dentate line can be felt with the examining finger. The mucosa above is more slippery to the examining finger than is the skin of the pecten (just as the mucosa of the inside of the mouth is more slippery than the skin of the lip). This difference in slipperiness can be appreciated with the examining finger, which allows a much more meaningful relationship of the lower border of the tumour to be assessed.

What actually matters in the critical case is not the measured height of the lower border of the tumour to the dentate line, but rather whether in the case in question there is a sufficient margin either for a clamp to be placed below the tumour and above the dentate line or for the dentate line to be divided transanally (see **Fig. 4.3**) without going too close to any palpably indurated tongue of tumour projecting downwards towards the dentate line. Added to this is a general assessment of the bulk of the tumour, the accessibility of the pelvis, the quality of the anus, and the potential for improving tumour characteristics by the application of preoperative radiotherapy.

QUALITY OF THE ANUS

A woman with a prior history of multiple vaginal deliveries, particularly if there has been a forceps delivery or a complication of episiotomy, has a fairly high chance of an occult sphincter injury, detectable by anal ultrasonography.[52] In practice, one is usually guided to the quality of a good anus by a history of flatus continence and an absence of episodes of faecal incontinence in the past. In more recent times the tumour itself may have contributed to a sense of urgency and thereby may lead to unreasonable pessimism as to the true state of the anus.

Nevertheless, a patient with an undoubtedly poor-quality anus will not be well served by an ultra-low anastomosis and would be very much better off with a colostomy. When the tumour itself is reasonably high in the rectum, then a low Hartmann's operation will avoid the complications of a perineal wound, but with a lower tumour an abdominoperineal excision would seem safest.

ABDOMINOPERINEAL EXCISION OF THE RECTUM

Even in the best hands abdominoperineal excision gives worse results than perhaps it should. Surgeons familiar with deep pelvic dissection and total mesorectal excision are now far less familiar with the bottom end of an abdominoperineal excision, particularly in the male. The scope for technical error is high as there is no clear anatomical plane from below, except anteriorly, where it is difficult. When performing total mesorectal excision the rectosacral fascia should be divided in order to dissect the rectum anteriorly, thereby exposing the anal canal, whereas this may compromise the lateral clearance margin when performing abdominoperineal excision. Pathologists report 'coning' or 'waisting' of the specimen at the level of the levators.

To some extent this is to be expected, as any cut voluntary muscle will contract and naturally give some impression of 'coning', but it is probable that surgeons are not excising the pelvic floor widely enough. Unless tumour is in the distal anal canal, when there will be a threat of inguinal lymphatic spread, wide excision of ischiorectal fat is probably unnecessary, although it is important to excise widely at the level of the pelvic floor, particularly as this is the point where any cancer is likely to be situated (if it were not, then total mesorectal excision would likely be feasible). It is possible that the more modern tendency of not routinely excising the coccyx at the time of abdominoperineal excision for cancer lessens the muscle clearance and should be reconsidered.

Whatever the technical issues, it is my practice now to offer preoperative radiotherapy to all patients scheduled for abdominoperineal excision, regardless of their tumour stage.

THE COLONIC POUCH

Straight coloanal anastomosis results in fairly poor function, certainly for a number of months and on occasion for a year or two. In a study of 84 cases treated at St Mark's Hospital by proctectomy with endoanal coloanal anastomosis, 8% went on to have a permanent colostomy constructed.[53]

A colonic pouch does not have the same objective as an ileal pouch. The consistency of the stool is different, the harder stool being much more difficult to expel than the semiliquid content of an ileal pouch. Early colonic pouches tended to copy ileal pouches in having a large capacity, but all the early authors had patients who had difficulty evacuating.[54-56] As experience has been gained, so the size of colonic pouches has fallen, now being recommended to be around 5–8 cm in length.[57-59]

There have been a number of reports that have confirmed that early function with a colonic pouch is superior to a straight coloanal anastomosis.[54-60] This is particularly important in elderly patients, in those with a slightly compromised anus and in those with a relatively short life expectancy.

The more difficult group to evaluate is the young. This is because the results of a straight coloanal anastomosis improve quite markedly with time, and nobody knows to what extent colonic pouches will dilate and decompensate over time. We do not know whether good function in the first few years might be followed by increasing problems with evacuation later as colonic pouches become floppy and dilated.

One recent argument in favour of the routine use of a colonic pouch is the possible lower anastomotic leak rate from side-to-end rather than end-to-end anastomosis in these circumstances.[27] Should this suggestion be borne out, it will prove a strong argument in favour of the routine use of a small colonic pouch in all cases after total mesorectal excision. The study in question found a clinical anastomotic leak in 15% of patients having a straight coloanal anastomosis and in only 2% with a pouch ($P = 0.03$). However, radiotherapy had been used more frequently (27% vs. 16%) and a covering stoma less frequently (59% vs. 71%). As radiotherapy may be damaging to anastomotic healing, and as a stoma protects against the clinical manifestations of an anastomotic leak, the question of safer anastomoses when a colonic pouch is constructed remains undecided.

Recently, an alternative has been to use a coloplasty instead of a colon pouch. An 8–10 cm incision is made, which is 4–6 cm proximal to the divided end of the colon, vertically along the antemesenteric border of the colon. The incision is then closed transversely,[61] forming the pouch. End-to-end coloanal anastomosis is then performed.

Sexual and urinary disturbance

The presacral nerves give rise to ejaculation in the male. They lie like a wishbone, joined at the sacral promontory and parting as they run distally on either pelvic side wall.[62] They can be identified at the start of the posterior dissection and preserved in most cases.

Erection in the male is innervated through the nervi erigentes. These nerves lie anterolaterally in the angle between the seminal vesicles and the prostate. Control of bleeding in this area may be followed by erectile failure subsequently, even when only unilateral damage has occurred.[63] With a posteriorly situated tumour early division of Denonvillier's fascia will protect the nerves, but in an anteriorly placed tumour it is important to remove as much Denonvillier's fascia as possible, as it acts as a barrier to tumour penetration, and it is in these circumstances that the nerves are at risk of damage.[64]

Patients should be warned that urinary and sexual difficulties may follow rectal excision, whether for benign or malignant disease.[65]

Temporary stomas

Anastomotic leakage after ultra-low anastomosis is regrettably quite common, occurring in 10–20% of cases.[23] One can either take the view that an elective stoma would be a burden to the 80–90% of patients unlikely to develop a leak or one can consider that the risks to health and subsequent function from an unprotected anastomotic leak are such that a stoma should be employed in all cases. I favour the latter argument.

The choice then lies between using a loop transverse colostomy or a loop ileostomy. The right upper quadrant is a poor place for siting a stoma, but it is a simple matter to mobilise the hepatic flexure and place a transverse loop colostomy in the right iliac fossa. However, even if this is done, a transverse loop colostomy is a bulky stoma that is prone to prolapse.

In many ways a loop ileostomy after rectal cancer surgery is a better stoma to have. After ileal pouch surgery for inflammatory bowel disease or familial adenomatous polyposis, the small bowel mesentery is pulled taut across the posterior abdominal wall to allow the ileal pouch to reach the anus. Thus it is often difficult to get a loop of small bowel to reach the anterior abdominal wall, making a loop ileostomy in these circumstances at times a pretty poor stoma to experience.

The situation when using a loop ileostomy to defunction a distal colonic anastomosis is entirely different. There is no difficulty in achieving a tension-free spout as the small bowel is freely mobile within the peritoneal cavity. However, a loop ileostomy can be a more difficult stoma to close than a loop transverse colostomy.

In my view, the point that swings the whole debate in favour of a loop ileostomy relates to the blood supply of the distal colon. After coloanal anastomosis, effectively a sine qua non of total mesorectal excision, a high vascular ligation is necessary in order for the descending colon to reach the anus. This means that the blood supply of the distal colon is from the middle colic artery via the marginal artery. The marginal artery is potentially at risk when a loop transverse colostomy is closed, particularly if the colostomy is resected at the time of closure. Any damage would lead to ischaemic necrosis of the distal colon, an avoidable complication if a loop ileostomy is used as a routine.

ROLE OF RADIOTHERAPY

This issue is covered in more detail in Chapter 5. Nevertheless, it is important to distinguish between radiotherapy as an adjuvant and radiotherapy as a treatment.

Radiotherapy as an adjuvant is taken to mean radiotherapy applied to a freely mobile tumour that could easily be removed technically without any radiotherapy. When using preoperative radiotherapy in these circumstances, there need be no delay between finishing the course of radiotherapy and embarking on surgery. When confronted by a fixed or tethered tumour, preoperative radiotherapy may allow tumour shrinkage and thus permit the tumour to be excised, but it will of course have no effect on the way the original stage of the tumour predicted the possibility of occult hepatic metastases, and therefore incurability. All it will do is from time to time permit local therapy that might otherwise prove technically impossible.

In these circumstances where radiotherapy is used as a treatment, it is important to leave a sufficient interval between the radiotherapy and the attempted surgery that will maximise any tumour shrinkage. This period is of the order of 2–3 months, when tumour shrinkage is beginning to be balanced by continuing tumour growth of resistant cells. An interval of only 1 month may deny the potential opportunity of tumour excision in some patients.

The lowest rates of local recurrence reported in the literature have come from surgeons who have not employed any radiotherapy. Indeed, although randomised trials have shown a significant reduction in local recurrence rates, these trials have been conducted against an unacceptably high rate of local recurrence in the control arms.[12]

> The Dutch total mesorectal excision radiotherapy trial has ostensibly addressed the question of whether routinely applied preoperative radiotherapy is an advantage when employing total mesorectal excision.[66] At first glance the case seems well established: at 2 years the radiotherapy group reported a 2.4% rate of local recurrence, statistically significantly better than the 8.2% for surgery alone. However, local recurrence rates have been shown to be constant until 4.5 years from surgery,[10] so the anticipated local recurrence rate at 5 years in the surgery-alone group may be of the order of 15%, far higher than that reported by others for total mesorectal excision alone. If one then takes into account the 108 different hospitals taking part, that only 77% of eligible cases ended up with tumour-free margins without tumour spillage, and that only 65% of cases actually had a low anterior resection (as opposed to abdominoperineal excision or Hartmann's operation), then the assertion that this was a trial of the application of radiotherapy to high-quality total mesorectal excision becomes somewhat suspect.

FOLLOW-UP

There are three issues that need to be considered during follow-up.

1. Was a synchronous tumour overlooked preoperatively?

2. How should metachronous tumours be looked for?

3. Is there any value at all to follow-up of this cancer?

Synchronous tumours

There is about a 3% chance of a synchronous cancer at the time of the original resection. Of these synchronous cancers, only about 10% are likely to be so small that they would be difficult to feel during a careful laparotomy. Perhaps 1 in 3 of these small and difficult-to-feel tumours might be amenable to removal at colonoscopy using a snare. Preoperative barium enema or colonoscopy is thus seeking to identify these 2 in 1000 cases where the original surgical management might have involved a more extensive or even an additional resection.

The problem is that preoperative investigation is often incomplete and may also be inaccurate. An obstructing tumour in the rectum may make proximal visualisation impossible. Even where it is possible to attempt complete colonic examination, preparation may be poor, thereby masking in particular any smaller synchronous tumours, or colonoscopy may be less than total. Against this background, intraoperative colonoscopy has been attempted. One study showed that even this was inaccurate, missing lesions as large as 2 cm detected at postoperative colonoscopy 3 months later.[67]

For all these reasons, postoperative colonoscopy at about 3 months after resection (and anyway within the first year) will start follow-up with the knowledge that the remaining colon does not already harbour an overlooked polyp or cancer.

Metachronous tumours

The risk of a metachronous tumour is again about 3%, although it will be higher in cases where there is a family history. It would seem sensible to screen the colon at intervals by colonoscopy, perhaps every 3 years in cases where there have been prior polyps and every 5 years otherwise. As any screening examination should 'protect' for about 5 years, a final screen at the age of 75 should protect the patient until at least the age of 80 years, when the risks of routine surveillance colonoscopy will start to outweigh any benefit. Nevertheless, such an approach has never been shown to be worthwhile and many colonoscopies will need to be performed for a very small return.

Surveillance for local and distant recurrence

Surgeons are divided between those who feel follow-up is worthwhile, if only for the emotional health of the patient and to allow an accurate and long-term audit to be kept, and those who are not so convinced.

Before the advent of safe liver resection, the issue of intensive vs. symptomatic follow-up was addressed in a number of studies that failed to show any real benefit for intensive follow-up.[68,69] More recently, a randomised trial of intensive follow-up using monthly carcinoembryonic antigen (CEA) monitoring failed to show any survival benefit to those screened, although it did show a lead time in the diagnosis of recurrence of about 1 year in those screened with CEA. The problem was that this average of 1-year lead time did not translate into lives saved by reoperative surgery (J.M.A. Northover, personal communication). CEA monitoring may yet allow patients with recurrence to be treated earlier with chemotherapy, and this may itself lead to longer survival.

From an examination of first principles, it would seem unlikely that pelvic recurrence after a properly conducted total mesorectal excision would be amenable to reoperative surgery anyway. After all, what is there left to remove that was not removed originally at the time of the first operation? Clearly, anastomotic recurrence might be treated by salvage abdominoperineal excision, but true anastomotic recurrence is rare. Furthermore, anastomotic recurrence, particularly after rectal cancer surgery, is likely to present with symptoms that would make screening for it largely unnecessary.

Sometimes after restorative surgery for a very low rectal cancer there may be recurrence on the lateral pelvic side wall, for example in obturator lymph nodes. Salvage abdominoperineal excision may be technically possible with removal of these lymph nodes, but overall salvage surgery for local recurrence has disappointing results, most patients still ultimately dying from their cancer.[70]

This really leaves the issue of the liver as the only area where follow-up might be beneficial. The problem is that even here it is not known whether regular screening will identify the particular sorts of liver recurrence amenable to curative resection, or whether these more biologically favourable tumours might not present symptomatically, regardless of screening.

The natural history of even solitary hepatic metastases will see a few survivors untreated at 5 years, but probably no more than 16%.[71] The results of liver resection are substantially better, with a low operative mortality[72] and around 40% living for 5 years.[73] Despite this, many surgeons remain unconvinced of the value of regular ultrasound examination of the liver during follow-up. Perhaps, by recognising that chemotherapy for advanced unresectable disease improves quality of life and is more effective when applied early, more surgeons will undertake regular liver surveillance after colorectal cancer surgery.

Against this background, two recent meta-analyses of all randomised trials of follow-up have shown improved survival for those followed-up intensively.[74–76] To address this important question the FACS (Follow-up After Colorectal Surgery) trial has been launched.

• **Key points**

- Most fit patients with rectal cancer should have total mesorectal excision.
- Endorectal ultrasound assesses the advisability of local excision by gauging invasive depth and thus the chance of occult lymph node involvement.
- MRI assesses the circumferential margin and helps decide whether preoperative chemoradiotherapy is worthwhile and whether pelvic exenteration in a young male with an anterior tumour is called for.
- The Dutch trial of total mesorectal excision with and without radiotherapy supports radiotherapy. However, there are still doubts as to whether the surgical standard, although better than in the past, was really good enough.
- After decades of doubt about the value of intensive follow-up, meta-analysis suggests benefit, spawning the FACS trial.

REFERENCES

1. Finlay IG, Meek DR, Gray HW, Duncan JG, McArdle CS. The incidence and detection of occult hepatic metastases in colorectal carcinoma. Br Med J 1982; 284:803–5.

2. Beynon J, Foy DMA, Roe AM, Temple LN, Mortensen NJMcC. Endoluminal ultrasound in the assessment of local invasion in rectal cancer. Br J Surg 1986; 73:474–7.

3. Blenkinsopp WK, Stewart-Brown S, Blesovsky L, Kearney G, Fielding LP. Histopathology reporting in large bowel cancer. J Clin Pathol 1981; 34:509–13.

4. Williams NS, Durdey P, Quirke P et al. Preoperative staging of rectal neoplasm and its impact on clinical management. Br J Surg 1985; 72:868–74.

5. Wood DA, Robbins GF, Zippin C, Lum D, Stearns MW. Staging cancer of the colon and rectum. Cancer 1979; 43:961–8.

6. Dukes CE. The classification of cancer of the rectum. J Pathol Bacteriol 1932; 35:323–32.

7. Jass JR, Love SB, Northover JMA. A new prognostic classification of rectal cancer. Lancet 1987; i:1303–6.

8. Fielding LP, Phillips RKS, Fry JS, Hittinger R. Prediction of outcome after curative surgery for large bowel cancer. Lancet 1986; ii:904–6.

9. Fielding LP, Stewart-Brown S, Blesovsky L, Kearney G. Anastomotic integrity after operations for large bowel cancer: a multicentre study. Br Med J 1980; 281:411–14.

10. Phillips RKS, Hittinger R, Blesovsky L, Fry JS, Fielding LP. Local recurrence after 'curative' surgery for large bowel cancer. 1. The overall picture. Br J Surg 1984; 71:12–16.

11. Heald RJ, Husband EM, Ryall D. The mesorectum in rectal cancer surgery: the clue to recurrence? Br J Surg 1982; 69:613–16.

12. McFarlane JK, Ryall RD, Heald RJ. Mesorectal excision for rectal cancer. Lancet 1993; i:457–60.

13. Brown G, Richards CJ, Newcombe RG et al. Rectal carcinoma: thin-section MR imaging for staging in 28 patients. Radiology 1999; 211:215–22.

14. Beets-Tan RG, Beets GL, Vliegen RF et al. Accuracy of magnetic resonance imaging in prediction of tumour-free resection margin in rectal cancer surgery. Lancet 2001; 357:497–504.

15. Shirouzu K, Isomoto H, Kakegawa T. Total pelvic exenteration for locally advanced colorectal carcinoma. Br J Surg 1996; 83:32–5.

16. Enker WE, Philipshen SJ, Heilwell ML et al. En bloc pelvic lymphadenectomy and sphincter preservation in the surgical management of rectal cancer. Ann Surg 1986; 293:426–33.

17. Moriya Y, Hojo K, Sawada T, Doyama Y. Significance of lateral node dissection for advanced rectal carcinoma at or below the peritoneal reflection. Dis Colon Rectum 1989; 32:307–15.

18. Surtees P, Ritchie J, Phillips RKS. High versus low ligation of the inferior mesenteric artery in rectal cancer. Br J Surg 1990; 77:618–21.

19. Corder AP, Karanjia ND, Williams JD, Heald RJ. Flush aortic tie versus selective preservation of the ascending left colic artery in low anterior resection for rectal carcinoma. Br J Surg 1992; 79:680–2.

20. Longmire WP. Gastric carcinoma: is radical gastrectomy worthwhile? Ann R Coll Surg Engl 1980; 62:25–30.

21. Scott N, Jackson P, Al-Jaberi T, Dixon MF, Quirke P, Finan PJ. Total mesorectal excision and local recurrence: a study of tumour spread in the mesorectum distal to rectal cancer. Br J Surg 1995; 82:1031–3.

22. Karanjia ND, Schache DJ, Heald RJ. Function of the distal rectum after low anterior resection for carcinoma. Br J Surg 1992; 79:114–16.

23. Karanjia ND, Corder AP, Bearn P, Heald RJ. Leakage from stapled low anastomosis after total mesorectal excision for carcinoma of the rectum. Br J Surg 1994; 81:1224–6.

24. Gilbert JM, Jeffrey I, Evans M, Kark AE. Sites of recurrent tumour after 'curative' colorectal surgery: implications for adjuvant therapy. Br J Surg 1984; 71:203–5.

25. Hojo K, Vernava AM, Sugihara K, Katumata K. Preservation of urine voiding and sexual function after rectal cancer surgery. Dis Colon Rectum 1991; 34:532–9.

26. Pezim MF, Nicholls RJ. Survival after high and low ligation of the inferior mesenteric artery during curative surgery for rectal cancer. Ann Surg 1984; 200:729–33.

27. Hallbook O, Paholman L, Krog M, Wexner SD, Sjodahl R. Randomized comparison of straight and colonic J pouch anastomosis after low rectal excision. Ann Surg 1996; 224:58–65.

28. Griffiths JD. Surgical anatomy of the blood supply of the distal colon. Ann R Coll Surg Engl 1956; 19:241–56.

29. Coverlizza S, Risio M, Ferrari A, Fenoglio-Preiser CM, Rossini FP. Colorectal adenomas containing invasive carcinoma: pathologic assessment of lymph node metastatic potential. Cancer 1989; 64:1937–47.

30. Huddy SP, Husband EM, Cook MG, Gibbs NM, Marks CG, Heald RJ. Lymph node metastases in early rectal cancer. Br J Surg 1993; 80:1457–8.

31. Nivatvongs S, Rojanasakul A, Reiman H et al. The risk of lymph node metastasis in colorectal polyps

with invasive adenocarcinoma. Dis Colon Rectum 1991; 34:323–8.

32. Lock MR, Ritchie JK, Hawley PR. Reappraisal of radical local excision for carcinoma of the rectum. Br J Surg 1993; 80:928–9.

33. Temple LFF, Naimark D, McLeod RS. Decision analysis as an aid to determining the management of early low rectal cancer for the individual patients. J Clin Oncol 1999; 17: 312–18.

34. Porter GA, Soshkolne CL, Yakimets WW, Newman SC. Surgeon-related factors and outcome in rectal cancer. Ann Surg 1998; 227:157–67.

35. Rouanet P, Saint Aubert B, Fabre JM et al. Conservative treatment for low rectal carcinoma by local excision with or without radiotherapy. Br J Surg 1993; 80:1452–6.

36. Chakravarti A, Compton CC, Shellito PC et al. Long term follow-up of patients with rectal cancer managed by local excision with and without adjuvant irradiation. Ann Surg 1999; 230:49–54.

37. Wagman R, Minsky BD, Cohen AM, Saltz L, Paty PB, Guillem JG. Conservative management of rectal cancer with local excision and postoperative adjuvant therapy. Int J Radiat Oncol Biol Phys 1999; 44:841–6.

38. Dahlberg M, Glimelius B, Graf W, Pahlman L. Preoperative irradiation affects functional results after surgery for rectal cancer. Results from a randomised study. Dis Colon Rectum 1998; 41:543–51.

39. Hershman MJ, Sun Myint A, Makin CA. Multimodality approach in curative local treatment of early rectal carcinomas. Colorectal Dis 2003; 5:445–50.

40. Umpleby HC, Fermor B, Symes MO, Williamson RCN. Viability of exfoliated colorectal carcinoma cells. Br J Surg 1984; 71:659–63.

41. O'Dwyer PJ, Martin EW. Viable intraluminal tumour cells and local/regional tumour growth in experimental cancer. Ann R Coll Surg Engl 1989; 71:54–6.

42. Leather AJM, Yiu CY, Baker LA, Boulos PB, Northover JMA, Phillips RKS. Passage of shed intraluminal colorectal cancer cells across a sealed anastomosis. Br J Surg 1991; 78:756.

43. Umpleby HC, Williamson RCN. The efficacy of agents employed to prevent anastomotic recurrence in colorectal carcinoma. Ann R Coll Surg Engl 1984; 66:192–4.

44. Docherty JG, McGregor JR, Purdie CA, Galloway DJ, O'Dwyer PJ. Efficacy of tumouricidal agents in vitro and in vivo. Br J Surg 1995; 82:1050–2.

45. Cole WH. Recurrence in carcinoma of the colon and proximal rectum following resection for carcinoma. Arch Surg 1952; 65:264–70.

46. Tiret E, Poupardin B, McNamara D, Debini N, Parc R. Ultralow anterior resection with intersphincteric dissection: what is the limit of safe sphincter preservation? Colorectal Dis 2003; 5:454–7.

47. Phillips RKS. Adequate distal margin of resection for adenocarcinoma of the rectum. World J Surg 1992; 16:463–6.

48. Williams NS, Dixon M, Johnston D. Reappraisal of the 5cm rule of distal excision for carcinoma of the rectum: a study of distal intramural spread and of patients' survival. Br J Surg 1983; 70:150–4.

49. Karanjia ND, Schache DJ, North WRS, Heald RJ. 'Close shave' in anterior resection. Br J Surg 1990; 77:510–12.

50. Phillips RKS, Hittinger R, Blesovsky L, Fry JS, Fielding LP. Local recurrence after 'curative' surgery for large bowel cancer. 2. The rectum and rectosigmoid. Br J Surg 1984; 71:17–20.

51. Quirke P, Durdey P, Dixon MF, Williams NS. Local recurrence of rectal adenocarcinoma due to inadequate surgical resection. Lancet 1986; ii:996–9.

52. Sultan AH, Kamm MA, Hudson CN, Bartram CI. Anal sphincter disruption during vaginal delivery. N Engl J Med 1993; 329:1905–11.

53. Sweeney JL, Ritchie JK, Hawley PR. Resection and sutured peranal anastomosis for carcinoma of the rectum. Dis Colon Rectum 1989; 32:103–6.

54. Lazorthes F, Fages P, Chiotasso P, Lemozy J, Bloom E. Resection of the rectum with construction of a colonic reservoir and colo-anal anastomosis for carcinoma of the rectum. Br J Surg 1986; 73:136–8.

55. Parc C, Tiret E, Frileux P, Moszkowski E, Loygue J. Resection and colo-anal anastomosis with colonic reservoir for rectal carcinoma. Br J Surg 1986; 73:139–41.

56. Nicholls RJ, Lubowski DZ, Donaldson DR. Comparison of colonic reservoir and straight colo-anal reconstruction after rectal excision. Br J Surg 1988; 75:318–20.

57. Seow-Choen F, Goh HS. Prospective randomised trial comparing J colonic pouch–anal anastomosis and straight coloanal reconstruction. Br J Surg 1995; 82:608–10.

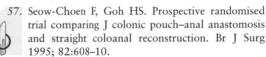

One of a number of randomised controlled trials showing the benefits of colonic pouch reconstruction.

58. Ho YH, Tan M, Seow-Choen F. Prospective randomized controlled study of clinical function and anorectal physiology after low anterior resection: comparison of straight and colonic J pouch anastomosis. Br J Surg 1996; 83:978–80.

59. Seow-Choen F. Colonic pouches in the treatment of low rectal cancer. Br J Surg 1996; 83:881–2.

60. Mortensen NJM, Ramirez JM, Takeuchi N, Smiglin Humphreys MM. Colonic J pouch–anal anastomosis

after rectal excision for carcinoma: functional outcome. Br J Surg 1995; 82:611–13.

61. Fazio VW, Mantyh CR, Hull TL. Colonic 'coloplasty'. Novel technique to enhance low colorectal or coloanal anastomosis. Dis Colon Rectum 2000; 43:1448–50.

62. Havenga K, De Ruiter MC, Enker WE, Welvaart K. Anatomical basis of autonomic nerve-preserving total mesorectal excision for rectal cancer. Br J Surg 1996; 83:384–8.

63. Heald RJ. Total mesorectal excision is optimal surgery for rectal cancer: a Scandinavian consensus. Br J Surg 1995; 82:1297–9.

64. Heald RJ, Moran BJ, Brown G, Daniels IR. Optimal total mesorectal excision for rectal cancer is by dissection in front of Denonvilliers' fascia. Br J Surg 2004; 91:121–3.

65. Banerjee AK. Sexual dysfunction after surgery for rectal cancer. Lancet 1999; 353:1900–1.

66. Kapiteijn E, Marijnen CAM, Nagtegaal ID et al. Preoperative radiotherapy combined with total mesorectal excision for resectable rectal cancer. N Engl J Med 2001; 345:638–46.

On the face of it, a most important trial showing radiotherapy improves results of even total mesorectal excision. Let down by increasing concerns of how good the total mesorectal excision really was.

67. Finan PJ, Donaldson DR, Allen-Mersh T, Northover J, Hawley PR, Williams CB. Experience with perioperative colonoscopy in patients with primary colorectal cancer. Gut 1988; 29:A730.

68. Cochrane JPS, Williams JT, Faber RG, Slack WW. Value of outpatient follow-up after curative surgery for carcinoma of the large bowel. Br Med J 1980; 280:593–5.

69. Tornquist A, Ekelund G, Leandder L. The value of intensive follow-up after curative resection for colorectal carcinoma. Br J Surg 1982; 69:725–8.

These two early studies (68, 69) cast major doubts on the value of intensive follow-up.

70. Gagliardi G, Hawley PR, Hershman MJ, Arnott SJ. Prognostic factors in surgery for local recurrence of rectal cancer. Br J Surg 1995; 82:1401–5.

71. Greenway B. Hepatic metastases from colorectal cancer: resection or not. Br J Surg 1988; 75:513–19.

72. Rees M, Plant G, Wells J, Bygrave S. One hundred and fifty hepatic resections: evolution of technique towards bloodless surgery. Br J Surg 1996; 83:1526–9.

73. Sugihara K, Hojo K, Moriya Y, Yamasaki S, Kosuge T, Takayama T. Patterns of recurrence after hepatic resection for colorectal metastases. Br J Surg 1993; 80:1032–5.

74. Renehan AG, Egger M, Saunders MP, O'Dwyer ST. Impact on survival of intensive follow-up after curative resection for colorectal cancer: systematic review and meta-analysis of randomised trials. Br Med J 2002; 324:813.

This meta-analysis has readdressed the value of intensive follow-up and finds significant benefit. The FACS trial should help decide this issue.

75. Jeffrey GM, Hickey BE, Hider P. Follow-up strategies for patients treated for non-metastatic colorectal cancer. Cochrane Library, Issue 1. Oxford: Update Software, 2002.

76. Renehan AG, O'Dwyer ST, Whynes DK. Cost effectiveness analysis of intensive versus conventional follow-up after curative resection for colorectal cancer. Br Med J 2004; 328:81–4.

CHAPTER
Five
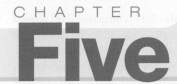

Adjuvant therapy for colorectal cancer

Paul Hatfield and
David Sebag-Montefiore

INTRODUCTION

At present, only chemotherapy and radiotherapy have an established role as adjuvant treatment for colorectal cancer. They are given, either before or after definitive surgical treatment, to specific groups of patients in an attempt to improve the outcome of the group as a whole. As with other adjuvant treatments in cancer, the majority of patients receiving the treatment will not actually benefit, either because surgery alone would be curative or because the disease will ultimately relapse despite the additional treatment. The policy is justified, however, because in a common cancer, with a significant rate of relapse, small improvements in absolute survival translate into many hundreds or thousands of lives saved. Nevertheless, large numbers of patients who ultimately will not benefit are exposed to the toxicity and inconvenience of additional treatment. Unfortunately, despite a large research effort, accurate methods of prospectively identifying those patients who will benefit are not currently available. When counselling individual patients it is important to outline some of these uncertainties, and to carefully evaluate any comorbid factors, which may increase the risks of treatment.

CHEMOTHERAPY

Chemotherapy based on 5-fluorouracil (5FU) is widely used as an adjuvant treatment in stage III colon cancer. This is based on a considerable body of published evidence from the last 15–20 years. Many uncertainties remain, however, such as the optimum regimen, the benefit of adding other chemotherapeutic agents, the best route of administration and the role of chemotherapy in stage II disease. The current international standard is 6 months of 5FU and folinic acid (FA). A number of different regimens are used, based on the results of clinical trials, including the Mayo Clinic regimen that is given on five consecutive days every month. However, in the UK, weekly bolus treatment is also widely practised and appears less toxic based on the result of a very large non-randomised comparison within a British study.[1] Overall, adjuvant chemotherapy appears to confer a 5–10% improvement in absolute survival.[2]

The largest evidence base exists in patients with colon cancer and its applicability to patients with rectal cancer remains controversial. Nonetheless, in routine clinical practice, it is common to use the same criteria to select patients irrespective of the primary site within the large bowel.

Why 5FU?

Various trials performed prior to 1990 attempted to show a benefit with adjuvant chemotherapy in colon cancer. Many included 5FU, which had a long history in metastatic colorectal cancer dating back to the 1950s.[3] However, a meta-analysis of 25 such studies in 1988 failed to show any significant survival benefit,[4] although the overall quality of studies was poor.

In 1989 and 1990 two important studies were published which changed the situation.[5,6] These large randomised trials clearly showed a survival benefit for 12 months of 5FU plus levamisole over observation alone. The results from INT-0035[6] were updated in 1995,[7] with similar results. The US National Institutes of Health therefore recommended this combination strategy in stage III colon cancer patients.[8]

Levamisole is an antihelmintic with various immunostimulatory properties. This led to the hypothesis that its use would enhance the efficacy of 5FU, although its mechanism of action remained unclear and there was little evidence for an effect when used as a single agent. Nevertheless, it was for this reason that trials from this period tested the role of levamisole combined with 5FU. Subsequently,

other studies (Table 5.1) compared 5FU-based regimens with observation alone[9–12] and showed an absolute improvement in survival of nearly 10%. Many of these used 5FU with FA, which potentiates the action of 5FU on its target enzyme thymidylate synthase. A meta-analysis in 1992 had shown this combination to have an increased effect in metastatic disease.[13]

Which 5FU-based regimen?

Important questions that then arose included the following.

1. Is 12 months necessary or would a shorter course be equivalent?
2. Is FA modulation better than levamisole?
3. Should FA and levamisole be given together?
4. What dose of FA is necessary?

Several trials (Table 5.2) addressed these issues using 12 months of 5FU/levamisole as a control.[14–18] In summary, these trials concluded that 6 months of chemotherapy with 5FU/FA was equivalent to 12 months of 5FU/levamisole, and superior to 6 months of 5FU/levamisole. Furthermore, combining 5FU/FA with levamisole gave no extra benefit.

Table 5.1 • Randomised trials of adjuvant 5-fluorouracil-based chemotherapy vs. observation following surgical resection in colon cancer since 1989

Study	N	Stage	Chemotherapy	5-year survival (%)		P
				Chemotherapy	Control	
NSABP C-01[9]	1166	II/III	MOF 12 months	67	60	0.005
Laurie et al.[5]	401	II/III	5FU/LEV 12 months	55	42	0.03*
INT-0035[7]	929	II/III	5FU/LEV 12 months	60	47	0.007*
Francini et al.[10]	239	II/III	5FU/FA 12 months	79	65	0.0044
IMPACT 1[11†]	1526	II/III	5FU/FA 6 months	83‡	78‡	0.029
O'Connell et al.[12]	309	II/III	5FU/FA 6 months	74	63	0.02

*Results for stage III only.
†Pooled results of three studies.
‡3-year survival.
FA, folinic acid; 5FU, 5-fluorouracil; IMPACT, International Multicentre Pooled Analysis of Colon Cancer Trials; INT, Intergroup; LEV, levamisole; MOF, semustine, vincristine, 5FU; NSABP, National Surgical Adjuvant Breast and Bowel Project.

Table 5.2 • Randomised trials of adjuvant chemotherapy in colon cancer comparing combinations of 5-fluorouracil and folinic acid with or without levamisole with 12-months of 5-fluorouracil/levamisole as a control

Study	N	Stage	Control arm	Experimental arm(s)
INT 89-46-51[14]	891	II/III	5FU/LEV 12 months	5FU/LEV 6 months 5FU/LEV/FA 6 months* 5FU/LEV/FA 12 months*
INT 0089[15]	3759	II/III	5FU/LEV 12 months	5FU/LDFA 6 months* 5FU/HDFA 7 months† 5FU/LDFA/LEV 6 months*
NSABP C-04[16]	2151	II/III	5FU/LEV 12 months	5FU/HDFA 11 months† 5FU/HDFA/LEV 11 months†
AdjCCA-01[17]	680	III	5FU/LEV 12 months	5FU/FA 12 months‡
FOGT-1[18]	813	II/III	5FU/LEV 12 months	5FU/FA/LEV 12 months 5FU/LEV/IFN 12 months

*5FU/FA given on five consecutive days and repeated every 4–5 weeks; FA dose 20 mg/m^2.
†5FU/HDFA given weekly for 6 of 8 weeks; FA dose 500 mg/m^2.
‡5FU/FA given on five consecutive days and repeated every 4 weeks; FA dose 100 mg/m^2.
FA, folinic acid; FOGT, Forschungsgruppe Onkologie Gastrointestinaler Tumoren; 5FU, 5-fluorouracil; HDFA, high-dose FA; IFN, interferon; INT, Intergroup; LDFA, low-dose FA; LEV, levamisole; NSABP, National Surgical Adjuvant Bowel Project.

The Quick and Simple and Reliable (QUASAR) study[1] compared high- and low-dose FA with or without levamisole. Nearly 5000 patients were recruited and no significant difference was shown between groups, suggesting that levamisole is not necessary and that low-dose FA provides adequate modulation of 5FU. In this study patients were given chemotherapy either as a weekly bolus or for five consecutive days every 4 weeks. Although not randomly allocated, the weekly schedule appeared much less toxic, with equivalent efficacy. This very large trial encouraged widespread adoption of the weekly regimen in the UK.

Toxicity

5FU can cause a number of adverse effects, such as fatigue, nausea, vomiting, diarrhoea, stomatitis, plantar–palmar erythema, epistaxis and sore eyes. Alopecia and significant myelosuppression are uncommon. The severity and site specificity of the adverse effects are dependent on the regimen used. A rare complication is angina, which may be related to coronary artery spasm and is commoner in those receiving continuous infusions of 5FU. This does not necessarily occur in patients with known coronary artery disease, although there is some evidence that this slightly increases the risk.[19]

A small proportion of people are deficient for the enzyme dihydropyrimidine dehydrogenase, which is important in metabolising 5FU. Such individuals will be otherwise healthy but have extremely severe and early toxicity with standard doses of 5FU. When such toxicity is observed, it is normally within the first 2–3 weeks of treatment and patients usually experience severe manifestations of all the listed adverse effects. Such cases require emergency admission to the oncology centre.

Although most of these toxicities can be controlled symptomatically or by reducing the dose by around 50% after recovery from toxicity, each patient clearly needs to be evaluated carefully before embarking on further treatment.

Patient selection

While the decision to treat a fit, fully informed patient with stage III disease is relatively straightforward, more difficult scenarios can arise. For instance, most trials have not included elderly patients and yet such patients form the majority of patients in clinic. What evidence there is seems to suggest that the magnitude of benefit in the elderly is the same as in younger patients,[20,21] but clearly this is a decision that needs to be individualised.

Another area of considerable debate is the role of chemotherapy in stage II colorectal cancer. Such patients already have a reasonable prognosis and very large studies are required to detect the likely size of any benefit from chemotherapy. Eight trials with mature follow-up have been published addressing this issue, of which five were combined to form the International Multicentre Pooled Analysis of Colon Cancer Trials (IMPACT) B2 study.[9,10,22,23] When combined, the benefit seen with adjuvant treatment in these trials is only 1.5% and this does not reach statistical significance.[2] However, other studies have been contradictory[24,25] and the controversy continues. It is known that some stage II tumours have a worse prognosis, such as those presenting with perforation, obstruction, extramural vascular invasion, peritoneal involvement or poorly differentiated histology.[26–31] Many clinicians would offer such patients adjuvant chemotherapy, on the basis that their absolute risk of relapse is higher and therefore the likely benefit is greater. However, there is little hard evidence for this practice and this should be reflected in the discussion with such patients in clinic.

Many patients are referred for chemotherapy with a defunctioning stoma after resection of the primary. Despite their obvious desire to have stoma reversal as soon as possible, this is commonly deferred till after chemotherapy. This is to allow chemotherapy to commence as soon as possible after surgery, as most of the clinical trials have required chemotherapy to commence within 6–8 weeks of surgery. The evidence base for benefit is much less clear if chemotherapy is commenced at a later time or if chemotherapy is interrupted to allow reversal.

Can current treatments be improved?

There are three ways that treatments could be improved. Firstly, patients could derive the same benefit with less toxicity and inconvenience. Secondly, the overall results could be improved by the integration of an additional agent or strategy with acceptable levels of toxicity. Finally, a way of avoiding overtreatment of patients who do not benefit could be discovered. Various possibilities exist for each of these.

INCREASING TOLERABILITY

Current treatment extends over 6 months and can adversely affect quality of life. A recent study has suggested that a 12-week course of infusional 5FU may be as effective as standard treatment with less toxicity.[32] A further approach would be the use of oral fluoropyrimidines, such as capecitabine, avoiding the need for indwelling venous access. Capecitabine is not currently licensed for adjuvant therapy but phase III trials in this setting have been completed and the results are awaited to determine whether capecitabine is equivalent to intravenous 5FU/FA with acceptable toxicity.

IMPROVING RESULTS

In metastatic disease the combination of irinotecan or oxaliplatin with 5FU/FA has been shown to improve various outcome measures, although usually with increased toxicity.[33,34] Several studies using such combinations in the adjuvant setting have completed recruitment and results can be expected in the near future.

Given that colorectal cancer commonly recurs in the liver, there has been considerable interest over the years in the role of infusional chemotherapy given directly into the portal circulation. Theoretically, this could maximise the dose at the site of greatest risk and reduce systemic toxicity. However, a large recent trial (AXIS)[35] has shown only marginal benefit to a 7-day portal infusion of 5FU postoperatively, and given the superiority of systemic therapy this is unlikely to change current practice.

Another approach would be to utilise our increasing knowledge of the molecular biology of colorectal cancer with targeted biological therapies. Theoretically, these could avoid the toxicity of classical cytotoxics and hopefully improve outcome. However, despite much progress in this field no such approach has yet shown proven benefit in the adjuvant setting.

BETTER TARGETING

Various molecular markers have been examined as potential predictive factors for response to adjuvant treatment. Examples include thymidylate synthase (the target enzyme of 5FU), the *DCC* (deleted in colorectal cancer) gene, microsatellite instability, as well as markers of angiogenesis or cellular proliferation. Others have performed sensitive assays for the detection of micrometastases to try to identify high-risk individuals. However, none of these strategies is sufficiently accurate to use in clinical practice at the present time.

RADIOTHERAPY

There has been a considerable effort over the last three decades to investigate the role of radiation in rectal cancer. Until the mid-1990s, randomised controlled trials included a standard arm of surgery alone.

 Today, however, there is unequivocal evidence that adjuvant radiation reduces the risk of local recurrence in resectable rectal cancer, outlined in two recent overviews.[36,37]

There is less certainty about whether there is a benefit in overall survival. Preoperative radiotherapy seems more effective than postoperative radiotherapy of higher or similar biological equivalent dose (a parameter that models the effect of total dose and fraction size). Current controversy relates to the sequence with respect to surgery, the choice of radiation schedule and the benefits of concurrent chemotherapy. At the same time there have also been important improvements in pelvic preoperative imaging, surgical technique and histopathological analysis of the resected specimen that will require further randomised trials in order to refine the role of radiation in this new era.

When prescribing radiotherapy the clinician seeks to define a volume of tissue within the patient and deliver a therapeutic dose of radiation to it. At the same time, surrounding normal tissues are spared as much as possible to reduce both acute and chronic complications.

Toxicity is related to treatment volume, total dose, fraction size (the dose given on each day of treatment), treatment time, beam energy and technique. It can also be increased by other factors such as comorbid conditions (e.g. diabetes mellitus, hypertension, connective tissue diseases or inflammatory bowel disease), prior surgery or the use of concurrent chemotherapy. In colorectal cancer, adjuvant radiotherapy tends to be confined to the pelvis because the large volumes of small bowel elsewhere in the abdomen and the difficulty of defining a suitable target volume generally preclude its use. Even in the pelvis every effort is given to minimising the treatment volume and avoiding structures such as the anal sphincter or pelvic bones where possible (**Fig. 5.1**).

Indications

There are three main indications for adjuvant radiation in rectal cancer. The greatest interest has focused on reducing the risk of local recurrence in patients with resectable rectal cancer. The second

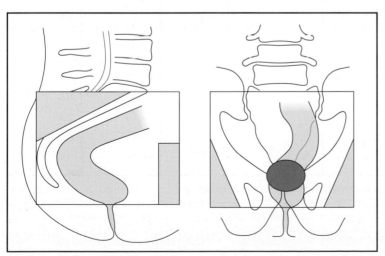

Figure 5.1 • Radiotherapy plan for SCPRT to the pelvis in resectable rectal cancer. Lateral and posterior radiotherapy portals are shown for a mid-rectal cancer (shown in black) with normal tissue shielding of bony pelvis (grey). The anal sphincter has been spared.

indication is to shrink locally advanced rectal cancer to facilitate successful resection, although this is confused by a lack of agreement about how to define the local extent of disease. Finally, there is an increasing interest in the use of radiation to shrink or 'downsize' resectable disease to achieve sphincter-preserving surgery.

PREOPERATIVE RADIOTHERAPY TO REDUCE LOCAL RECURRENCE IN RESECTABLE DISEASE

The advantage of preoperative radiotherapy is that the pelvic anatomy is undisturbed. Consequently, there is usually less small bowel in the radiation field and this results in less gastrointestinal acute toxicity and high compliance. The tissues are likely to be well oxygenated and tumour radiosensitivity may be increased. Disadvantages include overtreatment when a routine policy of preoperative radiotherapy is used, exposing some patients to the risks of late radiation damage without benefit.

Table 5.3 outlines some of the main trials that have used preoperative radiotherapy.[38–50]

Development of the '25 Gy in five fractions' schedule

The potential use of preoperative radiation was approached cautiously. One key requirement was the development of a short accelerated schedule that minimised any delay in definitive (surgical) treatment. This led to a number of trials that used 5 Gy per fraction, including two in the UK and three in Sweden.[40,44,48,49,51] Overall, this approach was well tolerated.

 The Swedish Rectal Cancer Trial was the largest of these studies and particularly influential, since it showed improved survival as well as reduced local recurrence rates.[51]

However, it has become clear that careful planning using a three- or four-field arrangement and a

Table 5.3 • Randomised trials of preoperative radiotherapy vs. surgery alone

Trial	N*	Total dose (Gy)	No. of fractions	BED	LR (P value)	Survival
MRC I[38]	564	5	1	7.5	n.s.	n.s.
MRC I	557	20	10	20.4	n.s.	n.s.
VASOG I[39]	700	20/25	10	21.0/28.3	n.s.	n.s.
St Mark's RCG[40]	475	15	3	22.5	<0.05	n.s.
Essen[41]	142	25	13	24	n.s.	n.s.
Bergen[42]	309	31.5	18	26.8	n.s.	n.s.
VASOG II[43]	359	31.5	18	26.8	–	n.s.
NWRCG[44]	284	20	4	30.0	<0.001	n.s.
SGSTCIRC Japan[45]	166	30	15	30.6	n.s.	n.s.
EORTC 76-81[46]	466	34.5	15	34.6	0.003	n.s.
MRC II[60]	279	40	20	36.0	0.04	n.s.
Stockholm I/II[48,49]	1019	25	5	37.5	<0.01	n.s.
Swedish RCT[51]	1165	25	5	37.5	<0.001	P = 0.004
Dutch TME trial[50]	1861	25	5	37.5	<0.001	n.s.

*Number of patients considered evaluable in a recent overview,[36] where applicable.
BED, biologically effective dose; EORTC, European Organisation for the Research and Treatment of Cancer; LR, local recurrence rate; MRC, Medical Research Council; n.s., not significant; NWRCG, North Western Rectal Cancer Group; RCG, Rectal Cancer Group; SGSTCIRC, Study Group of Surgical Therapy and Combined Irradiation in Rectal Cancer; Swedish RCT, Swedish Rectal Cancer Trial; TME, total mesorectal excision; VASOG, Veterans Association Surgical Oncology Group. Gy, gray (unit of absorbed radiation dose).

superior border no higher than the L4/5 junction is required to reduce toxicity (see **Fig. 5.1**).

'Long-course' preoperative radiation schedules

The alternative approach is to use a longer course of radiation with a lower dose per fraction. Most current long-course schedules use 45–50.4 Gy over 5–5.5 weeks using 1.8–2.0 Gy per fraction. Despite evidence for improved local control, there is no trial evidence for improved survival using this strategy. The main reason for the use of such schedules relates to the trials of postoperative radiation and chemoradiation and the translation of radiation schedules developed in unresectable disease to patients with resectable disease. The neoadjuvant concurrent chemoradiotherapy (cCRT) schedules are discussed in the section on locally advanced disease.

The use of cCRT preoperatively in resectable disease has increased significantly despite a very small evidence base of randomised controlled trials. The current EORTC 22921 trial in resectable disease compares preoperative radiotherapy with cCRT and also tests the benefit of postoperative adjuvant chemotherapy (aCT) against control. The German CAO/ARO/AI094 trial compares preoperative and postoperative cCRT. A recent Polish trial has completed recruitment comparing short-course preoperative radiotherapy (SCPRT) with preoperative cCRT.[52]

Preoperative long-course cCRT is used particularly in mainland Europe. However, the indications may include macroscopic tumour shrinkage to facilitate successful resection, reduction of local recurrence risk and to increase the probability of sphincter preservation.

POSTOPERATIVE RADIATION

The main advantage of postoperative radiation is the ability to select patients considered at increased risk of local recurrence based on histopathological examination of the resected specimen. This avoids the inevitable overtreatment that comes with a policy of routine SCPRT. Disadvantages are that a higher dose of radiation is required (which may relate in part to hypoxia within the field of surgery) and small bowel acute toxicity is increased. This is due to the presence of larger volumes of bowel within the radiation field and adhesions that may

reduce its mobility. There is also the problem of compliance (ability to receive the planned total dose of radiation) because of either inadequate recovery from surgery prior to receiving radiation or acute toxicity curtailing treatment before the planned total dose has been reached.

Randomised controlled trials using postoperative radiation

The systematic overview[36] identifies eight evaluable randomised trials[53–60] that assessed postoperative radiation and included surgery alone as a control arm (**Table 5.4**). Medical Research Council (MRC)3 is the only trial that demonstrated a statistically significant reduction in local recurrence, with no impact on overall survival. However, the systematic overview[36] demonstrates that there is a significant reduction in local recurrence and cancer-specific mortality, although the proportional reduction of these events is smaller than that found for preoperative radiation. Most of the postoperative trials are small and therefore underpowered to detect small improvements.

Development of postoperative chemoradiation

The relatively disappointing results of the trials of postoperative radiation alone, with the aim of improving overall survival, led to trials that integrated chemotherapy. Interpretation is difficult mainly due to trial design. It is important to distinguish between cCRT, when chemotherapy is delivered during the radiation phase of treatment, and aCT, when chemotherapy alone at systemically effective doses is delivered either prior to or after the radiation phase of treatment.

At least seven randomised trials[61–67] have tested the role of postoperative chemoradiation (**Table 5.5**). Of these, only three have included a surgery-alone arm and three a chemotherapy-alone arm. There is therefore considerable heterogeneity within the trials, which makes interpretation difficult. Most of these studies are from North America and the results of three[55,61,62] led to a consensus statement from the National Institutes of Health in 1990 that made postoperative chemoradiation (aCT plus cCRT) for patients with pT3/4 or N-positive disease (TNM stage II and III) the standard of care.[8] This policy is more selective than routine preoperative radiotherapy but only spares patients with stage I

Table 5.4 • Randomised trials comparing postoperative radiotherapy with surgery without radiotherapy

Trial	N*	Dose (Gy)	Fractions	LR (P value)	Survival
GITSG[53]	227	40–48	20–28	n.s.	n.s.
ECOG[54]	208	45	25	–	n.s.
NSABP R-01[55]	381	46/47	26/27	0.06	n.s.
Odense[56]	495	50	25	n.s.	n.s.
EORTC 81-86[57]	172	46	23	n.s.	n.s.
Rotterdam[58]	172	50	25	n.s.	n.s.
ANZ Study[59]	33	45	25	n.s.	n.s.
MRC3[60]	469	40	20	0.001	n.s.

*Number of patients considered evaluable in recent overview.[36]
ANZ, Australia/New Zealand; ECOG, Eastern Cooperative Oncology Group; EORTC, European Organisation for Research and Treatment of Cancer; GITSG, Gastrointestinal Tumour Study Group; LR, local recurrence rate; MRC, Medical Research Council; n.s., not significant; NSABP, National Surgical Adjuvant Breast and Bowel Project.

Table 5.5 • Important randomised trials involving postoperative chemoradiotherapy

Trial	N	Treatment arms	Results
GITSG 7175[61]	227	Surgery alone MF RT + MF RT	5-year survival: RT + MF 59%, control 43% (P <0.01)
Mayo/NCCTG 79-47-51[62]	204	MF + 5FU/RT + MF RT	7-year survival: combined arm 63%, RT alone 48% (P = 0.04)
GITSG 7189[63]	210	5FU/RT + 5FU MF/RT + MF	3-year disease-free survival: 45% MF vs. 69% 5FU
Mayo/NCCTG 86-47-51[64]	453	MF + RT/5FU + MF (bolus vs. infusional 5FU) 5FU + RT/5FU + 5FU (bolus vs. infusional 5FU)	MF not better than 5FU alone Infusion superior to bolus 5FU
Norway[65]	144	Surgery Surgery + 5FU/RT	Local recurrence: 32% vs. 11% (P <0.05) Survival: 49% vs. 63% (P <0.05)
NSABP R-02[66]	694	Chemotherapy vs. chemo/RT (men MOF or 5FU/FA; women 5FU/FA)	Radiotherapy did not improve overall survival but did reduce local recurrence
INT 0114[67]	1792	5FU + RT/5FU + 5FU with LEV, FA or both	No significant difference between arms

5FU, 5-fluorouracil; GITSG, Gastrointestinal Tumour Study Group; INT, Intergroup; LEV, levamisole; FA, folinic acid; MF, methyl CCNU + 5FU; MOF, MF plus vincristine (Oncovin); NCCTG, North Central Cancer Treatment Group; NSABP, National Surgical Adjuvant Breast and Bowel Project; RT, pelvic radiotherapy.

disease the morbidity of treatment. Furthermore, the acute toxicities are more severe and it may not be applicable to the population at large. There is particular concern about older patients.[68]

PREOPERATIVE VERSUS POSTOPERATIVE RADIATION

One randomised trial[69] comparing routine SCPRT and 'selective' postoperative radiotherapy has been performed. Although the postoperative regimen can be criticised radiobiologically for being 'split course', SCPRT produced a local recurrence rate of 13% compared with 22% using 'selective' postoperative radiotherapy. There was no difference in overall survival.

The recent overview demonstrates clear evidence that adjuvant radiation significantly reduces the risk of local recurrence and is effective when used preoperatively or postoperatively. The randomised controlled trials have significantly influenced clinical practice. In Sweden, a policy of routine SCPRT is the preferred approach, whereas in North America the National Institutes of Health standard of care has been widely adopted using 'selective' postoperative chemoradiation for stage II and III patients.

A NEW ERA OF CLINICAL TRIALS OF ADJUVANT THERAPY IN RECTAL CANCER

With the widespread adoption of total mesorectal excision (TME) for rectal cancer, the outcome of surgery alone has improved significantly. The evidence comes directly from individual surgical series,[70] population-based studies[71,72] and indirectly from a recently published randomised controlled trial.[50] This development alone is sufficient to make a distinction between the randomised trial evidence discussed above, where local recurrence rates following surgery alone were commonly greater than 20%, and the proponents of sharp mesorectal dissection who report local recurrence rates of 10% or less. Furthermore, the strong evidence supporting the hypothesis that local recurrence of rectal cancer is predicted by the presence of microscopic cancer cells within 1 mm of the circumferential resection margin (CRM)[72–74] has also been very influential. Therefore, the question in this new era

is how to define a routine policy for adjuvant therapy when several choices exist, e.g. routine SCPRT, selective SCPRT, neoadjuvant chemoradiotherapy or selective postoperative (chemo)radiotherapy.

The Dutch and MRC CR07 trials

To establish the role of SCPRT in this new era, the Dutch Colorectal Cancer Study Group trial[50] and the ongoing MRC CR07 trial have both been designed to compare SCPRT with a selective post-operative approach based on CRM status. Early results from the Dutch trial have shown a reduction in local recurrence with preoperative radiotherapy (2% vs. 8% at 2 years), which is associated with minimal complications. The overall rate of recurrence in both arms is relatively low at 2 years after standardised training in TME for participating surgeons. However, 5-year rates are likely to be higher and it is currently too early to detect any effect on survival.

In the UK, SCPRT is widely used but not routinely in every case as in Scandinavia or the Netherlands. It is likely that the results of CR07 will have a major impact on practice in this country. Undoubtedly there will be an increasing requirement on multi-disciplinary teams to have an established policy governing their choice of adjuvant treatment.

Locally advanced disease

A major problem is the lack of an agreed definition of 'locally advanced' disease. The development of preoperative imaging assessment has focused on prediction of T and N stage, with transrectal ultra-sound accepted as the reference investigation. The recognition of the importance of CRM has led to increased interest in cross-sectional imaging, particularly magnetic resonance imaging (MRI), for demonstrating the relationship of the tumour to the mesorectal fascia, the intended 'CRM' for a mesorectal excision. Digital rectal examination performed by experienced coloproctologists can also identify patients with a poor outcome after surgery alone.[75]

DEVELOPMENT OF PELVIC MRI

A number of studies[76–81] report the value of high-resolution pelvic MRI using phased-array surface coils in the preoperative staging of rectal cancer. There is early promise that this approach can identify patients where local disease extent invades beyond the mesorectal fascia (commonly described as T4 disease) and where the primary tumour extends close to the mesorectal fascia (**Fig. 5.2**). Prospective studies are in progress to try to confirm these findings. Pelvic MRI may be a future method of defining the local disease extent and may facilitate further randomised controlled trials.

RANDOMISED CONTROLLED TRIALS IN LOCALLY ADVANCED DISEASE

Two trials from the UK have evaluated the addition of preoperative radiation to surgery alone.[44,47] Both demonstrated a significant reduction in local recurrence but no difference in overall survival. A small trial from Uppsala[82] randomised 70 patients with fixed unresectable disease between 46 Gy radiation alone and a complex chemoradiotherapy schedule using 40 Gy and methotrexate, FA and 5FU over 8 weeks. There was a statistically significant reduction in local recurrence with chemoradiotherapy but no difference in overall survival.

PHASE II STUDIES

In recent years neoadjuvant cCRT has become a standard treatment for locally advanced rectal cancer, because of increased response rates seen in the very large number of phase II studies that have been performed. Many have used either infusional 5FU[83] or bolus 5FU with FA[84–86] but no direct comparison has been performed and there remains considerable uncertainty as to how to derive the optimum regimen.[87]

Currently, there is considerable interest in the use of other drugs such as capecitabine, oxaliplatin and irinotecan in chemoradiation schedules. The majority of these studies are dose-finding combination chemotherapy regimens added to radiation. The role of subsequent adjuvant chemotherapy after surgery in this setting remains uncertain and is the subject of clinical trials.

THE FUTURE

Radiotherapy has a well-established role in the adjuvant treatment of rectal cancer. The next few years are likely to see increased refinement of our current techniques. For instance, we may be able to

(a)
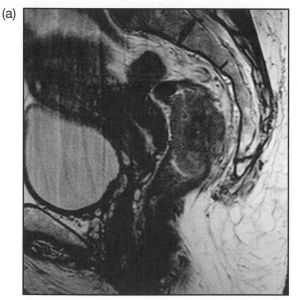
(b)
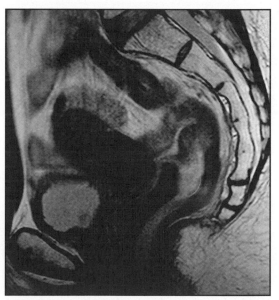

Figure 5.2 • MRI appearances of a locally advanced rectal cancer **(a)** before and **(b)** after neoadjuvant chemoradiotherapy. Prior to treatment there is a bulky mid-rectal tumour (seen in sagittal view) extending to the mesorectal fascia posteriorly. After treatment there has been a significant response, with the mesorectal fascia no longer threatened.

achieve better patient selection through the use of imaging or even molecular markers. More effective regimens of chemoradiotherapy are likely to be developed and trials designed to show when they should be used. More targeted use of SCPRT in the TME era may also be possible with maturing evidence from the Dutch trial and the results of CR07.

Key points

- Six months of adjuvant chemotherapy with 5-FU/FA is currently standard treatment for patients with stage III colorectal cancer.
- There is controversy around the use of chemotherapy in stage II disease, although many clinicians would treat selected 'high-risk' patients.
- The role of additional agents in adjuvant chemotherapy remains to be clarified.
- Adjuvant radiotherapy is widely used in rectal cancer to reduce the risk of local recurrence.
- SCPRT is widely used in resectable disease, although its precise role in the era of TME surgery remains to be clarified. In North America, selective postoperative chemoradiotherapy remains standard.
- Neoadjuvant chemoradiotherapy is frequently used in fit patients with unresectable rectal cancer to try to downstage the disease prior to surgery and allow complete resection.

REFERENCES

1. QUASAR Collaborative Group. Comparison of fluorouracil with additional levamisole, higher-dose folinic acid, or both, as adjuvant chemotherapy for colorectal cancer: a randomised trial. Lancet 2000; 355:1588–96.

   Influential UK study that showed that low-dose FA was equivalent to high-dose FA. Also showed no benefit for levamisole. Led to weekly bolus 5FU/FA becoming widely used in the UK.

2. Haydon A. Adjuvant chemotherapy in colon cancer: what is the evidence? Intern Med J 2003; 33:119–24.

3. Moertel CG. Chemotherapy for colorectal cancer. N Engl J Med 1994; 330:1136–42.

4. Buyse M, Zeleniuch-Jacquotte A, Chalmers TC. Adjuvant therapy of colorectal cancer. Why we still don't know. JAMA 1988; 259:3571–8.

5. Laurie JA, Moertel CG, Fleming TR et al. Surgical adjuvant therapy of large-bowel carcinoma: an evaluation of levamisole and the combination of levamisole and fluorouracil. The North Central Cancer Treatment Group and the Mayo Clinic. J Clin Oncol 1989; 7:1447–56.

   Large randomised study that was important in proving the principle of adjuvant chemotherapy.

6. Moertel CG, Fleming TR, Macdonald JS et al. Levamisole and fluorouracil for adjuvant therapy of resected colon carcinoma. N Engl J Med 1990; 322:352–8.

   Along with reference 5 led to the NIH Consensus State-ment recommending adjuvant chemotherapy for stage C colon cancer.

7. Moertel CG, Fleming TR, Macdonald JS et al. Fluorouracil plus levamisole as effective adjuvant therapy after resection of stage III colon carcinoma: a final report. Ann Intern Med 1995; 122:321–6.

   An update of the trial patients in reference 6 that continued to show ongoing benefit to adjuvant treatment.

8. NIH consensus conference. Adjuvant therapy for patients with colon and rectal cancer. JAMA 1990; 264:1444–50.

   Remains a very influential guide to practice in North America

9. Wolmark N, Fisher B, Rockette H et al. Post-operative adjuvant chemotherapy or BCG for colon cancer: results from NSABP protocol C-01. J Natl Cancer Inst 1988; 80:30–6.

10. Francini G, Petrioli R, Lorenzini L et al. Folinic acid and 5-fluorouracil as adjuvant chemotherapy in colon cancer. Gastroenterology 1994; 106:899–906.

11. International Multicentre Pooled Analysis of Colon Cancer Trials (IMPACT) investigators. Efficacy of adjuvant fluorouracil and folinic acid in colon cancer. Lancet 1995; 345:939–44.

    Pooled analysis of three randomised trials containing 1526 patients that demonstrated a clear benefit to adjuvant 5FU/FA over control.

12. O'Connell MJ, Mailliard JA, Kahn MJ et al. Controlled trial of fluorouracil and low-dose leucovorin given for 6 months as postoperative adjuvant therapy for colon cancer. J Clin Oncol 1997; 15:246–50.

13. Advanced Colorectal Cancer Meta-Analysis Project. Modulation of fluorouracil by leucovorin in patients with advanced colorectal cancer: evidence in terms of response rate. J Clin Oncol 1992; 10:896–903.

14. O'Connell MJ, Laurie JA, Kahn M et al. Prospec-tively randomized trial of postoperative adjuvant

chemotherapy in patients with high-risk colon cancer. J Clin Oncol 1998; 16:295–300.

15. Haller DG, Catalano PJ, MacDonald JS, Mayer RJ. Fluorouracil (FU), leucovorin (LV) and levamisole (LEV) adjuvant therapy for colon cancer: five-year final report of INT-0089 (abstract). Proc Am Soc Clin Oncol 1998; 17:256a.

16. Wolmark N, Rockette H, Mamounas E et al. Clinical trial to assess the relative efficacy of fluorouracil and leucovorin, fluorouracil and levamisole, and fluorouracil, leucovorin, and levamisole in patients with Dukes' B and C carcinoma of the colon: results from National Surgical Adjuvant Breast and Bowel Project C-04. J Clin Oncol 1999; 17:3553–9.

17. Porschen R, Bermann A, Loffler T et al. Fluorouracil plus leucovorin as effective adjuvant chemotherapy in curatively resected stage III colon cancer: results of the trial adjCCA-01. J Clin Oncol 2001; 19:1787–94.

18. Staib L, Link KH, Beger HG. Toxicity and effects of adjuvant therapy in colon cancer: results of the German prospective, controlled randomized multicenter trial FOGT-1. J Gastrointest Surg 2001; 5:275–81.

19. Labianca R, Beretta G, Clerici M, Fraschini P, Luporini G. Cardiac toxicity of 5-fluorouracil: a study on 1083 patients. Tumori 1982; 68:505–10.

20. Sargent DJ, Goldberg RM, Jacobson SD et al. A pooled analysis of adjuvant chemotherapy for resected colon cancer in elderly patients. N Engl J Med 2001; 345:1091–7.

21. Iwashyna TJ, Lamont EB. Effectiveness of adjuvant fluorouracil in clinical practice: a population-based cohort study of elderly patients with stage III colon cancer. J Clin Oncol 2002; 20:3992–8.

22. International Multicentre Pooled Analysis of B2 Colon Cancer Trials (IMPACT B2) Investigators. Efficacy of adjuvant fluorouracil and folinic acid in B2 colon cancer. J Clin Oncol 1999; 17:1356–63.

23. Moertel CG, Fleming TR, Macdonald JS et al. Intergroup study of fluorouracil plus levamisole as adjuvant therapy for stage II/Dukes' B2 colon cancer. J Clin Oncol 1995; 13:2936–43.

24. Mamounas E, Wieand S, Wolmark N et al. Comparative efficacy of adjuvant chemotherapy in patients with Dukes' B versus Dukes' C colon cancer: results from four National Surgical Adjuvant Breast and Bowel Project adjuvant studies (C-01, C-02, C-03, and C-04). J Clin Oncol 1999; 17:1349–55.

25. Taal BG, Van Tinteren H, Zoetmulder FA. Adjuvant 5FU plus levamisole in colonic or rectal cancer: improved survival in stage II and III. Br J Cancer 2001; 85:1437–43.

26. Wolmark N, Wieand HS, Rockette HE et al. The prognostic significance of tumor location and bowel obstruction in Dukes B and C colorectal cancer. Findings from the NSABP clinical trials. Ann Surg 1983; 198:743–52.

27. Steinberg SM, Barkin JS, Kaplan RS, Stablein DM. Prognostic indicators of colon tumors. The Gastrointestinal Tumor Study Group experience. Cancer 1986; 57:1866–70.

28. Steinberg SM, Barwick KW, Stablein DM. Importance of tumor pathology and morphology in patients with surgically resected colon cancer. Findings from the Gastrointestinal Tumor Study Group. Cancer 1986; 58:1340–5.

29. Shepherd NA, Baxter KJ, Love SB. Influence of local peritoneal involvement on pelvic recurrence and prognosis in rectal cancer. J Clin Pathol 1995; 48:849–55.

30. Talbot IC, Ritchie S, Leighton M, Hughes AO, Bussey HJ, Morson BC. Invasion of veins by carcinoma of rectum: method of detection, histological features and significance. Histopathology 1981; 5:141–63.

31. Talbot IC, Ritchie S, Leighton MH, Hughes AO, Bussey HJ, Morson BC. Spread of rectal cancer within veins. Histologic features and clinical significance. Am J Surg 1981; 141:15–17.

32. Saini A, Norman AR, Cunningham D et al. Twelve weeks of protracted venous infusion of fluorouracil (5-FU) is as effective as 6 months of bolus 5-FU and folinic acid as adjuvant treatment in colorectal cancer. Br J Cancer 2003; 88:1859–65.

33. Douillard JY, Cunningham D, Roth AD et al. Irinotecan combined with fluorouracil compared with fluorouracil alone as first-line treatment for metastatic colorectal cancer: a multicentre randomised trial. Lancet 2000; 355:1041–7.

34. Giacchetti S, Perpoint B, Zidani R et al. Phase III multicenter randomized trial of oxaliplatin added to chronomodulated fluorouracil–leucovorin as first-line treatment of metastatic colorectal cancer. J Clin Oncol 2000; 18:136–47.

35. James RD, Donaldson D, Gray R, Northover JM, Stenning SP, Taylor I. Randomized clinical trial of adjuvant radiotherapy and 5-fluorouracil infusion in colorectal cancer (AXIS). Br J Surg 2003; 90:1200–12.

36. Colorectal Cancer Collaborative Group. Adjuvant radiotherapy for rectal cancer: a systematic overview of 8,507 patients from 22 randomised trials. Lancet 2001; 358:1291–304.

Very important overview of the many trials of adjuvant radiotherapy in rectal cancer that clearly demonstrated a reduction in local recurrence and also suggested a reduction in cancer-related mortality.

37. Camma C, Giunta M, Fiorica F, Pagliaro L, Craxi A, Cottone M. Preoperative radiotherapy for resectable rectal cancer: a meta-analysis. JAMA 2000; 284:1008–15.

38. MRC Working Party–Second Report. The evaluation of low dose pre-operative X-ray therapy in the management of operable rectal cancer: results of a randomly controlled trial. Br J Surg 1984; 71:21–5.

39. Higgins GA Jr, Conn JH, Jordan PH Jr, Humphrey EW, Roswit B, Keehn RJ. Preoperative radiotherapy for colorectal cancer. Ann Surg 1975; 181:624–31.

40. Goldberg PA, Nicholls RJ, Porter NH, Love S, Grimsey JE. Long-term results of a randomised trial of short-course low-dose adjuvant pre-operative radiotherapy for rectal cancer: reduction in local treatment failure. Eur J Cancer 1994; 30A:1602–6.

41. Niebel W, Schulz U, Ried M et al. Five-year results of a prospective and randomized study: experience with combined radiotherapy and surgery of primary rectal carcinoma. Recent Results Cancer Res 1988; 110:111–13.

42. Dahl O, Horn A, Morild I et al. Low-dose pre-operative radiation postpones recurrences in operable rectal cancer. Results of a randomized multicenter trial in western Norway. Cancer 1990; 66:2286–94.

43. Higgins GA, Humphrey EW, Dwight RW, Roswit B, Lee LE Jr, Keehn RJ. Preoperative radiation and surgery for cancer of the rectum. Veterans Administration Surgical Oncology Group Trial II. Cancer 1986; 58:352–9.

44. Marsh PJ, James RD, Schofield PF. Adjuvant pre-operative radiotherapy for locally advanced rectal carcinoma. Results of a prospective, randomized trial. Dis Colon Rectum 1994; 37:1205–14.

45. Kimura K, Tuchiya S, Yasutomi M et al. Comparison of surgical therapy and combined irradiation in rectal cancer: first report, effect of irradiation on the tumor. Study Group of Surgical Therapy and Combined Irradiation in Rectal Cancer. [In Japanese] Gan To Kagaku Ryoho 1989; 16:3161–72.

46. Gerard A, Buyse M, Nordlinger B et al. Preoperative radiotherapy as adjuvant treatment in rectal cancer. Final results of a randomized study of the European Organization for Research and Treatment of Cancer (EORTC). Ann Surg 1988; 208:606–14.

47. Medical Research Council Rectal Cancer Working Party. Randomised trial of surgery alone versus radiotherapy followed by surgery for potentially operable locally advanced rectal cancer. Lancet 1996; 348:1605–10.

48. Cedermark B, Johansson H, Rutqvist LE, Wilking N. The Stockholm I trial of preoperative short term radiotherapy in operable rectal carcinoma. A prospective randomized trial. Stockholm Colorectal Cancer Study Group. Cancer 1995; 75:2269–75.

49. Stockholm Colorectal Cancer Study Group. Randomized study on preoperative radiotherapy in rectal carcinoma. Ann Surg Oncol 1996; 3:423–30.

50. Kapiteijn E, Marijnen CA, Nagtegaal ID et al. Preoperative radiotherapy combined with total mesorectal excision for resectable rectal cancer. N Engl J Med 2001; 345:638–46.

A very important study which will help to define the role of SCPRT in the era of TME surgery and pathological evaluation based on CRM.

51. Swedish Rectal Cancer Trial. Improved survival with preoperative radiotherapy in resectable rectal cancer. N Engl J Med 1997; 336:980–7.

A large randomised study of 1168 patients that demonstrated both a reduction in local recurrence and an improvement in overall survival for routine SCPRT in resectable rectal cancer.

52. Bujko K, Nowacki M, Nasierowska-Guttmejer A et al. Sphincter preservation following preoperative radiotherapy for rectal cancer: report of a randomised trial comparing short-term radiotherapy vs. conventionally fractionated radiochemotherapy. Radiother Oncol 2004; 72:15–24.

53. Thomas PR, Lindblad AS. Adjuvant post-operative radiotherapy and chemotherapy in rectal carcinoma: a review of the Gastrointestinal Tumor Study Group experience. Radiother Oncol 1988; 13:245–52.

54. Mansour E, Lefkopoulou M, Johnson R. A comparison of post-operative chemotherapy, radiotherapy or combination therapy in potentially curable rectal carcinoma: an ECOG Study EST4276. Proc Am Soc Clin Oncol 1991; 154:A484.

55. Fisher B, Wolmark N, Rockette H et al. Post-operative adjuvant chemotherapy or radiation therapy for rectal cancer: results from NSABP protocol R-01. J Natl Cancer Inst 1988; 80:21–9.

56. Balslev I, Pedersen M, Teglbjaerg PS et al. Post-operative radiotherapy in Dukes' B and C carcinoma of the rectum and rectosigmoid. A randomized multicenter study. Cancer 1986; 58:22–8.

57. Arnaud JP, Nordlinger B, Bosset JF et al. Radical surgery and postoperative radiotherapy as combined treatment in rectal cancer. Final results of a phase III study of the European Organization for Research and Treatment of Cancer. Br J Surg 1997; 84:352–7.

58. Treurniet-Donker AD, van Putten WL, Wereldsma JC et al. Postoperative radiation therapy for rectal cancer. An interim analysis of a prospective, randomized multicenter trial in The Netherlands. Cancer 1991; 67:2042–8.

59. Marneghan H, Gray B, de Zwart J. Adjuvant post-operative radiotherapy in rectal cancer: results from the ANZ bowel cancer trial (protocol 8202). Australas Radiol 1991; 35:61–5.

60. Medical Research Council Rectal Cancer Working Party. Randomised trial of surgery alone versus surgery followed by radiotherapy for mobile cancer of the rectum. Lancet 1996; 348:1610–14.

61. Gastrointestinal Tumor Study Group. Prolongation of the disease-free interval in surgically treated rectal carcinoma. N Engl J Med 1985; 312:1465–72.

62. Krook JE, Moertel CG, Gunderson LL et al. Effective surgical adjuvant therapy for high-risk rectal carcinoma. N Engl J Med 1991; 324:709–15.

63. Gastrointestinal Tumor Study Group. Radiation therapy and fluorouracil with or without semustine for the treatment of patients with surgical adjuvant adenocarcinoma of the rectum. J Clin Oncol 1992; 10:549–57.

64. O'Connell MJ, Martenson JA, Wieand HS et al. Improving adjuvant therapy for rectal cancer by combining protracted-infusion fluorouracil with radiation therapy after curative surgery. N Engl J Med 1994; 331:502–7.

65. Tveit KM, Guldvog I, Hagen S et al. Randomized controlled trial of postoperative radiotherapy and short-term time-scheduled 5-fluorouracil against surgery alone in the treatment of Dukes B and C rectal cancer. Norwegian Adjuvant Rectal Cancer Project Group. Br J Surg 1997; 84:1130–5.

66. Wolmark N, Wieand HS, Hyams DM et al. Randomized trial of postoperative adjuvant chemotherapy with or without radiotherapy for carcinoma of the rectum: National Surgical Adjuvant Breast and Bowel Project Protocol R-02. J Natl Cancer Inst 2000; 92:388–96.

67. Tepper JE, O'Connell MJ, Petroni GR et al. Adjuvant postoperative fluorouracil-modulated chemotherapy combined with pelvic radiation therapy for rectal cancer: initial results of intergroup 0114. J Clin Oncol 1997; 15:2030–9.

68. Neugut AI, Fleischauer AT, Sundararajan V et al. Use of adjuvant chemotherapy and radiation therapy for rectal cancer among the elderly: a population-based study. J Clin Oncol 2002; 20:2643–50.

69. Pahlman L, Glimelius B. Pre-operative and post-operative radiotherapy and rectal cancer. World J Surg 1992; 16:858–65.

70. Heald RJ, Moran BJ, Ryall RD, Sexton R, MacFarlane JK. Rectal cancer: the Basingstoke experience of total mesorectal excision, 1978–1997. Arch Surg 1998; 133:894–9.

71. Martling AL, Holm T, Rutqvist LE, Moran BJ, Heald RJ, Cedermark B. Effect of a surgical training programme on outcome of rectal cancer in the County of Stockholm. Stockholm Colorectal Cancer Study Group, Basingstoke Bowel Cancer Research Project. Lancet 2000; 356:93–6.

72. Wibe A, Rendedal PR, Svensson E et al. Prognostic significance of the circumferential resection margin following total mesorectal excision for rectal cancer. Br J Surg 2002; 89:327–34.

73. Adam IJ, Mohamdee MO, Martin IG et al. Role of circumferential margin involvement in the local recurrence of rectal cancer. Lancet 1994; 344:707–11.

74. Birbeck KF, Macklin CP, Tiffin NJ et al. Rates of circumferential resection margin involvement vary between surgeons and predict outcomes in rectal cancer surgery. Ann Surg 2002; 235:449–57.

75. Nicholls RJ, Mason AY, Morson BC, Dixon AK, Fry IK. The clinical staging of rectal cancer. Br J Surg 1982; 69:404–9.

76. Botterill ID, Blunt DM, Quirke P et al. Evaluation of the role of pre-operative magnetic resonance imaging in the management of rectal cancer. Colorectal Dis 2001; 3:295–303.

77. Blomqvist L, Machado M, Rubio C et al. Rectal tumour staging: MR imaging using pelvic phased-array and endorectal coils vs endoscopic ultra-sonography. Eur Radiol 2000; 10:653–60.

78. Brown G, Richards CJ, Newcombe RG et al. Rectal carcinoma: thin-section MR imaging for staging in 28 patients. Radiology 1999; 211:215–22.

79. Bissett IP, Fernando CC, Hough DM et al. Identification of the fascia propria by magnetic resonance imaging and its relevance to preoperative assessment of rectal cancer. Dis Colon Rectum 2001; 44:259–65.

80. Beets-Tan RG, Beets GL, Vliegen RF et al. Accuracy of magnetic resonance imaging in prediction of tumour-free resection margin in rectal cancer surgery. Lancet 2001; 357:497–504.

81. Brown G, Radcliffe AG, Newcombe RG, Dallimore NS, Bourne MW, Williams GT. Pre-operative assessment of prognostic factors in rectal cancer using high-resolution magnetic resonance imaging. Br J Surg 2003; 90:355–64.

82. Frykholm GJ, Pahlman L, Glimelius B. Combined chemo- and radiotherapy vs. radiotherapy alone in the treatment of primary, nonresectable adenocarcinoma of the rectum. Int J Radiat Oncol Biol Phys 2001; 50:427–34.

83. Rich TA, Skibber JM, Ajani JA et al. Preoperative infusional chemoradiation therapy for stage T3 rectal cancer. Int J Radiat Oncol Biol Phys 1995; 32:1025–9.

84. Minsky B, Cohen A, Enker W et al. Preoperative 5-fluorouracil, low-dose leucovorin, and concurrent

radiation therapy for rectal cancer. Cancer 1994; 73:273–80.

85. Minsky BD, Kemeny N, Cohen AM et al. Preoperative high-dose leucovorin/5-fluorouracil and radiation therapy for unresectable rectal cancer. Cancer 1991; 67:2859–66.

86. Bosset JF, Pavy JJ, Hamers HP et al. Determination of the optimal dose of 5-fluorouracil when combined with low dose DL-leucovorin and irradiation in rectal cancer: results of three consecutive phase II studies. EORTC Radiotherapy Group. Eur J Cancer 1993; 29A:1406–10.

87. Glynne-Jones R, Sebag-Montefiore D. Chemoradiation schedules: what radiotherapy? Eur J Cancer 2002; 38:258–69.

CHAPTER
Six

Anal cancer

John H. Scholefield

INTRODUCTION

Anal cancer is rare, accounting for approximately 4% of large bowel malignancies; however, there is some evidence that its incidence is increasing. Most anal cancers arise from the squamous epithelium of the anal margin or anal canal, although a few arise from anal glands and ducts.

Traditionally, the anal region is divided into the anal canal and the anal margin or verge. The natural history, demography and surgical management differ between these areas. There has been controversy regarding the exact definition of the anal canal. Anatomists see it as lying between the dentate line and the anal verge, whereas surgically it is defined as lying between the anorectal ring and the anal verge. For pathologists, the canal has been defined as corresponding to the longitudinal extent of the internal anal sphincter.[1] The canal above the dentate line is lined by rectal mucosa, except for a small zone immediately above the line called the transitional or junctional zone.[2] Inferiorly, the canal is covered by stratified squamous epithelium. Further confusion relates to the definition of the anal canal and anal margin as sites for cancer. The anal margin is variously described as the visible area external to the anal verge, or as the area below the dentate line. This argument has become less important as surgery plays a lesser role in treatment, but reports of surgical results from past decades are confused by this variation in definition.

Over 80% of anal cancers are of squamous origin, arising from the squamous epithelium of the anal canal and perianal area; 10% are adenocarcinomas arising from the glandular mucosa of the upper anal canal, the anal glands and ducts. A very rare and particularly malignant tumour is anal melanoma. Lymphomas and sarcomas of the anus are even less common but have increased in incidence in recent years, particularly among patients with human immunodeficiency virus (HIV) infection. There has also been a rise in the incidence of other anal epidermoid tumours among patients with HIV.

EPIDERMOID TUMOURS

Aetiology and pathogenesis

Anal squamous cell carcinomas are relatively uncommon tumours; there are between 250 and 300 new cases per year in England and Wales. Based on these figures each consultant general surgeon might expect to see one anal carcinoma every 3–4 years. However, anal cancers are probably under-reported, since some anal canal tumours are misclassified as rectal tumours and some perianal tumours as squamous carcinomas of skin.

The Office of Population Censuses and Surveys' Cancer Statistics for England and Wales recorded 289 cases of anal cancer in 1988.[3] The average age was 57 years for both sexes, although canal tumours were more common in women and margin tumours more common in men. However, these figures must be interpreted with caution since the distinction between anal canal and anal margin is poorly defined.

There is wide geographical variation in the incidence of anal cancers around the world,[4] but again these figures must be interpreted with caution for the reasons given above. Nevertheless, a low incidence (0.2 per 100 000 of population) is reported by Rizal in the Philippines, while the highest incidence (3.6 per 100 000 of population) is in Geneva, Switzerland. Other areas of high incidence are Poland (Warsaw) and Brazil (Recife). It is notable that these areas also have a high incidence of cervical, vulval and penile tumours (possibly reflecting the common proposed aetiological agent, i.e. papillomaviruses). The UK incidence of anal cancer lies between these extremes.

The increasing incidence of HIV infection in the USA has resulted in a rise in the incidence of anal cancer,[5] areas such as San Francisco, with a large gay population, reportedly seeing a dramatic increase. A recent study from Denmark has reported a doubling in the incidence of anal cancer over the last ten years, particularly in women.[6] No other countries have reported similar increases to date, but the Cancer Registry data in Denmark are renowned for their remarkable accuracy and completeness.

Cooper et al.[7] observed four cases of anal cancer arising in homosexual men with long histories of anoreceptive intercourse. The occurrence of a disproportionately high incidence of anal cancer among male homosexual communities was reported from San Francisco and Los Angeles. Daling et al.[8] identified risk factors for the development of squamous cell carcinoma of the anus, a history of receptive anal intercourse in males increasing the relative risk of developing anal cancer by 33 times compared with controls with colon cancer. A history of genital warts also increased the relative risk of developing anal cancer (27-fold in men and 22-fold in women). These studies suggest that a sexually transmissible agent may be an aetiological factor in anal squamous cell carcinoma.

Similarly, epidemiological and molecular biological data have shown an association between a sexually transmissible agent and female genital cancer. Using nucleic acid hybridisation techniques, human papillomavirus (HPV) type 16 DNA, and less commonly types 18, 31 and 33 DNA, were consistently found to be integrated into the genome in genital squamous cell carcinomas.[9] The same HPV DNA types have also been identified in a similar proportion of anal squamous cell carcinomas.[10] HPVs, which are DNA viruses, comprise more than 60 types capable of causing a wide variety of lesions on squamous epithelium. Common warts can be found on the hands and feet of children and young adults, and are caused by the relatively infectious HPV types 1 and 2. Anogenital papillomaviruses are less infective than types 1 and 2 and are exclusively sexually transmissible. The epidemiology of genital papillomavirus infection is poorly understood, largely due to the social and moral taboos surrounding sexually transmissible infections. Anogenital papillomavirus-associated lesions range from condylomas through intraepithelial neoplasia to invasive carcinoma. The most common HPV types causing genital warts are types 6 and 11, which may also be isolated from low-grade intraepithelial neoplasia. HPV types 16, 18, 31 and 33 are much less commonly associated with genital condylomas but are more commonly found in high-grade intraepithelial neoplasias and invasive carcinomas. Once one area of the anogenital epithelium is infected, spread of papillomavirus infection throughout the rest of the anogenital area probably follows, but remains occult in the majority of individuals.[11] Therefore the commonly held belief that anal cancer occurs only in individuals who practise anal intercourse is probably unfounded.

Premalignant lesions

Anal and genital papillomavirus-associated lesions may be identified clinically either by naked eye inspection or more usually with an operating microscope (colposcope) and the application of acetic acid to the epithelium, resulting in an 'aceto-white' lesion. Colposcopic examination may suggest the degree of dysplasia and permits targeted biopsy of a lesion, but histological examination remains the diagnostic standard. Although the natural history of cervical papillomavirus infection and intraepithelial neoplasia is reasonably well understood, the same is not true for anal lesions, probably because they have been diagnosed only over the last 5–10 years. Consequently, the natural history and malignant potential of anal intraepithelial neoplasia are both uncertain.

Anogenital intraepithelial neoplasia of the cervix (CIN), vulva (VIN), vagina (VAIN) and anus (AIN) is graded from I to III, according to the number of thirds of epithelial depth that appear dysplastic on histological section. Thus in grade III the cells of the whole thickness of the epithelium appear dysplastic, being synonymous with carcinoma in situ.

High-grade anal intraepithelial lesions may be characterised by hyperkeratosis or changes in the pigmentation of the epithelium. Thus carcinoma in situ may appear white, red or brown, the pigmentation commonly being irregular. The lesions may be flat or raised; ulceration, however, is suggestive of invasive disease. It is important that any suspicious area is biopsied and examined histologically. The terms 'Bowen's disease of the anus' and 'leucoplakia' are best avoided as they are confusing and convey no specific information, the malignant potential of both being uncertain.

At present, multifocal genital intraepithelial neoplasia represents a difficult clinical problem, which may be further complicated by the occurrence of synchronous or metachronous AIN.[12] The management of these patients is controversial as the natural history of these lesions remains poorly understood.[13]

Cocarcinogens

Carcinogenesis is a multistep process, papillomaviruses probably being only one of a number of factors in the pathogenesis of these tumours. Other potential cocarcinogens are being investigated, including other sexually transmissible infective agents such as herpes simplex type II and chlamydia.

There are few published data on the prevalence of HPV infection among HIV-infected patients, but it appears that anogenital HPV infection is particularly common in this group. The dramatic increase in the incidence of anal cancer in areas where HIV infection is prevalent suggests that suppression of cell-mediated responses to HPV infection may be relevant to the pathogenesis of anal cancer; this is further supported by the prevalence of squamous carcinomas in patients receiving systemic immunosuppression following organ transplantation.

Histological types

Included within the category of epidermoid tumours are squamous cell, basaloid (or cloacogenic) carcinomas and muco-epidermoid cancers. The different morphological types of anal cancer do not appear to have different prognoses.[14] Tumours arising at the anal margin tend to be well differentiated and keratinising, whereas those arising in the canal are more commonly poorly differentiated. Basaloid tumours arise in the transitional zone around the dentate line and form 30–50% of all anal canal tumours.

Patterns of spread

Anal canal cancer spreads locally, mainly in a cephalad direction, so that the tumour may appear to have arisen in the rectum. The tumour also spreads outwards into the anal sphincters and into the rectovaginal septum, perineal body, scrotum or vagina in more advanced cases (**Fig. 6.1**; see also Plate 2, facing p. 22). Lymph node metastases occur frequently, especially in tumours of the anal canal.[15] Spread occurs initially to the perirectal group of nodes and thereafter to inguinal, haemorrhoidal and lateral pelvic lymph nodes. The frequency of nodal involvement is related to the size of the primary tumour together with its depth of penetration.[16] Approximately 14% of patients will present with inguinal lymph node involvement, but this rises to approximately 30% when the primary tumour is greater than 5 cm in diameter.[17,18] Only 50% of patients with enlarged nodes at presentation will subsequently be shown to contain tumour. Synchronously involved nodes carry a particularly poor prognosis, whereas when metachronous spread develops the salvage rate is much higher.

Haematogenous spread tends to occur late and is usually associated with advanced local disease. The principal sites of metastases are the liver, lung and bones.[19] However, metastases have been described in the kidneys, adrenals and brain.

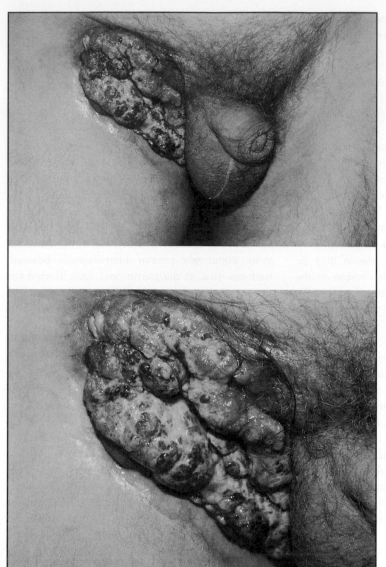

Figure 6.1 • Locally advanced anal cancer involving the anal canal, perianal skin, perineal skin and base of scrotum. Treatment with chemo-irradiation failed to control the disease and the patient underwent a salvage abdominoperineal excision.

Clinical presentation

Since anal cancer is rare but anal and rectal bleeding are common symptoms, it is not surprising that 75% of anal cancers are misdiagnosed as benign conditions initially.[20] The predominant symptoms of epidermoid anal cancer are pain and bleeding, which are present in about 50% of cases.[21] The presence of a mass is noted by a minority of patients, around 25%. Pruritus and discharge occur in a similar proportion. Advanced tumours may involve the sphincter mechanism, causing faecal incontinence.

Invasion of the posterior vaginal wall may cause a discharging fistula through the vagina.

Cancer of the anal margin usually has the appearance of a malignant ulcer, with a raised, everted, indurated edge. Lesions within the canal may not be visible, though extensive lesions spread to the anal verge, or can extend via the ischiorectal fossa to the skin of the buttock.[22] Digital examination of the anal canal is usually painful, and may reveal the distortion produced by the tumour. Since anal cancer tends to spread upwards, there may be involvement of the distal rectum, perhaps giving the impression that the lesion has arisen there. Involvement of the perirectal lymph nodes may be palpable on digital examination, rather more than may be apparent in disseminating rectal cancer. If the tumour has extended into the sphincter muscles, the characteristic induration of a spreading malignancy may be felt around the anal canal.

Although up to one-third of patients will have inguinal lymph nodes that are enlarged, biopsy will confirm metastatic spread in only 50% of these; the rest are due to secondary infection.[21] Biopsy or fine-needle aspiration is recommended by many to confirm involvement of the groin nodes if radical block dissection is contemplated. Distant spread is unusual in anal cancer, so hepatomegaly, though it must be looked for, is very uncommon. Frequently, other benign perianal conditions will exist in association with anal cancer, such as fistulas, condylomas or leucoplakia.

Investigation

The most important investigation in the management of anal cancer is examination under anaesthetic. Ideally, this should be carried out jointly by the surgeon and radiotherapist. Examination under anaesthesia permits optimum assessment of the tumour in terms of size, involvement of adjacent structures and nodal involvement, and also provides the best opportunity to obtain a biopsy for histological confirmation. Sigmoidoscopic examination is probably best performed at this examination.

Clinical staging

No one system of staging for anal tumours has been adopted universally. However, that of the UICC is the most widely used.[23] For anal canal lesions this system has been criticised as it has required assessment of involvement of the external sphincter. To overcome this a system has been suggested by Papillon et al.[24] as follows:

T1   <2 cm;
T2   2–4 cm;
T3   >4 cm, mobile;
T4a   invading vaginal mucosa;
T4b   extension into structures other than skin, rectal or vaginal mucosa.

Although insertion of the probe may be difficult or impossible due to discomfort, ultrasound can provide accurate information regarding sphincter involvement.[25] Computed tomography and magnetic resonance imaging may provide information on spread beyond the anal canal.

Serum tumour markers and other measures of biological activity such as DNA ploidy are generally unhelpful as they do not provide reliable information.

Treatment

HISTORICAL

Traditionally, anal cancer has been seen as a 'surgical' disease. Anal canal tumours were treated by radical abdominoperineal excision and colostomy, whereas anal margin lesions were treated generally by local excision. Over the past decade, non-surgical radical treatments, i.e. radiotherapy with or without chemotherapy, have taken over as primary treatments of choice in most cases.

Overall, the results of surgery for anal cancer are disappointing for what is essentially a locoregional disease. For decades radical abdominoperineal excision of the rectum and anus was the preferred method of treatment at most centres around the world. Abdominoperineal excision for anal canal cancer differs little from the procedure used for rectal cancer, but particular care is taken to clear the space below the pelvic floor.

Although extended pelvic lymphadenectomy in addition to abdominoperineal excision has been practised, such extensive operations did not appear to improve 5-year survival rates.[26] Compared with margin cancer, anal canal cancer is more likely to be locally advanced at presentation and to be associated with subsequent metastasis,[27] perhaps explaining the general preference for radical surgery. Around 20% of cases are incurable surgically at presentation. Results published since the mid-1980s reporting series collected over the previous several decades have varied widely in their survival outcome, but on average the 5-year survival has been around 55–60%.[15,21,28] Most postsurgical relapses occur locoregionally.

Around 75% of cancers at the anal margin have been treated in the past by local excision.[21,29] The rationale for this was based on the perception that margin lesions rarely metastasise, though this has not always been confirmed by prolonged follow-up. It may be postulated that disappointing 5-year survival rates (around 50–70%) might have been better if radical surgery had been applied more frequently, but this must remain a matter for speculation.

CURRENT

Radiotherapists have been treating anal tumours for many years, achieving equivalent survival rates but with the advantage of stoma avoidance in the majority of cases which might otherwise have required radical surgery. Ironically it was a surgeon, Norman Nigro, reporting the use of combined chemotherapy and radiotherapy to try to turn inoperable cases into candidates for surgical salvage, who began to turn surgeons away from operation as first-choice therapy.[30]

Radiation-alone therapy

The initial treatment for anal cancer was radiotherapy because the mortality and morbidity of surgical treatment of anal carcinoma were unacceptable. By the 1930s, however, it was recognised that the low-voltage radiotherapy used frequently produced severe radionecrosis. As surgery became safer, abdominoperineal excision for invading lesions, and local excision for small growths, became the standard treatment for the next four decades.

The development in the 1950s of equipment that could deliver high-energy irradiation by the cobalt source generator or, more recently, by linear accelerators enabled radiotherapists to deliver higher penetrating doses to deeper placed structures with less superficial expenditure of energy. Radiation damage to surrounding tissues was consequently reduced while simultaneously delivering an enhanced tumoricidal effect. Interstitial irradiation alone may produce local tumour control rates of 47%.[31] Improved results have been described using a technique of external beam irradiation, combined with interstitial therapy:[32] two-thirds survived for 5 years, the majority maintaining adequate sphincter function. An alternative is high-dose external beam radiotherapy alone, for which 5-year survival rates of 75% at 3 years have been described.[33]

Chemo-irradiation therapy (combined modality therapy)

Combined modality therapy for anal cancer was championed by Norman Nigro. Nigro chose to use 5-fluorouracil (5FU) and mitomycin C empirically as a preoperative regimen aimed at improving the results of radical surgery.[30] The radiotherapy then consisted of 30 Gy of external beam irradiation over a period of 3 weeks. A bolus of mitomycin C was given on the first day of treatment, and 5FU was delivered in a synchronous continuous 4-day infusion during the first week of radiotherapy. After completion of radiotherapy, a further infusion of 5FU was administered and patients later proceeded to abdominoperineal excision. It was evident to Nigro that the majority had quite dramatic tumour shrinkage: in his 1974 publication the tumour was reported to have disappeared completely in all three patients. No tumour was found in the surgical specimen in both of the patients who underwent abdominoperineal excision; the third refused surgery. Nigro's experience over the ensuing 10 years bore out his early enthusiasm. As he became more confident, he no longer routinely pressed his patients to undergo radical surgery, initially confining himself to excising the site of the primary tumour after combined modality therapy. Later, he dropped even this relatively minor surgical step if the primary site looked and felt normal after treatment.[34]

A variety of similar techniques have subsequently been described. With wider experience, it became clear that higher doses of radiotherapy (45–60 Gy) could be applied, usually split into two courses to minimise morbidity. Chemotherapy comprised intravenous infusion of 5FU at the beginning and end of the first radiotherapy course, and a single bolus of mitomycin C given on the first day of treatment. Modifications of chemotherapy dosage and prophylactic antibiotic therapy were necessary in elderly or frail patients, and those with extensive ulcerated tumours.

All the reported series describe excellent results, but it has yet to be determined whether similar levels of local tumour control and survival can be achieved without chemotherapy, perhaps thereby avoiding some morbidity. The only analysis comparing patients treated with the combined regimen and those receiving radiotherapy alone has suggested that initial local tumour control may be achieved in about 90% of the patients receiving various combined treatment protocols compared with 56% with radiotherapy alone.[35] This retrospective review compared patients who had received a combined treatment programme with historical controls treated by radiotherapy alone in the same institution. The overall uncorrected 5-year survival of the two groups of patients was similar at 58%. This group also looked at the role of mitomycin C in the treatment regimen and concluded from non-control data that this contributes to optimum local tumour control.[36]

The most recent data on combined modality therapy from the UK Coordinating Committee on Cancer Research compared chemo-irradiation with radiotherapy alone in a randomised multicentre study.[37] This study randomised 585 patients, making it the largest single trial in anal cancer. The trial showed that combined modality therapy gave superior local control of disease compared with radiotherapy alone. Only 36% of patients receiving combined therapy had 'local failure' compared with 59% of those receiving radiotherapy alone. Although there was no significant overall survival advantage for either treatment regimen, the risk of death from anal cancer was significantly less in the group receiving combined modality therapy (**Fig. 6.2**). As a result of this trial it seems that the standard treatment for anal squamous carcinoma should be a combination of radiotherapy and intravenous 5FU with mitomycin.

Surgery may then be reserved for those who fail.[37] New trials using alternative chemotherapeutic regimens including cisplatin instead of mitomycin C are currently under way.[37]

Role of surgery today

Although surgeons no longer play the central therapeutic role, they nevertheless have important contributions to make.

INITIAL DIAGNOSIS

Most patients present to surgeons, who are best suited to perform examination under anaesthesia to confirm diagnosis and assess local extent.

LESIONS AT THE ANAL MARGIN

Small lesions at the anal margin may still best be treated by local excision alone, obviating the need for protracted courses of non-surgical therapy.[38] There is some evidence that the risk of regional lymph node metastasis is not related to primary tumour size, which may explain the disappointing results sometimes reported after local excision; this conflicts with the view that tumour size is related to

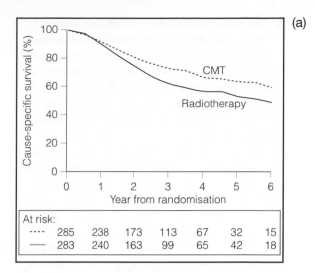

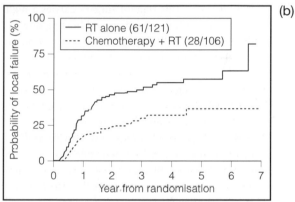

Figure 6.2 • (a) Deaths from anal cancer. Number of events: radiotherapy 105, combined modality therapy (CMT) 77 (RR = 0.71, 95% CI 0.53–0.95, P = 0.02). UKCCCR Anal Cancer Trial Working Party. The Lancet, 1996; 348:1055, Figure 5, with permission. Number at risk = number alive. **(b)** UKCCCR Anal Cancer trial: risk of local failure (T1–2 and N0). Northover J, Meadows A, Ryan C, Gray R, on behalf of UKCCCR Anal Cancer Trial Working Party. The Lancet, 1996; 349:206, UKCCCR, with permission.

stage, which explains the excellent results of local excision in small tumours.[15]

TREATMENT COMPLICATIONS AND DISEASE RELAPSE

Surgeons retain an important role in the treatment of anal cancer after failure of primary non-surgical therapy, either early or late.[39] Four situations may require surgery after primary non-surgical treatment: residual tumour, complications of treatment, incontinence or fistula after tumour resolution, and subsequent tumour recurrence.

1. The appearance of the primary site is often misleading after radiotherapy. In most patients complete remission is indicated by the tumour disappearing completely. In some, however, a lump may remain, occasionally looking like an unchanged primary tumour. Only generous biopsy will reveal whether the residual lump contains tumour or consists merely of inflammatory tissue.[40] Thus histological proof of residual disease is mandatory before radical surgery is recommended to the patient. For patients with proven residual disease, a salvage abdominoperineal resection may be the only option. In fit patients with extensive pelvic disease extending around the vagina or bladder, pelvic exenteration may need to be considered. In both cases, this type of surgery carries a high morbidity with impaired wound healing due to the radiotherapy.[41] A primary reconstruction of the perineal area is strongly recommneded in these cases. A rectus abdominis myocutaneous flap is my preferred option.

2. Complications of non-surgical treatment for anal cancer do occur in a proportion of patients, including radionecrosis, fistula and incontinence. Severe anal pain due to radionecrosis of the anal lining may necessitate either a colostomy, in the hope that the lesion may heal after faecal diversion, or radical anorectal excision.

3. Occasionally, a tumour is so locally extensive that the patient will be rendered incontinent as a consequence of primary tumour shrinkage. Although rectovaginal fistula may be amenable to repair, sphincter damage is unlikely to improve with local surgery, necessitating abdominoperineal excision of the anorectum. In my experience, abdominoperineal excision of the rectum under these circumstances is usually best undertaken in conjunction with a rectus abdominis myocutaneous flap to aid perineal wound revascularisation and facilitate healing of the perineal wound.

4. Should clinical evidence of recurrent disease develop after initial resolution, biopsy is again mandatory prior to surgical intervention. These biopsies need to be of reasonable size, number and depth as the histological appearances following radiotherapy can make histopathological interpretation difficult. If high-dose radiotherapy was used for primary treatment, further non-surgical therapy for recurrence is usually contraindicated, making radical surgical removal necessary.

INGUINAL METASTASES

Inguinal lymph nodes are enlarged in 10–25% of patients with anal cancers. Although inguinal lymph node involvement may be treated by radiotherapy, some argue in favour of surgery; however, histological confirmation is advisable before radical groin dissection as up to 50% of cases of inguinal lymphadenopathy may be due to inflammation alone.[21] Enlargement of groin nodes some time after primary therapy is most likely to be due to recurrent tumour; radical groin dissection is indicated in this situation, with up to 50% 5-year survival.[19]

Treatment of intraepithelial neoplasia

HPV infection of the anogenital area is very common and it has been reported that over 70% of sexually active adults have at some time had occult or overt genital HPV infection. In most individuals the infection remains occult, but in a minority, for reasons which are currently uncertain, the infection may manifest itself as either condylomas or intraepithelial neoplasia. As with other viral infections, it is impossible to eradicate HPV infection by surgical excision; for this reason, surgical excision of condylomas is effectively performed more for relief of symptoms and cosmesis.

Similarly, the natural history of low-grade AIN (I and II) seems to be relatively benign and therefore a policy of observation alone is probably adequate. This is likely to be particularly advisable when large areas of the anogenital epithelium are affected. However, for high-grade AIN (III) the advice is more circumspect as we do not know the natural history of this condition. If the area of AIN III is small, it is probably prudent to excise it locally and then to observe the patient. If the area of AIN III is too large for local excision without risk of anal stenosis, then a careful observational policy with 6-monthly review may be an option. Aggressive surgical excision of the whole perianal skin and anal canal and resurfacing with split skin has been performed in some patients but this usually requires the use of a defunctioning colostomy to permit the grafts to take. This sort of surgery necessitates multiple procedures and carries significant morbidity, which for a condition of uncertain malignant potential may make the treatment worse than the disease. Brush cytology has recently been shown to be of value in assessing perianal lesions and may be particularly valuable in patient follow-up.[42]

The use of immunomodulators in AIN has been investigated as a potential therapeutic option. While some authors report encouraging results,[43] these are all small studies of short duration. In my limited experience the disease recurs as soon as the treatment ceases.

Photodynamic therapy using photosensitisers may hold some promise for the future. It may be particularly suitable for use on the perianal skin with topically applied photosensitisers, but is still very much under investigation.[44]

RARER TUMOURS

Adenocarcinoma

Adenocarcinoma in the anal canal is usually simply a very low rectal cancer that has spread downwards to involve the canal; however, true adenocarcinoma of the anal canal does occur, probably arising from the anal glands which arise around the dentate line and pass radially outwards into the sphincter muscles. This is a very rare tumour, quite radiosensitive, but usually still treated by radical surgery.

Malignant melanoma

Another very rare tumour, this accounts for just 1% of anal canal malignant tumours. The lesion may mimic a thrombosed external pile due to its colour, although amelanotic tumours also occur. It has an even worse prognosis than at other sites. As the chances of cure are minimal, radical surgery as primary treatment has been all but abandoned at some centres.[45]

CURRENT AREAS OF RESEARCH

Natural history of AIN

The natural history of AIN is as yet uncertain. Evidence accumulated from several clinical studies

suggests that although it may have malignant potential, this is likely to be much less than that of CIN (approximately 35% malignant progression from CIN III to invasive carcinoma over 20 years) and more comparable with VIN (approximately 10% malignant progression from VIN III to invasive carcinoma over 20 years).

Until more is known about the natural history of the condition it is difficult to offer advice about treatment. However, patients with multifocal anogenital intraepithelial neoplasia seem to be an increasing clinical problem and therefore the following strategy may be helpful.

Modalities for the treatment of AIN

Given that AIN probably carries a relatively low risk of malignant progression, radical treatment risks overtreating the disease. Furthermore, logical management of AIN lesions is difficult because of the limited knowledge of their natural history. The evidence available suggests that AIN I and II lesions do not progress rapidly to AIN III. The current treatment strategy for CIN I and II is one of observation rather than excision; since AIN probably has a lower malignant potential than CIN, a similar strategy is currently advocated for AIN I and II. However, confirmation of the histological diagnosis is advisable before embarking on this policy. Six-monthly observation is currently used.

For AIN III lesions, confirming the diagnosis histologically and identifying the extent of the disease by multiple biopsies seems unreasonable. Observation of extensive lesions is the currently preferred option, although in patients who are poor attenders, and for smaller lesions that occupy less than 50% of the anal margin or canal circumference, excision appears to be a reasonable option. Provided the lesion is completely excised, a 5-mm or 1-cm margin may not be important. For extensive lesions a policy of observation at 3-monthly intervals is current practice. Before embarking on extensive excisional treatment it is wise to advise the patient of the significant morbidity associated with excision of the whole anal canal and perianal skin in these cases. However, there have been several cases of micro-invasive anal cancers identified at histopathological examination of resected AIN III lesions. For this reason ablative modalities of treatment such as laser ablation or cryotherapy cannot be recommended as these destroy the lesions, making histological examination impossible.

Brush cytology may offer opportunities for following patients with AIN in a less invasive manner than traditional biopsy under local anaesthetic. However, the reporting of cytological preparations is even more complicated than for cervical preparations as the cell yield is lower and the contamination greater. Further research in this area is under way.

Although a multicentre study of AIN is desirable in order to determine the natural history of this condition, it would have to be a long-term study and would therefore be prohibitively expensive for such a rare tumour.

• **Key points**

- HPV is an aetiological factor in anal squamous cell carcinomas. Women with previous gynaecological lesions on the cervix and vulva and the immunosuppressed (transplant recipients and HIV patients) are at risk for AIN. These premalignant lesions may be rapidly progressive in immunocompromised patients.

- The management of anal squamous carcinoma has changed dramatically in the last few years. Chemo-irradiation is the treatment of first choice for most lesions.

- Surgery may be the primary treatment modality for small perianal lesions that can be locally excised.

- Melanoma of the anus is very rare but difficult to treat as surgery is rarely effective in controlling the disease, chemotherapy is largely ineffective and the tumour is not sensitive to radiotherapy.

REFERENCES

1. Morson B, Dawson I. Morson and Dawson's gastrointestinal pathology. Oxford: Blackwell, 1990.

2. Fenger C. The anal transitional zone. Location and extent. Acta Pathol Microbiol Immunol Scand 1979; 87:379–86.

3. Office of Population Censuses and Surveys. Cancer Statistics Registrations. London: HMSO, 1988.

4. Muir C, Waterhouse J. Cancer in five continents (V). Lyons: IARC Scientific Publications, 1987.

5. Wexner S, Milsom J, Dailey T et al. The demographics of anal cancers are changing. Identification of a high risk population. Dis Colon Rectum 1987; 30:942–6.

6. Frische M, Melbye M. Trends in the incidence of anal carcinoma in Denmark. Br Med J 1993; 306:419–22.

7. Cooper H, Patchefsky A, Marks G. Cloacogenic carcinoma of the anorectum in homosexual men: an observation of four cases. Dis Colon Rectum 1979; 22:557–8.

 8. Daling J, Weiss N, Hislop T et al. Sexual practices, sexually transmitted diseases and the incidence of anal cancer. N Engl J Med 1987; 317:973–7.

   Excellent epidemiological paper on anal squamous cell carcinoma.

9. zur Hausen H. Papilloma viruses in human cancers. Mol Carcinog 1989; 1:147–50.

 10. Palmer JG, Scholefield JH, Shepherd N et al. Anal cancer and human papillomaviruses. Dis Colon Rectum 1989; 32:1016–22.

    Very relevant paper reporting the association between anal cancer and papillomaviruses.

11. Syrjanen K, Syrjanen S, von Krogh et al. Anal condylomas in homosexual/bisexual and heterosexual males. II. Histopathological and virological assessment. In: VII International Papillomavirus Workshop, 1988, p. 127.

12. Scholefield J, Hickson W, Smith J et al. Anal intraepithelial neoplasia: part of a multifocal disease process. Lancet 1992; 340:1271–3.

13. Cleary RK, Schaldenbrand JD, Fowler JJ, Schuler JM, Lampman RM. Perianal Bowen's disease and anal intraepithelial neoplasia. Dis Colon Rectum 1999; 42:945–51.

14. Morson B. The pathology and results of treatment of squamous cell carcinoma of the anal canal and anal margin. Proc R Soc Med 1960; 53:22–6.

15. Boman B, Moertel C, O'Connell M et al. Carcinoma of the anal canal. A clinical and pathologic study of 188 cases. Cancer 1984; 54:114–25.

16. Loygue J, Laugier A. Cancer epidermoide de l'anus. Chirurgie 1980; 6:710–16.

17. Klotz R, Pamukcoglu T, Souillard D et al. Transitional cell cloagenic carcinoma of the anal canal. Cancer 1967; 20:1724–45.

18. Stearns M, Urmacher C, Sternberg SS et al. Cancer of the anal canal. Curr Probl Cancer 1980; 4:1–44.

19. Greenall M, Magill G, Sternberg SS, Quan S et al. Recurrent epidermoid cancer of the anus. Cancer 1986; 57:1437–41.

20. Edwards A, Morus L, Foster ME et al. Anal cancer: the case for earlier diagnosis. J R Soc Med 1991; 84:395–7.

21. Pintor MP, Northover JM, Nicholls J et al. Squamous cell carcinoma of the anus at one hospital from 1948 to 1984. Br J Surg 1989; 76:806–10.

22. Nelson R, Prasad M, Abcarian H et al. Anal carcinoma presenting as a perirectal abscess or fistula. Arch Surg 1985; 120:632–5.

23. UICC. TNM classification of malignant tumours, 4th edn. Geneva: World Health Organization, Springer-Verlag, 1985.

24. Papillon J, Mayer M, Mountberon J et al. A new approach to the management of epidermoid carcinoma of the anal canal. Cancer 1987; 51:1830–7.

25. Goldman S, Norming U, Svenson C et al. Transanorectal ultrasonography in the staging of anal epidermoid carcinoma. Int J Colorectal Dis 1991; 6:152–7.

26. Paradis P, Douglass HJ, Hoylake E et al. The clinical implications of a staging system for carcinoma of the anus. Surg Gynecol Obstet 1975; 141:411–16.

27. Jensen S, Hagen K, Harling H et al. Long term prognosis after radical treatment for squamous call carcinoma of the anal canal and anal margin. Dis Colon Rectum 1988; 31:273–8.

28. Greenall M, Quan S, Stearns M et al. Epidermoid cancer of the anal margin. Pathologic features, treatment and clinical results. Am J Surg 1985; 149:95–101.

29. Greenall M, Quan S, Urmacher C et al. Treatment of epidermoid carcinoma of the anal canal. Surg Gynecol Obstet 1985; 161:509–17.

30. Nigro N, Vaitkevicius V, Considine B Jr et al. Combined therapy for cancer of the anal canal. A preliminary report. Dis Colon Rectum 1974; 27:354–6.

31. James R, Pointon R, Martin S et al. Local radiotherapy in the management of squamous carcinoma of the anus. Br J Surg 1985; 72:282–5.

32. Papillon J. Rectal and anal cancers. Berlin: Springer-Verlag, 1982.

33. Green J, Schaupp W, Cantrill S et al. Anal carcinoma: therapeutic concepts. Am J Surg 1980; 140:151–5.

34. Nigro N. An evaluation of combined therapy for squamous cell cancer in the anal canal. Dis Colon Rectum 1984; 27:763–6.

35. Cummings B, Keane T, O'Sullivan B et al. Epidermoid anal cancer: treatment by radiation alone or by 5-fluorouracil with or without mitomycin C. Radiat Oncol 1991; 21:1115–25.

36. Cummings B, Keane T, O'Sullivan B et al. Mitomycin in anal canal carcinoma. Oncology 1993; 50(suppl. 1):63–9.

37. UKCCCR Anal Cancer Trial Working Party. Epidermoid anal cancer: results from the UKCCCR randomised trial of radiotherapy alone versus radiotherapy, 5-fluorouracil, and mitomycin. Lancet 1996; 348:1049–54.

    A large well-run randomised trial that changed the management of this cancer in the UK.

38. Klas JV, Rothenberger DA, Wong WD, Madoff RD. Malignant tumours of the anal canal. Cancer 1999; 85:1686–93.

39. Salmon R, Zafrani B, Habib A et al. Prognosis of cloacogenic and squamous cancers of the anal canal. Dis Colon Rectum 1986; 29:336–40.

40. Northover J. The non-surgical management of anal cancer. Br J Radiol 1988; 61:755.

41. Nilsson PJ, Svensson C, Goldman S, Glimelius B. Salvage abdominoperineal resection in anal epidermoid cancer. Br J Surg 2002; 89:1425–9.

42. Scholefield JH, Johnson J, Hitchcock A et al. Guidelines for anal cytology: to make cytological diagnosis and follow up much more reliable. Cytopathology 1998; 9:15–22.

43. Corona R. Systematic review of imiquimod for the treatment of genital warts: all that glitters is not gold. Arch Dermatol 2002; 138:1599–601.

44. Martin-Hirsch PL, Whitehurst C, Buckley CH, Moore JV, Kitchener HC. Photodynamic treatment for lower genital tract intra-epithelial neoplasia. Lancet 1998; 351:1403–4.

45. Quan S. Anal cancers. Squamous and melanoma. Cancer 1992; 70(suppl. 5):1384–9.

Seven

Diverticular disease

Zygmunt H. Krukowski

INTRODUCTION

Although right-sided colonic diverticula are common in the Orient,[1] in Western society the problem is predominantly that of left-sided and particularly sigmoid diverticula. In relative terms sigmoid diverticular disease is a common condition, with a prevalence in excess of 60% in the population aged over 70 years,[2] while symptomatic complications occur in 10–30% of patients.[3–5] In view of the prevalence in an ageing Western population it is remarkable how relatively infrequently patients are admitted with inflammatory complications of this common disorder. Accurate documentation of the magnitude of the clinical problem may be obscured by the lack of sustained and determined efforts to document outcomes prospectively.[6] There are in addition major problems in relation to the elective management of patients with symptomatic diverticular disease[7] and those convalescing after an episode of sepsis requiring hospitalisation.

Morbidity and death in diverticulitis relate to the degree of sepsis at presentation compounded by coincidental degenerative disease in often elderly patients. The mortality may be reduced but cannot realistically be eliminated by optimal operative and supportive treatment in a non-selected large population of patients. In a condition in which the great majority of patients do not require surgery, the challenge in management is directed towards timely identification of patients who will benefit from operation. This will not only minimise the frequency of unnecessary and inappropriate interventions but also the morbidity and mortality that may follow a colonic resection. The traditional ethos of emergency surgery favours action, but unsupervised or inexperienced decision-making may mean morbidity from bad surgery exceeds that of conservatively managed disease. In the emergency situation, a conservative approach to operation appears to be the favoured option. Indiscriminate translation of this policy to the elective management of diverticular disease may deny patients with continuing symptoms, or those at risk of recurrent sepsis, an appropriate operation.[8,9] Forces other than clinical considerations may impact on management. Competition for scarce resources compounded by political pressure favouring the management of malignant disease may lead to major differences in both the rate and type of surgery for diverticular disease between countries. The differences in the application of laparoscopic surgery to the management of diverticular disease between the UK, USA and some European countries illustrate this point. Despite this, the two main challenges in managing diverticular disease, whether elective or emergency, remain those of decision for surgery and selection of the appropriate operation.

EVIDENCE BASE IN SURGERY FOR DIVERTICULAR DISEASE

Although there is substantial literature, the quality is poor.[10]

There are only two published randomised controlled trials in the management of complicated diverticulitis[11,12] and two consensus documents from the American Society of Colon and Rectal Surgeons[13] and the European Association of Endoscopic Surgeons.[14]

However, the latter is based on the expert synthesis of this indifferent evidence base. Although there are an increasing number of prospective observational studies, the vast majority of papers published between 1965 and 2003 are retrospective (**Fig. 7.1**).

PATHOLOGY

Aetiology

The pathogenesis of colonic diverticula has been the subject of recent comprehensive review,[15] which concurred with the concept that acquired sigmoid diverticular disease is a consequence of a deficiency in vegetable fibre in the diet.[1] Structural changes in the colonic wall with hyperelastosis,[16] altered collagen structure[17] related to ageing and disordered motility are all contributory factors. An active lifestyle and reduced intraluminal pressure associated with a high-fibre diet together reduce the incidence of diverticular disease.[18] Segmentation of the narrow-calibre sigmoid colon predisposes to high intraluminal pressure (Laplace's law) with characteristic protrusion of the colonic mucosa. The protrusion occurs at weak points where the terminal arterial branches penetrate the circular muscle adjacent to the taenia. The presence of a complete layer of longitudinal muscle and a larger diameter may account for the rarity of diverticula in the rectum. Colonic diverticula comprise mucosa and serosa, except within the mesocolon when they may also be surrounded by fat (**Fig. 7.2**).

Complications

Increased tension in the wall and pressure in the colonic lumen aggravated by visceral hypersensitivity account for the pain experienced by patients with uncomplicated diverticular disease.[7]

The major complications of sigmoid diverticular disease are a consequence of bacterial infection with local or generalised sepsis. Subsequent fibrosis complicating previous muscular contraction and mural thickening may cause stricture formation and obstruction. Fistula formation between the sigmoid

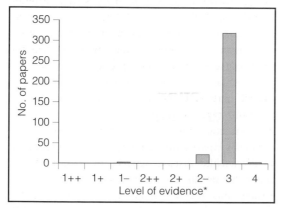

Figure 7.1 • Quality of published evidence in sigmoid diverticulitis. *Level of evidence as defined by SIGN (Scottish Intercollegiate Guidelines Network).

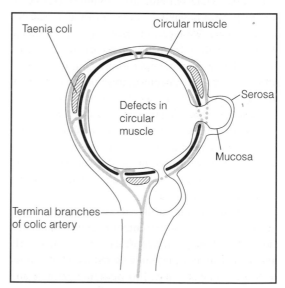

Figure 7.2 • Diagrammatic cross-section of colon showing sites of diverticulum formation.

colon and any contiguous structure is possible. Infrequently, profuse bleeding may arise from a diverticulum. Both smoking[19] and ingestion of non-steroidal anti-inflammatory drugs (NSAIDs)[20] have been implicated as aggravating factors in the development of complicated diverticulitis. Occasionally, the clinical and pathological diagnosis may be confusing because of the concurrence of other pathologies. For example, gangrenous sigmoiditis, which has been considered a consequence of prolonged muscular spasm, may reflect a vascular occlusive problem, and inflammatory bowel disease may coexist with diverticular disease.

Obstruction of a diverticular ostium promotes bacterial proliferation in a sealed space with the risk of abscess formation. Minor episodes with surrounding cellulitis may be self-limiting, but progression occurs in a variable and unknown proportion. Infection may involve a length of colon and spread into surrounding tissue to produce an inflammatory phlegmon. The rate of progression of sepsis and the initial site dictate the degree of localisation that occurs, a diverticulum within the mesocolon being more confined than one on the antimesenteric aspect. Slow development of infection allows adherence of inflamed adjacent structures, production of fibrinous exudate and localisation of peritoneal infection. At its worst a complex suppurative mass incorporating colon, small bowel, bladder, uterus, ovaries, tubes and occasionally ureter may develop. The extent of peritonitis associated with diverticular masses varies, and although there may be extensive fibrinous exudate and inflammatory peritoneal fluid this may contain few bacteria.

When an uninflamed diverticulum ruptures, a punched-out defect communicating directly with the colonic lumen may result, although such free perforation resulting in faecal peritonitis is uncommon. Normally, purulent peritonitis is the result of rupture of a previously contained abscess. Large communicating perforations occasionally release faecal boluses directly into the peritoneal cavity, but this sort of faecal peritonitis is probably due to stercoral ulceration secondary to pressure necrosis. Whether such a perforation is inappropriately attributed to the diverticular disease which often coexists is a moot point. Equally, when a single perforation due to a scyballous mass in the colon is

encountered, this may be included or excluded in a series on the whim of the surgeon with an eye to influencing subsequent analysis.

The highly variable inflammatory response and extent of peritoneal contamination that is a feature of diverticulitis may result in inaccurate classification. A considerable inflammatory exudate may be present, which on Gram staining shows scant bacterial contamination. While appearing dramatic, such reactive peritonitis has a different prognosis from a purulent generalised peritonitis resulting from the rupture of a previously localised abscess, for here the peritoneal fluid will be highly contaminated with millions of bacteria per millilitre of fluid. Similarly, although faecal peritonitis is notoriously associated with the highest mortality, early intervention may allow removal of solid faecal masses before peritoneal inflammatory changes become established. This will mean that residual contamination after peritoneal toilet is minor. However, when treatment is delayed, faecal contamination of the general peritoneal cavity is lethal.

Occasionally, a diagnosis of Crohn's disease is made in conjunction with that of sigmoid diverticular disease. This may be suggested by a preoperative barium enema showing sigmoid diverticula and one or more fistulous tracks, which often run along the length of the bowel, or by the presence of granulomatous changes on histological examination of sigmoid colon resected for diverticula. While this may indeed be the coincidence of two relatively common diseases, there is some evidence that a granulomatous reaction, histologically similar to Crohn's disease, can occur in association with diverticular disease that is limited to the sigmoid colon and which is not associated with any other current or subsequent manifestations of Crohn's disease (granulomatous sigmoiditis).[21,22]

Classification of contamination

Comparison between series is difficult because of the inconsistent description of peritoneal contamination encountered. Killingback's classification of the pathology permits accurate description (**Box 7.1**).[23,24] The importance of defining the nature and extent of the inflammatory process is well illustrated by Haglund et al.[25] Of 392 patients admitted with

Box 7.1 • Classification of pathology of 'acute diverticulitis'

Abscess
• Peridiverticular
• Mesenteric
• Pericolic (pelvic)
Perforation
• Free
• Concealed (indirect)
Gangrenous sigmoiditis
Peritonitis
• Serous, purulent or faecal
• Local, pelvic or generalised (diffuse)

Adapted from Killingback M. Management of perforated diverticulitis. Surg Clin North Am 1983; 63:97–115, with permission.

acute diverticulitis, 97 (25%) underwent emergency operation. Within the operative group, 31 patients had phlegmonous inflammation with no evidence of suppuration or perforation and the mortality was 3%. In contrast, in 66 patients with evidence of perforation the mortality was 33%. The relevance of this observation is that if the threshold for operation is inappropriately low, more patients with mild disease and an intrinsically good prognosis are subjected to surgery and a spuriously low mortality for surgery is reported. The overall number of emergency admissions, the number undergoing surgery and an accurate classification of the extent of sepsis must be recorded in any systematic analysis of the outcome of management of acute diverticular disease. Furthermore, the declining rate of autopsy in the UK must mean that some elderly patients dying with 'peritonitis' in whom surgery was considered inappropriate will have perforated diverticulitis.

PRESENTATION

The spectrum of pathology encountered in sigmoid diverticular disease results in a wide variety of clinical presentations.

Elective

Many patients who present with symptoms of lower abdominal pain, distension and altered bowel habit are shown to have diverticular disease during the course of exclusion of neoplastic disease by endoscopy and contrast radiology. In the majority of patients, advice to increase dietary soluble fibre coupled with reassurance will suffice. Failure of medical management with continuing symptoms over a number of years may justify surgery in the absence of other specific complications of diverticular disease. In a study of 261 patients with a radiological diagnosis of diverticular disease, only 6.5% subsequently required antibiotics for presumed diverticulitis, although 36% experienced recurrent episodes of pain.[26] Unfortunately, elective resection of the colon does not relieve the pain in all these patients,[27] and by inference this is because of a persisting underlying functional bowel problem.

Emergency

ACUTE DIVERTICULITIS

The typical presentation of acute diverticulitis is with a few days' history of increasing lower abdominal pain that localises in the left iliac fossa,[28] variably accompanied by nausea, altered bowel habit and irritation of pelvic viscera. However, depending on the disposition of the sigmoid colon, pain and tenderness can be maximal to the right of the midline – this is a trap for the unwary.

In the majority, left iliac fossa signs suggest a working diagnosis of acute diverticulitis, although there is a differential diagnosis that includes processes affecting the large or small bowel, the genitourinary system, major arteries and abdominal wall. Initial clinical assessment of the extent of peritoneal inflammation may be misleading and may overestimate the extent. Once patient anxiety is relieved following resuscitation and analgesia, an apparently diffuse process often becomes more localised. In a minority of patients there are unequivocal and persisting signs of generalised peritonitis and systemic sepsis, and it is in these that the indications for operation are overwhelming and further investigations are inappropriate. However, in the majority of patients a vigorous trial of conservative therapy is initially more appropriate.

FISTULA

The potential exists for fistulation between an inflamed diverticulum and any abutting viscus. Although fistulas have been described between colon and appendix, ovarian tube, uterus, ureter, skin and both large and small bowel, the most common are colovesical and colovaginal.[29] The latter may be more common after hysterectomy.[30] When a pericolic abscess, usually at the apex of the sigmoid colon, adheres to and subsequently ruptures into the vault of the bladder, a vesicocolic fistula results, with the typical symptoms of urinary tract infection and pneumaturia. In these circumstances diagnostic effort is directed at determining the site of communication and the underlying pathology. Sigmoid diverticular disease is the most likely cause, but Crohn's disease, colon cancer and even bladder cancer must all be excluded.

ABSCESS

Patients with pericolic, pelvic or mesocolic abscesses secondary to diverticular disease usually present with signs of localised lower abdominal sepsis and systemic upset. Although a classical pelvic abscess palpable through the anterior rectal wall may be clinically obvious, most diverticular abscesses are detected on contrast enema (**Fig. 7.3**), ultrasound or computed tomography (CT). In some patients the development of an abscess is more insidious and identified only in retrospect by outpatient barium enema.

HAEMORRHAGE

Bleeding from colonic diverticular disease is characteristically painless and profuse, with the colour depending on the level of bleeding in the colon. Bleeding from the left side of the colon presents as bright red blood with clots, whereas that arising on the right side is often darker and plum-coloured. Colonic bleeding is rarely exsanguinating, although it may be repeated or persistent requiring transfusion and ultimately operation.[31]

OBSTRUCTION

Patients with left-sided colonic obstruction due to fibrous stricturing in the sigmoid colon present in a manner identical to that due to the progressive obstruction developing in a carcinoma. Investigation and management are essentially identical and depend on the demonstration of typical features on plain abdominal radiographs, with confirmation of the site of the obstruction on an urgent contrast study. The differentiation between a malignant and a benign stricture may be suspected on the radiological features but is normally confirmed only after resection, examination of the opened bowel and subsequent histology.

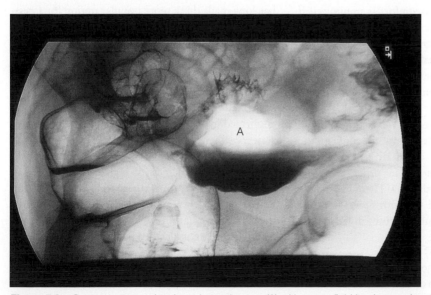

Figure 7.3 • Contrast enema showing a large abscess (A) with a gas–fluid level secondary to diverticular disease.

Intestinal obstruction also results from adhesion of loops of small bowel to an inflammatory mass in the pelvis and occasionally the features of small bowel obstruction are more striking than those of the initiating colonic pathology.[32]

INVESTIGATION

Acute diverticulitis/abscess

The value of a careful history and physical examination must never be underestimated. The clinical features in patients with mild disease may be sufficient to define management with minimal investigation.[33,34] Plain radiography of the abdomen and chest often provides indirect evidence of major inflammation, the most obvious being a pneumoperitoneum. However, the demonstration of a small amount of subdiaphragmatic gas, a traditional sign of generalised peritonitis, is not an absolute indication for operation, and management should be based on the clinical assessment of the patient not the radiology. Occasionally soft tissue changes, including evidence of obstruction, thickening of bowel wall and extraluminal masses, suggest acute diverticulitis.

Digital rectal examination but not sigmoidoscopy is essential before an emergency contrast study. However, sigmoidoscopy is mandatory before laparotomy and patient discomfort is minimised if this is performed under general anaesthesia before opening the abdomen. Sigmoidoscopy is necessary to exclude those anorectal conditions that might influence the proposed operation, the most important of which is a coincidental rectal neoplasm or a defective anal sphincter.

When the clinical features do not require immediate laparotomy, it is necessary to confirm the provisional diagnosis of acute diverticulitis and exclude alternative diagnoses in order to avoid prolonging inappropriate therapy. There has been a major shift towards spiral CT with bowel contrast when investigating possible acute diverticulitis (**Figs 7.4** and **7.5**).

The arguments in favour of this preference for CT over ultrasound or single contrast enema are persuasive,[35] despite the increased exposure to ionising radiation, particularly if usage is 'early and frequent'.[36] This concern should be set against the quality of images and their impact on management.

If access to spiral CT is limited, then water-soluble contrast enema remains a practical alternative. Although dilute barium gives superior mucosal definition, it is undesirable if perforation may be present and it is more difficult to eliminate from the bowel lumen in the event of operation. A contrast enema may show thickening, mucosal oedema, irregularity and occasional extravasation of contrast. Extravasation, if present, is usually localised, but free perforation into the peritoneal cavity may be seen. The examination should be limited to confirming the diagnosis, and possible synchronous pathology must subsequently be excluded by formal colonoscopy or barium enema in the convalescent period. It is important to remember that the information derived from an urgent enema, although valuable in determining management, cannot be considered definitive. The possibility of carcinoma coexistent with the inflammatory mass or elsewhere in the colon must be excluded after resolution of the acute episode (**Fig. 7.6**). Indeed, when the left colon is excised as an emergency for presumed diverticular disease, a colon cancer may be found within the mass in 20–25% of cases.[24]

Easier access to CT scanning in North America has long made this a more popular option for assessing the acute abdomen. While there are advantages over a single contrast enema in demonstrating extraluminal changes secondary to acute diverticular disease and also alternative diagnoses, it is clear that the threshold for requesting CT varies. The suspected diagnosis of acute diverticulitis was confirmed in only 43% (64 of 150 patients) in one series,[36] whereas perhaps more discriminating use in other series has shown 66–77% of patients with the disease.[37,38] Specificity is high, greater than 97% in most series,[35,36] and alternative pathology can be shown, which is why spiral CT should now be the first investigation when imaging is indicated. Radiologists are undecided about the relative merits of rectal or oral contrast. The former can be performed rapidly and will confirm extravasation, whereas the latter requires a 48-hour delay but yields extra information as it opacifies the small bowel.

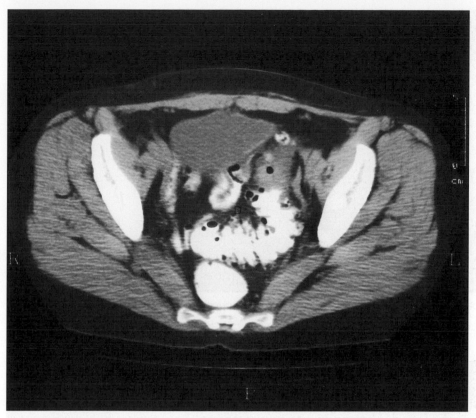

Figure 7.4 • CT scan of pelvis showing contrast in the colonic lumen and sigmoid diverticula.

While the improved imaging and diagnostic yield of routinely employed CT is an advantage in terms of diagnosis, the impact on early management may not be so striking. Demonstration of extravasation of contrast on either enema[39] or CT[40] increases the likelihood that operation will be required during the acute admission, but it is not an absolute indication for operation. Between 1990 and 1999 the routine first investigation in our unit was water-soluble contrast enema, with CT reserved for patients for whom management was not adequately clarified: the overall operation rate was 15% (**Fig. 7.7**). This is somewhat less than the 24% reported when CT is used as a routine[35] or the national average of 23% for England and Wales.[41] CT does detect more abscesses than would otherwise be diagnosed, but only a minority of these require intervention.[40]

Ultrasound has been employed effectively in some centres, but the variability of interpretation and dependence on operator skill reduces its general applicability as the first investigation. When the surgical staff themselves have received training in this modality, then it significantly enhances diagnostic accuracy.[42] Sonography has a role in monitoring the progression of known abscesses or masses.

Contrast enema, CT and ultrasound are looking for different things in acute diverticulitis. A contrast enema will show intraluminal changes and leakage of contrast, but may underestimate extramural disease; even so, sensitivity is high (approximately 90%).[35,43] CT and ultrasound are better at demonstrating bowel wall thickening, non-communicating abscesses and extraluminal disease than a contrast enema. Nevertheless, the overall impact on patient management should be similar, so the selection of imaging modality can justifiably reflect local expertise and facilities. All imaging investigations must be interpreted within the patient's clinical context to minimise unnecessary intervention.

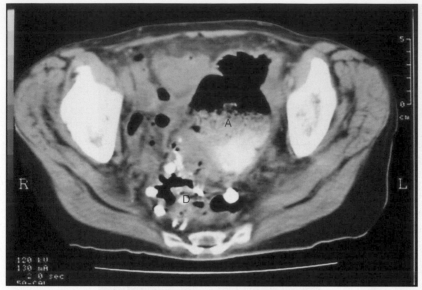

Figure 7.5 • CT scan showing large abscess (A) secondary to sigmoid diverticular disease (D).

(a)

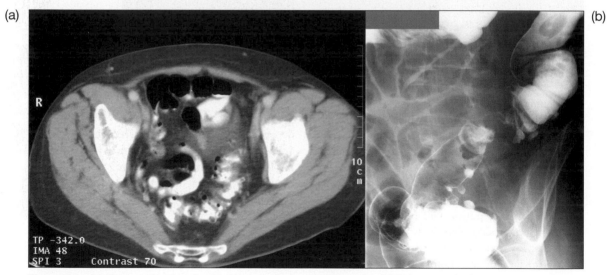

(b)

Figure 7.6 • **(a)** CT scan showing diverticulitis and colonic wall abnormality. **(b)** Subsequent barium enema showing carcinoma within diverticular disease.

Obstruction

If left-sided colonic obstruction is suspected on plain abdominal radiography, a single contrast enema will help determine the level of obstruction and exclude pseudo-obstruction.

Fistula

Barium enema is often sufficient to diagnose the underlying pathology in patients with a colovesical fistula, although to exclude carcinoma may require biopsy, necessitating flexible endoscopy and

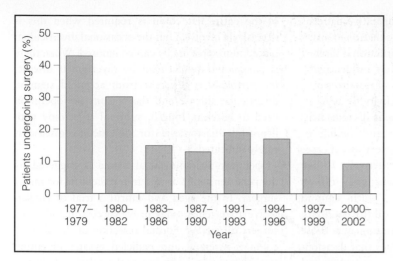

Figure 7.7 • Percentage of patients admitted with acute diverticulitis undergoing surgery during their emergency admission.

cystoscopy. Increasingly, CT is used as the first investigation and may reveal some of the rarer fistulas. Colovaginal fistula is much commoner if a patient has had a prior hysterectomy and a vaginal fistulogram may be more sensitive.[30]

Haemorrhage

Continuing or repeated episodes of bleeding require urgent mesenteric angiography, which should include visualisation of both the superior and inferior mesenteric circulation. Demonstration of a bleeding point (**Fig. 7.8**) permits targeted resection[31] limited to one half of the colon rather than blind subtotal colectomy. When angiography fails to identify the source of bleeding or has not been possible to arrange before surgery, on-table colonic irrigation with colonoscopy may identify the source and avoid subtotal colectomy. Passage of the colonoscope per anum and advancement to the caecum are straightforward when the abdomen is open and the instrument can be directed by the operating surgeon. Furthermore, transillumination of the colon may show the characteristic features of angiodysplasia. In a debilitated patient unfit for resectional therapy there may be a role for endoscopic haemostasis in some cases, but only if the bleeding diverticulum can be identified.[44] Embolisation of bleeding colonic lesions risks infarction of the colonic wall and thus is a procedure I distrust.

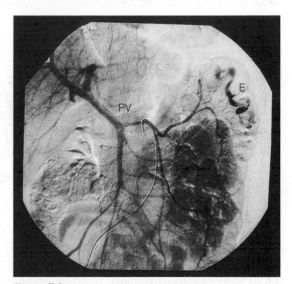

Figure 7.8 • Venous phase of inferior mesenteric angiography with the portal vein (PV) labelled and extravasation of contrast into the colonic lumen (E) secondary to bleeding from a diverticulum at the splenic flexure.

MANAGEMENT

The management of acute diverticulitis continues to evolve, there being more discriminating attitudes to operation, improved supportive therapy and increasing confidence in single-stage definitive surgery in the emergency situation. Yesterday's heresy evolves into current convention. There are many influences on interventional and operative patterns in both the elective and emergency situation in diverticular disease. Individual and institutional interest and, possibly, wealth can positively influence the rate of treatment. Conversely, lack of resources may be a subtle negative pressure on activity for what is, after all, a benign condition. There is disagreement about optimal patient selection and timing of surgery, so surgeons vary in the proportions of cases operated on as emergencies or electively. Unlike colonic cancer, where surgery automatically follows diagnosis, relatively few patients with sigmoid diverticular disease need surgery, and the boundary between those who need an operation and those who do not is imprecise. This means that decision-making is difficult, requiring experience and judgement.

Although diverticular disease is often perceived to be a common problem, a recent prospective audit from 30 UK hospitals indicated that on average only ten patients with complicated diverticular disease were admitted to each unit over a 4-year period.[6]

An individual consultant general surgeon is therefore unlikely to admit more than two or three patients with the most severe forms of acute diverticulitis in a year. Accumulating and maintaining experience is difficult for both trainee and consultant.

Elective

In the absence of prior emergency admissions with complications, elective surgery is reserved for so-called failed medical treatment. However, careful follow-up after elective resection for uncomplicated sigmoid diverticular disease reveals continuing symptoms in one-quarter of patients,[27] which probably reflects an underlying problem in gut motility, sigmoid diverticula simply being the most easily demonstrated abnormality. This possibility of postoperative symptoms should be explained to patients before surgery is considered. The extent of resection depends on the extent of the diverticular disease, but should never be less than a formal sigmoid colectomy with anastomosis of the colon to the upper rectum. The distal resection must include all the affected colon, for without this the incidence of recurrent disease is unacceptably high. Resection

of the entire left colon is required when this is extensively involved, but the occasional diverticulum placed more proximally can be ignored. When there is pancolonic involvement by diverticular disease, the aetiology is different from acquired sigmoid diverticular disease and the reasons for operation need to be clear. Indeed, subtotal colectomy with ileorectal anastomosis for diverticular disease is rarely indicated.

Operation for colovesical fistula is triggered by the persistence of a fistula in a patient fit for major surgery. In the aged and infirm a trial of conservative management may prove successful and avoid surgery altogether. Formal resection of the affected colon is essential and pedicled greater omentum should be interposed between the colorectal anastomosis and the bladder defect. The fistulous opening in the bladder wall is usually too small to require suture, catheter drainage being all that is required. Fistula recurrence is rare, except when the sigmoid colon is not resected but simply detached with repair of the fistulous opening, in which case there is an unacceptably high recurrence rate of the order of 30–50%.

Emergency

The surgical management of acute diverticulitis seeks to control peritoneal sepsis that is too extensive or which has failed to respond to best medical management (Box 7.2). Emergency management

Box 7.2 • Surgical options in perforated diverticulitis

Conservative
• Suture of perforation, with or without drainage, with or without transverse colostomy

Exteriorisation
Radical
• Resection without anastomosis
• Resection plus anastomosis
• Resection plus anastomosis plus colostomy

From Krukowski ZH, Matheson NA. Emergency surgery for diverticular disease complicated by generalized and faecal peritonitis: a review. Br J Surg 1984; 71:921–7, with permission.

may be summarised by answering three questions: when to operate, when to resect and when to anastomose?

WHEN TO OPERATE

This is the most difficult of the three questions. When abdominal signs are localised to the left lower quadrant and systemic upset is limited, few would advocate urgent surgery. At the other extreme, when there is widespread evidence of peritonitis and free gas, urgent operation for generalised peritonitis of unknown origin is indicated. For the remainder a policy of vigorous resuscitation and antibiotic therapy is appropriate. It is remarkable how rapidly patients with sometimes quite extensive signs of peritoneal contamination can improve on such a regimen. We have on occasion successfully managed patients with radiological evidence of free perforation without an operation either because clinical improvement was rapid or the risk of surgery unacceptable.

Optimal management demands serial assessment, ideally by the same observer. A trial of conservative management requires a readiness to review the decision not to operate in the light of the evolving clinical response. In my unit, a trial of conservative management is allowed for 3 days before deciding on surgery. In contrast to North American practice, abscesses are rarely drained percutaneously, the majority of those less than 5 cm in diameter resolving on conservative measures.[40] Extravasation of contrast increases the likelihood of surgery during the emergency admission but is not of itself

an absolute indication for urgent operation.[39,40] Laparoscopy has been described in the evaluation and treatment of acute diverticulitis. Although we have diagnosed phlegmonous inflammation of the sigmoid colon during diagnostic laparoscopy for suspected appendicitis, it seems unnecessarily invasive in diverticulitis when management can be determined by alternative methods. Such a conservative policy has resulted in a substantial reduction in the frequency of urgent operation for sigmoid diverticular disease over the last 25 years, with no apparent detriment (see **Fig. 7.7**).

WHEN TO RESECT

The indication for operation is generalised or faecal peritonitis or, more commonly, failure to resolve with conservative management. Surgery seeks to control sepsis in the peritoneal cavity and in the circulation by removal of the source. Critical analysis of published data confirms an increased survival rate in severe sepsis if emergency resection is employed as opposed to more conservative procedures that do not resect colon and which depend on drainage and proximal colostomy[24] (**Fig. 7.9**). This is why the clear recommendation is to resect the sigmoid colon.

More problematic is the situation where the operation has been performed prematurely or where the diagnosis is unexpected, the latter usually resulting from misdiagnosis as gynaecological or appendicular sepsis. Increasingly, however, with the wider use of laparoscopy in the assessment of the acute abdomen, an inflamed left colon may be found

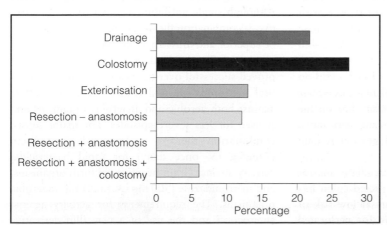

Figure 7.9 • Mortality following conservative and radical surgery for generalised and faecal peritonitis. Adapted with permission from Krukowski ZH, Matheson NA. Emergency surgery for diverticular disease complicated by generalized and faecal peritonitis: a review. Br J Surg 1984; 71:921–7.

with a variable degree of peritoneal inflammatory response. In these circumstances it is reasonable to avoid resection and rely on postoperative antibiotics. This has been needed only rarely, but has invariably resulted in rapid resolution without reoperation. The alternative choices of stoma formation, drainage or resection are unwarranted. Some surgical dogma might dictate resection to eliminate the source of peritoneal contamination, but an elderly or compromised patient is thereby subjected to a prolonged procedure with a major bowel resection and often a stoma, which itself may prove permanent. Although perceived as life-saving by some, the mortality, morbidity, inconvenience and potential for a second major laparotomy for re-anastomosis makes me favour a non-resectional approach in these cases.

Using a policy of conservative management with urgent investigation whenever possible, the problem of operating on an inflamed but non-perforated colon rarely arises. Every surgeon with an emergency commitment should be aware that such a conservative option is not only available but is usually preferable.

WHEN TO ANASTOMOSE

Given the above decisions on when to operate and when to resect, when to anastomose requires experience and judgement. In the last quarter of the twentieth century, considerations of safety led to advocacy of Hartmann's procedure as the safest option in managing left-sided colonic emergencies. Immediate resection without anastomosis eradicates the source of sepsis but without the risk of anastomotic leakage. However, it brings with it its own peculiar set of problems. Anastomotic avoidance means that a stoma will be required along with closure or exteriorisation of the rectal stump. These manoeuvres demand similar levels of technical skill to anastomosis in unfavourable circumstances. A left iliac fossa colostomy brought out under tension can result in complications as problematic as a poor anastomosis. Breakdown of the suture line on the rectal stump can lead to significant peritonitis, particularly if the intraperitoneal portion is long and packed with stool.

Widespread experience with immediate anastomosis after resection for the obstructed colon has led to its increasing use in patients at low risk of anastomotic failure after resection for perforated

diverticulitis. Anastomosis should be performed only in a fully resuscitated patient, with competent anaesthesia and a surgeon proficient in colorectal anastomoses. Good postoperative care and supervision will allow cardiovascular instability and hypoxaemia to be anticipated and treated, promoting anastomotic healing. In other circumstances considerations of safety should override surgical enthusiasm and anastomosis should be deferred.

HAEMORRHAGE

Strenuous efforts should be made preoperatively to localise the site either by angiography if actively bleeding or by labelled red cell scan if less acute. When this fails, peroperative colonoscopy should be attempted. If a bleeding point still cannot be found and thus targeted resection is not possible, then 'blind' subtotal colectomy must be performed. When this is necessary the patient's condition is usually parlous and it is unwise to perform an ileo-rectal anastomosis.[31] Completion of the operation by ileostomy and closure of the rectal stump is the prudent option. The possibility of subsequent restoration of bowel continuity can be considered later.

RECOMMENDATIONS

Conservative management

Rapid resolution of apparently extensive peritoneal contamination follows vigorous conservative management with fluid resuscitation, appropriate monitoring and systemic antibiotics and represents routine practice for most patients in my unit. Although single antibiotic agents may be as effective as combination therapy, none has been shown to be superior and most are more expensive. A tailored response reflecting the degree of contamination has proved successful over the years. A combination of oral metronidazole and trimethoprim is effective against both aerobic and anaerobic organisms and is used for less severe episodes. For major sepsis, combination therapy is favoured: gentamicin (7 mg/kg i.v. once daily) for rapid bactericidal activity against Gram-negative coliform organisms, and metronidazole (500 mg i.v. t.i.d.) for anaerobic organisms. The requirements for activity against enterococci and the use of a penicillin derivative remain unconvincing and is not essential in first-line therapy.

> Suitable alternative combinations include metronidazole and cefuroxime/cefotaxime or single agents like co-amoxiclav, imipenem or cefoxitin.[28]

Although antibiotics are the mainstay of conservative therapy, they must always be instituted before operation: the dramatic impact of systemic antibiotics on reducing the viable bacterial population in peritonitis is well documented.[45]

Operative strategy

Preparation of the patient undergoing laparotomy for advanced intraperitoneal sepsis requires thorough clinical assessment, fluid resuscitation and antibiotics supplemented by appropriate monitoring, which must continue through to the postoperative period.

INCISION

A midline incision is used because of its simplicity, reliable closure and low wound infection rate.[46] I prefer making the skin incision to the right of the umbilicus so as not to interfere with any left-sided stoma. Mechanical precautions that minimise contamination of the abdominal parietes from infected intraperitoneal material include wound towels, plastic ring wound protector and institution of a 'red danger towel' technique. Contamination of the abdominal parietes should be minimised by elevating the abdominal wall and aspirating pus and contaminated peritoneal fluid through a small incision in the peritoneum before it percolates over and inoculates the wound.

There are only disadvantages to a short incision in this situation, not least of which is failure to appreciate and document accurately the extent of peritoneal and colonic disease. Restricted exposure and access lead to inadequate surgery with incomplete peritoneal toilet and lavage and limited colonic mobilisation. Thorough access to all quadrants of the abdomen permits accurate assessment and classification of contamination. Inexperience, a desire to justify the decision to operate and anticipation of an unfavourable outcome are common reasons for overreporting the severity of peritoneal sepsis.

Although the operation is for presumed benign disease, there is little place for wedge excision of a few centimetres of sigmoid colon. Mobilisation of the left colon should be equivalent to a radical cancer operation with routine (although not invariable) mobilisation of the splenic flexure for tension-free formation of a stoma or anastomosis. The extent of resection of the colon is dictated by the extent of inflammation and adequacy of arterial pulsation at the point of division.

If there is gross faecal loading of the colon, this should be evacuated, even when Hartmann's procedure is chosen, in order to avoid stercoral perforation and obstruction proximal to a stoma. Access to the rectum is required in emergency left-sided colonic procedures. The rectum should be routinely washed out per anum as a prophylactic measure to reduce the risk of leakage from a closed rectal stump and in case a cancer has been unknowingly resected.

HARTMANN'S PROCEDURE

If conditions preclude safe anastomosis, the divided left colon is brought out through a trephined wound in the left lower quadrant, selecting a flat area of the abdomen and preferably emerging through the rectus abdominis muscle. Parastomal herniation may thereby be reduced. Avoiding closure of the lateral space simplifies both the operation and subsequent reconstitution of bowel continuity. Closure of the rectal stump can be accomplished by cross-stapling or suturing, although my experience (including closure of the rectal stump after total colectomy for inflammatory bowel disease) suggests fewer leaks in sutured cases. A single layer of continuous 2/0 or 3/0 serosubmucosal monofilament absorbable suture is supplemented with two long non-absorbable sutures at the lateral ends to aid future identification of the rectal stump.

IMMEDIATE ANASTOMOSIS

Although there is debate about the need for mechanical preparation of the colon, on-table colonic irrigation achieves near-perfect cleansing and has aesthetic if unproven clinical appeal. The appendix, or if absent the terminal ileum, is intubated with a Foley catheter. In the absence of a custom collection device, corrugated anaesthetic tubing is inserted into the colon proximal to the diseased area and tied in place with nylon tape. The rigid corrugated tube may result in siphoning with suction of the bowel wall into the tube when irrigation proceeds. This is prevented by inserting a 16 FG needle into the tubing to abolish the low pressure inducing the siphon.

The advantages of radical resection are that unexpected malignancy has been appropriately treated and healthy bowel is obtained for potential anastomosis. After irrigation and division of the rectum between the sacral promontory and peritoneal reflection, and after division of the proximal colon, an open single layer serosubmucosal end-to-end colorectal anastomosis is made with interrupted 3/0 sutures. There seems no place for proximal 'defunctioning' stomas in anastomoses at this level.

ANTIBIOTIC POLICY

For many years it was the practice to lavage the peritoneal cavity and abdominal parietes with tetracycline solution because of the low wound and intraperitoneal infection rates.[46] Difficulty obtaining a suitable parenteral preparation of tetracycline forced a change to cefotaxime as the lavage agent (1 mg/mL 0.9% saline). This has been used for many years in local paediatric practice with comparable results and continuing audit has confirmed equivalence in adults. The midline incision is closed with a continuous mass suture with 1-polydioxanone and further lavage of the subcutaneous space precedes primary skin closure. This strategy, even in such 'dirty' surgery, is associated with a low wound infection rate and delayed primary closure is not required at a first laparotomy. Postoperative antibiotics are continued for only 3 days, provided peritoneal contamination has been eliminated. Gentamicin levels are checked once daily and if systemic sepsis persists beyond 3 days, bacteriology and sensitivities from cultures taken at operation will be available to direct a change of antibiotics.

CONTROVERSY

Timing of emergency surgery

If all patients with sigmoid diverticular disease were destined to come to operation, a case could be made for early scheduled intervention with, preferably, a single-stage procedure during the acute admission. However, urgent operation is required in less than one-quarter of patients and the majority of patients without 'severe diverticulitis' do not experience significant recurrent complications over the next ten years.[47] An excessively interventional approach, whether born of enthusiasm or inexperience, can result in the accumulation of a large series of patients treated surgically with low mortality and morbidity and a high rate of single-stage procedures. It is likely that substantial numbers of patients with moderate diverticular inflammation are subjected to surgery in the belief, albeit misplaced, that this is life-saving. In these circumstances data may be produced that appear to support conservative surgery in the management of complicated diverticulitis, but current thinking suggests that not performing an operation at all may have been just as effective. Interpretation of such accounts would be aided by reporting the number of patients managed non-operatively during the study period.

Radical versus conservative procedures

It is noteworthy that although indirect evidence supports the concept that elimination of the source of sepsis (by resection) in the most severe forms of peritonitis is historically associated with lower mortality,[24] the two randomised comparative trials comparing primary resection with proximal stoma formation and drainage showed a lower mortality in the conservative group.[11,12]

Primary anastomosis

The role of primary resection and anastomosis during an emergency admission is increasingly being reported as an option, even in the presence of diffuse or faecal peritonitis.[48] It remains controversial and can be used selectively, but only when circumstances are favourable.

Subsequent elective surgery

Opinion is divided on the need for surgery following conservative management of an acute episode of diverticulitis.

Ambrosetti has refined the argument by demonstrating a relationship between the severity of the episode as judged on CT and the risk of delayed complications. Patients categorised as 'mild' have a risk of recurrent episodes of 14%, while 'severe' forms have a risk of 39%.[40,47]

However, the corollary of this useful observation is that the majority of patients do not suffer a further attack. The unanswered question is whether this level of risk merits subsequent colectomy. The variability of the acute disease and the wide spectrum of patients affected precludes categorical statements and exercise of clinical judgement remains appropriate. For example, an aged and infirm patient with a mild attack settling rapidly on antibiotics should simply be observed in anticipation that recurrence is unlikely.

There is consensus that the risk of subsequent episodes in younger patients (flexibly defined as less than 40 or 50 years of age) is of the order of 25%, but this is then variably interpreted as confirming the need for elective surgery[8] or indicating that the majority of patients will not require operation and all should be managed conservatively.[49] Ambrosetti reported a recurrence rate of 60% for young patients with an initial severe episode of sepsis, with even the mild form carrying a 23% risk of further complications.[40] Although such a high risk of recurrence is not universal and the severity of the presenting episode may be more important than the age,[50] there is an emerging consensus that any patient under the age of 50 years admitted with a severe episode of diverticulitis that settles should be offered elective resection.

Any patient admitted twice with acute sepsis, even if of limited extent, should be considered for operation, having taken account of coincidental risk factors. Elective surgery in a young patient is just as much a matter of judgement, but majority opinion favours operation after a single attack.

There is some evidence that long-term administration of a poorly absorbed antibiotic and mesalazine may reduce the frequency and severity of episodes of diverticular inflammation,[51] which might be an option to consider in a poor-risk patient. Similarly, increased admission rates in patients on NSAIDs implies critical reassessment of their need in the elderly.

Role of laparoscopic surgery

Laparoscopy has been advocated in the diagnosis and management of acute diverticulitis,[52] but the arguments for and against remain anecdotal for the present. Reservations about accurate description of case selection apply just as much to series of laparoscopic as they do to open operations. There is an accumulating body of published evidence attesting to the applicability of laparoscopically assisted techniques for elective colectomy (**Table 7.1**). Although some papers have addressed the comparative costs of laparoscopic surgery for diverticular disease, there has been no sophisticated health economic analysis to support or refute a wholesale change to this approach. Furthermore, publication bias may present a more favourable picture of laparoscopic surgery in terms of morbidity and conversion rates than actually pertains. Nevertheless, when successful, a laparoscopic resection for sigmoid diverticular disease appears to be associated with short-term benefits in terms of duration of hospitalisation and convalescence.

CONCLUSION

The management of complicated acute diverticulitis demands thoughtful clinical appraisal, appropriate imaging and a surgical strategy that combines conservatism before operation with a radical approach once committed if low mortality and morbidity are to be achieved.

Table 7.1 • Laparoscopic surgery for sigmoid diverticular disease: review of published series comprising more than 50 procedures

Reference	Year	Number	Conversion	Died
Dwivedi et al.[53]	2002	66	13 (19.7%)	0
Bouillot et al.[54]	2002	179	25 (13.9%)	0
Senegaore et al.[55]	2002	61	4 (6.4%)	0
Trebuchet et al.[56]	2002	170	7 (4.1%)	0
Tuech et al.[57]	2001	77	13 (16.8%)	0
Vargas et al.[58]	2000	69	18 (26.1%)	0
Burgel et al.[59]	2000	56	8 (14.3%)	0
Kockerling et al.[60]	1999	304	22 (7.2%)	3 (1.0%)
Schlacta et al.[61]	1999	92	6 (6.5%)	0
Siniser[62]	1999	65	3 (4.6%)	0
Smadja et al.[63]	1999	54	5 (9.2%)	0
Berthou & Charbonneau[64]	1999	110	9 (8.2%)	0
Petropoulos et al.[65]	1998	171	18 (10.5%)	1 (0.6%)
Schiedeck et al.[66]	1998	57	8 (14.0%)	1 (1.8%)
Overall		1531	159 (10.4%)	5 (0.3%)

• Key points

- Sigmoid diverticular disease is common.
- Emergency admission is uncommon.
- Contrast CT is the best emergency investigation.
- Urgent operation is required in less than 25% of admissions.
- Abscesses less than 5 cm in diameter resolve with antibiotics.
- If operation is required, resection is the best option.
- Primary anastomosis is safe in selected cases.
- Elective resection should be offered to patients less than 50 years old after a single emergency admission and after two admissions if over 50 years old.

REFERENCES

1. Chia JG, Wilde CC, Ngoi SS, Goh PM, Ong CL. Trends of diverticular disease of the large bowel in a newly developed country. Dis Colon Rectum 1991; 34:498–501.

2. Painter NS, Burkitt DP. Diverticular disease of the colon, a 20th century problem. Clin Gastroenterol 1975; 4:3–22.

3. Pohlman T. Diverticulitis. Gastrointest Clin North Am 1988; 17:357–85.

4. Almy TP, Howell DA. Diverticular disease of the colon. N Engl J Med 1980; 302:325–31.

5. Parks TG. Natural history of diverticular disease of the colon. Clin Gastroenterol 1975; 4:53–69.

6. Tudor RG, Farmakis N, Keighley MRB. National audit of complicated diverticular disease: analysis of index cases. Br J Surg 1994; 81:730–2.

7. Simpson J, Scholefield JH, Spiller RC. Origin of symptoms in diverticular disease. Br J Surg 2003; 90:899–908.

Good review.

8. Farmakis N, Tudor RG, Keighley MRB. The 5-year natural history of complicated diverticular disease. Br J Surg 1994; 81:733–5.

9. Schoetz DJ. Uncomplicated diverticulitis: indications for surgery and surgical management. Surg Clin North Am 1993; 73:965–74.

10. O'Kelly TJ, Krukowski ZH. Acute diverticulitis. Non-operative management. In: Schein M, Wise L (eds) Crucial controversies in surgery. Basel: Karger Landes Systems, 1999; vol. 3, pp. 109–16.

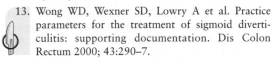11. Kronborg O. Treatment of perforated sigmoid diverticulitis: a prospective randomised trial. Br J Surg 1993; 80:505–7.

First randomised trial with some methodological concerns.

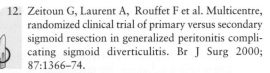12. Zeitoun G, Laurent A, Rouffet F et al. Multicentre, randomized clinical trial of primary versus secondary sigmoid resection in generalized peritonitis complicating sigmoid diverticulitis. Br J Surg 2000; 87:1366–74.

Second randomised trial showing reduced morbidity with primary resection.

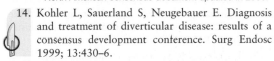13. Wong WD, Wexner SD, Lowry A et al. Practice parameters for the treatment of sigmoid diverticulitis: supporting documentation. Dis Colon Rectum 2000; 43:290–7.

North American consensus document updated in 2000.

14. Kohler L, Sauerland S, Neugebauer E. Diagnosis and treatment of diverticular disease: results of a consensus development conference. Surg Endosc 1999; 13:430–6.

15. Simpson J, Scholefield JH, Spiller RC. Pathogenesis of colonic diverticula. Br J Surg 2002; 89:546–54.

16. Whiteway J, Morson BC. Elastosis in diverticular disease of the sigmoid colon. Gut 1985; 26:258–66.

17. Wess L, Eastwood MA, Wess TJ, Busuttil A, Miller A. Cross linkage of collagen is increased in colonic diverticulosis. Gut 1995; 37:91–4.

18. Aldoori WH, Giovannucci EL, Rimm EB et al. Prospective study of physical activity and the risk of symptomatic diverticular disease in men. Gut 1995; 36:276–82.

19. Papagrigoriadis S, Macey L, Bourantas N, Rennie N. Smoking may be associated with complications of diverticular disease. Br J Surg 1999; 86:923–6.

20. Campbell K, Steele RJ. Non-steroidal anti-inflammatory drugs and complicated diverticular disease: a case control study. Br J Surg 1991; 78:190–1.

21. Burroughs SH, Bowrey DJ, Morris-Stiff GJ, Williams GT. Granulomatous inflammation in sigmoid diverticulitis: two diseases or one? Histopathology 1998; 33:349–53.

22. Gledhill A, Dixon MF. Crohn's-like reaction in diverticular disease. Gut 1998; 42:392–5.

23. Killingback M. Management of perforated diverticulitis. Surg Clin North Am 1983; 63:97–115.

24. Krukowski ZH, Matheson NA. Emergency surgery for diverticular disease complicated by generalized and faecal peritonitis: a review. Br J Surg 1984; 71:921–7.

Historic basis for recommending radical over conservative surgery for severe diverticulitis.

25. Haglund U, Hellberg R, Johnsen C, Hulten L. Complicated diverticular disease of the sigmoid colon: an analysis of short and long term outcome in 392 patients. Ann Chir Gynaecol 1979; 68:41–6.

26. Simpson J, Neal KR, Scholefield JH, Spiller RC. Patterns of pain in diverticular disease and the influence of acute diverticulitis. Eur J Gastroenterol Hepatol 2003; 15:1005–10.

27. Munson KD, Hensien MA, Jacob LN, Robinson AM, Liston WA. Diverticulitis: a comprehensive follow-up. Dis Colon Rectum 1996; 39:318–22.

28. Kellum JM, Sugerman HJ, Coppa JF et al. Randomized prospective comparison of cefoxitin and gentamicin/clindamycin in the treatment of acute colonic diverticulitis. Clin Ther 1992; 14:376–84.

Randomised trial showing that single antibiotics are equivalent to combination.

29. Vasilevsky CA, Belliveau P, Trudel JL, Stein BL, Gordon BH. Fistulas complicating diverticulitis. Int J Colorectal Dis 1998; 13:57–60.

30. Tancer ML, Veridiano NP. Genital fistulas caused by diverticular disease of the sigmoid colon. Am J Obstet Gynecol 1996; 174:1547–50.

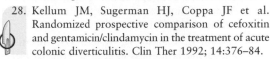31. McGuire HH. Bleeding colonic diverticula. A reappraisal of natural history and management. Ann Surg 1994; 220:653–6.

Good all-round review of diverticular haemorrhage.

32. Kim AY, Bennett GL, Bashist B et al. Small bowel obstruction associated with sigmoid diverticulitis. Am J Roentgenol 1998; 170:1311–13.

33. Rege RV, Nahrwold DL. Diverticular disease. Curr Probl Surg 1989; 26:128–32.

34. Thompson DA, Bailey HR. Management of acute diverticulitis with abscess. Semin Colon Rectal Surg 1990; 1:74–80.

35. Ambrosetti P, Becker P, Terrier F. Colonic diverticulitis: impact of imaging on surgical management. A prospective study of 542 patients. Eur Radiol 2002; 12:1145–9.

Excellent report from leading centre on impact of imaging on surgical management.

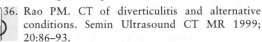36. Rao PM. CT of diverticulitis and alternative conditions. Semin Ultrasound CT MR 1999; 20:86–93.

37. Eggesbo HB, Jacobsen T, Kolmannskog F et al. Diagnosis of acute left sided colonic diverticulitis by three radiological modalities. Acta Radiol 1998; 39:315–21.

38. Brengman ML, Otchy DP. Timing of computed tomography in acute diverticulitis. Dis Colon Rectum 1998; 41:1023–8.

39. Kourtesis GL, Williams RA, Wilson SE. Acute diverticulitis. Safety and value of contrast studies in predicting need for operation. Aust NZ J Surg 1988; 58:801–4.

40. Ambrosetti P. Diverticulitis of the left colon. In: Taylor I, Johnson CD (eds) Recent advances in surgery. Edinburgh: Churchill Livingstone, 1997; vol. 20, pp. 145–60.

41. Kang JY, Hoare J, Tinto A et al. Diverticular disease of the colon on the rise: a study of hospital admissions in England between 1989/1990 and 1999/2000. Aliment Pharmacol Ther 2003; 17:1189–95.

42. Schwerk WB, Schwarz S, Rothmund M. Sonography in acute colonic diverticulitis: a prospective study. Dis Colon Rectum 1992; 35:1077–84.

43. Smith TR, Cho KC, Morehouse HT, Kratka PS. Comparison of computed tomography and contrast enema evaluation of diverticulitis. Dis Colon Rectum 1990; 33:1–6.

44. Prakash C, Chokshi H, Walden DT, Alberti G. Endoscopic hemostasis in acute diverticular bleeding. Endoscopy 1999; 31:460–3.

45. Krukowski ZH, Al Sayer HM, Reid TMS, Matheson NA. Effect of topical and systemic antibiotics on bacterial growth kinesis in generalized peritonitis in man. Br J Surg 1987; 74:303–6.

46. Krukowski ZH, Matheson NA. A ten-year computerised audit of infection after abdominal surgery. Br J Surg 1988; 75:857–61.

47. Chautems RC, Ambrosetti P, Ludwig A et al. Long term follow-up after first acute episode of sigmoid diverticulitis: is surgery mandatory? A prospective study of 118 patients. Dis Colon Rectum 2002; 45:962–6.

   Cohort study quantifying risk of late complications and requirement for surgery after successful conservative management of acute diverticulitis.

48. Schilling MK, Maurer CA, Kollmar O, Buchler MW. Primary vs. secondary anastomosis after sigmoid colon resection for perforated diverticulitis (Hinchey Stage III and IV): a prospective outcome and cost analysis. Dis Colon Rectum 2001; 44:699–703.

   Non-randomised comparison confirming relative safety of single-stage treatment.

49. Vignati V, Welch JP, Cohen JL. Long-term management of diverticulitis in young patients. Dis Colon Rectum 1995; 38:627–9.

50. Biondo S, Pares D, Marti Rague J et al. Acute colonic diverticulitis in patients under 50 years of age. Br J Surg 2002; 89:1137–41.

51. Tursi A, Brandimarte G, Daffina R. Long-term treatment with mesalazine and rifaximin versus rifaximin alone for patients with recurrent attacks of acute diverticulitis of colon. Digest Liver Dis 2002; 34:510–15.

52. Franklin ME, Dorman JP, Jacobs M, Plasencia G. Is laparoscopic surgery applicable to complicated colonic diverticular disease? Surg Endosc 1997; 11:1021–5.

53. Dwivedi A, Chahin F, Agrawal S et al. Laparoscopic colectomy vs open colectomy for sigmoid diverticular disease. Dis Colon Rectum 2002; 45:1309–14.

54. Bouillot JL, Berthou JC, Champault G et al. Elective laparoscopic colonic resection for diverticular disease: results of a multicenter study in 179 patients. Surg Endosc 2002; 16:1320–3.

55. Senagore AJ, Duepree HJ, Delaney CP et al. Cost structure of laparoscopic and open sigmoid colectomy for diverticular disease: similarities and differences. Dis Colon Rectum 2002; 45:485–90.

56. Trebuchet G, Lechaux D, Lecalve JL. Laparoscopic left colon resection for diverticular disease. Surg Endosc 2002; 16:18–21.

57. Tuech JJ, Regenet N, Hennekinne S et al. Laparoscopic colectomy for diverticulitis in obese and non-obese patients: a prospective comparative study. Surg Endosc 2001; 15:1427–30.

58. Vargas HD, Ramirez RT, Hoffman GC et al. Defining the role of laparoscopic-assisted sigmoid colectomy for diverticulitis. Dis Colon Rectum 2000; 43:1726–31.

59. Burgel JS, Navarro F, Lemoine MC et al. Elective laparoscopic-assisted sigmoidectomy for diverticulitis. Prospective study of 56 cases. Ann Chirurg 2000; 125:231–7.

60. Kockerling F, Schneider C, Reymond MA et al. Laparoscopic resection of sigmoid diverticulitis. Results of a multicenter study. Surg Endosc 1999; 13:567–71.

61. Schlachta CM, Mamazza J, Poulin EC. Laparoscopic sigmoid resection for acute and chronic diverticulitis. An outcomes comparison with laparoscopic resection for nondiverticular disease. Surg Endosc 1999; 13:649–53.

62. Siniser F. Laparoscopic assisted colectomy for diverticular sigmoiditis. A single-surgeon prospective study of 65 patients. Surg Endosc 1999; 13:811–13.

63. Smadja C, Sbai Idrissi M, Tahrat M et al. Elective laparoscopic sigmoid colectomy for diverticulitis. Results of a prospective study. Surg Endosc 1999; 13:645–8.

64. Berthou JC, Charbonneau P. Elective laparoscopic management of sigmoid diverticulitis. Results in a series of 110 patients. Surg Endosc 199; 13:457–60.

65. Petropoulos P, Nassiopoulos K, Chanson C. Laparoscopic therapy of diverticulitis. Zentralbl Chir 1998; 123:1390–3.

66. Schiedeck TH, Schwander O, Bruch HP. Laparoscopic sigmoid resection in diverticulitis. Chirurg 1998; 69:846–53.

Eight

Ulcerative colitis

R. John Nicholls and
Paris P. Tekkis

INTRODUCTION

Ulcerative colitis is a disease of unknown aetiology confined to the large intestine. It is characterised by mucosal inflammation with definable histological features. Medical treatment can control the disease in most cases but about 30% of patients will come to surgery. Criteria for the management of acute and chronic disease are now well established.

EPIDEMIOLOGY

The disease affects the young, has an equal sex distribution and is rare in the tropics. The annual incidence per 100 000 population is shown in **Table 8.1**, which demonstrates similar rates for males and females up to the fourth decade of life. Thereafter, the incidence in females declines whereas it remains much the same in males. Incidence rates of Crohn's disease are lower. As a rule of thumb, it is useful to remember incidences of 10 and 5 per 100 000 for ulcerative colitis and Crohn's disease respectively. The incidence of ulcerative colitis has changed little over the last 30 years, whereas that for Crohn's disease has increased about fivefold, although this may now be stabilising and is possibly in decline.

The prevalence of ulcerative colitis is about 160 per 100 000 population (compared with about 50 per 100 000 for Crohn's disease). This means that there are around 100 000 people affected in the UK. There is an increased incidence of ulcerative colitis among Jews and Indian immigrants to the UK.[1,2]

Table 8.1 • Annual incidence of ulcerative colitis and Crohn's disease in Europe per 100 000 population

	Men			Women		
Age group (years)	15–44	45–64	65+	15–44	45–64	65+
Ulcerative colitis	11.2	12.1	10.8	10.7	6.4	5.3
Crohn's disease	6.0	3.2	2.9	7.7	3.0	2.0

From Guidelines in Gastroenterology. Inflammatory Bowel Disease. London: British Society of Gastroenterology, September 1996, with permission.

AETIOLOGY

Although unknown, the aetiology is clearly influenced by genetic and environmental factors that almost certainly interact.

Genetic

Kirsner and Spencer[3] considered the possibility that inflammatory bowel disease (IBD) may have a genetic aetiology. There is a higher prevalence among Ashkenazi than Sephardic Jews,[4] and also an increased familial incidence unrelated to race. Between 10 and 20% of affected individuals have a first-degree relative with IBD.[5,6] The relative risk of a first-degree relative of a proband is 10–20 fold.[7] Although such associations may not distinguish between environmental and genetic influences, the importance of the latter is indicated by the higher concordance within Jewish families, the low incidence in spouses and the non-existence of IBD in families of adopted probands.[7] In the Swedish twin study of ulcerative colitis, there was no case in 20 dizygotic pairs of affected individuals compared with one case of 26 monozygotic probands.[8] This association is weak, particularly when compared with the concordance observed for Crohn's disease of 1 of 26 dizygotic and 8 of 18 monozygotic twin pairs.[8] In a study of 150 twin pairs by questionnaire, concordance was reported in 5 of 25 monozygotic and 3 of 46 dizygotic twin pairs for Crohn's disease and in 6 of 38 monozygotic and 1 of 34 dizygotic twin pairs for ulcerative colitis.[9]

Any genetic influence is clearly not Mendelian in nature. Crohn's disease and ulcerative colitis can occur in the same family,[10] and the overlap of features of the two diseases (indeterminate colitis) of 10–15% and the change of diagnosis from one to the other in a further 10% may be a feature of genetic heterogeneity. While it has been suggested that both diseases share some similar gene loci with other genes defining each condition, it is noteworthy that there are no reports of mixed Crohn's disease and ulcerative colitis among monozygotic twins.

Serum perinuclear antineutrophil cytoplasmic antibody (p-ANCA) occurs much more frequently in ulcerative colitis than in Crohn's disease.[11] Its positivity is associated with the HLA-DR2 subtype and its negativity with the HLA-DR4 subtype.[12] However, studies of twins have not shown increased p-ANCA in the healthy twin of affected p-ANCA-positive probands. Extra-alimentary manifestations, including ankylosing spondylitis and primary sclerosing cholangitis, are more common in first-degree relatives of affected propositi; both have HLA associations, including HLA-B27 and HLA-B8 respectively.[5]

Ulcerative colitis is more common in whites than in blacks or Arabs.[5] However, it is not possible to conclude that this is a manifestation of genetic susceptibility over environmental influences. IBD has a low incidence in underdeveloped countries but there is evidence that it increases with increasing wealth.

Environmental factors

Epidemiological work suggests that the incidence of ulcerative colitis rises about 10 years ahead of Crohn's disease.[13] This observation points to changes in environmental factors.

Non-steroidal anti-inflammatory drugs have a direct cellular toxic effect and lead to increased mucosal permeability. There is evidence that they precipitate IBD in humans.[14] It has long been recognised that some patients with ulcerative colitis have a history of infective proctocolitis.[15] Smoking is protective in ulcerative colitis[16] but not in Crohn's disease, where it is associated with an increased incidence of recurrence.[17] Cessation increases the risk of developing ulcerative colitis, and in patients in remission increases the risk of an exacerbation. This also appears to be true for pouchitis.[18]

Data are conflicting on the influence of oral contraceptives and most of the information relates to Crohn's disease. No causative dietary factor has been identified in humans. However, lactose intolerance can accompany ulcerative colitis, although this is rare.

Possible mechanisms

The large bowel lumen contains substantial amounts of potentially damaging substances, including bacteria, bacterial toxins and dietary antigens. Mucosal permeability measured by transmucosal passage of intraluminal EDTA or polyethylene glycol increases when inflammation is present and is normal when it is not.[19] The increase may be due to an epithelial abnormality resulting from damage by drugs or bacterial infection (see above) or from a genetic susceptibility. Passage of luminal pro-inflammatory molecules across the epithelial barrier produces an inflammatory response characterised by polymorphonuclear neutrophils and activation of both B- and T-cell compartments. There appears to be a failure of downregulation of the immune response, leading to continuing inflammation and tissue damage. Under normal conditions macro-molecules are absorbed across the columnar epithe-lium, and transported by microfold (M) cells that are in direct contact with macrophages and lymphocytes in the underlying lamina propria. In active ulcerative colitis epithelial cells express major histocompatibility complex (MHC) class II antigens, which present antigen to CD4[+] rather than CD8[+] T cells,[20] suggesting a defect of cell–cell interaction. There is also evidence that mucosal mononuclear cells lose the tolerance to autologous antigen that occurs in normal mucosa.[21] Study of mucosal cytokines has suggested a profile of the Th2 type,[22] but others[23] have demonstrated normal interleukin-4 production from isolated lamina propria CD4[+] T cells in active ulcerative colitis.

At present, it is not known whether ulcerative colitis is a primary immune disorder in a genetically susceptible individual, whether the primary abnor-mality is outside the immune system but accom-panied by an excessive immunological response, or whether it is a combination of both.

Changes in colonic mucin have been observed in ulcerative colitis[24] and also in ileoanal pouches,[25] but their significance is not clear. There may be a possible role for defective metabolism of short-chain fatty acids in the aetiology.[26] Pouchitis occurs in patients who originally had ulcerative colitis but rarely, if ever, familial adenomatous polyposis (FAP). The ileoanal pouch offers a model for the prospective study of IBD in humans. Whether this is the same or analogous to mechanisms that occur in ulcerative colitis is not yet known. There are, however, many similarities between pouchitis and ulcerative colitis itself.

CLINICAL PRESENTATION

The large intestine includes the colon, rectum and anal canal. The mucosal columnar glandular epithelium extends into the anal canal to the anal transitional zone, which varies in longitudinal length from a few millimetres to over a centimetre.[27] The anatomical extent of ulcerative colitis varies from involvement of the upper anal canal and rectum alone (proctitis) to the colon more proximally (proctocolitis). The rectum is always involved for all practical purposes, although relative rectal sparing can occur in patients receiving local anti-inflammatory treatment.

At presentation, approximately 50% of cases have disease confined to the rectum; in 30% this extends to the left colon (proctosigmoiditis) and in a further 20% disease extends beyond the splenic flexure (extensive colitis) (**Fig. 8.1**). Proximal extension may go no further than the splenic flexure or it may extend to the ileocaecal junction.

The disease is diffuse without any intervening segment of normal mucosa. A spared rectum not relatable to local treatment should raise the sus-picion of Crohn's disease. Backwash ileitis occurs only in cases with colonic extension to the ileocaecal junction, while anal disease occurs in ulcerative colitis in about 10% of cases coming to procto-colectomy. The lesion is usually minor, e.g. a low fistula or fissure. Rectovaginal fistula can occasion-ally occur in ulcerative colitis.

The disease can present with local symptoms with or without systemic disturbance. The severity of the former and the presence of the latter depend largely on the anatomical extent of the disease.

Proctitis

The disease is limited to the rectum. Inflammation results in bleeding and mucus secretion. Sometimes patients may become constipated but more often there is an increased frequency of defecation. Rectal irritability may result in urgency of defecation.

Systemic symptoms are very uncommon. Patients do not suffer from disturbances of growth, and only rarely from extra-alimentary manifestations or subsequent cancer. There is, however, a tendency for proctitis to extend proximally with time.

Proctocolitis

Proximal extension of the disease leads to worsen-ing of local symptoms and to systemic disturbances. Frequency of defecation with urgency associated with a bloody loose stool is the hallmark of colitis. Urgency is the most incapacitating local symptom.

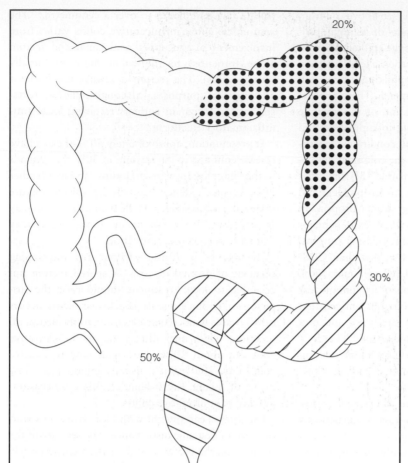

Figure 8.1 • Extent of disease at presentation.

When severe, patients may have warning of impending defecation of a few seconds only. In such cases, urge incontinence can occur. Urgency to this degree will dominate the patient's life and seriously affect work and family life. A protein-losing enteropathy is often associated with bleeding, which may lead to malnutrition with loss of lean body mass and anaemia. Retardation of growth in children may be a feature of extensive ulcerative colitis. In acutely ill patients, water and electrolyte loss may cause hypovolaemia and breakdown of the mucosal barrier may lead to toxicity.

The disease is characterised by exacerbations and remissions. Exacerbations may be precipitated by anxiety or stress but usually there is no recognisable causative factor. The disease may be of the acute relapsing type, with acute episodes interspersed by periods of complete resolution. Alternatively it may take the form of persisting chronic disease. Such patients may develop acute exacerbations that settle only partially on treatment.

Patients with extensive disease are more likely to have associated extra-alimentary manifestations and are at greater risk of developing malignancy. These complications can occur in patients with disease confined to the left side of the colon but are much more frequent with extent beyond the splenic flexure.

ACUTE PRESENTATION

About 5–10% of patients present with acute severe colitis. The patient will be ill with severe local symptoms, weight loss, anorexia, and water and sodium depletion. Intensive medical treatment has a high chance of inducing remission, although about 30% of such patients will come to urgent surgery.

Acute severe colitis may progress to toxic dilatation and perforation. The former is recognised by distension of the colon to a diameter greater than 6 cm on the plain radiograph. Abdominal signs including distension, sometimes with localised tenderness, and rigidity may be present. The latter suggests localised peritonitis due to either irritation of the parietal peritoneum in contact with the inflamed colon or a confined perforation.

In severely ill patients on high doses of steroids, perforation may display few symptoms or signs, although usually the normal features of generalised peritonitis are present. Perforation is a grave complication, with a mortality of over 40% even with surgery and modern intensive care. Bleeding is a rare indication for emergency surgery. When it occurs, the source is usually from ulceration in the rectum and the standard emergency operation of colectomy may need to be modified to include removal of part or all of the rectum.

EXTRA-ALIMENTARY MANIFESTATIONS

About one-quarter to one-third of patients with ulcerative colitis will develop at least one extra-alimentary manifestation during the course of the illness. These can be divided into those related to disease activity and those that are not. Some such as amyloid or hypertrophic osteoarthropathy can be ascribed to the consequences of long-standing chronic illness.

Arthropathy

Arthropathy is the commonest extra-alimentary manifestation. It can be divided into three broad groups.

ACTIVITY-RELATED POLYARTHROPATHY

This occurs in up to 20% of patients and is more likely in those with extensive disease. It is the commonest extra-alimentary manifestation, affecting predominantly the large joints of the limbs, the knees being the most common. The arthropathy is fleeting and asymmetrical and is rheumatoid-factor negative, being related to activity. It disappears when medical treatment induces a remission or after proctocolectomy. It can develop in patients with pouchitis after restorative proctocolectomy.

ANKYLOSING SPONDYLITIS

This axial arthropathy involving the sacroiliac joints and one or more vertebrae occurs in up to 5% of patients. The majority of such cases are HLA-B27 positive. The disease is unrelated to the activity of colitis and does not respond to proctocolectomy. There may be a genetic basis.

ASYMPTOMATIC SACROILEITIS

This is an arthropathy limited to the sacroiliac joint and is HLA-B27 negative. It occurs more frequently than ankylosing spondylitis and is also unaffected by treatment for the colitis.

Liver

Associated hepatic and extrahepatic disorders occur in up to 5% of cases. These are predominantly those with extensive anatomical involvement. Fatty degeneration is commonly seen. This may simply be a manifestation of chronic illness, malnutrition and steroid medication. It has no obvious clinical importance. Parenchymal liver disease of the chronic active hepatitis type and cirrhosis can occur. The latter may lead to portal hypertension.

Primary sclerosing cholangitis is more often seen in ulcerative colitis than in Crohn's colitis. Pathologically, the disease is characterised by a fibrous inflammatory reaction within the biliary tree leading to irregularity with multiple stenoses and biliary obstruction. The diagnosis is made on endoscopic retrograde cholangiopancreatography or magnetic resonance imaging (MRI). There is no apparent relationship between duration of disease and disease activity, although patients with primary sclerosing cholangitis undergoing restorative proctocolectomy have a higher subsequent incidence of pouchitis.[28]

Treatment by steroids, colectomy or antibiotics is ineffectual. Ultimately the disease progresses to liver failure. Such patients may be considered for liver transplantation.

Cholangiocarcinoma is a rare association with ulcerative colitis. There may be an induction period of many years and the risk appears to continue even after proctocolectomy.

Skin

Erythema nodosum is the commonest cutaneous manifestation of IBD. It occurs more often in Crohn's disease than in ulcerative colitis. The condition is activity related and can accompany the activity-related polyarthropathy. Pyoderma gangrenosum is more often associated with ulcerative colitis than Crohn's disease. It usually occurs in the lower limb as a circumscribed area of erythema with a punched-out ulcerated centre. Lesions may be multiple and in severe cases may be very extensive and occur elsewhere, including the face. In about 50% of cases, proctocolectomy seems to be associated with healing, a process that may take weeks to months.

Eyes

Uveitis is rare and is not related to disease activity. The condition can lead to scarring with visual impairment and ophthalmological management is essential. Episcleritis is activity related and occurs more often in Crohn's disease than in ulcerative colitis. It does not lead to chronic changes.

CANCER

There is a huge literature on the cancer risk in ulcerative colitis. The occurrence of malignant transformation has been known for years but it was not until 1967 that dysplasia was recognised as a histopathological marker for impending or actual malignancy.[29] The introduction of colonoscopy led to the strategy of histopathological surveillance of the entire large bowel.

Ulcerative colitis rarely presents with primary cancer but the diagnosis should always be considered in any patient presenting at an early age with adenocarcinoma of the large bowel.

The incidence of cancer in patients with ulcerative colitis depends on the duration of the disease. This is estimated to be zero within 10 years of onset, increasing to 10–15% in the second decade and to over 20% in the third. These rates were higher than those observed in practice by Lennard Jones et al.,[30] with incidences of zero below 10 years, 5% at 20 years and 9% at 25 years. In this longer follow-up group cancer has been reported in 10–25% of cases.[31–33]

Colonoscopic surveillance relies on the microscopic identification of dysplasia. There is general agreement among pathologists on the criteria for its diagnosis.[34] The presence of low-grade dysplasia is as likely as high-grade dysplasia (54% vs. 67%) to be associated with an already established cancer.[35] Based on the application of surgery for low-grade dysplasia, a cost-effective programme can be devised.[36]

INVESTIGATION

Investigations are used to make the diagnosis and to assess the severity of disease.

Diagnosis

A classification of IBD is shown in **Box 8.1**. In the tropics, infective causes comprise the vast majority of cases but in temperate regions these are rare.

Box 8.1 • Classification of inflammatory bowel disease

Infective
Virus
• Cytomegalovirus
Bacteria
• *Campylobacter*
• *Escherichia coli*
• *Shigella*
• *Clostridium difficile*
• *Chlamydia*
• Gonococcus
Protozoa
• Amoebiasis
• *Cryptosporidium**
• *Giardia**
Non-infective
• Ulcerative colitis
• Crohn's disease
• Radiation enteritis
• Drug induced

*Especially in immunocompromised patients.

Nevertheless, infective causes must be considered and excluded. The diagnosis of IBD is suspected by the history and confirmed by physical examination including endoscopy and biopsy.

Endoscopy

The earliest mucosal abnormality is loss of the vascular pattern. This is due to mucosal oedema which obscures the submucosal vessels. Epithelial oedema leads to the macroscopic change described as fine granularity. More severe changes include erythema, contact bleeding and occasionally frank ulceration. Where previous acute attacks have been followed by repair, mucosal regeneration nodules (coarse granularity) or pseudopolyps may be seen. Pseudopolyps represent tags of mucosa that have been partially detached during the active episode and remain as projections after healing of the ulcers. Rigid rectoscopy will only visualise the rectum. Colonoscopy allows assessment of the anatomical extent of more proximal disease.

Bacteriology

A specimen of stool should be sent for microbiological examination. If amoebiasis is suspected, the specimen should be examined by the laboratory within a few hours. In addition, diagnosis of amoebiasis requires a biopsy that the pathologist examines for cysts. Other causes of infective proctocolitis include *Shigella* and *Campylobacter* infection. The latter is the commonest cause of infective colitis in the British Isles. The microscopic appearances in *Campylobacter* infection are identical to those observed in ulcerative colitis. Special microbiological techniques are required to identify the organism and the microbiologist should be warned on the request form that *Campylobacter* infection is suspected. Bacillary dysentery, for example due to *Shigella* infection, should also be excluded.

Pseudomembranous colitis is a specific form of infective colitis associated with hospitalised patients receiving antibiotics. It is rare but should be suspected in a patient who develops severe diarrhoea after large bowel surgery. Endoscopy shows the pseudomembrane as an off-white slough of the mucosa consisting of necrotic mucosa and exudate. Again the microbiologist needs to be informed that the diagnosis is suspected since special techniques are required to identify the organism *Clostridium difficile* or its toxin.

Proctitis can be due to gonorrhoeal and chlamydial infection. The inflammation is catarrhal and consists of an erythematous flare associated with a purulent exudate. It rarely extends proximally beyond a few centimetres from the anal verge. When suspected, a rectal swab should be combined with urethral and vaginal swabs. Again the microbiologist should be forewarned. Opportunistic infection may cause proctocolitis in immunocompromised patients (e.g. those with human immunodeficiency virus infection) or those on immunosuppressive drugs. Examples include cytomegalovirus, *Mycobacterium avium-intracellulare* and cryptosporidia (see also Chapter 15).

Radiology

Radiological investigation is necessary only in cases with inflammation extending beyond the range of the rigid sigmoidoscope. Most clinicians prefer endoscopy to assess the extent of disease, but barium enema examination gives a permanent record that is easily interpreted. In most hospitals, this is carried out with full bowel preparation. Although there is no evidence that bowel preparation disturbs the patient, this is avoided by using the instant barium enema that can be carried out during the patient's first outpatient visit and then immediately followed by a biopsy. Using this approach the diagnosis and assessment of anatomical extent are made in one visit.

The radiological features will show the proximal extent and also the severity of mucosal damage (**Fig. 8.2**). This ranges from granularity to deep ulceration and pseudopolyp formation. Haustra are absent and the bowel calibre has a so-called 'lead pipe' appearance. Stricture is uncommon but may indicate malignancy.

Histopathology

Histopathological examination of a mucosal biopsy is the basis of diagnosis.

BIOPSY TECHNIQUE

A biopsy is obligatory and is most easily obtained during rigid rectoscopy. Colonoscopy used for surveillance allows multiple biopsies to be taken.

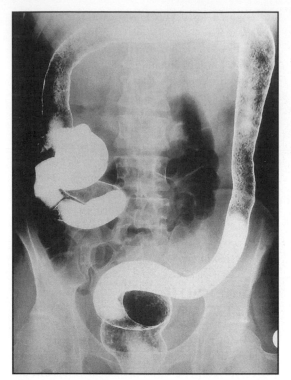

Figure 8.2 • Unprepared barium enema in a patient with extensive colitis. Note the narrowed bowel lacking in haustra.

Perforation and bleeding are potential complications. The patient must be asked whether anticoagulants or immunosuppressive drugs are being taken before a biopsy is performed. The biopsy taken during rigid rectoscopy itself should be obtained with forceps with a circular cusp that minimises the depth of penetration. The optimal site is about 7 cm from the anal verge in the posterior quadrant of the rectum. Adequate vision during rectoscopy must be assured and the jaws of the forceps are firmly closed, taking a bite of mucosa and submucosa. After the biopsy has been taken, the site must be inspected for bleeding. If this is significant, then local application of a topical solution of adrenaline (epinephrine) 1 in 1000 should be performed. If the clinician is concerned about bleeding, the patient should be re-examined about 20 minutes later. The biopsy should be carefully oriented onto a ground glass slide and placed in formalin (10%).

HISTOPATHOLOGICAL FEATURES

The disease is confined to the mucosa except in fulminant colitis, where penetration of the inflam-matory process into the muscularis propria may be observed. The disease itself may be in a state of acute exacerbation or remission. Fulminant colitis shows exaggerated features of those seen in acute disease.

ACTIVE DISEASE

In active disease (**Fig. 8.3**), there is mucosal thickening with heavy infiltration of plasma cells and lymphocytes into the lamina propria. These are accompanied by neutrophils, eosinophils and mast cells. Mucin within goblet cells is discharged so that these are less evident or absent. The extent of neutrophil infiltration is the best histopathological marker of the severity of inflammation. In mild disease, neutrophils are distributed within the lamina propria. When they are extruded into the crypt lumen, a crypt abscess is said to be present. The number of crypt abscesses significantly correlates with the severity of disease. Ulceration may be present and to some extent this is the result of rupture of crypt abscesses leading to mucosal destruction. Areas of residual epithelium between zones of ulceration are referred to as pseudopolyps. Damage to the crypt basal epithelium leads to loss of crypts. Attempts at regeneration may be mistaken for dysplasia but the presence of more normal cells towards the luminal surface allows these two conditions to be distin-guished. There may be branching of crypts owing to regeneration following crypt epithelial damage.

FULMINANT COLITIS

Progression of these acute changes occurs in cases with fulminant colitis. Ulceration can be very exten-sive, leaving large areas of exposed muscularis propria covered with granulation tissue. This may be associated with thinning of the musculature and colonic dilatation. Inflammation may be transmural and fissure formation may be seen.

REMISSION

Colitis in remission may leave a distorted archi-tectural pattern with crypt depletion. Mucosal cells that remain often regain normal function and show retained mucin as identifiable goblet cells. A chronic inflammatory cell exudate in the lamina propria is likely to be present, although this may be very mild in patients in remission for long periods of time. Paneth cell metaplasia indicates episodes of previous colitis.

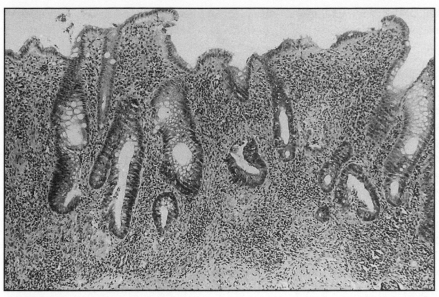

Figure 8.3 • Microscopic appearances of active colitis. Note the white cell infiltration of the lamina propria, goblet cell depletion and crypt abscess formation.

ULCERATIVE COLITIS OR CROHN'S DISEASE

Diagnostic difficulties in differentiating ulcerative colitis and Crohn's disease have been recognised for many years. The pathological criteria distinguishing them have been defined and are shown in **Box 8.2.**

INDETERMINATE COLITIS

In some cases insufficient numbers of these diagnostic attributes are present or there is considerable overlap and atypical features are seen. Thus it may be impossible for the pathologist to separate the two diseases, which may be reported as unclassified

Box 8.2 • Histopathological distinction between ulcerative colitis and Crohn's disease

	Ulcerative colitis	**Crohn's disease**
Macroscopic		
Distribution	Colon and rectum	Gastrointestinal tract
Rectum	Involved	Often spared
Anal disease	Rare	Common
Malignant risk	10% at 20 years	Probably similar (large bowel disease)
Intestinal fistula	Never	Common
Stricture (non-neoplastic)	Rare	Common
Microscopic		
Bowel wall involvement	Mucosa and submucosa	Full thickness
Granulomas	None	60–70%
Mucus secretion	Impaired (goblet cell depletion)	Slightly impaired
Fissuring	Absent	Common
Crypt abscess	Common	Rare

colitis or as unclassified colitis with additional indication of the possible or probable presence of Crohn's disease or ulcerative colitis. In about 10% of cases, however, the pathologist will be able to state only that the colitis is indeterminate.[37]

Indeterminate colitis is not necessarily a disease entity. It is more a diagnostic label which indicates that the histopathologist is unable to come to a firm diagnosis. Usually the dilemma arises in specimens removed during the acute stage of disease where the severity of inflammation may be combined with features of both ulcerative colitis and Crohn's disease.

The first step in resolving the diagnostic dilemma should be to obtain more tissue for histopathological examination. If the patient has had a colectomy for acute disease, then a biopsy from the rectal stump should be carried out. Further help may be obtained by endoscopy or radiology, which may show normal areas separated by abnormal segments suggestive of Crohn's disease. The presence of anal or small bowel disease would be further evidence.

When histopathological, radiological and clinical features are considered together, patients with indeterminate colitis can usually be judged to incline more to Crohn's disease or ulcerative colitis. Where they cannot, the natural history tends to incline to that of ulcerative colitis.[38]

MANAGEMENT

The unit

The management of IBD requires teamwork involving collaboration between various professionals. Best care is now no longer achieved by the medical staff alone. Input from nurses, nutritionists and stomatherapists should combine to achieve optimal management. The psychosocial consequences of IBD can be devastating. The social worker may offer vital support to the patient and family and as much attention as possible should be given to assist the patient in school or at work. The creation of an IBD unit will give the best opportunity to achieve best care. There must be a close working relationship between gastroenterologist and surgeon. Patient-sharing where appropriate, joint outpatient consultations for difficult cases, and early involve-

ment of the surgeon in acute disease are situations in which such collaboration can be most helpful.

Assessment of severity

Treatment is related to the severity of the disease, which is also related to the anatomical extent as assessed by endoscopy and radiology. Rigid sigmoidoscopy will identify those with disease confined to the rectum but more proximal examination is indicated in all other cases. The severity of symptoms, the presence of extra-alimentary disease and evidence of chronic ill health, such as malnutrition or anaemia, must all be ascertained.

TREATMENT

The classification of Truelove[39] that divided patients into those with mild, moderate and severe disease can roughly be correlated with anatomical extent and the choice of treatment. However, today it is more convenient to divide patients into those with distal disease or those with more proximal extension.

Distal disease

Disease is limited to the rectum or distal sigmoid as determined by endoscopy with biopsy confirmation. Treatment is medical in almost all cases. It involves the combination of steroids with 5-aminosalicylic acid preparations. The former is intended to induce a remission, the latter to maintain a remission once achieved. Local steroids can be given as suppositories (e.g. prednisolone 5 mg) or as an enema. Suppositories are effective against inflammation of the lower and mid rectum, whereas enemas extend proximally well into the left colon. Steroid preparations such as budesonide have a lesser tendency for absorption. An oral 5-aminosalicylic acid preparation should also be prescribed from the beginning. Salazopyrin is the cheapest of these and well tolerated by most patients, although about 20% will reject it owing to nausea, headache or skin eruptions. Rarely, marrow toxicity and oligospermia can occur. A dose of 500–1000 mg three times daily should be prescribed.

The sulphonamide–aspirin bond in Salazopyrin protects the aspirin element from degradation in the upper intestine. On arrival in the caecum, the aspirin is liberated through fracture of the bond by microbiological enzymes. The adverse effects of sulfasalazine are mostly due to the sulphonamide component. Modern 5-aminosalicylic drugs (Asacol, Pentasa and Dipentum) no longer contain this and have been formulated to protect the aspirin from degradation before it arrives in the colon. There are no convincing data to guide the clinician on the duration of 5-aminosalicylic acid treatment but it is generally felt that this should be continued indefinitely.

Some patients do not respond to this regimen and the proctitis is then said to be refractory. Other preparations, including bismuth, nicotine and witch hazel, have been used. It is worth adding a topical 5-aminosalicylic acid preparation to any of the above and this may sometimes be effective.

Most patients with distal disease can be satisfactorily treated in this manner, but in some cases progressive inflammation extends proximally with a corresponding worsening of symptoms.

Proximal extension

Medical treatment can be divided into anti-inflammatory, nutritional, symptomatic and psychological. Steroids are used to induce remission and 5-aminosalicylic acid preparations should be given to maintain a remission.

Except for the small group of patients who require admission for acute severe colitis (see below), prednisolone is given in an initial dose of 30 mg, gradually reducing this as remission occurs over the next few weeks. Azathioprine can be tried in patients who do not respond to steroids or in those who are steroid-dependent in the hope of avoiding long-term steroid treatment. Ciclosporin can be effective in inducing remission in patients suffering from acute severe colitis but its role in chronic disease is not established. The nutritional state should be monitored. There is no specific diet that influences the activity of the disease but a high protein and calorie intake should be encouraged. Specific replacement treatment such as iron may be necessary. Antidiarrhoeal agents including codeine phosphate and loperamide are usually effective in reducing frequency and urgency. Maximal doses are 60 mg four times daily and 8 mg four times daily

respectively. Lomotil (atropine and diphenoxylate) is occasionally effective where there has been a poor response.

ACUTE SEVERE COLITIS

Patients with severe acute colitis require admission to hospital. Initial treatment is medical but about 30% of patients will come to surgery. Surgery is absolutely indicated in cases with acute toxic dilatation or perforation.

Management

Management consists of monitoring and treatment.

MONITORING

Monitoring is essential to assess improvement or deterioration. The pulse rate, temperature and blood pressure are regularly recorded. The patient should be weighed on admission and twice weekly thereafter. Blood should be sent for haemoglobin, albumin and electrolyte estimations. A stool chart is essential. This should record every defecation with an assessment of volume and consistency of stool and the presence of blood on each occasion. The patient should be examined regularly to determine general condition and the state of the abdomen. Abdominal distension is an important physical sign suggesting that toxic megacolon may be developing. It may be evident clinically but a plain radiograph will enable an assessment of colonic diameter (**Fig. 8.4**). The development of abdominal tenderness and rigidity suggests local or general peritonitis. The presence of intramural gas on the plain abdominal radiograph is a sign of imminent perforation and is therefore an indication for immediate surgery.

MEDICAL TREATMENT

Treatment involves bed rest and the correction of water and electrolyte depletion by intravenous infusion of normal saline. Severely anaemic patients should be given blood. Where there is no immediate indication for surgery, the patient should be encouraged to eat a high protein and calorie diet. Intravenous nutrition may be indicated in severely malnourished patients, as judged by decrease in lean body mass and serum albumin, but there is no

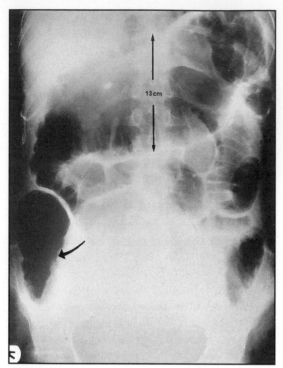

Figure 8.4 • Plain abdominal radiograph of toxic dilatation. Note the bowel diameter (>6 cm), absence of caecal faecal shadowing and widening of the bowel wall shadow (lower left arrow).

Table 8.2 • Urgent surgery for ulcerative colitis 1976–90

Main reason for surgery	No. of patients
Failed medical treatment for severe colitis	71
Toxic dilatation	23
Perforation	9
Bleeding	2
Other	1
Total	**106**

From Melville DM, Ritchie JK, Nicholls RJ et al. Surgery for ulcerative colitis in the area of the pouch: the St Mark's Hospital experience. Gut 1994; 35:1076–80, with permission.

evidence that 'bowel rest' with intravenous nutrition will specifically lead to improvement of the inflammatory component.

Anti-inflammatory treatment is given in the form of intravenous prednisolone in a dose of 60 mg daily. It is doubtful that 5-aminosalicylic drugs are of value in acute disease. Some gastroenterologists recommend an H_2 receptor antagonist or a proton pump inhibitor to protect against upper gastrointestinal ulceration. Ciclosporin has been reported to induce remission in over 50% of patients unresponsive to steroids but early relapse may occur, resulting in the same clinical situation within a short period.[40]

Surgery

INDICATIONS

Surgery has a major role in the management of acute colitis. The relative frequency of the main indications for surgery are shown in **Table 8.2**.

Acute severe colitis occurs in about 10% of patients with ulcerative colitis and is the initial presentation of 30% of patients with ulcerative colitis.[41]

Failure to respond to medical treatment should be recognised early during the course of management. The gastroenterologist and surgeon should confer at least daily to decide whether there has been improvement, stagnation or deterioration. Deterioration despite adequate medical treatment should be an indication for surgery. Stagnation over several days with no sign of improvement should also be an indication for operation. The patient's recent history of general health and previous exacerbations should be taken into account.

Clinical indicators that surgery is more likely to be necessary at the time of admission include a frequency of defecation of over ten times per 24 hours, with the passage of blood at every defecation attempt. A low albumin, low haemoglobin and a fall in lean body mass of more than 10% are other risk factors for surgery. The number and severity of any previous acute attack should also be taken into account. Recurrent attacks of acute severe colitis may be an indication that maintenance treatment has failed and if so it may be preferable to decide on early surgery during such an exacerbation. The need for surgery is highest during the first year after onset of the disease (**Fig. 8.5**).

Megacolon is an indication for surgery. If signs of peritonism are present, operation should not be delayed. Perforation is a grave development, with a mortality of around 40%. It may be silent in a

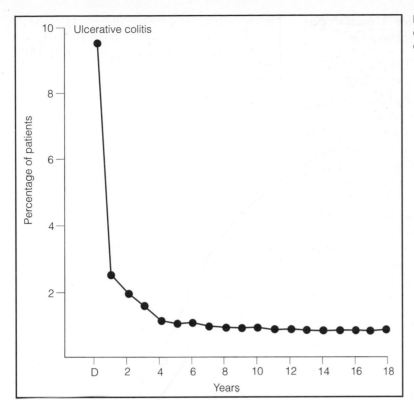

Figure 8.5 • Colectomy rates in different years after the diagnosis of ulcerative colitis.

patient on large doses of steroids, and may become evident only by the presence of free gas on the plain abdominal radiograph. When surgery is performed prior to perforation, the mortality can be reduced to 2–8%.[42] Perforation is usually associated with toxic colitis or megacolon or as a result of colonoscopic surveillance.[43] Its occurrence without megacolon is rare and should raise the possibility of Crohn's disease.[44] Intestinal obstruction occurs more commonly in patients with Crohn's disease but in ulcerative colitis it may suggest malignancy. Severe gastrointestinal bleeding is a rare presentation but may account for up to 10% of all urgent colectomies.[45,46]

CHOICE OF OPERATION

The operation of choice is colectomy with ileostomy and preservation of the rectal stump. Proctocolectomy used as an emergency has become less frequent owing to the introduction of restorative proctocolectomy, which offers the patient the subsequent prospect of avoiding ileostomy.

TECHNIQUE: GENERAL ASPECTS

Certain basic principles apply to all surgery for ulcerative colitis. These include the following.

Position of the patient

This should always be the Lloyd-Davies position, thereby allowing access to the rectum. The bladder is routinely catheterised.

Ileostomy

When an ileostomy forms part of the procedure, the trephine for this should be made before opening the abdomen. This enables division of layers of the anterior abdominal wall directly to the peritoneal cavity before the distortion created by the incision.

Incision

This should be routinely midline. The anterior abdominal wall is preserved for the construction of an ileostomy on either side if necessary in the future. A paramedian incision is no longer appropriate. A few surgeons use a laparoscopically facilitated technique, which may include a manual port introduced through a Pfannenstiel incision.

COLECTOMY WITH ILEOSTOMY AND PRESERVATION OF THE RECTUM

In carrying out an emergency colectomy, particularly if dilatation is present, it is helpful to insert a proctoscope before starting to deflate the bowel. On opening the abdomen, great care must be taken to avoid perforation. Where adhesions have formed between the colon and the parietes, dissection should be made within the latter.

Mobilisation should start in the right colon. Once freed, it is useful to divide the bowel at the ileocaecal junction before proceeding further. This manoeuvre allows the surgeon to control the specimen manually to prevent tension on the ileocolic and right colic vessels, enabling their safe division. There is no evidence that preservation of the greater omentum is desirable. The splenic flexure is often easy to mobilise owing to contraction and shortening of the bowel due to the disease.

The level of division of the distal colon is important. It should be made in the sigmoid to allow exteriorisation of the distal stump, whether this is formed into a mucous fistula or closed (**Fig. 8.6**). Division at the level of the peritoneal reflection should not be routinely carried out. It leaves a distal stump that is too short to be exteriorised in the uncommon event of breakdown of the suture line and also makes identification of the rectum at a subsequent operation difficult. A long rectosigmoid stump should therefore be aimed for. However, this is not applicable in cases with bleeding from rectal ulceration. Here the resection should be made as far distally as is necessary to include the site of haemorrhage. The sphincter complex should be preserved so that an ileoanal pouch can be constructed at a later date should the patient so wish.[47]

Whether the stump is closed or brought out as a mucous fistula depends on clinical judgement during the operation. In a series of 147 consecutive cases there was a mortality of 3% and only 2% experienced leakage of the stump.[48] However, if the patient's condition is poor and the state of the bowel is deemed too fragile to take sutures or staples, then a mucous fistula is obligatory. The surgeon should ensure that the ileostomy and mucous fistula are sufficiently apart to allow placement of a stoma

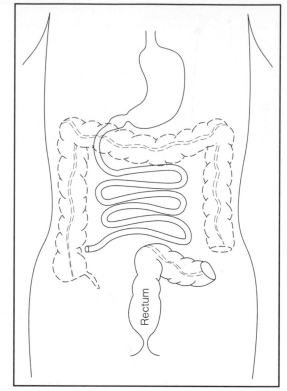

Figure 8.6 • Emergency colectomy: level of division of the sigmoid allowing adequate mobility for exteriorisation.

appliance to each. The outcome after subcutaneous rectal stump closure has been reported in 31 patients undergoing emergency colectomy for IBD.[49] Complications developed in 22% of patients, of which two required surgical intervention. The rectal stump was always readily located at the time of subsequent restorative surgery and any leakage from the stump could easily discharge through the wound.

The incidence of continued bleeding from the rectum has been reported to be 0–12%.[46] The majority of patients can be managed conservatively by packing the rectal stump with adrenaline-soaked gauze.[45]

POSTOPERATIVE OUTCOME

In the immediate postoperative period, it is advisable to drain the rectum (particularly if the stump is closed) by daily insertion of a proctoscope. Complications include intestinal obstruction and sepsis. The former usually resolves spontaneously.

Sepsis may occur as a result of an intra-abdominal collection or leakage from a closed rectosigmoid stump. This will usually require reoperation and exteriorisation of the distal bowel if possible. Rarely, rectal excision preserving the anal canal will be necessary.

In one study, there were three (3%) postoperative deaths out of 106 patients undergoing urgent surgery.[50] Recovery usually occurs within a few weeks to a couple of months, during which steroids are gradually withdrawn. Occasionally, persisting inflammation in the rectal stump may be so severe despite local treatment that rectal excision is required.

CHRONIC COLITIS

Indications for elective surgery

Most patients requiring surgery are those with anatomically extensive disease. They are more likely to have severe symptoms and systemic illness than patients with limited disease. There is a greater risk of developing acute severe colitis and malignant transformation and they are more prone to extra-alimentary manifestations. Very occasionally, a patient with distal disease may come to surgery, usually because of severe local symptoms. Indications for elective surgery include (i) failed medical treatment, (ii) retardation of growth in the young and (iii) malignant transformation.

FAILED MEDICAL TREATMENT

This is difficult to define. Correct judgement requires clinical experience. The indications for surgery in acute severe colitis are largely determined by the disease itself, but in the elective situation the patient's view is an important component in the decision. A close relationship between gastroenterologist and surgeon is essential. Although there may be considerable overlap, the term 'failed medical treatment' includes the following clinical situations.

Chronic disease

The patient continues to suffer from a combination of systemic and local symptoms despite adequate medical treatment. Chronic anaemia associated with general weakness, poor energy levels, amenorrhoea and extra-alimentary manifestations may leave the patient unable to lead a normal life. Multiple hospitalisations, periods off work, disruption of family life and other social effects of chronic illness will support the decision for surgery. Patients who have never experienced a complete remission from medical treatment are included in this group.

Steroid dependence

A response to steroids may be maintained only by continuing the therapy. Conversely, a relapse occurs on withdrawal. If alternative medication such as immunosuppression is unsuccessful, then surgery is indicated unless there are particular reasons against. Thus the dangers of surgery must be offset against those of long-term steroid medication. Bone densitometry should be carried out where steroid medication has been prolonged.

Recurrent acute exacerbations

Patients with acute colitis who respond to medical treatment are at risk of developing recurrent episodes. The decision for surgery will depend on the perceived severity of attacks and their frequency. It should be remembered that surgery during an acute attack will usually take the form of a colectomy with ileostomy and preservation of the rectal stump. In contrast, an elective decision during remission may allow a definitive procedure such as restorative proctocolectomy as the first operation.

Severe symptoms

The patient may be systemically well but severely inconvenienced by frequency and urgency of defecation. The latter may be incapacitating, particularly if associated with urge incontinence. Urgency is the cardinal symptom of proctocolitis, and is due to severe distal inflammation resulting in rectal irritability and low capacitance. Failure to control it medically is an indication for surgery.

Extra-alimentary manifestations

Not all symptoms will respond to removal of the large bowel; liver manifestations and sacroiliitis do not. However, the activity-related polyarthropathy does respond, as will some cases of pyoderma gangrenosum, although the response of the latter may be slow, occurring over several months.

RETARDATION OF GROWTH

Ulcerative colitis, if extensive, has an inhibitory effect on growth and the development of secondary sexual characteristics. Steroid medication itself leads to early fusion of epiphyses, resulting in permanent stunting of growth. Patients in this category are usually under the care of a paediatrician expert in the assessment of growth. However, within the years of puberty a delay in surgery may occur, partly because of the antipathy of the paediatrician and/or of the patient (or parents) to an ileostomy.

MALIGNANT TRANSFORMATION

The presence of high- or low-grade dysplasia or an established invasive tumour is an indication for surgery. The surgical technique should be as though invasion had occurred since this can be determined only by examination of the resected specimen.

Choice of operation: general considerations

There are four surgical options:

1. colectomy with ileostomy and rectal preservation;
2. colectomy and ileorectal anastomosis;
3. conventional proctocolectomy and permanent ileostomy;
4. restorative proctocolectomy and ileal reservoir.

Conservative proctocolectomy is now little used. It consists of removal of the colon and rectum with preservation of the pelvic floor and anal canal. The operation was followed by a high incidence of pelvic infection as a result of poor drainage resulting from an intact sphincter. Furthermore, a second-stage ileoanal procedure was rendered difficult because of the distal level of division of the gut tube.[51]

In patients having a permanent ileostomy, a Kock pouch (see below) may be possible in certain circumstances. All these operations involve total removal of the colon. There is no place for partial colectomy, even in cases with a normal right colon, where experience has shown a high frequency of recurrence in the remaining colon.

The choice of operation is based on medical criteria and the wishes of the patient. Assessment of the large bowel by radiology, endoscopy and rectal capacitance studies may assist the clinical assessment in deciding whether the rectum and the anus are suitable for conservation. Colectomy with ileorectal anastomosis should be considered only where the rectum is minimally inflamed and distensible and where there is no evidence of dysplasia anywhere in the large bowel. Most patients do not fulfil these criteria, leaving the alternative of conventional or restorative proctocolectomy. The latter is excluded, however, if the anal sphincter is inadequate or the anus is diseased. Much will depend on the wishes of the patient. Here, it is essential for the clinician to give detailed information on the morbidity, function, late complications and likely duration of treatment of the various options. Input from the stomatherapist and patient-support groups should be obtained. The introduction of restorative proctocolectomy[52] has resulted in this operation being the most commonly used,[50] as shown in **Fig. 8.7**.

COLECTOMY WITH ILEOSTOMY AND PRESERVATION OF THE RECTUM

This operation, normally used for acute severe colitis, has a place in elective treatment. A few patients with chronic colitis or steroid dependence may be considered too unfit for a restorative proctocolectomy (if that is the patient's ultimate desire). Patients incapacitated by severe frequency and urgency may have lost their self-confidence. Under such circumstances it may be preferable to carry out a colectomy with ileostomy and preservation of the rectal stump. The advantages include a well-tolerated procedure with low morbidity that allows the recovery of general health and the withdrawal of medication. The patient can return to normal life within a few weeks. The experience of an end-ileostomy may be invaluable to the patient in deciding on subsequent surgery. In cases where the diagnosis of ulcerative colitis is in doubt, an initial colectomy allows the histopathologist more material with which to make a decision. The disadvantage is the need for a further operation, whether removal of the rectum or some form of reconstruction. There is, however, no particular hurry for reoperation in most cases. Dysplasia is extremely rare within 10 years of the onset of colitis and any pressure for surgery usually comes from the patient.

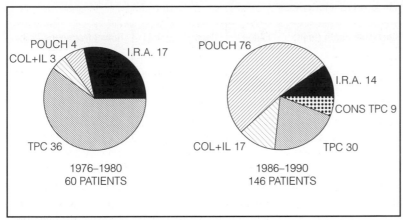

Figure 8.7 • Change in choice of elective operation for ulcerative colitis during the 5-year periods 1976–80 and 1986–90 at St Mark's Hospital.

COLECTOMY WITH ILEORECTAL ANASTOMOSIS

Indications

The rectum should be regarded as being able to act as a reservoir. If endoscopy shows relative mucosal sparing with distensibility on insufflation of air, if proctography shows the same and provided the sphincter is adequate and there is no dysplasia, colectomy with ileorectal anastomosis should be seriously considered. An inflamed contracted rectum detected by any of the above methods of assessment is a contraindication for rectal conservation. The patient must also be prepared to be followed up because of the risk of malignancy in the rectal stump. Annual rectoscopy with biopsy supported by competent histopathology should be carried out. If this is not available, then the operation should not be advised.

Before the introduction of restorative procto-colectomy the operation was used in 10–90% of patients coming to surgery. This huge variation was largely the result of surgeon preference. The fear of cancer in the rectal stump and the possibility of a poor functional result persuaded some surgeons[53,54] to advise the operation in only a small minority of patients. Others used the operation in almost all cases.[55]

Since the introduction of restorative procto-colectomy, colectomy with ileorectal anastomosis has gradually declined in frequency (see **Fig. 8.7**). Nevertheless, it still has a place since it is easy to carry out, complications are infrequent, and in correctly selected cases long-term results are satisfactory in many patients.

Technique

The technique is identical to that of colectomy with ileostomy and preservation of the rectal stump up to the point of removal of the specimen. The anastomosis is very accessible for hand suturing and there is no evidence that any particular technique has any advantage over any other. Stapled ileorectal anastomosis carried out by many surgeons is more expensive, and clinical trials offer no proof that it is more secure than a manual anastomosis.

Results

Colectomy with ileorectal anastomosis is a compromise operation. Residual disease in the rectal stump can lead to failure because of two factors. The first is persisting inflammation causing poor function; in one study, 20% of patients had a frequency of defecation of six or more times per 24 hours.[56] The second is the development of malignancy. The results of five large series (**Table 8.3**) demonstrate a low mortality and morbidity but considerable differences in failure requiring removal of the rectum. The cancer rate is low, although in a series of 384 patients there were 12 deaths of the 22 cancers that developed during follow-up.[57]

Patients who fail are candidates for either rectal excision with permanent ileostomy or restorative proctectomy, provided in this instance that any cancer can be adequately cleared without having to

Table 8.3 • Results of colectomy with ileorectal anastomosis

Reference	N	Operative death (leak)	Failed	Cancer (death)	Bowel frequency/24 h
Baker et al. (1978)[57]	384	10 (5)	11	22 (12)	–
Gruner et al. (1975)[58]	57	– (6)	40	–	–
Hawley (1985)[59]	125	0 (–)	26	4 (1)	4.2
Oakley et al. (1985)[60]	145	0 (3)	23	5 (2)	4.3

sacrifice the anal canal and pelvic floor and provided there is no dissemination.

CONVENTIONAL PROCTOCOLECTOMY WITH PERMANENT ILEOSTOMY

The introduction of the everted ileostomy[61] established this operation as the standard procedure for ulcerative colitis until the description of restorative proctocolectomy. Ulcerative colitis is cured, with the only disadvantage being a permanent ileostomy.

Indications

The operation is indicated where the rectum and anus are not suitable for a restorative procedure. The decision between conventional and restorative proctocolectomy depends on medical factors and on the wishes of the patient. In discussing the relative merits, the patient should appreciate the possibility of ileostomy-related complications requiring further surgery and delayed healing of the perineal wound. These are offset by those of pelvic sepsis and long-term developments such as pouchitis after restorative proctocolectomy.

Technique

Creating the ileostomy trephine before the midline incision has already been discussed. The technique of mobilisation of the colon and rectum will depend on whether carcinoma or dysplasia is present. Where it is, the dissection should be as for any carcinoma, with wide clearance and high ligation of the lympho-vascular pedicle. The rectum should be mobilised in the anatomical plane outside the fascia propria, taking care to preserve the presacral nerves. In cases without neoplastic transformation the rectum may be removed by close (perimuscular) dissection. Although this manoeuvre is not practised by many

surgeons, it has the merit of resulting in an exceedingly low incidence of pelvic nerve damage, which might cause urinary or sexual dysfunction.[62] However, no statistically significant difference was found in a non-randomised comparison between this and conventional dissection.[63] Whatever technique is adopted, the dissection should be kept close to the rectal wall in the region of the lateral ligaments where the autonomic pelvic nerves are mostly at risk. In patients with dysplasia or an already established carcinoma in the large bowel, a meso-rectal dissection should be carried out.

In the absence of carcinoma in the low anorectal region, the perineal dissection should be by the inter-sphincteric technique.[64] The anal skin is circumcised close to the orifice and the plane between internal and external sphincters developed. The perineal wound is closed with pelvic drainage via a suction drain brought out through the lower abdomen. Good ileostomy technique may avoid some of the complications. Before division of the ileocaecal junction, the ileocolic vessels should be ligated to leave the terminal 5 cm of the ileum supplied only by the marginal vessel present in this part of the small bowel (**Fig. 8.8**). This will facilitate eversion of the stoma by having a minimal bulk of mesentery. The bowel is brought out through the trephine and the edge of the mesentery sutured to the peritoneum on the anterior abdominal wall in the sagittal plane from the trephine itself over a distance of 5–10 cm superiorly. The stoma itself is created by muco-cutaneous interrupted sutures using a subcuticular technique. It will evert spontaneously, a projection of 2.5 cm being ideal.

Results

Obstruction and pelvic sepsis are the most likely complications in the immediate postoperative period.

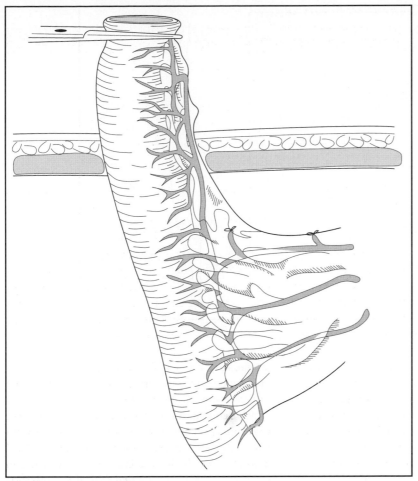

Figure 8.8 • Formation of terminal ileostomy. Division of mesenteric vessels with preservation of the 'marginal' vessels to the terminal ileum.

Obstruction may occasionally require reoperation but usually settles spontaneously. Rarely it is due to herniation of the small bowel into the space lateral to the ileostomy. A haematoma in the cavity left by the rectum may become infected. Drainage with resolution of the acute problem may be followed by a perineal sinus. This may require subsequent surgery with curettage and rarely in refractory cases the need for a perineal myocutaneous rectus abdominus flap. Delayed healing of the perineal wound at 6 months has been reported to occur in 20 to over 50% of cases.[65,66]

Phillips et al.[51] have reviewed the long-term outcome of proctocolectomy at one hospital and showed considerable morbidity. Ileostomy complications were common. Stricture formation, prolapse and retraction may cause difficulty in maintaining a watertight appliance, as may parastomal herniation. Corrective surgery is often required, with a reported cumulative ileostomy revision rate of around 25% at 5 years. It is usually possible to carry out a local revision, but in some cases, particularly with herniation, resiting is required. This is a major undertaking.

THE CONTINENT ILEOSTOMY

Kock[67] developed this operation to create a continent abdominal stoma. It involves the construction of a reservoir from 30 cm of small bowel with the distal terminal ileum (15 cm) invaginated into the reservoir to form a nipple valve (**Fig. 8.9**). In patients with an intact pelvic floor the operation has been superseded

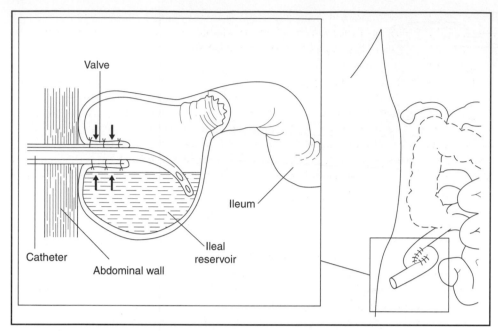

Figure 8.9 • The Kock continent ileostomy.

by restorative proctocolectomy but it still has a place in patients in whom this is absent. Kock originally regarded Crohn's disease as a contraindication. The cumulative 10-year recurrence rate in 49 patients with Crohn's disease was 48%, with excision of the pouch required in only eight.[68]

The abdomen is opened and any small bowel adhesions are divided. The terminal 45 cm is measured and the two proximal 15-cm segments are sutured to form a U-shape, which is then opened. The apex of the opened loops of bowel is then sutured to the base to form a reservoir. Before completing the closure, the proximal two-thirds of the terminal 15 cm of ileum are invaginated into the reservoir and fixed with four rows of staples applied longitudinally. The mesentery included in the invagination is stripped of peritoneum and staple lines are applied to the nipple as close as possible on each side of the mesentery. After closing the reservoir, the terminal ileum is brought out flush onto the anterior wall through a trephine placed about 5 cm above the mid-inguinal point below the bikini-line. Non-absorbable interrupted sutures are placed on the inside between the reservoir and anterior abdominal wall around the site of invagination. The competence of the valve is tested and a large catheter (Medina) is passed into the reservoir

via the stoma and left in situ for 2–3 weeks. Post-operatively, the patient is taught intermittent catheterisation after 10 days.

Early complications include leakage from the reservoir causing peritonitis or fistulation. The most important late complication is subluxation of the nipple valve. It is suggested by the onset of incontinence of the stoma and difficulty in inserting the catheter. Contrast radiology may show partial or complete prolapse of the valve. Valve slippage occurs in 17 to over 40% of cases,[69–71] and is the most common cause of failure. Reported fistula rates range from 10 to 26%. Of 330 patients treated at a single institution between 1974 and 2001, pouch survival at 10 and 20 years was 87% and 77% respectively.[72] Patients with indeterminate colitis or Crohn's disease were 4.5 times more likely to lose the pouch than those without. Long-term continence rates of over 90% have been reported.[70,71,73] Pouchitis occurs in up to 40% of patients by 4 years and dysplasia has been reported in 3 of 40 patients followed for a median of 30 years.[74,75] A case of carcinoma in the pouch has been reported.[76]

Despite the possibility of complications, continent ileostomy may be indicated in motivated patients in whom restorative proctocolectomy is not an option and in patients who already have a permanent ileostomy and desire an improved quality of life. While technically possible after failed restorative proctocolectomy, the risk of complications with failure following a Kock reservoir may further worsen the patient's condition.

RESTORATIVE PROCTOCOLECTOMY WITH ILEAL RESERVOIR

The strategy of complete removal of the large bowel with sphincter preservation was first described fully by Ravitch and Sabiston.[77] The 'straight' ileoanal anastomosis was adopted by a few surgeons at the time and the functional results were subsequently reviewed by Valiènte and Bacon.[78] Function was often poor due largely to urgency and frequency. An ileoanal ileal reservoir was developed in dogs but was not applied to humans.

The introduction of the continent ileostomy showed that a small bowel reservoir could function in humans and this led Parks and Nicholls[52] to combine this with their own endoanal anastomotic technique to create the ileoanal ileal reservoir procedure. Despite reports indicating that the straight ileoanal operation could result in acceptable function,[79] there are now data to show that capacitance of the neorectum is inversely related to frequency, irrespective of whether the neorectum is constructed using straight ileum,[80] ileal reservoir[81] or colonic reservoir.[82]

Indications

The only reason for the operation is to avoid a permanent ileostomy. A conventional proctocolectomy gives excellent results except for this. The indications can be divided into medical and personal. Any severely ill patient should have an initial colectomy. Where a cancer is present, it must be possible to achieve locoregional clearance, an assessment similar to that made when considering neoadjuvant chemoradiotherapy or anterior resection or total rectal excision for 'ordinary' rectal carcinoma. The operation is not indicated in patients with disseminated disease.

The anal sphincter should be adequate. A low preoperative resting pressure is related to subsequent anal leakage.[83,84] However, there is no agreement whether preoperative manometry can predict frequency of defecation.[84,85] Manometry should be performed where there is clinical uncertainty of sphincter function.

There are several clinical circumstances in which the indication for restorative proctocolectomy is controversial.

Age Failure, complication rates and function are similar in paediatric patients to the overall series.[86–88] General health and quality of life is similar to that of healthy children in those patients with a functioning pouch.[89] However, fertility in females is reduced after restorative proctocolectomy (see below) and careful counselling of patient and parents is essential.

There is some evidence that incontinence, usually minor, is more common in patients over 45 years old.[90,91]

There is, however, no absolute contraindication in older patients[92] and the indication should depend on the assessment of the individual patient, particularly regarding sphincter function.

Crohn's disease Patients with Crohn's disease experience a higher failure rate than the general pouch population (**Table 8.4**) and Crohn's disease has therefore been regarded as a contraindication to restorative proctocolectomy. However, a group of patients has been reported with a failure rate at 10 years of 10%.[97,98] These patients were characterised by the combination of large bowel involvement with small bowel and anal sparing.

Table 8.4 • Outcome of restorative proctocolectomy in Crohn's disease

Reference	N	Ileostomy	Failed*
Galanduik et al. (1990)[93]	16	9	4
Deutsch et al. (1991)[94]	9		4
Hayman et al. (1991)[95]	25	1	7
Grobler et al. (1993)[96]	20		8
Panis et al. (1996)[97]	31		2
Regimbeau et al. (2001)[98]	41		3
Tulchinsky et al. (2003)[99]	13		6

*Failure is defined as removal of pouch and permanent ileostomy.

In large general series followed over a similar period, failure rates for ulcerative colitis and Crohn's disease were 10% and 50% respectively.[99,100] Thus great care in patient selection should be exercised when considering the operation for Crohn's disease.

Indeterminate colitis Indeterminate colitis without radiological or clinical evidence of Crohn's disease tends to behave like ulcerative colitis. Failure rates in large series followed for 10 or more years are around 10%.[99,100] Complications and function also appear to be similar to ulcerative colitis.[101] In a patient with indeterminate colitis it is essential to examine the small bowel radiologically and to identify past or present anal disease.

Sclerosing cholangitis Patients with sclerosing cholangitis have double the incidence of pouchitis after restorative proctocolectomy.[28] While not a contraindication, the patient should be carefully counselled. Liver function tests should be performed routinely preoperatively.

Prior anal pathology A history of anal disease may suggest the possibility of Crohn's disease. The presence of an anal lesion increases the risk of anastomotic leakage.[102] Carefully selected patients with an unequivocal diagnosis of ulcerative colitis may have a satisfactory result but anal disease increases the risk of pouch–perineal fistulas and subsequent failure.[103]

Fertility

Female fertility is reduced by more than 50% following restorative proctocolectomy.[104,105]

This applies to both ulcerative colitis and FAP but more so in the former. Fertility is not affected by colectomy and it appears that the pelvic dissection is the factor responsible. Fertility is therefore a major consideration of medicolegal importance when advising females who may wish to have children. After counselling, the patient may decide to have a colectomy with ileostomy as the best strategy for recovery of health and preservation of fertility, leaving a restorative proctectomy for a later date convenient to the patient.

The patient's wishes The personal component is very important. Where there is no medical objection, the choice lies between a restorative or conventional proctocolectomy and is almost entirely the patient's to make. This is possible only if the disadvantages are fully discussed. These include failure and complication rates, total treatment time, the possibility of pouchitis occurring and the likely functional outcome. A pouch support nurse, stomatherapist and patient-support group can offer valuable advice but in the end the patient must decide.

Technique

The technique (**Fig. 8.10**) is identical to conventional proctocolectomy up to the point following mobilisation of the rectum. This is taken down to the anorectal junction and the bowel is divided at this level after cleaning the anal canal with an antiseptic solution. If a stapled ileoanal anastomosis is intended, a transverse stapler is applied at this level. Where a hand-sutured anastomosis is to be carried out, the bowel is divided, leaving an open anal stump.

Having removed the surgical specimen, dissection of the small bowel mesentery should be carried out to achieve full mobility. It is very helpful to perform a trial descent to the anal canal level of the point on the ileum selected for the ileoanal anastomosis. If it reaches at this stage, it will do so after the reservoir is constructed. If it does not, mesenteric vessels that appear to restrain mobility may be divided. They should be carefully selected to avoid ischaemia.

Various types of reservoir have been described. The arguments in favour of any particular design can be resolved into capacitance and emptying characteristics. The two-loop (J) reservoir[106] is easy to make by hand or by stapling. The original three-loop (S) reservoir of Parks often led to evacuation difficulty due to the short segment of ileum distal to the pouch. The four-loop (W) reservoir[107] achieves a capacitance generally greater than that of the J reservoir and similarly has no distal segment. In general, the larger the reservoir, the lower the frequency.

There is controversy concerning the preferred method of ileoanal anastomosis, whether manual or stapled. Two randomised trials have shown no important difference in morbidity or function of hand-sutured versus stapled ileoanal anastomosis.[108,109]

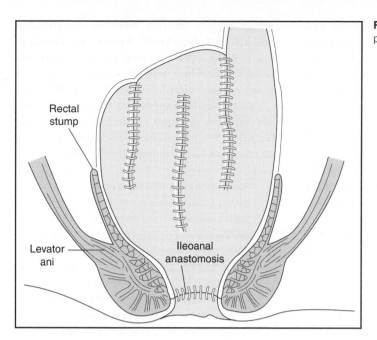

Figure 8.10 • Restorative proctocolectomy.

Rectal stump

Levator ani

Ileoanal anastomosis

The manual technique allows a precise level for the anastomosis and avoids the possibility of leaving rectal mucosa behind. Although there are techniques available to permit the accurate placement of the transverse stapler within the anal canal,[110] routine stapling per abdomen may sometimes result in the creation of an ileal pouch–rectal anastomosis (**Fig. 8.11**). The residual inflamed mucosa may cause continuing bleeding, discomfort and urgency. Emptying may be incomplete, leading to frequent passage of small volumes of stool. Even when the anastomosis is performed at the correct level, persisting columnar epithelium in the anal stump may give troublesome symptoms such as bleeding, anal burning and frequent evacuation of small-volume stool. 'Strip proctitis' has been reported in around 10–15% of cases having a stapled anastomosis.[111,112] There is a small cumulative risk of dysplasia of 3% over a mean follow-up of 16 months.[113]

Both manual and stapled anastomoses are followed by a fall in resting anal canal pressure.[109] This is greater with the former but has not affected continence significantly in clinical trials. Where descent of the small bowel to the anal canal level might result in excessive tension in the mesentery, a stapled anastomosis at the anorectal junction is preferable. The learning curve in ileal pouch surgery was recently evaluated using ileal pouch failure as

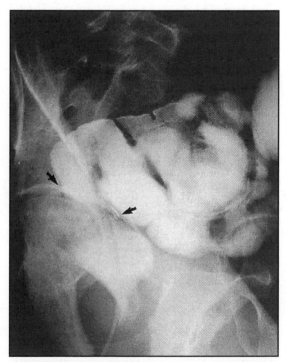

Figure 8.11 • Restorative proctocolectomy. Radiograph of pouch showing faulty technique by creation of anastomosis between ileal reservoir and rectal stump.

the primary endpoint. Having adjusted for case mix, trainee staff undertaking stapled anastomosis showed an improvement in the pouch failure rate following an initial training period of 23 cases. The learning curve for hand-sewn anastomoses was quantified only for senior staff who attained adequate results following an initial period of 31 procedures.[114] The surgeon should be capable of performing either technique.

Most surgeons include a defunctioning ileostomy routinely. It is thought to mitigate the effects of any pelvic sepsis should it occur and allows recovery from this major operation without the functional difficulties that may follow initially. The ileostomy can cause morbidity, however, both in its formation and its closure and this may account for 20% of complications. The operation has been carried out without ileostomy[115] with excellent results, and a randomised trial showed that pelvic sepsis was no different in the group without ileostomy (1/22) compared with the group with ileostomy (1/23).[116]

However, there is a price to pay, namely the need to create an ileostomy in 10–20% of patients in the immediate postoperative period, sometimes as an emergency. The clinician has to balance a successful 'one-stage' procedure in the majority against the potentially serious complication of faecal pelvic sepsis or peritonitis in the minority.

Results

Failure Failure is defined as the need to remove the pouch and establish a permanent ileostomy. Some authors include patients who are defunctioned without any prospect of having the ileostomy closed. Early reports focused on the failure rate during the first year after ileostomy closure, with figures ranging from 5 to over 15% (**Table 8.5**). It is now apparent that failure continues to occur over 15 years or more at much the same rate[99] (**Fig. 8.12**). The reasons include pelvic sepsis (50%), poor function (30%) and pouchitis (10%).

Pelvic sepsis in the early postoperative period confers a threefold increase in the chance of subsequent failure[122] and about 30% of patients who develop pelvic sepsis will ultimately fail. In a series of 1965 patients treated in a single centre between 1983 and 2001, four preoperatve and four postoperative factors were found to be associated with ileal pouch failure. Using a multifactorial survival analysis, each factor was assigned appropriate weights to form a scoring system for quantifying the risk of pouch failure in individual patients. The risk of ileal pouch failure at 1, 5 and 10 years of follow-up is shown in **Table 8.6**.[103]

Removal of the pouch has a significant morbidity, with delayed healing of the perineal wound in 30% of patients.[123]

Complications All reports indicate a high morbidity, ranging from 20 to 50% (**Table 8.7**). Many complications resolve spontaneously but some may require active intervention. The most important is pelvic

Table 8.5 • Failure after restorative proctocolectomy

Reference	N	Follow-up (months)*	Pouch excision	Indefinite diversion	Overall failure (%)
Gemlo et al. (1992)[117]	253	>12	–	–	9.9
Foley et al. (1995)[118]	460	–	7	9	3.5
MacRae et al. (1997)[119]	551	>30	49	9	10.5
Korsgen & Keighley (1997)[120]	180	>24	23	8	17.2
Meagher et al. (1998)[121†]	1310	24–180 (77)	84	50	10
Tulchinsky et al. (2003)[99†]	634	36–288 (85)	41	20	9.7
Fazio et al. (2003)[103]	1975	1–228 (49)	38	39	4.1

*Numbers in parentheses indicate mean values.
†Patients with ulcerative colitis only.

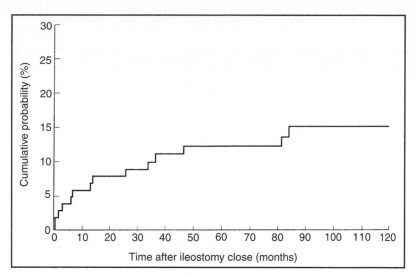

Figure 8.12 • Long-term failure after restorative proctocolectomy.

sepsis due to breakdown of the ileoanal anastomosis or an infected haematoma, or both. Authors may vary in the rigour with which they define pelvic sepsis and this may account for the wide variance of its reported incidence, from less than 5 to 20%. A pyrexia develops within a few days and digital examination per anum may reveal an anastomotic defect or an extraluminal swelling indicating the presence of haematoma. Passage of fresh blood is highly significant. An examination under anaesthesia should be performed and any collection drained into the lumen.

Stricture of the anastomosis requiring active intervention (either dilatation or a more major procedure) is common. Intestinal obstruction occurs in 5–20% of patients and surgery may be necessary to treat it, although most cases resolve spontaneously.

Pouch–vaginal fistula (the male equivalent is pouch–perineal fistula) occurs in 5–10% of (female) patients and is an important reason for late failure. In a large survey of patients the incidence was 7.5%.[129] Patients with indeterminate colitis or Crohn's disease have significantly worse outcomes in comparison with ulcerative colitis patients (hazard ratio 1.4, 2.2 respectively). Prior anal pathology has also been associated with the development of pouch–vaginal fistula. The presence of perianal abscess or fistula-in-ano before the construction of the ileal pouch reserviour is associated with 3.7- and 6-fold increases in the risk of developing pouch–vaginal fistula. It often occurs well after closure of the ileostomy, with an 8-month interval reported in one study.[130]

Function Frequency ranges from a median of four to seven defecations per 24 hours but 20–30% have a frequency of eight or more. Surprisingly, this is often regarded by the patient as acceptable, probably because urgency is present in less than 5% of patients. Nocturnal defecation is probably the most sensitive indicator of function. Frequency varies spontaneously and is also influenced by diet. Continence rates also vary but faecal incontinence is rare (5%). The need for antidiarrhoeal medication ranges from 20 to 50%. There is a tendency for function to improve with time.[107,121,124,125,127,128]

Long term

General In the absence of chronic complications such as sepsis, general health is good. Deficiencies of iron and vitamin B_{12} occur in less than 10% over a follow-up of 2–3 years. These may be associated with anaemia.

Reservoir morphology The small bowel mucosa changes when a pouch is constructed. There is a degree of villous atrophy in almost all cases (including those with FAP). This is associated with a dramatic rise in the concentration of bacteria in the pouch. Bacterial counts in the normal terminal ileum are in the range 10^4–10^6 colony-forming units

Table 8.6 • **(a)** Ileal pouch failure model and **(b)** conversion chart for the prediction of ileal pouch failure following restorative proctocolectomy

(a)	Points
Preoperative risk factors	
Diagnosis	
Familial adenomatous polyposis	0
Ulcerative colitis or indeterminate colitis	1
Crohn's disease	1.5
Patient comorbidity	
No comorbid conditions	0
One comorbid condition	0.5
Two or more comorbid conditions	1.0
Prior anal pathology	
No prior anal pathology	0
Prior anal pathology	1
Anal sphincter manometry	
Normal manometry	0
Abnormal manometry	1
Postoperative risk factors	
Anastomotic separation	
No anastomotic separation	0
Anastomotic separation	1
Anastomotic stricture	
No stricture or asymptomatic stricture	0
Symptomatic stricture	1
Pelvic sepsis	
No sepsis	0
One episode of pelvic sepsis	1
Two or more episodes of pelvic sepsis	2
Fistula formation	
No fistula	0
Pouch–perineal fistula	1
Pouch–vaginal fistula	2

(b) Score	Follow-up (years)		
	1	5	10
0	0.1%	0.4%	0.8%
1	0.3%	1.1%	2.0%
2	0.8%	2.9%	5.0%
3	2.0%	7.2%	12.3%
4	5.0%	17.4%	28.5%
5	12.4%	38.7%	57.7%
6	28.7%	71.5%	89.0%

(a) from Fazio VV, Tekkis PP, Remzi F et al. Quantification of risk for pouch failure after ileal pouch anal anastomosis surgery. Ann Surg 2003; 238:605–14, with permission.

per gram of faeces. In the ileal pouch these counts rise to 10^{10}–10^{12}, with a predominance of anaerobes.

Pouchitis In some patients acute inflammation occurs that may be associated with symptoms of frequency, urgency, liquid stool and extra-alimentary manifestations. This condition is known as pouchitis. The aetiology is unknown but pouchitis is related to the original disease. It occurs in ulcerative colitis but is exceedingly rare in FAP.[131] It appears to be more common in non-smokers[18] and in those with sclerosing cholangitis.[28] No specific microbiological association has been found but the response to antibacterials and probiotics suggests a bacterial cause in susceptible individuals. This has been demonstrated objectively in vivo by polymorphonuclear leucocyte scanning.[132]

The diagnosis depends on clinical, endoscopic and histopathological features. The last is essential and must show acute inflammation. The natural history is similar to ulcerative colitis, with some cases showing an acute relapsing and others a chronic persisting behaviour. The latter causes significant debility but occurs in only about 5% of all cases having restorative proctocolectomy. Grading systems to assess severity have been described.[131,133,134] There is evidence that pouchitis occurs early after closure of the ileostomy.[135,136] Marked acute inflammation over several years may be associated with dysplasia, with this occurring in 3 of 87 patients followed for a median of 6 years.[137] Others have found a lower incidence over 12 or more years of follow-up[138] and dysplasia appears therefore to be rare, but continued surveillance by endoscopy with multiple biopsies at 5-year intervals is recommended.[76]

Table 8.7 • Morbidity after restorative proctocolectomy

Reference	N	Operative death (%)	Pelvic sepsis (%)	Stenosis (%)	SBO (total/reoperated)
Schoetz et al. (1986)[124]	104	0	11 (11)	3 (3)	25/21
Pemberton et al. (1987)[125]	390	1	10 (3)	– (86/50)	
Nicholls & Lubowski (1987)[107]	152	1	26 (17)	– (18)	NS/19
Oresland et al. (1989)[126]	100	0	10 (10)	4 (4)	6/6
Wexner et al. (1989)[127]	180	–	7 (4)	NS/NS	
Keighley et al. (1993)[128]	168	0	21 (12.5)	25/15	31/14

NS, not stated; SBO, small bowel obstruction.

Treatment consists of antibiotics or anti-inflammatory therapy. The role of 5-aminosalicylic acid drugs and steroids is uncertain. Xanthine oxidase inhibitors (allopurinol) and short-chain fatty acids have been tried without convincing benefit. Antibacterial drugs, including metronidazole, ciprofloxacin and Augmentin, can induce a response in over 80% of patients.

 Maintainence of remission by daily administration of the probiotic VSL3 has been shown to be effective in 85% of patients compared with controls (0%) when taken over a 9-month period.[139,140] However, withdrawal is followed by recurrence.

Probiotics also appear to be useful when given as prophylaxis.[141] If oral metronidazole fails, topical administration may be successful. Long-term metronidazole should be avoided due to the risk of peripheral neuropathy.

Removal of the reservoir for pouchitis is uncommon, with reported rates of 1–2%. Defunctioning does not affect the degree of inflammation, and excision with construction of a new reservoir is followed by pouchitis.

Carcinoma There are now several reports of carcinoma associated with restorative procto-olectomy. This may be due to pre-existing cancer in the rectum[142] or to carcinoma in the residual distal large bowel mucosa below the ileoanal anastomosis.[143] Carcinoma in the pouch itself has been reported in a Kock reservoir[76] and in five patients

Box 8.3 • Differential diagnosis of poor function after restorative proctocolectomy

Sepsis
- Chronic pelvic abscess
- Abdominal fistula from pouch
- Pouch–vaginal (perineal) fistula

Mechanical
- Partial intestinal obstruction
  - Ileostomy reversal site
  - Pre-pouch ileal segment
  - Other sites
- Pouch outlet obstruction
  - Ileoanal stricture
  - Distal ileal segment S-pouch
  - Retained distal rectum
- Weak sphincter
- Small reservoir

Inflammatory
- Pouchitis
- Retained distal rectum
- Crohn's disease

Functional
- Malabsorption
- Increased motility
- Short bowel syndrome

after restorative proctocolectomy.[144] Long-term follow-up is therefore essential.

ILEAL POUCH SALVAGE

Where failure is threatened by sepsis or poor function, salvage surgery may be considered. Such patients often have functional difficulties, which should be investigated by contrast radiology including evacuation pouchography, anal manometry, pouch volumetry, MRI and histopathological examination of biopsy material. Action will depend on the diagnosis (**Box 8.3**).

Pelvic sepsis with or without abdominal fistulation has been treated successfully by abdominal salvage in 80% of patients,[145,146] while others have reported less satisfactory results of 50% or lower.[122,93,147,148]

Pouch–vaginal fistula should be treated by defunctioning followed by an attempt at repair. In most patients this will require a local approach via the endoanal or transvaginal route. Successful closure has been reported in about 60% of patients by either technique,[149,150] although late recurrence can occur. Where the fistula is more proximal (usually associated with a stapled ileoanal anastomosis), abdominal advancement of the anastomosis with mucosectomy has achieved success in over 70%.[146,151] Pouch–perineal fistula, which usually occurs in males, is difficult to close and patients are often successfully managed by a long-term seton.

Mechanical outflow obstruction due to stricture of the ileoanal anastomosis or a retained rectal stump may require abdominal revision. Success rates of 70–90% have been reported.[99,152–154] There is little information on pouch augmentation procedures for small-volume reservoir. One study reported marked reduction in frequency after conversion to a W reservoir in five patients.[155]

• Key points

- The prevalence of ulcerative colitis is about 160 per 100 000 population compared with about 50 per 100 000 for Crohn's disease.
- At presentation, 50% of cases have disease confined to the rectum, in 30% this extends to the left colon and, in a further 20%, disease extends beyond the splenic flexure.
- About 25% of patients with UC will develop at least one extra-alimentary manifestation during the course of the illness such as arthropathy, primary sclerosing cholangitis, erythema nodosum or uveitis.
- The incidence of cancer in patients is estimated to be 0% within 10 years of onset of UC, 10–15% in the second decade and over 20% in the third.
- Histopathological examination of a mucosal biopsy is the basis for the diagnosis of UC.
- The initial treatment of acute severe acute colitis is medical but about 30% of patients will require surgery. Surgery is absolutely indicated in cases with acute toxic dilatation or perforation.
- The operation of choice for acute severe colitis is subtotal colectomy with ileostomy and preservation of the rectal stump.
- Indications for elective surgery for chronic UC include failure of medical treatment, growth retardation in the young and neoplastic transformation.
- Restorative proctocolectomy is the procedure of choice for the majority of patients with chronic UC.
- Contraindications to restorative proctocolectomy include Crohn's disease, indeterminate colitis favouring Crohn's disease, weak sphincter and patient choice.
- The choice of ileal pouch reservoir (J vs. W) or type of anastomosis (handsewn vs. stapled) has similar postoperative outcomes and bowel function.
- One-third of patients undergoing RPC develop at least one adverse event, which include anastomotic separation, pelvic sepsis, anastomotic stricture, fistula, small bowel obstruction, bleeding or pouchitis.
- Ileal pouch failure is a time-dependent outcome with an estimate 5–10% pouch excision rate or indefinite diversion at 10 years following RPC.
- Patients who are threatened with pouch failure salvage surgery may be considered, with successful outcome in 80% of patients.

REFERENCES

1. Probert CSJ, Jayanthi V, Pinder D et al. Epidemiological study of ulcerative proctocolitis in Indian migrants and the indigenous population of Leicester. Gut 1992; 33:687–93.

2. Guidelines in Gastroenterology. Inflammatory Bowel Disease. London: British Society of Gastroenterology, September 1996.

3. Kirsner JB, Spencer JA. Family occurrences of ulcerative colitis, regional enteritis and ileocolitis. Ann Intern Med 1963; 59:133–44.

4. Roth MP, Petersen GM, McElree C et al. Geographic origins of Jewish patients with inflammatory bowel disease. Gastroenterology 1989; 97:900–4.

5. Calkins BM, Mendeloff AI. Epidemiology of inflammatory bowel disease. Epidemiol Rev 1986; 8:60–91.

6. Monsen U, Bernell O, Johansson C et al. Prevalence of inflammatory bowel disease among relatives of patients with Crohn's disease. Scand J Gastroenterol 1991; 26:302–6.

7. Satsangi J, Jewell DP, Rosenberg WMC et al. Genetics of inflammatory bowel disease. Gut 1994; 35:696–700.

8. Tysk C, Linkberg E, Jarnesot G et al. Ulcerative colitis and Crohn's disease in an unselected population of monozygotic and dizygotic twins: a study of heritability and the influence of smoking. Gut 1988; 29:990–6.

9. Thompson NP, Driscoll R, Pounder RE et al. Genetics versus environment in inflammatory bowel disease: results of a British twin study. Br Med J 1996; 312:95–6.

10. Orholm M, Munkholm P, Longholz E et al. Familial occurrence of inflammatory bowel disease. N Engl J Med 1991; 324:84–8.

11. Yang H, Jarnerot G, Danielsson D et al. p-ANCA in monozygotic twins with inflammatory bowel disease. Gut 1995; 36:887–90.

12. Yang H, Rotter JI, Toyoda H et al. Ulcerative colitis: a genetically heterogeneous disorder defined by genetic (HLA Class II) and subclinical (antineutrophil cytoplasmic antibodies) markers. J Clin Invest 1993; 92:1080–4.

13. Calkins BM, Mendeloff AI. The epidemiology of idiopathic inflammatory bowel disease. In: Kirsner JB, Shorter BG (eds) Inflammatory bowel disease, 4th edn. Baltimore: Williams and Wilkins, 1995.

14. Bjorson I, Macpherson AJS, Teahon K. Non steroidal anti-inflammatory drugs and inflammatory bowel disease. Can J Gastroenterol 1993; 7:160–9.

15. Powell SJ, Wilmont AJ. Ulcerative post-dysenteric colitis. Gut 1966; 7:438–43.

16. Calkins BM. A meta-analysis of the role of smoking in inflammatory bowel disease. Dig Dis Sci 1989; 34:1841–54.

17. Sutherland LR, Ramcharan S, Bryant H et al. Effect of cigarette smoking in recurrence of Crohn's disease. Gastroenterology 1990; 98:1123–8.

18. Merrett MN, Mortensen NJ, Kettlewell M et al. Smoking may prevent pouchitis in patients with restorative proctocolectomy for ulcerative colitis. Gut 1996; 38:362–4.

19. Almet S, Frauzen L, Olaison G et al. Increased absorption of polyethylene glycol 600 deposited in the colon in active ulcerative colitis. Gut 1993; 34:507–13.

20. Mayer L, Eisenhardt D, Salomon P et al. Expression of class II molecules on intestinal epithelial cells in humans. Differences between normal and inflammatory bowel disease. Gastroenterology 1991; 100:3–12.

21. Duchmann R, Kaiser I, Hermann E et al. Tolerance exists towards resident intestinal flora but is broken in active inflammatory bowel disease (IBD). Clin Exp Immunol 1995; 102:448–55.

22. Sartor RB. Cytokines in intestinal inflammation: pathophysiological and clinical considerations. Gastroenterology 1994; 106:533–9.

23. Fuss I, Neurath M, Boirivant M et al. Disparate CD4+ lamina propria (LP) lymphokine secretion profiles in inflammatory bowel disease. J Immunol 1996; 157:1261–70.

24. Chapman MA, Grahn MF, Boyle MA et al. Butyrate oxygenation is impaired in the colonic mucosa of sufferers of quiescent ulcerative colitis. Gut 1994; 35:73–6.

25. Shepherd NA, Jass JR, Duvall I et al. Restorative proctocolectomy with ileal reservoir: pathological and histochemical study of mucosal biopsy specimens. J Clin Pathol 1987; 40:601–7.

26. Roediger WE, Duncan A, Kapaniris O et al. Reducing sulphur compounds of the colon impair colonocyte nutrition: implications for ulcerative colitis. Gastroenterology 1993; 104:802–9.

27. Thomson-Fawcett MW, Mortensen NJ. Anal transitional zone and columnar cuff in restorative proctocolectomy. Br J Surg 1996; 83:1047–55.

28. Penna C, Dozois RR, Tremaine W et al. Pouchitis after ileal pouch anal anastomosis for ulcerative colitis occurs with increased frequency in patients with associated primary sclerosing cholangitis. Gut 1996; 38:234–9.

29. Morson BC, Pang LSC. Rectal biopsy as an aid to cancer control. Gut 1967; 8:423–34.

30. Lennard Jones JE, Melville DM, Morsom BC et al. Pre-cancer and cancer in extensive ulcerative colitis: findings among 401 patients over 22 years. Gut 1990; 31:800–6.

31. Edwards FC, Truelove SC. Course and prognosis of ulcerative colitis. Part IV. Cancer of the colon. Gut 1964; 5:15–22.

32. Greenstein AJ, Sachar DB, Smith H et al. Cancer in universal and left sided ulcerative colitis: factors determining risk. Gastroenterology 1979; 77:290–4.

33. Brostom O, Loftberg, Ost A et al. Cancer surveillance of patients with long-standing ulcerative colitis: a clinical, endoscopical and histological study. Gut 1986; 27:1408–13.

34. Riddell RH, Goldman H, Ransohoff DF et al. Dysplasia in inflammatory bowel disease: standardised classification with provisional clinical applications. Hum Pathol 1983; 4:931–68.

35. Connell WR, Lennard Jones JE, Williams CB et al. Factors affecting the outcome of endoscopic surveillance for cancer in ulcerative colitis. Gastroenterology 1994; 107:934–44.

36. Provenzale D, Kowdley KV, Asora S et al. Prophylactic colectomy or surveillance for chronic ulcerative colitis: a decision analysis. Gastroenterology 1995; 109:1188–96.

37. Price AB. Overlap in the spectrum of non-specific inflammatory bowel disease: 'colitis indeterminate'. J Clin Pathol 1978; 31:567–77.

38. Wells AD, McMillan I, Price AB et al. Natural history of indeterminate colitis. Br J Surg 1991; 78:179–81.

39. Truelove SC. Systemic and local corticosteroid therapy in ulcerative colitis. Br Med J 1960; 1:464–7.

40. Treen WR, Cohen J, Davis PM et al. Cyclosporine for the treatment of fulminant ulcerative colitis in children. Immediate response, long-term results and impact on surgery. Dis Colon Rectum 1995; 38:474–9.

41. Roy MA. Inflammatory bowel disease. Surg Clin North Am 1997; 77:1419–31.

42. Sheth SG, LaMont JT. Toxic megacolon. Lancet 1998; 351:509–12.

43. Keighley MRB. Acute fulminating colitis and emergency colectomy. In: Keighley MRB, Williams NS (eds) Surgery of the anus, rectum and colon. London: WB Saunders, 1993; pp. 1379–97.

44. Nicholls RJ, Dozois RR. Surgery for ulcerative colitis, Crohn's disease. In: Nicholls RJ, Dozois RR (eds) Surgery of the colon and rectum. New York: Churchill Livingstone, 1997; pp. 593–644.

45. Parc R, Roger V, Penna C. Management of hemorrhage. In: Michelassi F, Milsom JW (eds) Operative strategies in inflammatory bowel disease. New York: Springer-Verlag, 1999; pp. 229–33.

46. Robert JH, Sachar DB, Aufses AHJ et al. Management of severe hemorrhage in ulcerative colitis. Am J Surg 1990; 159:550–5.

47. Tjandra JJ. Toxic colitis and perforation. In: Michelassi F, Milsom JW (eds) Operative strategies in inflammatory bowel disease. New York: Springer-Verlag, 1999.

48. Wojdemann M, Weltergren A, Hartvigsen A et al. Closure of rectal stump after colectomy for acute colitis. Int J Colorectal Dis 1995; 10:197–9.

49. Ng RL, Davies AH, Grace RH et al. Subcutaneous rectal stump closure after emergency subtotal colectomy. Br J Surg 1992; 79:701–3.

50. Melville DM, Ritchie JK, Nicholls RJ et al. Surgery for ulcerative colitis in the era of the pouch: the St Mark's Hospital experience. Gut 1994; 35:1076–80.

51. Phillips RKS, Ritchie JK, Hawley PR. Proctocolectomy with ileostomy for ulcerative colitis: the longer term story. J R Soc Med 1989; 82:386–7.

52. Parks AG, Nicholls RJ. Proctocolectomy without ileostomy for ulcerative colitis. Br Med J 1978; 2:85–8.

53. Adson MA, Cooperman AM, Farrow GM. Ileorectostomy for ulcerative disease of the colon. Arch Surg 1972; 104:424–8.

54. Goligher JC. Procedures conserving continence in the surgical management of ulcerative colitis. Surg Clin North Am 1983; 63:49–60.

55. Aylett SO. Diffuse ulcerative colitis and its treatment by ileorectal anastomosis. Ann R Coll Surg Engl 1960; 27:160–5.

56. Baker WNW. Results of ileorectal anastomosis at St Mark's Hospital. Gut 1970; 11:235–9.

57. Baker WNW, Glass RE, Ritchie JK et al. Cancer of the rectum following colectomy and ileorectal anastomosis for ulcerative colitis. Br J Surg 1978; 65:862–8.

58. Gruner OPN, Flatmark A, Maas R et al. Ileorectal anastomosis in ulcerative colitis. Scand J Gastroenterol 1975; 10:641–6.

59. Hawley PR. Ileorectal anastomosis. Br J Surg 1985; 72(suppl.):575–82.

60. Oakley JR, Jagelman DG, Fazio VW et al. Complications and quality of life after ileorectal anastomosis for ulcerative colitis. Am J Surg 1985; 149:23–30.

61. Brooke B. The outcome of surgery for ulcerative colitis. Lancet 1956; ii:532–6.

62. Lee ECG, Truelove SC. Proctocolectomy for ulcerative colitis. World J Surg 1980; 4:195–201.

63. Lindsey I, George BD, Kettlewell MG et al. Impotence after mesorectal and close rectal dissection for inflammatory bowel disease. Dis Colon Rectum 2001; 44:831–5.

64. Lyttle JA, Parks AG. Intersphincteric excision of the rectum. Br J Surg 1977; 64:413–16.

65. Lee ECG, Dowling BL. Perimuscular excision of the rectum for Crohn's disease and ulcerative colitis: a conservative technique. Br J Surg 1972; 59:29–32.

66. Ritchie JK. Ileostomy and excisional surgery for chronic inflammatory disease of the colon: a survey of one hospital region. Br Med J 1971; 1:264–8.

67. Kock NG. Intra-abdominal 'reservoir' in patients with permanent ileostomy. Arch Surg 1969; 99:223–31.

68. Myrvold H. The continent ileostomy. World J Surg 1987; 11:720–6.

69. Fazio VW, Church JM. Complications and function of the continent ileostomy at the Cleveland Clinic. World J Surg 1988; 12:148–54.

70. Kock NG MH, Nilsson LO, Philipson BM. Continent ileostomy: an account of 314 patients. Acta Chir Scand 1981; 147:67–72.

71. Dozois RR, Kelly KA, Beart RW et al. Improved results with continent ileostomy. Ann Surg 1980; 192:319–24.

72. Nessar G, Fazio VW, Tekkis PP et al. Long-term outcomes of quality of life after continent ileostomy. Ann Surg 2004 (in press).

73. Jarvinen HJ, Makitie A, Sivala A. Long term results of continent ileostomy. Int J Colorectal Dis 1986; 1:40–3.

74. Duff SE, O'Dwyer ST, Hulten L et al. Dysplasia in the ileoanal pouch. Colorectal Dis 2002; 4:420–9.

75. Hulten L, Willen R, Nilsson O et al. Mucosal assessment for dysplasia and cancer in the ileal pouch mucosa in patients operated on for ulcerative colitis: a 30-year follow-up study. Dis Colon Rectum 2002; 45:448–52.

76. Cox CL, Butts DR, Roberts MP et al. Development of an invasive adenocarcinoma in a long-standing Kock continent ileostomy: report of a case. Dis Colon Rectum 1997; 40:500–3.

77. Ravitch MM, Sabiston DC. Anal ileostomy with preservation of the sphincter. Surg Gynecol Obstet 1947; 84:1095–109.

78. Valiènte MA, Bacon HE. Construction of pouch using pantaloon technique for pull-through ileum following total colectomy. Am J Surg 1955; 90:742–50.

79. Martin LW, Le Coutre C, Schubert WK. Total colectomy and mucosal proctectomy with preservation of continence in ulcerative colitis. Ann Surg 1977; 186:477–80.

80. Heppel J, Kelly KA, Phillips SF et al. Physiologic aspects of continence after colectomy, mucosal proctectomy and ileo-anal anastomosis. Ann Surg 1982; 195:435–43.

81. Nicholls RJ, Pezim ME. Restorative procto-colectomy with ileal reservoir for ulcerative colitis and familial adenomatous polyposis: a comparison of three reservoir designs. Br J Surg 1985; 72:470–4.

82. Lazorthes F, Fages P, Chiotasso P et al. Resection of the rectum with construction of colonic reservoir and coloanal anastomosis for carcinoma of the rectum. Br J Surg 1986; 73:136–8.

83. Halverson AL, Hull TL, Remzi F et al. Perioperative resting pressure predicts long-term postoperative function after ileal pouch–anal anastomosis. J Gastrointest Surg 2002; 6:316–20.

84. Lindquist K. Anal manometry with microtransducer technique before and after restorative procto-colectomy. Sphincter function and clinical correlations. Dis Colon Rectum 1990; 33:91–7.

85. Morgado PJJ, Wexner SD, James K et al. Ileal pouch–anal anastomosis: is preoperative anal manometry predictive of postoperative functional outcome? Dis Colon Rectum 1996; 37:224–8.

86. Alexander F, Sarigol S, Difiore J et al. Fate of the pouch in 151 pediatric patients after ileal pouch anal anastomosis. J Pediatr Surg 2003; 38:78–82.

87. Robb BW, Gang GI, Hershko DD et al. Restorative proctocolectomy with ileal pouch–anal anastomosis in very young patients with refractory ulcerative colitis. J Pediatr Surg 2003; 38:863–7.

88. Rintala RJ, Lindahl HG. Proctocolectomy and J-pouch ileo-anal anastomosis in children. J Pediatr Surg 2002; 37:66–70.

89. Odigwe L, Sherman PM, Filler R et al. Straight ileoanal anastomosis and ileal pouch–anal anastomosis in the surgical management of idiopathic ulcerative colitis and familial polyposis coli in children: follow-up and comparative analysis. J Pediatr Gastroenterol Nutr 1987; 6:426–9.

90. Delaney CP, Fazio VW, Remzi FH et al. Prospective, age-related analysis of surgical results, functional outcome, and quality of life after ileal pouch–anal anastomosis. Ann Surg 2003; 238:221–8.

91. Farouk R, Pemberton J, Wolff B et al. Functional outcomes after ileal pouch–anal anastomosis for chronic ulcerative colitis. Ann Surg 2000; 231:919–26.

A descriptive study of 1386 patients undergoing restorative proctocolectomy between 1981 and 1994 with a median follow-up of 8 years. Incontinence rates were significantly higher in older patients after ileal pouch–anal anastomosis for ulcerative colitis.

92. Lewis WG, Sagar PM, Holdsworth PJ et al. Restorative proctocolectomy with end to end pouch–anal anastomosis in patients over the age of fifty. Gut 1993; 34:948–52.

93. Galanduik S, Scott NA, Dozois RR et al. Ileal pouch–anal anastomosis. Re-operation for pouch-related complications. Ann Surg 1990; 212:446–54.

94. Deutsch AA, McLeod RS, Cullan J et al. Results of the pelvic pouch procedure in patients with Crohn's disease. Dis Colon Rectum 1991; 34:475–7.

95. Hayman NH, Fazio VW, Tuckson WB et al. The consequences of ileal pouch–anal anastomosis for Crohn's disease. Dis Colon Rectum 1991; 34:653–7.

96. Grobler S, Hosie KB, Affice E et al. Outcome of restorative proctocolectomy in patients when the diagnosis is suggestive of Crohn's disease. Gut 1993; 34:1384–8.

97. Panis Y, Poupard B, Nemeth J et al. Ileal pouch–anal anastomosis for Crohn's disease. Lancet 1996; 347:854–7.

98. Regimbeau JM, Panis Y, Pocard M et al. Long-term results of ileal pouch–anal anastomosis for colorectal Crohn's disease. Dis Colon Rectum 2001; 44:769–78.

99. Tulchinsky H, Hawley PR, Nicholls J. Long-term failure after restorative proctocolectomy for ulcerative colitis. Ann Surg 2003; 238:229–34.

Descriptive single-centre experience of 634 patients undergoing restorative proctocolectomy for ulcerative colitis between 1976 and 1997 with a mean follow-up of 85 months. Failure rate rose with time of follow-up from 9% at 5 years to 13% at 10 years. Pelvic sepsis and poor function were the main reasons for later failure.

100. Yu CS, Pemberton JH, Larson D. Ileal pouch–anal anastomosis in patients with indeterminate colitis: long-term results. Dis Colon Rectum 2000; 43:1487–96.

101. Delaney CP, Remzi FH, Gramlich T et al. Equivalent function, quality of life and pouch survival rates after ileal pouch–anal anastomosis for indeterminate and ulcerative colitis. Ann Surg 2002; 236:43–8.

102. Richard CS, Cohen Z, Stern HS et al. Outcome of the pelvic pouch procedure in patients with prior perianal disease. Dis Colon Rectum 1997; 40:647–52.

103. Fazio VW, Tekkis PP, Remzi F et al. Quantification of risk for pouch failure after ileal pouch anal anastomosis surgery. Ann Surg 2003; 238:605–14.

Descriptive single-centre study of 1965 patients undergoing primary restorative proctocolectomy between 1983 and 2001 with a median follow-up of 4.1 years. Four preoperative and four postoperative factors were found to be important predictors of ileal pouch failure.

104. Olsen KO, Juul S, Bulow S et al. Female fecundity before and after operation for familial adenomatous polyposis. Br J Surg 2003; 90:227–31.

105. Olsen KO, Joelsson M, Laurberg S et al. Fertility after ileal pouch–anal anastomosis in women with ulcerative colitis. Br J Surg 1999; 86:493–5.

An epidemiological study of fertility in females before and after the diagnosis of ulcerative colitis and surgery. Restorative proctocolectomy reduces fertility by more than 50% compared with the same colitic patients before this surgery.

106. Utsunomiya J, Iwama T, Imago M et al. Total colectomy, mucosal proctectomy and ileo-anal anastomosis. Dis Colon Rectum 1980; 23:459–66.

107. Nicholls RJ, Lubowski DZ. Restorative proctocolectomy: the four loop W reservoir. Br J Surg 1987; 74:564–6.

108. Hallgren T, Fasth S, Nordgren S et al. The stapled ileal pouch–anal anastomosis. A randomised study comparing two different pouch designs. Scand J Gastroenterol 1990; 25:1161–8.

109. Seow Choen P, Tsunoda A, Nicholls RJ. Prospective randomised trial comparing anal function after hand sewn ileoanal anastomosis with mucosectomy versus stapled ileoanal anastomosis without mucosectomy in restorative proctocolectomy. Br J Surg 1991; 78:430–4.

Thirty-two patients were randomised to hand-sewn ileoanal anastomosis with mucosectomy and compared with stapled ileoanal anastomosis without mucosectomy during restorative proctocolectomy. Complication rates and pouch function were assessed at a median of 11 months and were similar in both groups.

110. Brough WA, Schofield PF. An improved technique of J pouch construction and ileoanal anastomosis. Br J Surg 1989; 76:350–1.

111. Lavery IC, Sirimarco MT, Ziv Y et al. Anal canal inflammation after ileal pouch–anal anastomosis. The need for treatment. Dis Colon Rectum 1995; 38:803–6.

112. Thompson-Fawcett MW, Mortensen NJ, Warren BF. 'Cuffitis' and inflammatory changes in the columnar cuff, anal transitional zone, and ileal reservoir after stapled pouch–anal anastomosis. Dis Colon Rectum 1999; 42:348–55.

113. Ziv Y, Fazio VW, Sirmarco MT et al. Incidence risk factors and treatment of dysplasia in the anal transitional zone after ileal pouch–anal anastomosis. Dis Colon Rectum 1994; 37:1281–5.

114. Tekkis PP, Fazio VW, Remzi FH et al. Evaluation of the learning curve in ileal pouch–anal anastomosis surgery. Ann Surg 2004 (in press).

115. Everett WG, Pollard SG. Restorative proctocolectomy without temporary ileostomy. Br J Surg 1990; 77:621–2.

116. Grobler SP, Hosie KB, Keighley MRB. Randomised trial of loop ileostomy in restorative proctocolectomy. Br J Surg 1992; 79:903–6.

117. Gemlo BT, Wong WD, Rothenberger DA et al. Ileal pouch–anal anastomosis. Patterns of failure. Arch Surg 1992; 127:784–6; discussion 787.

118. Foley EF, Schoetz DJJ, Roberts PL et al. Reversion after ileal pouch–anal anastomosis. Causes of

failures and predictors of subsequent pouch salvage. Dis Colon Rectum 1995; 38:793–8.

119. MacRae HM, McLeod RS, Cohen Z et al. Risk factors for pelvic pouch failure. Dis Colon Rectum 1997; 40:257–62.

120. Korsgen S, Keighley MR. Causes of failure and life expectancy of the ileoanal pouch. Int J Colorectal Dis 1997; 12:4–8.

121. Meagher AP, Farouk R, Dozois RR et al. J ileal pouch–anal anastomosis for chronic ulcerative colitis: complications and long term outcome in 1310 patients. Br J Surg 1998; 85:800–3.

122. Heuschen UA, Allemeyer EH, Hinz U et al. Outcome after septic complications in J pouch procedures. Br J Surg 2002; XX:194–200.

A long-term follow-up of patients having early sepsis after restorative proctocolectomy. Failure was at least three times the rate of the general population.

123. Karoui M, Cohen CRG, Nicholls RJ. Results of surgical removal of the pouch after failed restorative proctocolectomy. Dis Colon Rectum 2004; (in press).

124. Schoetz DJ, Coller JA, Veidenheimer MC. Ileoanal reservoir for ulcerative colitis and familial polyposis. Arch Surg 1986; 121:404–9.

125. Pemberton JH, Kelly KA, Beart RW et al. Ileal pouch–anal anastomosis for chronic ulcerative colitis. Long term results. Ann Surg 1987; 206:504–13.

126. Oresland T, Fasth S, Nordgren S et al. The clinical and functional outcome after restorative proctocolectomy. A prospective study in 100 patients. Int J Colorectal Dis 1989; 4:50–6.

127. Wexner SD, Jensen L, Rothenberger DA et al. Long term functional analysis of the ileoanal reservoir. Dis Colon Rectum 1989; 32:275–81.

128. Keighley MRB, Grobler S, Bain I. An audit of restorative proctocolectomy. Gut 1993; 34:680–4.

129. Wexner SD, Rothenberger DA, Jensen L et al. Ileal pouch–vaginal fistulas: incidence, aetiology and management. Dis Colon Rectum 1989; 32:460–5.

130. Groom JS, Nicholls RJ, Hawley PR et al. Pouch–vaginal fistula. Br J Surg 1993; 80:936–40.

131. Moskowitz RL, Shepherd NA, Nicholls RJ. An assessment of inflammation in the reservoir after restorative proctocolectomy with ileoanal ileal reservoir. Int J Colorectal Dis 1986; 1:167–74.

132. Kmiot WA, Hesslewood SR, Smith N et al. Evaluation of the inflammatory infiltrate in pouchitis with ^{111}In-labeled granulocytes. Gastroenterology 1993; 104:981–8.

133. Shen B, Achkar JP, Connor JT et al. Modified pouchitis disease activity index: a simplified approach to the diagnosis of pouchitis. Dis Colon Rectum 2003; 46:748–53.

134. Sandborn WJ, Tremaine WJ, Batts KP et al. Pouchitis after ileal pouch–anal anastomosis: a Pouchitis Disease Activity Index. Mayo Clin Proc 1994; 69:409–15.

135. Apel R, Cohen Z, Andrews CW et al. Prospective evaluation of early morphological changes in pelvic pouches. Gastroenterology 1994; 107:435–43.

136. Setti Carraro P, Talbot IC, Nicholls RJ. A long term appraisal of the histological appearances of the ileal reservoir mucosa after restorative proctocolectomy for ulcerative colitis. Gut 1994; 35:1721–7.

137. Verres B, Reinholt FP, Linquist K et al. Mucosal adaption in the ileal reservoir after restorative proctocolectomy. A long term follow-up. Ann Chir 1992; 46:10–18.

138. Thompson-Fawcett MW, Marcus V, Redston M et al. Risk of dysplasia in long-term ileal pouches and pouches with chronic pouchitis. Gastroenterology 2001; 121:275–81.

139. Mimura T, Rizzello F, Helwig U et al. Once daily high dose probiotic therapy (VSL3) for maintaining remission in recurrent or refractory pouchitis. Gut 2004; 53:108–14.

140. Gionchetti P, Rizzello F, Venturi A et al. Oral bacteriotherapy as maintenance treatment in patients with chronic pouchitis: a double-blind, placebo-controlled trial. Gastroenterology 2000; 119:305–9.

Forty patients with pouchitis who were in clinical and endoscopic remission were randomised to receive a probiotic preparation (VSL3) or control preparation. Three patients (15%) in the VSL3 group had relapsed within the 9-month follow-up period, compared with 20 (100%) in the placebo group (P <0.001). The authors suggest that oral administration of probiotics is effective in preventing flare-ups of chronic pouchitis.

141. Gionchetti P, Rizzello F, Helwig U et al. Prophylaxis of pouchitis onset with probiotic therapy: a double-blind, placebo-controlled trial. Gastroenterology 2003; 124:1202–9.

142. Stern H, Walfisch S, Mullen B et al. Cancer in an ileoanal reservoir: a new late complication? Gut 1990; 31:473–5.

143. Ooi BS, Remzi FH, Gramlich T et al. Anal transitional zone cancer after restorative proctocolectomy and ileoanal anastomosis in familial adenomatous polyposis: report of two cases. Dis Colon Rectum 2003; 46:1418–23.

144. Heuschen UA, Heuschen G, Autshbach F et al. Adenocarcinoma in the ileal pouch: late risk of cancer after restorative proctocolectomy. Int J Colorectal Dis 2001; 16:126–30.

145. Fazio VW, Wu JS, Lavery IC. Repeat ileal pouch–anal anastomosis to salvage septic complications of pelvic pouches: clinical outcome and quality of life assessment. Ann Surg 1998; 228:588–97.

146. Cohen Z, Smith D, McLeod R. Reconstructive surgery for pelvic pouches. World J Surg 1998; 22:342–6.

147. Poggioli G, Marchetti F, Selleri S et al. Redo pouches: salvaging of failed ileal pouch–anal anastomosis. Dis Colon Rectum 1993; 36:492–6.

148. Paye F, Penna C, Chiche L et al. Pouch-related fistula following restorative proctocolectomy. Br J Surg 1996; 83:1574–7.

149. Shah NS, Remzi F, Massmann A et al. Management and treatment outcome of pouch–vaginal fistulas following restorative proctocolectomy. Dis Colon Rectum 2003; 46:911–17.

150. Burke D, van Laarhoven CJ, Herbst F et al. Transvaginal repair of pouch–vaginal fistula. Br J Surg 2001; 88:241–5.

151. Zinicola R, Wilkinson KH, Nicholls RJ. Ileal pouch–vaginal fistula treated by abdominoanal advancement of the ileal pouch. Br J Surg 2003; 90:1434–5.

152. Ogunbiyi OA, Korsgen S, Keighley MR. Pouch salvage. Long-term outcome. Dis Colon Rectum 1997; 40:548–52.

153. Herbst F, Sielszneff I, Nicholls RJ. Salvage surgery for ileal pouch outlet obstruction. Br J Surg 1996; 83:368–71.

154. Sagar PM, Dozois RR, Wolff BG et al. Disconnection, pouch revision and reconnection of the ileal pouch–anal anastomosis. Br J Surg 1996; 83:1401–5.

155. Klas J, Myers GA, Starling JR et al. Physiologic evaluation and surgical management of failed ileoanal pouch. Dis Colon Rectum 1998; 41:854–61.

Nine

Crohn's disease

Mark W. Thompson-Fawcett and
Neil J.McC. Mortensen

INTRODUCTION

Crohn's disease is a chronic transmural inflammatory process that can affect the gastrointestinal tract anywhere from mouth to anus and which may be associated with extraintestinal manifestations. The disease is commonly confined to various regions of the gut, frequent patterns observed including ileal, ileocolic and colonic. Perianal disease may coexist with any of these. Often there are discontinuous segments of disease with areas of normal mucosa intervening. Inflammation may cause ulceration, fissures, fistulas and fibrosis with stricturing. Histology reveals a chronic inflammatory infiltrate that is typically patchy and transmural, and may reveal classic granulomas with giant cell formation. Clinically, patients have abdominal pain and diarrhoea, and they may develop bowel obstruction or intestinal fistulas. A combination of the clinical, macroscopic, radiological and pathological features is required to make the diagnosis. In the past, Crohn's disease was also referred to as regional enteritis or granulomatous enteritis.

EPIDEMIOLOGY

Crohn's disease has a prevalence of around 0.1%. Peak age of onset is 15–25 years, with a slightly higher incidence in females. There is no association with socioeconomic status or occupation, but an urban environment, cooler climate and increased standards of domestic hygiene may increase the risk.

In northern Europe, Scandinavia and North America the annual incidence of Crohn's disease is 5–6 per 100 000 population. This has steadily increased over recent decades but has now possibly plateaued. Rates are lower in southern and eastern Europe, and especially in Japan. Evidence of environmental effects is seen from studies of migrant populations. Jews have a higher incidence of Crohn's disease than other North Americans in the USA but a similar incidence while living in Israel. In Britain, West Indian and Asian migrants have a higher incidence of disease than in their home country. Ethnic differences are seen, with a particularly high rate in Ashkenazi Jews and a low incidence in black Americans, native Americans, Latin Americans and Asians.[1]

AETIOLOGY

Crohn's disease involves an interplay between environmental and genetic factors. The specific cause of the exaggerated inflammatory response at the mucosal level remains unclear. There are a number of areas where much investigation has been focused.

Smoking and oral contraception

Smoking increases the relative risk of Crohn's disease by 2–2.4 times in contrast with ulcerative colitis, where smoking provides a protective effect. Oral contraception may be associated with a small increase in risk, but whether this is causal or by association is not clear. Evidence suggests that oral contraceptive use has no effect on disease activity.[1]

Infection

Mycobacterium paratuberculosis causes a granulomatous inflammatory disorder in the intestine of cattle (Johne's disease) and it has been hypothesised that Crohn's is the human form of this disease. The organism is difficult to culture but recently some investigators have isolated the DNA of *M. paratuberculosis* from human intestinal tissue in two-thirds of patients with Crohn's disease and only 10% of controls. However, immunological reactivity cannot be demonstrated to *M. paratuberculosis* in patients with Crohn's disease, and antituberculous therapy has been ineffective, so the role of *M. paratuberculosis* as an aetiological agent is in doubt.[2,3]

In situ hybridisation has demonstrated measles virus DNA within foci of granulomatous vasculitis and lymphoid follicles in the bowel of patients with Crohn's disease. It has been suggested that Crohn's disease results from a granulomatous vasculitis secondary to measles virus infection. This could be proved only if there was a specific antiviral agent to eliminate the infection,[4] and studies using nested reverse polymerase chain reaction have found no evidence of the virus.[5] To date, then, the role of measles virus remains unproven.[6]

Genetic

Genetic predisposition to dysregulation of the immune system when exposed to particular microbial antigens probably plays a key role in the aetiology of inflammatory bowel disease (IBD). Epidemiological studies have demonstrated familial aggregation, greater concordance for IBD in monozygotic than dizygotic twins, and ethnic aggregation in the Ashkenazim. Siblings of patients with Crohn's disease are about 25 times more likely to develop Crohn's than the general population.[7] This rate is even greater if disease onset is before the age of 21 years,[8] and disease concordance in monozygotic twins is nearly 50%.[9] The relatives of patients with Crohn's disease have an increased risk of developing not just Crohn's but also ulcerative colitis, and some of the susceptibility genes are likely to be shared. Clinical patterns of IBD in affected parent–child pairs are concordant for each of disease type, extent and extraintestinal manifestations in about 70% of cases, and for affected sibling pairs this figure is about 80%.[10] Inheritance of susceptibility probably involves a number of genes and is not of a simple Mendelian mode. A recessive gene with incomplete penetrance may be important in Crohn's disease. The *NOD2/CARD15* gene demonstrates recent progress. Genome-wide scans of affected sib-pairs with IBD have led to the publication of a number of linkage areas. The first of these susceptibility loci was IBD1 on chromosome 16. Further work on IBD1 identified variants in the *NOD2/CARD15* gene that were associated with Crohn's disease. *NOD2* is expressed on monocytes and plays a role in apoptosis and nuclear factor κB activation to bacterial lipopolysaccharides. A number of variants have been described and there is a dose effect for the strength of association with Crohn's disease, i.e. stronger association for homozygous than heterozygous, and stronger if an individual has an increasing number of variants. Crohn's disease *NOD2/CARD15* variants have been associated with ileal but not colonic disease. Genetic heterogeneity is likely to account for the varied clinical pattern or phenotype (e.g. fistulating, stenosing; described later in the chapter) of Crohn's disease. There are increasing associations being reported between genetic variants and disease phenotype in IBD. As this complex polygenetic disorder is unravelled, the hope is that further therapeutic and preventative strategies will be developed.[1]

PATHOGENESIS

Normally, the gut is able to suppress the inflammatory immune response to the stream of microbial, dietary and other antigens in contact with the mucosa, but the ability to suppress this is lost in IBD. There is increased mucosal permeability in Crohn's disease but this may be a primary abnormality or secondary to the inflammatory process.

Increased permeability allows an increased antigen load to cross the mucosal barrier. The resident microflora probably play an important role and bacteria can be proinflammatory or anti-inflammatory (*Lactobacillus* spp. and probiotics are an example of the latter). In Crohn's disease the cell-mediated response is predominant, with excessive activation of CD4+ T cells (Th1) by antigenic stimulus. The subsequent release of cytokines is responsible for both the local and systemic response, including fever, an acute-phase response, hypoalbuminaemia, weight loss, increased mucosal epithelial permeability, endothelial damage and increased collagen synthesis. A wide variety of these soluble inflammatory mediators, such as interleukin (IL)-1, IL-2, IL-6, tumour necrosis factor (TNF), platelet activating factor and transforming growth factor (TGF)-β1 and TGF-α, are released from cells of leucocyte lineage as well as endothelial cells, epithelial cells and fibroblasts. It appears there may be an inability to induce T-cell suppressor function to specific antigens and also a subpopulation of T cells with decreased ability to induce apoptosis. This allows the inflammatory response in the intestinal mucosa to proceed unchecked, producing a chronic inflammatory state. Imbalances between proinflammatory and anti-inflammatory cytokines in IBD have led to work investigating treatment by specific inhibition of proinflammatory cytokines and supplementation with anti-inflammatory cytokines.[1]

PATHOLOGY

Distribution

The macroscopic appearance of the disease and its distribution in the gut are the first important pathological considerations and may provide key information towards making the diagnosis and differentiating Crohn's disease from other forms of IBD, particularly ulcerative colitis. Frequencies of regions involved are:

1. small bowel alone, 30–35%;
2. colon alone, 25–35%;
3. small bowel and colon, 30–50% (usually ileocolic);
4. perianal lesions, over 50%;
5. stomach and duodenum, 5% (minor subclinical mucosal abnormalities in 50%).[11]

Skip lesions (areas of disease separated by normal bowel) are diagnostic for Crohn's disease, with the exception of distal ulcerative colitis, where occasionally ulceration may be seen in the appendix or caecum.[12,13]

Macroscopic appearance

The unmistakable appearance of Crohn's disease is of a stiff thick-walled segment of bowel with fat wrapping. There is creeping extension of mesenteric fat around the serosal surface of the bowel wall towards the antimesenteric border,[14] and this is part of the connective tissue changes that affect all layers of the bowel wall. As inflammation is full thickness, there can be fibrinous exudate and adhesions on the serosal surface. Narrow linear ulcers with intervening islands of oedematous mucosa give the mucosal surface its classically cobblestone appearance. Ulceration is discrete, and serpiginous linear ulcers usually run along the mesenteric aspect of the lumen. Deep fissuring from linear ulceration may lead to formation of fistulas through the bowel wall. Closer inspection may reveal multiple aphthous ulcers that usually develop on the surface of submucosal lymphoid nodules,[15] and this is the earliest macroscopic lesion in Crohn's disease to be seen before the classic appearances of more established disease. Inflammatory polyps are often found in the involved colon but are unusual in the small bowel. Enlarged lymph nodes may be present in the resected mesentery but are not caseated or matted together. Strictures can vary from 1 to 30 cm in length. These may be stiff like a hosepipe with turgid oedema, or tight fibrotic strictures from burnt-out inflammation. The narrowing of the lumen may be sufficient to produce obstruction and proximal dilatation, and there may be multiple dilated segments between multiple tight strictures. Fistulas, sinuses and abscesses are often present in the ileocaecal region but may arise from any segment of active disease and can communicate with other loops of bowel, stomach, bladder, vagina, skin or intra-abdominal abscess cavities.

Microscopy

Inflammation involves the full thickness of the bowel wall. Early mucosal changes show neutrophils attacking the base of crypts, causing injury and focal crypt abscesses. The formation of mucosal lymphoid aggregates followed by overlying ulceration produces aphthous ulcers. There is relative preservation of goblet cell mucin in comparison with ulcerative colitis, where there is usually mucin depletion. As the disease progresses, connective tissue changes occur in all layers of the bowel wall giving the stiff, thick-walled, macroscopic appearance. There is submucosal fibrosis and muscularisation. The muscularis mucosa and muscularis propria are thickened from increased amounts of connective tissue.[1] Typically, the chronic inflammatory infiltrate and the architectural changes in the mucosa are patchy. Transmural inflammation is in the form of lymphoid aggregates seen throughout the bowel wall, leading to the formation of a Crohn's 'rosary' on the serosal surface. The following three features are diagnostic hallmarks of Crohn's disease:

1. deep non-caseating granulomas (excluding those that are mucosal or related to crypt rupture) are present in 60–70% of patients and are commonly located in the bowel wall but may be in the mesentery, regional lymph nodes, peritoneum, liver or contiguously involved tissue;[11]
2. intralymphatic granulomas;
3. granulomatous vasculitis.[16]

Pitfalls of differentiating Crohn's colitis from ulcerative colitis

Sometimes it is difficult even for an experienced gastrointestinal pathologist to differentiate between Crohn's colitis and ulcerative colitis on histology, and considerable interobserver variation is reported among pathologists. There can be a lot of overlap between the diseases and this can lead to the diagnosis of indeterminate colitis in 5–10% of patients with colonic involvement alone. During the course of the disease subsequent disease behaviour may change, leading to a change in diagnosis, usually towards Crohn's disease. For difficult cases, consideration of the macroscopic, microscopic, radiological and endoscopic features and the history and clinical picture is essential, for it is often the cumulative evidence that makes the diagnosis. A definitive diagnosis is more likely if the resected colon is

available for assessment as opposed to mucosal biopsies. If only endoscopic biopsies are available, the endoscopic findings are important and must be discussed with, or shown to, the pathologist.[1]

Rectal sparing may be seen in ulcerative colitis, especially if topical preparations have been used. Patchy inflammation is a feature of Crohn's disease, but treated ulcerative colitis can itself show patchy mucosal inflammation. Perianal disease is very suggestive of Crohn's, although patients with ulcerative colitis can develop cryptoglandular fistulas and abscesses. Lymphoid follicles may be seen in the base of the mucosa in severe ulcerative colitis but they are a prominent feature of Crohn's disease, where they are transmural. In Crohn's disease there is relative preservation of goblet cell mucin, whereas mucin depletion is a feature of ulcerative colitis (with the exception of fulminant ulcerative colitis where there may be surprisingly little mucin depletion).

CLINICAL

Gastrointestinal symptoms

The clinical presentation varies depending on the site of disease. Acute first presentations of disease are uncommon, but ileal disease can mimic acute appendicitis and colonic disease may present as a fulminating colitis.

The majority of patients complain of diarrhoea (70–90%), abdominal pain (45–65%), rectal bleeding (30%) and perianal disease (10%). Diarrhoea may result from mucosal inflammation, fistulation between loops of bowel, a short bowel from previous resections, bacterial overgrowth from obstructed segments, or bile salt malabsorption from terminal ileal disease; these latter two causes also produce steatorrhoea. Distal colitis and proctitis, and decreased rectal compliance, produce tenesmus and frequent bowel motions. Abdominal pain may be of a colicky nature from obstructing lesions or from peritoneal irritation caused by acute inflammation. Terminal ileal disease is the most common site for obstructive lesions. Rectal bleeding is uncommon from terminal ileal disease, but does occur in 50% of patients with colonic disease. Massive bleeding occurs in 1–2%,[17,18] and though the site is often difficult to identify the distribution is similar to that of the disease. When perianal disease is present, patients often complain of purulent discharge and minor leakage of faecal material and the associated discomfort this brings. Fissures may be large, indolent and painless. Significant perianal pain suggests undrained sepsis and thus an abscess. Fistulas extending to the bladder can produce pneumaturia and recurrent urinary tract infection,[19] while those extending to the vagina cause the passing of wind or faeces per vaginam.

Systemic symptoms

Weight loss is reported by 65–75% of patients. This is usually in the order of 10–20% of body weight and is the result of anorexia, food fear, diarrhoea and, less often, malabsorption. The latter may be caused by inflammatory disease but more commonly is due to bacterial overgrowth as a result of colo-enteric fistulas, blind loops or stasis from chronic obstruction. If there is extensive small bowel disease, there may be poor absorption of fat-soluble vitamins leading to symptoms and signs of osteomalacia (vitamin D) or a bleeding tendency (vitamin K). Other deficiencies are uncommon, usually resulting from inadequate intake rather than increased losses, but may include deficiencies of magnesium, zinc, ascorbic acid and the B vitamins. Symptoms of anaemia are common and usually result from iron deficiency due to intestinal blood loss and, less commonly, from vitamin B_{12} or folate deficiency. After resection of more than 50 cm of terminal ileum, vitamin B_{12} absorption falls below normal. Malabsorption of bile salts and fats, which can cause diarrhoea, usually only follows an ileal resection of greater than 100 cm. The inflammatory process produces a low-grade fever in 30–49% of patients; where high and spiking, or the patient reports rigors, it is likely that there is a suppurative intra-abdominal complication.[1]

Extraintestinal manifestations

These are outlined in **Box 9.1** and are more common in association with Crohn's colitis than isolated small bowel disease. They are similar to those that occur in ulcerative colitis, and may precede, be independent of or accompany active IBD, and can cause significant morbidity. Gallstones are said to be common due to malabsorption of bile salts in the terminal ileum; however, symptomatic problems

Box 9.1 • Extraintestinal manifestations of Crohn's disease

Related to disease activity

- Aphthous ulceration (10%)
- Erythema nodosum (5–10%)
- Pyoderma gangrenosum (0.5%)
- Acute arthropathy (6–12%)
- Eye complications (conjunctivitis, etc.) (3–10%)
- Amyloidosis (1%)

Unrelated to disease activity

- Sacroiliitis (often minimal symptoms) (10–15%)
- Ankylosing spondylitis (1–2%)
- Primary sclerosing cholangitis (rare)
- Chronic active hepatitis (2–3%)
- Cirrhosis (2–3%)
- Gallstones (15–30%)
- Renal calculi (5–10%)

are not increased compared with the general population.[20] Steatorrhoea promotes increased absorption of oxalate, thereby increasing the incidence of oxalate renal stones. Patients may have a fatty liver as a result of malnutrition or from receiving total parenteral nutrition. Mild abnormalities of liver function are common with active disease, so this does not imply significant liver disease.

Thromboembolic complications occur with IBD and are usually associated with severe active colonic disease. Common sites are the lower extremities and pelvic veins, but cerebrovascular accidents are also reported. Metastatic Crohn's disease is an unusual complication in which nodular ulcerating skin lesions occur at distant sites including the vulva, sub-mammary areas and extremities. Biopsies of these show non-caseating granulomas. Clubbing is seen in some cases of extensive small bowel disease.

Amyloidosis is reported in 25% of patients with Crohn's disease at post-mortem but only 1% have clinical manifestations. It can occur in the bowel or within other organs, including the liver, spleen and kidneys. If renal function is affected, resection of the diseased bowel will result in regression of amyloid and improvement of renal function.[1]

Physical signs

Patients may appear well and have a normal physical examination. With more severe disease there may be evidence of weight loss, anaemia, iron deficiency, clubbing, cachexia, proximal myopathy, easy bruising, elevated temperature, tachycardia and peripheral oedema. Signs of extraintestinal manifestations may be present.

Abdominal examination can be normal but tenderness in the right iliac fossa is common. Thickened loops of bowel may be palpable and if matted together can produce an abdominal mass. A psoas or intra-abdominal abscess produces signs and occasionally there is free peritonitis. Enterocutaneous fistulas are most common when there has been previous surgery and usually presents through a scar. Acute or chronic strictures or carcinoma may produce signs of obstruction. There is a 3–5% risk of adenocarcinoma complicating Crohn's colitis and also an increased risk of small-bowel carcinoma. Perianal disease varies from an asymptomatic fissure or inflamed skin tag to severe disease that may look like a 'forest fire', with erythema, large fleshy skin tags, deep chronic fissures with bridges of skin and multiple fistulas creating the so-called 'watering-can perineum'. Fibrosis from chronic inflammation may have produced a woody, stiff anal canal or an anal or rectal stenosis.

Paediatric age group

In children and adolescents, the gastrointestinal manifestations are similar but extraintestinal and systemic manifestations of disease become more important. About 15% have arthralgia and arthritis that often precedes bowel symptoms by months or years. Diagnosis may be delayed by a non-specific presentation with systemic symptoms of weight loss, growth failure and unexplained anaemia and fever. If active disease is dealt with promptly by medical or surgical treatment and adequate nutrition is maintained, retardation of growth and sexual development can usually be reversed.[1]

Pregnancy

This issue is often of concern as the disease primarily affects young adults. For the majority of patients with IBD fertility is normal but in some subgroups fertility rates are slightly reduced. In the absence of active disease, the outcome of pregnancy equals that of matched controls. With active disease at conception, there is an increase in spontaneous abortions and premature delivery, and a greater than 50% chance of relapsing disease during pregnancy. The risk of relapse is only 20–25% if disease is inactive at conception. It is therefore advisable to avoid conception during an acute phase of disease. Pregnancy probably does not affect the long-term course of the disease. Aminosalicylates, steroids and azathioprine are safe in pregnancy, but the use of ciclosporin should generally be avoided and methotrexate is contraindicated.[1]

INVESTIGATIONS

Laboratory

In more severe or established disease, magnesium, zinc and selenium levels should be checked. Serum albumin is often low in active disease due to down-regulation of albumin synthesis by cytokines (IL-1, IL-2, TNF). Mild episodic elevations of liver function tests are common but persistent abnormalities require further investigation. Evidence of anaemia should be sought, and if present investigated. A neutrophil leucocytosis usually indicates active disease or septic complications. Of the serum protein markers for inflammation, C-reactive protein and orosomucoid most closely match clinical disease activity. Erythrocyte sedimentation rate is useful in Crohn's colitis but not in small-bowel disease. Faecal fat excretion may be increased if malabsorption is present. Severe ileocaecal involvement can cause right hydronephrosis or sterile pyuria, and an enterovesical fistula will lead to bacteria in the urine.[1]

Radiology

A small bowel barium study has traditionally been the key to confirming the presence of small-bowel disease. It remains debatable whether this is best done by barium meal and follow-through techniques or by a small-bowel enema; probably most important is a radiologist committed to producing good-quality images. More subtle features of small bowel Crohn's include thickening of the valvulae coniventes, a granular mucosal pattern and aphthous ulcers. As disease progresses features include wall thickening, cobblestoning and fissure-like ulcers, sinus tracts and fistulas. There may be stenosis causing obstructive symptoms, commonly in the terminal ileum (**Fig. 9.1**). Multiple tight stenoses with intervening dilated segments produce a 'chain of lakes' appearance (**Fig. 9.2**). With increased use of computed tomography (CT) to investigate abdominal pain, thickened small bowel loops, especially terminal ileum, may strongly suggest a diagnosis of Crohn's disease (**Fig. 9.3**). Capsule endoscopy may point to a diagnosis in difficult cases.

A double-contrast barium enema provides an overall picture of disease extent and severity, and a record for future comparison. Changes in the colon are similar to those seen in the small bowel. Fistulas are uncommon and there is frequently rectal sparing. Strictures, which must be differentiated from carcinoma, are seen in 25% of patients and

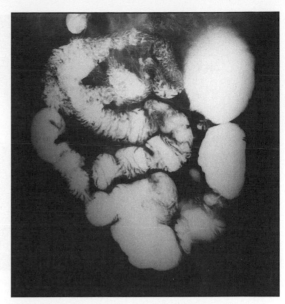

Figure 9.2 • Small-bowel barium enema showing multiple stenoses with intervening dilatation.

half of these are multiple. Chronic disease leads to shortening and loss of haustral folds. In severe cases plain abdominal films should be made initially to look for evidence of obstruction, mucosal oedema or dilatation.

Occasionally, if there is doubt about the barium studies or the degree of disease activity, there is a role for a radiolabelled white cell scan which highlights areas of active inflammation. Ultrasonography and CT can demonstrate thickened loops of bowel and are important for investigating complications of fistulating disease.[21] Magnetic resonance imaging (MRI) is the investigation of choice for complicated perianal sepsis, although endoanal ultrasound is also very useful in experienced hands. [22]

Endoscopy

Colonoscopy is complementary to barium enema. Its role is to assess areas that are equivocal on barium enema, to obtain biopsies that aid in the differential diagnosis, to assess and biopsy strictures and to clarify the situation where significant symptoms are not backed up by clinical evidence of disease. Intubation of the ileocaecal valve allows examination and biopsy of the terminal ileum. Small aphthous ulcers are the early features of

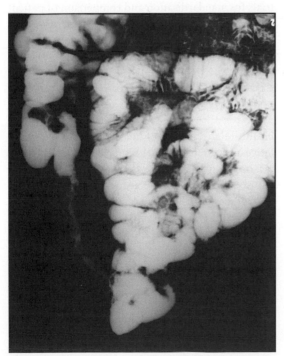

Figure 9.1 • Small-bowel enema with classic terminal ileal disease showing narrowing, cobblestone mucosa and fissures.

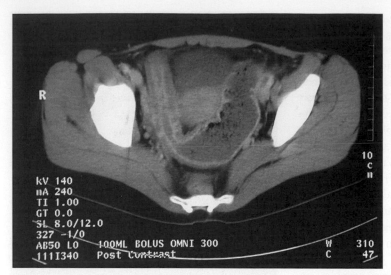

Figure 9.3 • CT scan showing thick-walled terminal ileum with proximal dilatation.

Crohn's disease, in contrast with the erythema and loss of vascular pattern in ulcerative colitis. In more severe disease the oedematous mucosa is penetrated by deep fissuring ulceration to give a cobblestone appearance. Multiple biopsies should be taken even if the mucosa appears normal as granulomas may be present that can confirm the diagnosis.[1] There is not usually a role for routine follow-up endoscopy and endoscopic findings correlate poorly with clinical remission.[23] However, there is a cancer risk in long-standing Crohn's colitis and most apply the same colonoscopic surveillance, despite various objections and limitations, as they do in cases of extensive ulcerative colitis.

Endoscopy of the oesophagus, stomach and duodenum is necessary if there are appropriate symptoms or abnormalities on a barium meal. Findings may include rugal hypertrophy, deep longitudinal ulcers and a cobblestone mucosa, the latter being the main differentiating feature from peptic ulcer disease. Biopsies should be taken but granulomas are often absent.[1]

Very occasionally, the diagnosis of Crohn's disease is made by capsule endoscopy; this is usually in the context of investigating obscure chronic gastro-intestinal bleeding when other investigations have been negative. One of the technical problems is that if there are areas of disease where the lumen is compromised, the capsule may get held up. If there is any significant concern that this may happen, a dummy dissolvable capsule can be used first.

Disease activity assessment

A number of indexes of disease activity have been developed for Crohn's disease, including the Crohn's Disease Activity Index and the Harvey–Bradshaw index, but their role is largely confined to clinical trials for standardisation and comparison of patient groups. For clinical purposes, disease activity is best assessed by clinical features and the investigations outlined above.

Health-related quality-of-life measures

Health-related quality of life (HRQOL) is a quantitative measurement of the subjective perception a person has of their health state, including emotional and social aspects. There are several well-validated 'instruments' or questionnaires to obtain these measures. In the past HRQOL data have been virtually absent from the surgical literature on Crohn's disease. However, if clinical trials are being conducted to compare different treatments, use of HRQOL instruments is essential for providing a valid and objective measure of outcome.[24]

Phenotyping

Phenotyping of Crohn's disease has arisen from the observation that presentation with disease varies with the site of disease and the behaviour of the disease (i.e. stricturing or fistulating). This is important for genetic studies investigating the correlation between phenotype and genotype, and for studying the outcome of therapy (medical or surgical) in different phenotypes. An international working party at the World Congress of Gastroenterology in 1998 produced the Vienna classification, to be tested in trials. At the time of diagnosis the following are recorded: age <40 years or ≥40 years, location of disease (terminal ileum, colon, ileocolon, upper gastrointestinal tract), behaviour (non-stricturing/non-penetrating, stricturing, penetrating), as well as data on sex, ethnicity, whether Jewish, family history of IBD, and extraintestinal manifestations.[1] To date it seems that the location of disease tends to be stable over time. However, the behaviour of Crohn's disease according to the Vienna classification varies dramatically over the course of the disease. At 10 years, 46% of patients exhibit different disease behaviour than at diagnosis. Therefore for phenotype–genotype analyses Crohn's disease should be studied in subgroups of patients defined by their disease behaviour after a fixed duration of disease.[25]

DIFFERENTIAL DIAGNOSIS

Small-bowel Crohn's disease

In most cases, after an appropriate work-up involving history and clinical, laboratory, radiological, endoscopic and pathological findings the diagnosis will be fairly clear-cut. **Box 9.2** shows the differential diagnoses of small-bowel Crohn's disease; perhaps the two that cause most difficulty are *Yersinia* and tuberculosis.

Large-bowel Crohn's disease

When there is no small-bowel or perineal involvement, there are two areas where the diagnosis may be difficult. An isolated segment of disease, especially if it is a short segment, has to be differentiated from carcinoma, ischaemia, tuberculosis and lymphoma; occasionally, severe diverticular disease can appear as or disguise a segment of Crohn's disease. Inflamed diverticular disease can mimic Crohn's disease, with the presence of granulomas, transmural inflam-

Box 9.2 • Differential diagnosis of small-bowel Crohn's disease

Differential diagnosis	Useful discriminating features
Appendicitis	History, CT scan
Appendix abscess	History, ultrasound/CTscan
Caecal diverticulitis	Older age, barium enema
Pelvic inflammatory disease	History
Ovarian cyst or tumour	Ultrasound
Caecal carcinoma	Barium enema/colonoscopy
Ileal carcinoid	Small-bowel enema
Behçet's disease	Painful ulceration of the mouth and genitalia
Systemic vasculitis affecting small bowel	Underlying systemic connective tissue disorder
Radiation enteritis	History of radiotherapy
Ileocaecal tuberculosis	History of tuberculosis, circulating antibodies to *Mycobacterium*, stool cultures
Yersinia enterocolitica ileitis	Self-limiting, stool cultures, serology
Eosinophilic gastroenteritis	Gastric involvement, peripheral eosinophilia
Amyloidosis	Biopsy
Small-bowel lymphoma	Radiological appearance
Actinomycosis	Microscopy of fine-needle aspirate
Chronic non-granulomatous jejunoileitis	Clinical picture and histology

mation and fissuring ulceration. Isolated involvement of the sigmoid colon is not common in Crohn's disease, so care should be taken before making this diagnosis in the presence of diverticular disease.[26] Differentiating Crohn's disease from ulcerative colitis has been discussed earlier.

MEDICAL TREATMENT

A summary of first-line medical treatment options for Crohn's disease is given in **Box 9.3**. The concept of treating Crohn's disease is to induce remission

Box 9.3 • Summary of first-line medical treatment options for Crohn's disease

Mild to moderate disease

- Appropriate salicylate compound
- Metronidazole 400 mg t.d.s.
- Prednisolone 20 mg daily for 4–6 weeks

Moderate disease

- Prednisolone 40–60 mg daily for 2–3 weeks, then tapering to 20 mg for 4 weeks

Severe disease

- Intravenous hydrocortisone 100 mg 6-hourly ± intravenous metronidazole
- Electrolyte and blood replacement and nutritional support

Chronic active disease

- Prednisolone
- Azathioprine or 6-mercaptopurine

Maintenance of remission

- Azathioprine

and then to maintain it. The most effective agents for inducing remission are corticosteroids and more recently, in highly selected cases, infliximab. For moderate to severe disease, steroids are commenced and at the same time immunosuppression, usually azathioprine, is commenced. After some weeks or months, when the therapeutic benefit of immunosuppression commences, steroids can be removed. Aminosalicylates have a role for less severe disease, but the degree of clinical benefit in small-bowel disease is being increasingly questioned.

Aminosalicylates

Sulfasalazine and 5-aminosalicylic acid (also known as mesalazine or mesalamine) are most commonly used to treat disease of mild to moderate severity. Sulfasalazine consists of a sulfapyridine carrier linked to 5-aminosalicylic acid. A small amount of sulfasalazine is absorbed in the small bowel but 90% passes to the colon, where bacteria cleave off the active 5-aminosalicylic acid, of which about 20% is absorbed. If 5-aminosalicylic acid is taken orally by itself, it is completely absorbed in the proximal small bowel; although it is the main active drug, the sulfapyridine produces most of the adverse effects, including nausea, vomiting, heartburn, headache, oligospermia and low-level haemolysis. These adverse effects are dose related. There are also a number of hypersensitivity reactions unrelated to drug levels, including worsening colitis. Adverse effects occur in 30% of people taking 4 g daily of sulfasalazine. Newer 5-aminosalicylic acid preparations use different carriers, or use pH- or time-dependent protective coatings that allow release to start in the jejunum, ileum or colon, thereby giving a much lower adverse effect profile and also small-bowel activity.[27]

Sulfasalazine has proven beneficial in the treatment of active colonic disease in doses of 1 g per 15 kg, but it is not superior to placebo for small-bowel disease or for maintenance. The newer 5-aminosalicylic acid compounds such as Pentasa have been shown to be as effective as sulfasalazine in the colon and have the added benefit of being effective in small-bowel disease, but adequate doses must be used (usually 4–5 g daily).

 Meta-analysis of a number of studies has also shown that these agents can be used prophylactically after medical or surgical remission to effect an absolute risk reduction of symptomatic recurrence by about 5–10%.[28–30]

The evidence is strongest for ileal disease in doses of at least 3 g daily. Topical rectal preparations are effective for distal disease and can be used with oral preparations. All the above compounds seem to be safe in pregnancy and breast-feeding.[27,31]

Steroids

Systemically absorbed corticosteroids are the most effective and commonly used drugs for moderate to severe Crohn's disease and will induce remission in 70–80% of cases, although they are less effective if only the colon is involved. Doses of prednisolone range from 20–40 mg/day orally for moderate disease to 60–80 mg/day intravenously for severe disease. Steroids should be used in short courses and must be tapered when a clinical response is achieved. They can be useful in resolving the obstructive symptoms in early disease caused by narrowing due to inflammatory oedema. Steroids will not help with obstructive symptoms caused by established fibrotic stenosis. Steroids are useful for maintaining a steroid-induced remission, which implies steroid-dependent disease, but they do not have a role in maintenance beyond this. There is no advantage in combining salicylate therapy with steroids.

Rectal administration of hydrocortisone and prednisolone is effective for left-sided colonic disease, but they are absorbed systemically, and prolonged therapy can cause adrenal suppression. 5-Aminosalicylic acid foam enemas are equally effective and can be used in combination with oral steroids in an exacerbation of disease.[27,31]

To avoid systemic adverse effects, topically active corticosteroids have been developed. Budesonide, formulated as a slow-release oral preparation, acts in the small bowel and colon or can be given as an enema. The systemic bioavailability of budesonide is only 10–15% because of rapid first-pass metabolism in the liver, but it can still produce some suppression of plasma cortisol levels.

In active Crohn's disease, budesonide produced remission in 51–60% of patients compared with 60–73% on systemic steroids, but with a halving of reported adverse effects from 60 to 30%. When budesonide 9 mg daily was compared with mesalamine 4 g daily for ileal and/or ascending colon disease, remission in the budesonide group at 16 weeks was 62% vs. 36% for mesalamine, and budesonide was better tolerated. Budesonide appears to have no role in maintenance therapy.[27,32,33] Budesonide was compared to placebo in a double-blind randomised controlled trial to assess its benefit for reducing endoscopic recurrence (at 3 and 12 months) after an ileal or ileocolic resection, with no benefit overall.[34]

Antibiotics

Metronidazole is the most frequently used antibiotic. Its mechanism of action is unclear, but may be by a variety of antibacterial effects or by its ability to suppress cell-mediated immunity. Its effectiveness was first reported in perianal disease, where it is commonly used with anecdotal success, although there are no controlled trials to support this practice.

In a randomised placebo-controlled trial[27] it has been shown to decrease disease activity in ileocolonic and colonic disease but not in small-bowel disease, and there was no change in the rate of remission. Other reports have shown it to have a similar efficacy to sulfasalazine. Long-term use of metronidazole in doses >10 mg/kg is contraindicated because of the risk of peripheral neuropathy.

Other antibiotics are used from time to time but there are few data on their efficacy. Ciprofloxacin has been popular in recent years and has been used for both perianal disease and ileitis.[27]

Nutrition for therapy

The rationale for nutritional therapy is that intraluminal dietary antigens may drive the inflammatory response and that removal of these and bowel rest will bring remission.

Total parenteral nutrition is effective in inducing remission in 60–80% of patients, which matches the effect of steroids, but combining both these therapies gives no added benefit over using only one. Total parenteral nutrition is less effective in isolated colonic disease. The relapse rate is high after a short course, and as long-term parenteral nutrition is not practicable its role is confined to nutritional support during periods of intestinal failure.

Total enteral nutrition is equally as effective as parenteral nutrition and has a similar relapse rate after cessation. Polymeric diets seem as effective as elemental and peptide-based diets, but polymeric diets are cheaper and more palatable and are therefore preferred.[27]

Immunomodulatory therapy

This is used to reduce steroid requirements, particularly after a remission has been achieved, and in refractory disease. Azathioprine and 6-mercaptopurine are purine analogues, azathioprine being quickly metabolised to 6-mercaptopurine. They inhibit cell proliferation and suppress cell-mediated events by inhibiting the activity of cytotoxic T cells and natural killer cells. The onset of a therapeutic effect takes 3–6 months. Toxicity is not uncommon and 3–15% of patients will develop pancreatitis, which will resolve on stopping the drug.

Fever, rash, arthralgias and hepatitis may occur and marrow suppression is dose related.

> In trials to improve disease or to decrease steroid requirements, there is a success rate of about 70–80%, and this applies equally to all disease sites, including perianal disease.

Methotrexate is used occasionally for treating Crohn's disease. Limited data suggest it is as effective as azathioprine or 6-mercaptopurine and it is prescribed for patients who do not tolerate or respond to the latter two drugs.[27]

Ciclosporin inhibits the T-cell-mediated amplification of the inflammatory cascade. It does not have the cytotoxic and marrow suppression of the above drugs, has a narrow therapeutic window, and oral bioavailability varies between patients. The most important adverse effect is nephrotoxicity, but others include paraesthesiae, hypertrichosis, tremor, hypertension, nausea, vomiting, headache and, occasionally, seizures and other neurotoxicities.[27] The evidence is conflicting but uncontrolled data report remission in up to 80% of patients within 2 weeks using intravenous administration, though remission may be limited to the course of therapy. It has also not proved effective for maintenance of remission. However, for fistulous perianal disease, several small case series report a dramatic response to a short course of intravenous ciclosporin, with some intermediate-term benefit.[35]

Clinical trials are ongoing with a number of monoclonal antibodies directed at specific mediators of the inflammatory response.

> The initial placebo-controlled trial with a mouse–human chimeric monoclonal antibody to TNF-α (infliximab) addressed induction of remission after a single dose. At 4 weeks after a single dose, an initial treatment response was seen in 65% (54 of 83) who received infliximab and 17% (4 of 24) in the placebo group; at 12 weeks this was 41% and 12% respectively.[36] The recent ACCENT I study addressed the maintenance of remission with a year of treatment with infliximab; 573 patients were recruited. After an initial infusion, 58% responded. The responders were then randomised to placebo or infliximab at 2 and 6 weeks and then 8 weekly up to 54 weeks. At week 54, of initial responders, about 15% in the placebo group and 35% in the treatment group were in clinical remission.[37]

> Similar results with initial moderate efficacy have been demonstrated using infliximab to treat fistulas. Present et al.[38] studied perianal and enterocutaneous draining fistulas, and defined their primary endpoint as a reduction in the number of fistulas by 50% or more. After three infusions at 0, 2 and 6 weeks, response was achieved in 26% of the placebo group and 62% of the treatment group. Complete closure of fistulas was seen in 13% of the placebo group and 46% of the treatment group. The ACCENT II study was an extension of this initial study with fistulas. The same selection criteria and initial dose were used and all patients received infliximab at the beginning. The study randomised responders at week 14 to placebo or infliximab infusions 8 weekly to week 54. The primary endpoint was loss of response, with fistulas reactivating or reappearing. Of 306 patients enrolled, 195 (64%) responders were randomised at week 14. At week 54, 23 of 98 patients receiving placebo maintained a response compared with 42 of 91 receiving infliximab. This means that of all 306 patients entered into the study, about 30% of patients treated with infliximab will maintain a response at 1 year, 22% having a complete response. In the placebo group after initial infliximab response, 19% (19 of 98) had a complete response.[39] The efficacy at 1 year judged by complete response is therefore modest.

Long-term safety data are not available yet but there are ongoing concerns about a potential increase in malignancies and reactivation of tuberculosis. Infliximab therapy is costly and not without adverse effects. In clinical practice it is best used short term as an agent to induce remission when conventional modalities have been ineffective, with a view to following on with conventional immunosuppression. Infliximab should only be used in the context of an experienced multidisciplinary team.

Other drugs

Antidiarrhoeal medication and anticholinergic agents to relieve colicky pain are useful in mild to moderate disease but should be avoided in severe exacerbations. Non-steroidal anti-inflammatory drugs should also be avoided as they may make the disease worse, and narcotics can increase bowel spasm. Cholestyramine is useful for treating bile salt diarrhoea.

SURGERY

Development of surgery

Crohn and colleagues initially described radical resection of involved segments of bowel, but high recurrence rates led to a vogue for bypassing affected segments. Frequent complications with the bypassed segments caused a return to resectional surgery.[40] Modern surgery for Crohn's disease involves resecting the least amount of bowel to re-establish satisfactory intestinal function.

 This is based on the concept that Crohn's is a gut-wide disease and that microscopic disease at the resection margin does not influence recurrence of disease.[41–44]

Furthermore, one small study has shown that asymptomatic endoscopic small-bowel lesions remaining after ileocolic resection did not correlate with clinical recurrence.[45] Although the term 'recurrence of disease' is widely used, a better term is 'recrudescence', implying a new outbreak of already present disease.

It is important to avoid any unnecessary sacrifice of gut as these patients may need resections of further segments for future disease recrudescence. In the move to conservatism, however, it is important not to procrastinate when there is an indication for surgery: when patients were questioned on the timing of their surgery, most would have preferred to have had the procedure 12 months earlier because of the benefits it gave.[46] Low quality-of-life scores with active disease improve to normal when remission is obtained, whether by surgery or medical treatment.[47–49] When medical treatment does not induce remission or the adverse effects of therapy are unacceptable, in most cases the best course of action for the patient is to proceed to surgery.

Laparoscopic surgery is feasible and safe for resection and diversion in uncomplicated Crohn's disease[50,51] and is increasingly being used for more complicated cases. The most time-efficient and cost-effective approach is an extracorporeal anastomosis and, where possible, extracorporeal ligation of the mesentery. For ileocolic resections this can usually be accomplished with relative ease, giving the patient a small 3–5 cm incision around the umbilicus. Patients generally prefer a laparoscopic approach, with its cosmetic advantage[52] and perceived quicker recovery. One small randomised study of 60 patients with terminal ileal disease showed slightly quicker recovery favouring laparoscopic surgery over open surgery, with discharge at a median of 5 vs. 6 days.[53]

Risk of operation and reoperation

Accurate population figures about patterns of disease and complications are not easy to obtain. It should be remembered that many of the data presented in this chapter are from specialist centres and these figures may not always apply to the Crohn's population at large. In perhaps the largest population-based cohort reported of 1936 patients from Sweden, the cumulative rate of intestinal resection was 44, 61 and 71% at 1, 5 and 10 years respectively after diagnosis; the subsequent risk of recurrence was 33 and 44% at 5 and 10 years respectively.[54] In another population-based study involving 210 patients with Crohn's disease at a mean of 11 years from disease onset, 56% required surgery; by life-table analysis the reoperation rate was 25% at 10 years and 56% at 20 years.[55]

In a tertiary referral centre experience of 592 patients with Crohn's disease, 74% required surgery at a median of 13 years' follow-up. The chance of surgery varied with the site of disease and was 65% in those with small-bowel involvement, 58% in those with colonic or anorectal disease, and 91% in those with ileocolic disease.[56] Half of the patients in a tertiary referral centre who have had one operation will require reoperation for further disease with follow-up of more than 10 years.[57,58] Most studies report the annual rate of symptomatic recurrence to be 5–15% and that of reoperation 2–10%. For patients presenting to a surgical service, the cumulative chance of a permanent stoma at 20 years is 14% and of a temporary stoma 40%.[59]

Risk factors for recurrence

Many studies have looked at risk factors for recurrence. Recurrence (or recrudescence) can be defined by radiological findings, endoscopic findings, the return of symptoms or the need for further surgery. Most studies have been retrospective, and although some claim to identify risk factors, others report no association for the same risk factor. There is no consistently robust evidence that age of onset of disease, gender, site of disease, number of resections, length of small bowel resection, proximal margin length, microscopic disease at the resection margin, fistulising vs. obstructive disease, number of sites of disease, presence of granulomas or blood transfusion are associated with recurrence.[41,60–66]

Although a recurrence frequently occurs immediately proximal to the previous anastomosis, there is no evidence that anastomotic technique (side-to-side, end-to-end, end-to-side, hand-sewn or stapled) affects recurrence.[67–70] (The randomised study included here is somewhat underpowered and the other studies are not randomised.)

However, there are two important factors that do alter recurrence rates.

It is now clear that continuing to smoke after a surgical resection doubles the risk of recurrence and patients must be urged to stop smoking.[67,71,72] Prophylactic use of 5-aminosalicylic acid after surgical resection showed a relative risk reduction of 0.62 (95% CI 0.40–0.97) in one trial, and a meta-analysis of three randomised trials showed an absolute risk reduction for symptomatic recurrence of 13.1% (95% CI 4.5–21.8%).[29,30] One study has suggested the effect is greater for small bowel disease and of marginal benefit for other sites.[73]

Some patients prefer to be free of medication after surgery and accept a small increase in risk of recurrence. Because of the limited ability of 5-aminosalicylic acid compounds to reduce recurrence after surgery, there is a trend in favour of azathioprine. Many believe azathioprine has improved efficacy, but good prospective data to support this are not available at present.[74,75]

Principles of surgery for Crohn's disease

PERIOPERATIVE CONSIDERATIONS

Excellent perioperative care is essential for a good outcome in patients with Crohn's disease. As there is always potential for colonic involvement with small bowel disease, in all elective cases adequate bowel preparation of the colon should be considered. Deep vein thrombosis prophylaxis is mandatory because patients with IBD are at increased risk of thrombotic complications.[76] Usually, low-dose subcutaneous heparin and compression stockings suffice but these measures are not necessarily adequate if there is a history of thrombosis. Patients will often be at risk of adrenal suppression and the need for intravenous steroid cover should be considered every time. Before elective surgery, significant malnutrition should be restored by either enteral or parenteral nutrition, all potential electrolyte problems corrected and sepsis controlled. If this is not possible, consideration should be given to a temporary stoma rather than an anastomosis. In the perioperative period, psychological factors and adequate counselling are important as these patients may face, or have already had, one or more major operations with a complication rate of 30%, one-third of these being major.[77] Joint management with a gastroenterologist is an essential principle in the decision-making and hospital care.

TECHNIQUE

Some patients with Crohn's disease will be among the most technically difficult cases a surgeon will face and any compromise of good technique can be unforgiving. Any part of the bowel can be affected or involved with Crohn's disease, so in most cases the patient should be placed in a modified lithotomy or Lloyd-Davies position. A midline infraumbilical incision gives good access, is more easily reopened in the future and will not interfere with stomas that may be needed on either side of the abdomen. At each operation a full laparotomy should be carried out to stage the disease and the length of remaining and resected bowel measured. In the event of recurrence it is helpful to have marked anastomotic sites with a metal clip. At the first abdominal operation for Crohn's disease, consideration should be given to removing the appendix to prevent future diagnostic problems and confusion.

Thick oedematous mesenteric pedicles require special mention. A standard tie may allow a vessel to retract into the mesentery, resulting in a mesenteric haematoma with potential to compromise the blood supply to large segments of bowel. Thick pedicles should be dealt with by a fail-safe technique and some recommend double suture ligation.[78] Spillage of gastrointestinal contents must be minimised and controlled, and meticulous haemostasis is important as there may be inevitable loss from oozing inflamed raw surfaces. Great care should be taken not to damage or perforate other loops of bowel or other organs in the presence of difficult adhesions and inflammation.

Hyaluronidase-impregnated methylcellulose membranes have been developed to reduce adhesions. Membranes have been effective in reducing adhesions between midline wounds and abdominal contents, and may have particular application to this group of patients who have a high rate of reoperation.[79]

There are a number of similar products available, including spray-on application and membranes that are easier to use than the above, with claimed similar efficacy. In addition, one of the benefits of laparoscopic surgery may be a decrease in adhesion formation.

Surgery for small-bowel and ileocolic Crohn's disease

INDICATIONS

Surgery for small-bowel Crohn's disease is aimed at treating complications not amenable to medical therapy. Surgical interventions are required for:

1. stenosis causing obstructive symptoms;
2. enterocutaneous or intra-abdominal fistulas to other organs;
3. draining intra-abdominal or retroperitoneal abscesses;
4. controlling acute or chronic bleeding;
5. free perforation.

Of these, obstruction is the most frequent indication.

GASTRODUODENAL DISEASE

Symptomatic gastroduodenal disease is present in 0.5–4% of patients and is usually associated with disease in other sites. The first and second parts of the duodenum are most commonly involved and the disease often extends into the gastric antrum. Most patients who require surgery require it for problems of stenosis or occasionally bleeding. Often it is difficult at endoscopy to differentiate Crohn's from peptic ulcer disease but a trial of medical ulcer therapy may be diagnostic. Gastrojejunostomy is the standard procedure for duodenal or pyloric stenosis. Many have added a vagotomy but it may not decrease the 25–40% risk of stomal ulceration;[1] truncal vagotomy may increase the chance of diarrhoea and a parietal cell vagotomy is preferable.[80] However, now that proton pump inhibitors are available, vagotomy is probably unnecessary.

If a pyloric or duodenal strictureplasty is feasible, this is preferable to a bypass as it will decrease the chance of gastric hypersecretion, diarrhoea and stomal ulceration. Results of a duodenal strictureplasty can be variable and the key is probably careful case selection.[81,82] Massive acute bleeding is rare, but if endoscopic methods are unsuccessful, bleeding should be controlled by under-running the bleeding vessel with a suture. Balloon dilatation of benign upper gastrointestinal tract strictures is safe, but the limited experience in Crohn's disease suggests dilatation has little long-term benefit.[83] Fistulas involving the duodenum occur in 0.5% of patients with Crohn's disease and generally arise from other diseased segments fistulating into the duodenum. Surgical therapy is usually successful and prognosis relates to the severity of disease in the primary segment.[84,85] Closure of secondary duodenal defects with a jejunal serosal patch or Roux-en-Y limb may be preferable to primary suture.[86]

ILEOCOLIC DISEASE

The cumulative operation rate for patients with distal ileal disease at 5 years from the time of diagnosis is 80% and with longer follow-up 91%.[56] Ileocaecal disease is treated with a limited ileocaecal resection, including a few centimetres of macroscopically normal bowel at each end, and using an end-to-end anastomosis seems satisfactory. Anastomotic configuration probably does not affect recurrence rates,[69,70] although some suggest that an end-to-side or side-to-side anastomosis is better.[87]

After a first operation the reoperation rate at 5 years is 20–25% and at 10 years 35–40%. Reoperation rates for second and subsequent operations are the same.[41,58,61] There is colonoscopic evidence of early recurrence in 72% at 1 year and in 88% with longer follow-up.[88] Further disease is usually on the ileal side of the anastomosis and it is important to stress that this is new disease and does not relate to an inadequate resection margin. Although recurrent disease rates are high and on average a patient will need an operation every 10 years, surgery is highly successful at relieving symptoms and restoring health when disease is refractory to medical treatment.

Balloon dilatation of selected symptomatic ileocolic strictures, usually short anastomotic strictures, is a treatment option with at least short-term benefit in 60–80% (with a risk of perforation of 2–11%) and with longer term benefit in 40–60%.[89–92]

ILEAL AND JEJUNAL MULTISITE DISEASE

If there is isolated small bowel disease, it is almost invariably in the terminal ileum and is usually suited to a limited resection. More extensive disease can produce obstructive strictures throughout the small bowel. In the past, these patients requiring surgery had multiple resections, with a risk of short bowel syndrome. In an endeavour to maximise conservation of bowel length the concept of strictureplasty was introduced,[93] and this technique is now preferred for all suitable lesions. It is ideally suited to short fibrotic strictures but it may be used for strictures up to 10–15 cm long. Generally, long strictures with active inflammation are usually better managed with resection unless there is concern about bowel length. In most series half the patients having a strictureplasty will also have a segmental resection.

Strictureplasty is carried out using the same methods as used for pyloroplasty. The Heineke–Mikulicz technique is usually used. In a small number of cases with longer strictures where bowel conservation is required, a Finney or a Jaboulay strictureplasty may be used.[94] For even longer narrowed segments a side-to-side isoperistaltic technique described by Michelassi may be used.[95] A modification to this was recently described where normal small bowel above the stricture is slid distally and anastomosed side to side to the diseased segment, with the claim of lessening the risk of further stenosis.[96] Most patients have three or four strictureplasties but in some cases there may be 10–15.[97] To ensure no strictures have been missed, the technique includes passing a Foley catheter along the small bowel through an enterotomy. The balloon is then inflated to a diameter of 25 mm and pulled back through the bowel, and strictures not easily seen externally will be identified. Alternatively, a marble or steel or wooden ball with a diameter of 25 mm can be traced through the bowel to identify strictures.

Results of strictureplasty have proved it to be a safe and effective technique. Postoperative abdominal septic complications occur in 4–5%, and overall 98–99% have symptomatic relief. Postoperative bleeding from a strictureplasty site occurs in 5–9% of patients, but this usually resolves with conservative measures.[98,99] Recurrence requiring reoperation has been reported as occurring in 13–20% at 40 months' follow-up,[100,101] in 35% at 54 months[102,103] and in 44% at 107 months.[104] Reoperation rates after a strictureplasty are similar whether or not a limited resection is included in the operation.[103,105] Only 2–4% of the strictureplasties themselves restricture, so most of the recurrent disease occurs at new sites.

Fistulas and abscesses

Enteric fistulas may affect up to 30% of patients with Crohn's disease and in a referral centre about 40% are internal, 40% external and 20% mixed. They may occur spontaneously or postoperatively, the latter usually being external. Fistula tracts have an associated abscess in 60% of cases. In expert hands surgical repair is successful in closing the fistula in more than 95% of cases, but failure after an attempt at definitive surgery can result in a mortality rate of 50%.[86]

ENTEROCUTANEOUS FISTULAS AND INTRA-ABDOMINAL ABSCESS

Enterocutaneous fistulas in Crohn's disease are a common cause of intestinal failure and patients who develop intestinal failure are best managed in a specialised unit[106] with a multidisciplinary approach. Intra-abdominal abscesses that are drained externally will usually result in a fistula. When abscesses complicate existing fistulas it is necessary to convert these fistula/abscess complexes into a well-draining fistula. Fistulas, whether postoperative or spontaneous, will drain along the line of least resistance, which is often previous scar tissue from incisions or drain sites.

Management principles

Although spontaneous and postoperative fistulas behave differently, the same management principles apply. The steps are outlined below.[107]

1. Resuscitate the patient, correcting electrolytes and restoring haemoglobin levels. Control sepsis by open or percutaneous drainage and antibiotics; occasionally, exteriorisation of the bowel ends will be required. Attempts at repair and anastomosis should never be made in a patient with significant nutritional compromise or sepsis. Protect the skin from the fistula output by expert application of stoma appliances.

 There has been a vogue for using somatostatin analogues to decrease fistula output but it has shown no benefit in a clinical trial.[108]

2. Establish nutrition by either enteral feeding or total parenteral nutrition.
3. Support morale as these patients are often emotionally very fragile. They are upset and angry about what has happened to them and often demoralised and frightened as well. The surgeon should at all times recognise this and be prepared directly to address these issues with the patient.
4. Mobilise the patient. If it is reasonable to anticipate closure with conservative measures, or the fistula is postoperative, wait for at least 6 weeks. If a fistula has not closed by 12 weeks, it probably never will. However, it will generally close spontaneously by 6 weeks unless it:
   (a) originates from a diseased segment of bowel;
   (b) arises from an anastomotic breakdown greater than 50% of the circumference of the bowel;
   (c) has a very short tract or communication between skin and mucosa;
   (d) has bowel obstruction distal to it.
5. Plan a definitive operation with:
   (a) complete enterolysis;
   (b) en bloc resection of the diseased or damaged bowel and the fistula tract with primary anastomosis.

The work-up includes radiological imaging to (i) define the extent of intestinal disease, (ii) exclude any obstructing lesions and (iii) delineate the fistula tracts. Avoid the temptation to carry out earlier and repetitive imaging unless the results will alter management.

Spontaneous enterocutaneous fistulas

In Crohn's disease this implies that there is a segment of diseased bowel that will require resection. This group generally benefits from earlier surgery for the following reasons.

1. The fistula will not heal spontaneously.
2. There is no concern about a more recent laparotomy making surgery difficult.
3. The bowel perforation occurs slowly and abdominal sepsis is usually localised, lessening the initial systemic insult.
4. Although the aim is to optimise the patient's general and nutritional state before surgery, active Crohn's disease will limit what is achievable.[109]

POSTOPERATIVE FISTULAS

In contrast to spontaneous fistulas, these will usually close with conservative measures as the diseased bowel has been removed, provided there is no downstream obstruction. However, the patient is often very ill and can have extensive abdominal contamination, which will usually drain by an incision or a drain site but may require added open or percutaneous drainage; rarely a laparostomy may be needed.[110]

INTRA-ABDOMINAL FISTULAS

These fistulas are usually spontaneous. The primary defect may arise from any segment of diseased bowel but is most commonly from the ileocaecal region. Similar management principles apply to these fistulas as to those described above, but the patients are generally in better health and less symptomatic. About half of the fistulas are diagnosed clinically, the remainder being asymptomatic and discovered at surgery.[111,112] A fistula should always be suspected between two loops of adherent bowel. The secondary defect can occur in the stomach, duodenum, vagina, fallopian tube, ureter or urethra, but the sigmoid colon, small bowel and bladder are the most common sites.[111] Most high vaginal fistulas are from the rectum but some are from the ileum.

Surgery involves en bloc resection of the primary defect and fistula with primary anastomosis and often only simple closure of the secondary defect, but with the exception of the duodenum. For suspected ileosigmoid fistulas, preoperative colonoscopy is wise to avoid the possibility of reoperation for missed Crohn's disease in the sigmoid colon, but resection of the secondarily involved sigmoid is not usually necessary.[113] If there is inflammation around the repair of a secondary defect in the colon, temporary proximal diversion is probably wise. Well-planned surgery gives good results with a low rate of fistula recurrence.[19,86,114]

SPONTANEOUS FREE PERFORATION IN THE SMALL BOWEL OR COLON

Free perforation occurs in about 1% of patients with Crohn's disease and involves the small bowel and colon with similar frequency, occurring at a mean of about 3 years from the onset of disease. Best results are from operation within 24 hours, with resection of the diseased segment and externalisation of the bowel ends.[115–118] Careful assessment is always needed for patients on steroids, as these may mask acute abdominal signs.

Surgery for colonic and rectal Crohn's disease

INDICATIONS

Whereas small-bowel surgery is most often directed towards treating complications, the most common indication for colonic surgery is intractable disease that is not well controlled with medical therapy. The need for surgery and the choice of operation will depend on the extent of the disease. Long-term follow-up of 507 patients with colorectal Crohn's showed the distribution of disease to be segmental in 40%, left sided in 26% and total in 31%, with perianal disease occurring in 37%. At 10 years from diagnosis half of the patients required a major operation, and 25% had a permanent ileostomy.[119] From other large series, 70% of patients with involvement of the entire colon needed surgery compared with only 29% of those with segmental

colonic or isolated anorectal disease.[56,120] Of those who have severe colitis, 60% will settle with initial medical management and of these remission can be maintained in about 60%, meaning that over 60% of patients with severe colitis will require colectomy within 1–2 years of the attack.[121]

EMERGENCY COLECTOMY

Acute colectomy for Crohn's disease constitutes 8% of all operations for acute Crohn's disease.[122] The indications for this include toxic dilatation, haemorrhage, perforation and severe colitis not responding to medical therapy. Toxic dilatation complicates 4–6% of cases of Crohn's colitis and 1% of cases of ileocolitis, with a mortality of 10%.[123,124] If medical treatment brings a response in 48–72 hours and urgent surgery is avoided, early elective colectomy is usually advisable as the chance of recurrent toxic colitis in the following years is 50% and symptomatic control is poor in nearly all patients.[125] Severe haemorrhage and perforation both occur in about 1% of patients with colitis. Treatment should usually be a total colectomy and ileostomy. The rectal stump has traditionally been exteriorised for safety but may be oversewn at the sacral promontory,[126] particularly if there is rectal sparing.

Completion proctectomy should usually be left until the patient is in good health, but on occasions it may be necessary sooner because of severe haemorrhage. After colectomy for acute disease, 60% will require subsequent proctectomy for troublesome anorectal disease.[122] Retaining the rectum does raise concern about the long-term risk of cancer in the rectal stump. In selected cases loop ileostomy can be used to defunction moderately severe colitis. This will allow clinical improvement in 87% and half will be able to have the stoma closed initially, but only 20% continued without relapse after medium-term follow-up.[127]

SEGMENTAL COLECTOMY

Segmental colonic disease occurs in less than 10% of patients with Crohn's disease, and segmental colectomies make up 4–10% of cases needing an operation.[55,56,120] It has become more popular in recent years. The usual indication for segmental resection is a symptomatic stricture. In some cases it may be required to establish the diagnosis. The

Table 9.1 • Long-term outcome of patients with segmental colonic Crohn's disease who have a segmental resection

Reference	N	Mean follow-up (years)	Clinical recurrence (%)	Reoperation rate at 10 years (%)	Permanent stoma avoided (%)
Allan et al.[128]	36	–	–	66	–
Makoweic et al.[129]	142	12	60	32	88
Prabhakar et al.[130]	48	14	77	33	86

The series by Prabhakar et al. includes 10 patients who had the majority of their colon removed.

pattern of recurrence is similar to that seen with segmental small bowel disease (**Table 9.1**).

TOTAL COLECTOMY AND ILEORECTAL ANASTOMOSIS

In 25% of patients needing a colectomy for Crohn's colitis there is rectal sparing, with a normally functioning rectum and sphincter mechanism. These patients are suitable for an ileorectal anastomosis, which can provide satisfactory function and avoid an ileostomy.[55,131] Generally, the distal resection line in the rectosigmoid region is just distal to where the disease finishes as determined by endoscopy. Patients may even achieve reasonable function with a degree of proctitis and mild perianal disease. In this situation it is important to conserve all the rectum as a better functional result is achieved with a greater maximum tolerated rectal volume; if the latter is below 150 mL, the functional result is often poor.[132] If there is uncertainty about the significance of rectal or perianal disease or the patient is in poor condition at the time of colectomy, the procedure can be done in two stages.[120]

Clinical recurrence is reported in 43–60% of cases at 10 years.[41] Of those who lose their ileorectal anastomosis, many will still have obtained 4–5 years of useful function, and this can be particularly important if a stoma is deferred for teenage and young adult years. Anastomotic leaks occur in about 5%, most patients have between two and six motions per day, and at 10 years 60% have managed to retain their rectum. The development of perianal disease usually leads to proctectomy.[133,134]

TOTAL COLECTOMY AND ILEOSTOMY

Other than the indications discussed above, this operation may be used in the presence of sub-stantial anorectal disease when there is concern about perineal wound healing. It is argued that if the rectum is defunctioned with a period of maximal medical therapy the disease may settle, facilitating better results with proctectomy, but doubt remains as to whether this is effective. Colectomy and ileostomy may also be used in patients who are unsuitable for a one-stage proctocolectomy because of operative risks. In a population-based series, 7% of patients with Crohn's disease had a colectomy and ileostomy and half of these later required a proctectomy for symptomatic anorectal disease.[55] If the rectum is retained, cancer surveillance is still required.

PANPROCTOCOLECTOMY

This operation is the gold standard for treating colorectal disease and is associated with the lowest recurrence rate, albeit at the price of a stoma. Local recurrence usually involves small-bowel disease, but it can be from perineal Crohn's after removal of the anorectum. Recurrence rates after panprocto-colectomy are in the order of 15–25% at 10 years; it is not clear whether these rates are affected by terminal ileal involvement at the time of colonic resection.[41] A second reoperation after the first will be needed in 20%.[120] Patients report a good quality of life after colectomy and ileostomy for disease confined to the colon.[57] About 5% will need revisional surgery for ileostomy complications.[59]

Removal of the rectum requires particular care not to damage the pelvic nerves, and a technique of intersphincteric and perimuscular dissection of the rectum has been popularised.[135] As there is no natural anatomic plane, the dissection is more vascular and time-consuming than dissection in the mesorectal plane. With increasing specialisation and awareness of the pelvic nerves from total mesorectal excision, it is probably safe for the specialist to carry out most of the dissection in the mesorectal plane, perhaps coming inside the mesorectal plane at the critical points in relation to the parasympathetic nerves. Whichever technique is preferred, the surgeon has to be prepared to modify this to take account of severe perineal or perirectal disease that can make the dissection very difficult. The perineal wound is best treated with primary closure and suction drainage (if desired) from above.[136] Delayed wound healing is frequently a problem; although 60–80% will have uncomplicated healing, up to 30% will take 4–6 months to heal completely. About 10% will have longer term problems with perineal sinuses, most of which settle with further surgical procedures.[131,136,137] These latter measures include several attempts at scraping the sinus tract to remove necrotic tissue and freshen the walls, and excluding an enteroperineal fistula (**Fig. 9.4**) and cutaneous Crohn's disease. In troublesome cases of active perineal disease after proctectomy, there is a role for wide excision and a rectus abdominis

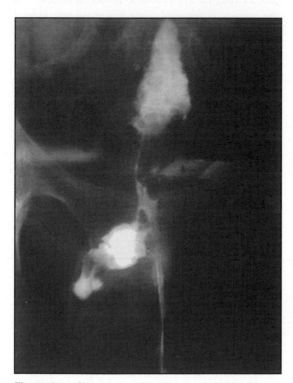

Figure 9.4 • Sinogram examination demonstrating an enteroperineal fistula.

transpelvic musculocutaneous flap reconstruction (**Fig. 9.5**).[138] Disappointingly, in a small number the flap of normal skin can also develop granulomatous cutaneous Crohn's disease.[139]

RESTORATIVE PROCTOCOLECTOMY

Ileal pouch–anal anastomosis has become the operation of choice for most patients with ulcerative colitis, but Crohn's disease has been regarded as a contraindication because of the risk of developing small-bowel or perianal disease that will lead to pouch excision. There has, however, been a softening of this view recently. It is now probably acceptable (although perhaps still controversial) to offer an ileal pouch to a well-informed patient who has isolated colonic Crohn's and requires a proctocolectomy. The risk of pouch failure (and excision) is in the range of 10–45%, and is higher than for ulcerative colitis. However, for Crohn's disease at other sites reoperation rates of 50% at 10 years are acceptable, and small-bowel recurrence probably involves a similar sacrifice of bowel to that of excising a pouch.[140–142] The group in Paris who controversially promoted pouches in selected patients with colorectal Crohn's disease have reported 10-year follow-up documenting Crohn's-related events in 35%, with 10% requiring pouch excision.[143]

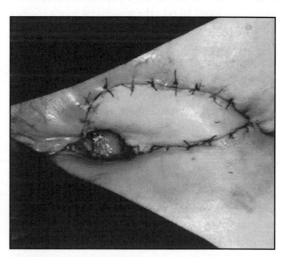

Figure 9.5 • A rectus abdominis myocutaneous flap used to reconstruct a severely diseased perineum complicated by a squamous carcinoma arising in a fistula tract.

CROHN'S COLITIS AND CANCER

With extensive Crohn's colitis an 8% risk of developing colon cancer at 22 years after disease onset has been reported, which is the same as the cancer risk with ulcerative colitis.[144] Although the absolute numbers are small because many patients with Crohn's colitis will have had colectomies, if one accepts the case for screening with colonoscopy in ulcerative colitis, then arguably this should also apply to Crohn's colitis.[145] This is further reinforced by the finding that nearly all Crohn's-related colonic carcinomas had adjacent dysplasia and half had distant dysplasia.[146] The long-term benefit of screening is not known for either disease. Particular care is needed in the presence of colonic strictures, which should always be regarded as malignant until proven otherwise; this may entail a resection to make the diagnosis.

Perianal disease

Some 30–70% of patients with Crohn's disease will have a degree of involvement of the anal canal, ranging from minor skin tags to severe disease.[1,147,148] However, only 3–5% will need surgical intervention for anal disease.[149] It is more frequent in association with colonic and, particularly, rectal disease.[150,151] A small percentage of patients have their initial presentation with anal disease, for example an anal fissure, and over 10 years half of these will develop disease at other intestinal sites. The activity of anal disease is unrelated to more proximal disease activity.

Generally, the prognosis is good, only 5–10% of patients with perianal Crohn's requiring a proctectomy at 10 years for perianal disease alone.[147,152,153] However, if rectal disease is also present, proctectomy will be needed in up to twice this number. Fissures or fistulas may be asymptomatic, and over a 10-year period about half will have healed spontaneously and a further 20–30% will heal after a surgical procedure.[152,154] Carcinoma is a rare but recognised complication,[155] and hidradenitis suppurativa may coexist.[156] The benign course of most perianal lesions caused by an incurable disease has led many (but not all surgeons) to a general policy of conservative treatment. More recent reports have shown that carefully selected cases without active disease can benefit from active

surgical management. Nevertheless, preserving a functioning sphincter must remain a paramount concern in these patients. **Box 9.4** outlines a useful classification of lesions described by Hughes and Taylor.[157] Surgery is most frequently indicated for secondary and incidental lesions.

INVESTIGATION

Careful examination, often under anaesthesia, is the most useful investigation and an essential part of the work-up. In complicated cases, MRI and/or endoanal ultrasound in combination with examination under anaesthesia allow accurate identification of obscure tracts and collections.[22]

MEDICAL TREATMENT

Metronidazole, azathioprine, ciclosporin and infliximab are probably effective at controlling or

Box 9.4 • Hughes' classification of perianal lesions in Crohn's disease

Primary lesions
- Anal fissure
- Ulcerated oedematous pile
- Cavitating ulcer
- Aggressive ulceration

Secondary lesions
- Skin tags
- Anal/rectal stricture
- Perianal abscess/fistula
- Anovaginal/rectovaginal fistula
- Carcinoma

Incidental lesions
- Piles
- Perianal abscess or fistula
- Skin tags
- Cryptitis
- Hidradenitis suppurativa

From Hughes LE, Taylor BA. Perianal lesions in Crohn's disease. In: Allan R, Keighley M, Alexander-Williams J, Hawkins C (eds) Inflammatory bowel disease, 2nd edn. Edinburgh: Churchill Livingstone, 1990; pp. 351–61, with permission.

improving perianal disease (see above), but most of the claims in the literature are anecdotal and the impact of medical therapy on reducing complications or the need for surgery is not known. In those with active disease, however, it seems reasonable to employ any measure that may help the symptomatic patient and avert proctectomy. Metronidazole is often used for septic problems and should be the first-line medical treatment, but be wary of the neurological adverse effects. Ciprofloxacin has also found recent favour.

ANAL FISSURE

Most fissures are in the midline posteriorly, one-third are multiple and two-thirds are asymptomatic. Anal canal pressures are similar to those in controls and 50–70% heal with conservative or concurrent medical therapy.[149,152,154] Most recommend a conservative approach to chronic fissures.[154] Newer treatment options include topical glyceryl trinitrate and diltiazem, and botulinum toxin injection. All efforts should be made to conserve the internal anal sphincter in Crohn's disease. However, if all else fails and the patient has significant symptoms, the fissure will usually heal after a lateral anal sphincterotomy without compromising continence. This should probably not be done in the presence of active proctitis. Healing the fissure may prevent future abscesses and fistulas arising from its base.[147,158]

ABSCESSES

Abscesses may arise from deep cavitating ulcers or distorted anal glands (**Fig. 9.6**). The first sign of an abscess is often increasing perianal pain. Careful examination under anaesthesia will usually reveal the problem and collections should be drained by removing a small area of overlying skin to allow drainage. In larger cavities it may be useful to insert a mushroom catheter to facilitate drainage and irrigation. It is usually inadvisable to lay open a primary tract at this stage. In complicated cases or where the cause of pain is not apparent, MRI is useful. Occasionally, abscesses may be above the levator muscles.

ANAL FISTULAS

Fistulous disease may range from an incidental fistula to a 'watering-can' perineum. If a fistula has been judged incidental or there is no active inflammation in the perianal region or rectum, it can be treated by standard techniques that preserve the sphincter muscle: identification of the track and preliminary seton drainage followed by a rectal advancement flap, giving a success rate as high as 50–70% at 2–3 years. A covering stoma is probably not of benefit for the majority of cases.[159–161] The lay open technique gives good results for superficial tracts.[149,153,162] In complicated fistulas or in the presence of active inflammation, the aim is to establish adequate drainage and this is best done with a loose silastic seton which may be left long term with a good functional result (**Fig. 9.7**).[149,153] Supralevator fistulas are a difficult problem and usually involve perforating disease from the rectum or even more proximal bowel. Again, the primary aim is drainage and identification of the internal origin, but these cases are more likely to need a proctectomy. Fistulas arising from deep cavitating ulcers are difficult to manage and proctectomy is often unavoidable in the long term.

RECTOVAGINAL FISTULAS

The distressing problem of passing faeces or wind per vaginam means that these fistulas usually

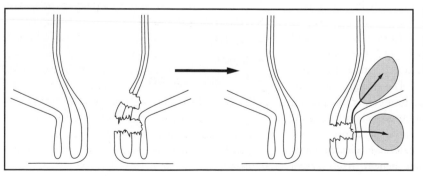

Figure 9.6 • Pathogenesis of anal suppurative disease. Deep cavitating ulcers give rise to extrasphincteric and supralevator abscesses.

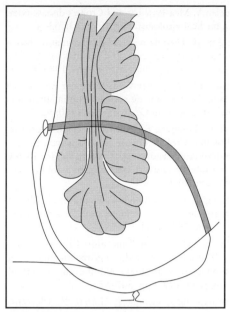

Figure 9.7 • Diagram of a seton placed for drainage of an anal fistula.

require surgical therapy. They occur in 10% of women presenting to specialist centres with Crohn's disease. In one series 37% had a proctectomy, but only one-third of these were primarily for the rectovaginal fistula.[163] Again, initial therapy is directed at identifying the tract and establishing drainage with a seton. Provided the vaginal opening is not in the introitus, the most effective radiological investigation to identify the tract is probably a vaginogram, which has a sensitivity of 79% compared with 60% for CT and only 34% for barium enema.[164] There is little specific information on MRI for rectovaginal fistulas.

If the local tissues are in reasonable condition, then a rectal advancement flap can be used, with a reported success rate of 30–70%.[160,161] Similar results have been reported with the use of anocutaneous advancement flaps[165] and vaginal flaps,[166] and these latter procedures may be more suitable if there is a degree of proctitis or anorectal scarring. Using vaginal flaps and ignoring the theoretical consideration that the flap should be on the high-pressure rectal side does not seem to compromise results.

Advancement flaps may not be the best operation for recurrent fistulas due to higher failure rates and consideration should be given to other procedures, such as a gracilis interposition or sphincteroplasty.[167]

DEFUNCTIONING ILEOSTOMY

A temporary ileostomy has a role in providing symptomatic relief to the desperate patient while more definitive treatment options are discussed or tried. In this situation, the majority will experience symptomatic improvement but with longer follow-up only a small number have intestinal continuity restored and following this an even smaller number remain in clinical remission.[127] Defunctioning also has a role in protecting local operations on the anus; however, it is not usually necessary with advancement flaps for example, and the approach should be selective.[159,161]

COMPLICATIONS

Longer term complications of perianal Crohn's disease may include rectal or anal strictures and incontinence due to fibrosis and sphincter damage. Symptomatic strictures should be gently dilated, remembering that with an impaired sphincter there is a risk of precipitating or worsening incontinence. About half the patients who develop an anal or rectal stricture will require proctectomy.[168] In some cases with defined sphincter defects good results can be obtained from sphincter repair.[168]

PROGNOSIS

It has often been said that patients can anticipate a normal life expectancy and that they do not die of Crohn's disease. However, standardised mortality rates are high for patients who have the onset of their disease before the age of 20 years and are particularly high early in the course of the disease, although the absolute numbers dying remain small. Causes of death include sepsis, perioperative complications, electrolyte disturbances and gastrointestinal tract cancers.

Quality-of-life issues are important to these patients and they express concerns over energy levels, fear of surgery and body image. Often, loss of energy and malaise contribute more to functional disability than specific gastrointestinal symptoms. In terms of academic success and advancement, patients are not hampered by the disease, and employment rates are the same as for matched healthy controls. However, patients frequently express impairment of employment, recreation, interpersonal and sexual relationships. Most patients continue to function optimistically and adapt successfully, but disease relapses produce considerable stress, and psychological support from counsellors, psychiatrists, non-medical and patient-support groups should be utilised.[23]

• **Key points**

- Patients with Crohn's disease usually enjoy reasonable health punctuated by periods of increased disease activity, initially managed medically.
- Many patients will require surgery at some stage and a multidisciplinary team is key to optimise management.
- Surgery is restricted to dealing with troublesome segments that cannot be managed medically.
- Surgery for small-bowel disease is usually necessary because of complications of disease such as strictures and fistulas.
- Surgery for large-bowel disease is usually necessary because of inability of medical treatment to control symptoms.

REFERENCES

1. Satsangi J, Sutherland LR (eds) Inflammatory bowel diseases. London: Elsevier, 2003.
2. Sartor RB. *Mycobacterium paratuberculosis* in Crohn's disease. In: Tytgat GNJ, Bartelsman JFWM, van Deventer SJH (eds) Inflammatory bowel disease. Lancaster: Kluwer Academic Publishers, 1995; pp. 425–8.
3. Rowbotham DS, Mapstone N, Trejdosiewicz LK et al. *Mycobacterium paratuberculosis* DNA not detected in Crohn's disease tissue by fluorescent polymerase chain reaction. Gut 1995; 37:660–7.
4. Pounder RE. Measles virus and Crohn's disease: research from the Royal Free Hospital in London. J Gastroenterol 1995; 8:48–51.
5. Haga Y, Funakoshi O, Kuroe K et al. Absence of viral genomic sequence in intestinal tissue from Crohn's disease by nested polymerase chain reaction. Gut 1996; 38:211–15.
6. Muelen V. Measles virus and Crohn's disease: view of a medical virologist. Gut 1998; 43:733–4.
7. Fielding JP. The relative risk of inflammatory bowel disease among patients and siblings of Crohn's disease patients. J Clin Gastroenterol 1986; 8:655.
8. Farmer RG, Michener WM, Mortimer EA. Studies of family history among patients with inflammatory bowel disease. Clin Gastroenterol 1980; 9:271–7.
9. Tysk C, Lindberg E, Jarnerot G et al. Ulcerative colitis and Crohn's disease in an unselected population of monozygotic and dizygotic twins. A study of heritability and the influence of smoking. Gut 1988; 29:990–6.
10. Satsangi J, Grootscholten C, Holt J et al. Clinical patterns of familial inflammatory bowel disease. Gut 1996; 38:738–41.
11. Gilmour PH. The small intestine: Crohn's disease. In: Whitehead R (ed.) Gastrointestinal and oesophageal pathology. Edinburgh: Churchill Livingstone, 1995; pp. 547–58.
12. Groisman GM, George J, Harpaz N. Ulcerative appendicitis in universal and nonuniversal ulcerative colitis. Mod Pathol 1994; 7:322–5.
13. Kroft SH, Stryker SJ, Rao MS. Appendiceal involvement as a skip lesion in ulcerative colitis. Mod Pathol 1994; 7:912–14.
14. Sheehan AL, Warren BF, Gear MW et al. Fat-wrapping in Crohn's disease: pathological basis and relevance to surgical practice. Br J Surg 1992; 79:955–8.
15. Fujimura Y, Kamoi R, Iida M. Pathogenesis of aphthoid ulcers in Crohn's disease: correlative findings by magnifying colonoscopy, electron microscopy and immunohistochemistry. Gut 1996; 38:724–32.
16. Wakefield AJ, Sankey EA, Dhillon AP et al. Granulomatous vasculitis in Crohn's disease. Gastroenterology 1991; 100:1279–87.
17. Robert JR, Sachar DB, Greenstein AJ. Severe gastrointestinal hemorrhage in Crohn's disease. Ann Surg 1991; 213:207–11.
18. Cirocco WC, Reilly JC, Rusin LC. Life-threatening hemorrhage and exsanguination from Crohn's disease. Report of four cases. Dis Colon Rectum 1995; 38:85–95.
19. McNamara MJ, Fazio VW, Lavery IC et al. Surgical treatment of enterovesical fistulas in Crohn's disease. Dis Colon Rectum 1990; 33:271–6.
20. Chew SSB, Ngo TQ, Douglas PR et al. Cholecystectomy in patients with Crohn's. Dis Colon Rectum 2003; 46:1484–8.
21. Olliff JFC. Radiology: CT, ultrasound and MRI. In: Allan R, Rhodes JM, Hanauer SB, Keighley MRB, Alexander-Williams J, Fazio VW (eds) Inflammatory bowel disease, 3rd edn. Edinburgh: Churchill Livingstone, 1997; pp. 249–59.

22. Schwartz DA, Wiersema MJ, Dudiak KM et al. A comparison of endoscopic ultrasound, magnetic resonance imaging, and exam under anesthesia for evaluation of Crohn's perianal fistulas. Gastroenterology 2001; 121:1064–72.

23. Kornbluth A, Salomon P, Sachar D. Crohn's disease. In: Feldman M, Scharschmidt BF, Sleisenger MH (eds) Sleisenger and Fordtran's gastrointestinal and liver disease, 6th edn. Philadelphia: WB Saunders, 1998; pp. 1708–34.

24. Maunder RG, Cohen Z, McLeod RS et al. Effect of intervention in inflammatory bowel disease on health-related quality of life: a critical review. Dis Colon Rectum 1995; 38:1147–61.

25. Louis E, Collard A, Oger AF et al. Behaviour of Crohn's disease according to the Vienna classification: changing pattern over the course of the disease. Gut 2001; 49:777–82.

26. Shephard NA. Pathological mimics of chronic inflammatory bowel disease. J Clin Pathol 1991; 44:726–33.

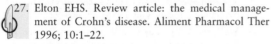

27. Elton EHS. Review article: the medical management of Crohn's disease. Aliment Pharmacol Ther 1996; 10:1–22.

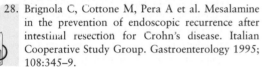

28. Brignola C, Cottone M, Pera A et al. Mesalamine in the prevention of endoscopic recurrence after intestinal resection for Crohn's disease. Italian Cooperative Study Group. Gastroenterology 1995; 108:345–9.

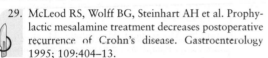

29. McLeod RS, Wolff BG, Steinhart AH et al. Prophylactic mesalamine treatment decreases postoperative recurrence of Crohn's disease. Gastroenterology 1995; 109:404–13.

30. Camma C, Giunta M, Roselli M et al. Mesalamine in the maintenance treatment of Crohn's disease: a meta-analysis adjusted for confounding variables. Gastroenterology 1997; 113:1465–73.

Meta-analysis of 15 randomised controlled trials for propylactic mesalamine to maintain remission; three studies are post surgery and are analysed as a subgroup.

31. Hanauer SB. Drug therapy: inflammatory bowel disease. N Engl J Med 1996; 334:841–8.

32. Scholmerich J. Topically active corticosteroids. In: Tytgat GNJ, Bartelsman JFWM, van Deventer SJH (eds) Inflammatory bowel disease. Lancaster: Kluwer Academic Publishers, 1995; pp. 631–2.

33. Thomsen O, Cortot A, Jewell D et al. A comparison of budesonide and mesalamine for active Crohn's disease. N Engl J Med 1998; 339:370–4.

34. Hellers G, Cortot A, Jewell D et al. Oral budesonide for prevention of postsurgical recurrence in Crohn's disease. Gastroenterology 1999; 116:294–300.

Budesonide does not have a role in prophylaxis after surgery.

35. Hanauer SB. Intravenous cyclosporine in severe IBD. In: Tytgat GNJ, Bartelsman JFWM, van Deventer SJH (eds) Inflammatory bowel disease. Lancaster: Kluwer Academic Publishers, 1995; pp. 581–4.

36. Targan SR, Hanauer SB, van Deventer SJ et al. A short-term study of chimeric monoclonal antibody cA2 to tumor necrosis factor alpha for Crohn's disease. Crohn's Disease cA2 Study Group. N Engl J Med 1997; 337:1029–35.

37. Hanauer SB, Feagan BG, Lichtenstein GR et al. Maintenance infliximab for Crohn's disease: the ACCENT I randomised trial. Lancet 2002; 359:1541–9.

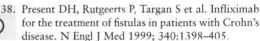

Many centres took part with small numbers each. There is drug company representation on the writing committee. Infliximab is moderately effective at inducing remission but at 12 months is only a little better than placebo. The data need to be interpreted carefully: infliximab is very expensive, has a poor cost–benefit ratio and there are concerns about serious long-term adverse effects. On the other hand, there are many anecdotes of dramatic clinical responses when other measures have failed. It has a role in inducing remission in refractory cases.

38. Present DH, Rutgeerts P, Targan S et al. Infliximab for the treatment of fistulas in patients with Crohn's disease. N Engl J Med 1999; 340:1398–405.

39. Sands BE, Anderson FH, Bernstein CN et al. Infliximab maintenance therapy for fistulizing Crohn's disease. N Engl J Med 2004; 350:876–85.

This study looks at the role of infliximab for fistulating Crohn's disease and is a similar design to ACCENT 1. Similar comments apply as for ACCENT 1 above.

40. Alexander-Williams J. Bypass, diversion and dilatation. In: Kumar D, Alexander-Williams J (eds) The surgical managment of Crohn's disease and ulcerative colitis. London: Springer-Verlag, 1993; pp. 85–8.

41. Williams JG, Wong WD, Rothenberger DA et al. Recurrence of Crohn's disease after resection. Br J Surg 1991; 78:10–19.

42. Kotanagi H, Kramer K, Fazio VW et al. Do microscopic abnormalities at resection margins correlate with increased anastomotic recurrence in Crohn's disease? Retrospective analysis of 100 cases. Dis Colon Rectum 1991; 34:909–16.

43. Fazio VW, Marchetti F, Church M et al. Effect of resection margins on the recurrence of Crohn's disease in the small bowel. A randomized controlled trial. Ann Surg 1996; 224:563–71.

From retrospective reviews and now a small randomised trial it seems highly likely that microscopic involvement of resection margin does not increase recurrence rates.

44. McLeod RS. Resection margins and recurrent Crohn's disease. Hepatogastroenterology 1990; 37:63–6.

45. Klein O, Colombel JF, Lescut D et al. Remaining small bowel endoscopic lesions at surgery have no influence on early anastomotic recurrences in Crohn's disease. Am J Gastroenterol 1995; 90:1949–52.

46. Scott NA, Hughes LE. Timing of ileocolonic resection for symptomatic Crohn's disease: the patient's view. Gut 1994; 35:656–7.

47. Thirlby RC, Land JC, Fenster LF et al. Effect of surgery on health related quality of life in patients with inflammatory bowel disease: a prospective study. Arch Surg 1998; 133:826–32.

48. Tillinger W, Mittermaier C, Lochs H et al. Health-related quality of life in patients with Crohn's disease: influence of surgical operation. A prospective trial. Dig Dis Sci 1999; 44:932–8.

49. Casellas T, Lopez-Vivancos J, Badia X et al. Impact of surgery for Crohn's disease on health related quality of life. Am J Gastroenterol 2000; 95:177–82.

50. Ludwig KA, Milsom JW, Church JM et al. Preliminary experience with laparoscopic intestinal surgery for Crohn's disease. Am J Surg 1996; 171:52–5.

51. Canin-Endres J, Salky B, Gattorno F et al. Laparoscopically assisted intestinal resection in 88 patients with Crohn's disease. Surg Endosc 1999; 13:595–9.

52. Dunker MS, Stiggelbout AM, van Hogezand RA et al. Cosmesis and body image after laparoscopic-assisted and open ileocolic resection for Crohn's disease. Surg Endosc 1998; 12:1334–40.

53. Milsom JW, Hammerhofer KA, Bohm B et al. Prospective, randomized trial comparing laparoscopic vs. conventional surgery for refractory ileocolic Crohn's disease. Dis Colon Rectum 2001; 44:1–8; discussion 8–9.

54. Bernell O, Lapidus A, Hellers G. Risk factors for surgery and postoperative recurrence in Crohn's disease. Ann Surg 2000; 231:38–45.

55. Shivananda S, Hordijk ML, Pena AS et al. Crohn's disease: risk of recurrence and reoperation in a defined population. Gut 1989; 30:990–5.

56. Farmer RG, Whelan G, Fazio VW. Long-term follow-up of patients with Crohn's disease. Relationship between the clinical pattern and prognosis. Gastroenterology 1985; 88:1818–25.

57. Halme LE. Results of surgical treatment of patients with Crohn's disease. Ann Chir Gynaecol 1992; 81:277–83.

58. Nordgren SR, Fasth SB, Oresland TO et al. Long-term follow-up in Crohn's disease. Mortality, morbidity, and functional status. Scand J Gastroenterol 1994; 29:1122–8.

59. Post S, Herfarth CH, Schumacher H et al. Experience with ileostomy and colostomy in Crohn's disease. Br J Surg 1995; 82:1629–33.

60. Borley NR, Mortensen NJ, Jewell DP. Preventing postoperative recurrence of Crohn's disease. Br J Surg 1997; 84:1493–502.

61. Michelassi F, Balestracci T, Chappell R et al. Primary and recurrent Crohn's disease. Experience with 1379 patients. Ann Surg 1991; 214:230–8.

62. Post S, Herfarth C, Bohm E et al. The impact of disease pattern, surgical management, and individual surgeons on the risk for relaparotomy for recurrent Crohn's disease. Ann Surg 1996; 223:253–60.

63. Wolff BG. Factors determining recurrence following surgery for Crohn's disease. World J Surg 1998; 22:364–9.

64. Aeberhard P, Berchtold W, Riedtmann HJ et al. Surgical recurrence of perforating and non-perforating Crohn's disease. A study of 101 surgically treated patients. Dis Colon Rectum 1996; 39:80–7.

65. Greenstein AJ, Lachman P, Sachar DB et al. Perforating and non-perforating indications for repeated operations in Crohn's disease: evidence for two clinical forms. Gut 1988; 29:588–92.

66. McDonald PJ, Fazio VW, Farmer RG et al. Perforating and nonperforating Crohn's disease. An unpredictable guide to recurrence after surgery. Dis Colon Rectum 1989; 32:117–20.

67. Moskovitz D, McLeod RS, Greenberg GR et al. Operative and environmental risk factors for recurrence of Crohn's disease. Int J Colorectal Dis 1999; 14:224–6.

68. Kusunoki M, Ikeuchi H, Yanagi H et al. A comparison of stapled and hand-sewn anastomoses in Crohn's disease. Dig Surg 1998; 15:679–82.

69. Cameron JL, Hamilton SR, Coleman J et al. Patterns of ileal recurrence in Crohn's disease. A prospective randomized study. Ann Surg 1992; 215:546–51.

70. Scott NA, Sue-Ling HM, Hughes LE. Anastomotic configuration does not affect recurrence of Crohn's disease after ileocolonic resection. Int J Colorectal Dis 1995; 10:67–9.

71. Cottone M, Rosselli M, Orlando A et al. Smoking habits and recurrence in Crohn's disease. Gastroenterology 1994; 106:643–8.

72. Sutherland LR, Ramcharan S, Bryant H et al. Effect of cigarette smoking on recurrence of Crohn's disease. Gastroenterology 1990; 98:1123–8.

The first of a number of papers that have shown the powerful effect of smoking on recurrence. Evidence is probably level 3 but the strength of the effect is such that there is little doubt.

73. 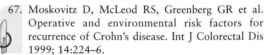 Lochs H, Mayer M, Fleig WE et al. Prophylaxis of postoperative relapse in Crohn's disease with mesalamine: European Cooperative Crohn's Disease Study VI. Gastroenterology 2000; 118:264–73.

74. Rutgeerts P. Strategies in the prevention of post-operative recurrence in Crohn's disease. Best Pract Res Clin Gastroenterol 2003; 17:63–73.

75. Travis S. Azathioprine for prevention of post-operative recurrence in Crohn's disease. Eur J Gastroenterol Hepatol 2001; 13:1277–9.

76. Hudson M, Chitolie A, Hutton RA et al. Thrombotic vascular risk factors in inflammatory bowel disease. Gut 1996; 38:733–7.

77. Heimann TM, Greenstein AJ, Mechanic L et al. Early complications following surgical treatment for Crohn's disease. Ann Surg 1985; 201:494–8.

78. Alexander-Williams J. Reducing the risks of operation. In: Kumar D, Alexander-Williams J (eds) The surgical managment of Crohn's disease and ulcerative colitis. London: Springer-Verlag, 1993; pp. 51–66.

79. Becker JM, Dayton MT, Fazio VW et al. Seprafilm biosorbable membrane in the prevention of post operative abdominal adhesions: a prospective, randomised, double blinded multicenter study. J Am Coll Surg 1996; 183:297–306.

Robust evidence that adhesion formation is reduced, but it is still not known if reoperation rates for small bowel obstruction or reoperation times are reduced with this expensive product.

80. Fazio VW, Strong AW. The surgical managment of Crohn's disease. In: Kirsner JB, Shorter RG (eds) Inflammatory bowel disease. Baltimore: Williams and Wilkins, 1995; pp. 830–87.

81. Worsey MJ, Hull T, Ryland L et al. Stricturoplasty is an effective operation in the operative management of duodenal Crohn's. Dis Colon Rectum 1999; 42:596–600.

82. Yamamoto T, Bain IM, Connolly AB et al. Outcome of stricturoplasty for duodenal Crohn's disease. Br J Surg 1999; 86:259–62.

83. Matsui T, Hatakeyama S, Ikeda K et al. Long-term outcome of endoscopic balloon dilation in obstructive gastroduodenal Crohn's disease. Endoscopy 1997; 29:640–5.

84. Klein S, Greenstein AJ, Sachar DB. Duodenal fistulas in Crohn's disease. J Clin Gastroenterol 1987; 9:46–9.

85. Pichney LS, Fantry GT, Graham SM. Gastrocolic and duodenocolic fistulas in Crohn's disease. J Clin Gastroenterol 1992; 15:205–11.

86. Pettit SH, Irving MH. The operative management of fistulous Crohn's disease. Surg Gynecol Obstet 1988; 167:223–8.

87. Caprilli R, Corrao G, Taddei G et al. Prognostic factors for postoperative recurrence of Crohn's disease. Dis Colon Rectum 1996; 39:335–41.

88. Rutgeerts P, Geboes K, Vantrappen G et al. Natural history of recurrent Crohn's disease at the ileocolonic anastomosis after curative surgery. Gut 1984; 25:665–72.

89. Blomberg B, Rolny P, Jarnerot G. Endoscopic treatment of anastomotic strictures in Crohn's disease. Endoscopy 1991; 23:195–8.

90. Couckuyt H, Gevers AM, Coremans G et al. Efficacy and safety of hydrostatic balloon dilatation of ileocolonic Crohn's strictures: a prospective long-term analysis. Gut 1995; 36:577–80.

91. Sabate JM, Villarejo J, Bouhnik Y et al. Hydrostatic balloon dilatation of Crohn's strictures. Aliment Pharmacol Ther 2003; 18:409–13.

92. Thomas-Gibson S, Brooker JC, Hayward CM et al. Colonoscopic balloon dilation of Crohn's strictures: a review of long-term outcomes. Eur J Gastroenterol Hepatol 2003; 15:485–8.

93. Lee EC, Papaioannou N. Minimal surgery for chronic obstruction in patients with extensive or universal Crohn's disease. Ann R Coll Surg Engl 1982; 64:229–33.

94. Fazio VW, Tjandra JJ. Strictureplasty for Crohn's disease with multiple long strictures. Dis Colon Rectum 1993; 36:71–2.

95. Michelassi F. Side-to-side isoperistaltic strictureplasty for multiple Crohn's strictures. Dis Colon Rectum 1996; 39:345–9.

96. Poggioli G, Laureti S, Pierangeli F et al. A new model of strictureplasty for multiple and long stenoses in Crohn's ileitis: side-to-side diseased to disease-free anastomosis. Dis Colon Rectum 2003; 46:127–30.

97. Tjandra JJ, Fazio VW, Lavery IC. Results of multiple strictureplasties in diffuse Crohn's disease of the small bowel. Aust NZ J Surg 1993; 63:95–9.

98. Gardiner KR, Kettlewell MGW, Mortensen NJM. Intestinal haemorrhage after strictureplasty for Crohn's disease. Int J Colorectal Dis 1996; 11:180–2.

99. Ozuner G, Fazio VW. Management of gastro-intestinal bleeding after strictureplasty for Crohn's disease. Dis Colon Rectum 1995; 38:297–300.

100. Ozuner G, Fazio VW, Lavery IC et al. How safe is strictureplasty in the management of Crohn's disease? Am J Surg 1996; 171:57–60.

101. Dehn TC, Kettlewell MG, Mortensen NJ et al. Ten-year experience of strictureplasty for obstructive Crohn's disease. Br J Surg 1989; 76:339–41.

102. Serra J, Cohen Z, McLeod RS. Natural history of strictureplasty in Crohn's disease: 9-year experience. Can J Surg 1995; 38:481–5.

103. Stebbing JF, Jewell DP, Kettlewell MG et al. Long-term results of recurrence and reoperation after strictureplasty for obstructive Crohn's disease. Br J Surg 1995; 82:1471–4.

104. Yamamoto T, Bain IM, Allan RN et al. An audit of strictureplasty for small-bowel Crohn's disease. Dis Colon Rectum 1999; 42:797–803.

105. Tjandra JJ, Fazio VW. Strictureplasty without concomitant resection for small bowel obstruction in Crohn's disease. Br J Surg 1994; 81:561–3.

106. Scott NA, Leinhardt DJ, O'Hanrahan T et al. Spectrum of intestinal failure in a specialised unit. Lancet 1991; 337:471–3.

107. Hill GL, Bourchier RG, Witney GB. Surgical and metabolic management of patients with external fistulas of the small intestine associated with Crohn's disease. World J Surg 1988; 12:191–7.

108. Scott NA, Finnegan S, Irving MH. Octreotide and postoperative enterocutaneous fistulae: a controlled prospective study. Acta Gastroenterol Belg 1993; 56:266–70.

109. Alexander-Williams J. The management of fistulae. In: Kumar D, Alexander-Williams J (eds) The surgical managment of Crohn's disease and ulcerative colitis. London: Springer-Verlag, 1993; pp. 103–10.

110. Mughal MM, Bancewicz J, Irving MH. 'Laparostomy': a technique for the management of intractable intra-abdominal sepsis. Br J Surg 1986; 73:253–9.

111. Glass RE, Ritchie JK, Lennard Jones JE et al. Internal fistulas in Crohn's disease. Dis Colon Rectum 1985; 28:557–61.

112. Heyen F, Ambrose NS, Allan RN et al. Enterovesical fistulas in Crohn's disease. Ann R Coll Surg Engl 1989; 71:101–4.

113. Saint Marc O, Vaillant JC, Frileux P et al. Surgical management of ileosigmoid fistulas in Crohn's disease: role of preoperative colonoscopy. Dis Colon Rectum 1995; 38:1084–7.

114. Greenstein AJ, Sachar DB, Tzakis A et al. Course of enterovesical fistulas in Crohn's disease. Am J Surg 1984; 147:788–92.

115. Greenstein AJ, Sachar DB, Mann D et al. Spontaneous free perforation and perforated abscess in 30 patients with Crohn's disease. Ann Surg 1987; 205:72–6.

116. Bundred NJ, Dixon JM, Lumsden AB et al. Free perforation in Crohn's colitis. A ten-year review. Dis Colon Rectum 1985; 28:35–7.

117. Greenstein AJ, Mann D, Sachar DB et al. Free perforation in Crohn's disease: I. A survey of 99 cases. Am J Gastroenterol 1985; 80:682–9.

118. Softley A, Clamp SE, Bouchier IA et al. Perforation of the intestine in inflammatory bowel disease. An OMGE survey. Scand J Gastroenterol Suppl 1988; 144:24–6.

119. Lapidus A, Bernell O, Hellers G et al. Clinical course of colorectal Crohn's disease, a 35 year follow-up study of 507 patients. Gastroenterology 1998; 114:1151–60.

120. Goligher JC. Surgical treatment of Crohn's disease affecting mainly or entirely the large bowel. World J Surg 1988; 12:186–90.

121. Kornbluth A, Marion JF, Salomon P et al. How effective is current medical therapy for severe ulcerative and Crohn's colitis? An analytic review of selected trials. J Clin Gastroenterol 1995; 20:280–4.

122. Mortensen NJ, Ritchie JK, Hawley PR et al. Surgery for acute Crohn's colitis: results and long term follow-up. Br J Surg 1984; 71:783–4.

123. Greenstein AJ, Sachar DB, Gibas A et al. Outcome of toxic dilatation in ulcerative and Crohn's colitis. J Clin Gastroenterol 1985; 7:137–43.

124. Grieco MB, Bordan DL, Geiss AC et al. Toxic megacolon complicating Crohn's colitis. Ann Surg 1980; 191:75–80.

125. Grant CS, Dozois RR. Toxic megacolon: ultimate fate of patients after successful medical management. Am J Surg 1984; 147:106–10.

126. McKee RF, Keenan RA, Munro A. Colectomy for acute colitis: is it safe to close the rectal stump? Int J Colorectal Dis 1995; 10:222–4.

127. Edwards CM, George BD, Jewell DP et al. Role of a defunctioning stoma in the management of large bowel Crohn's disease. Br J Surg 2000; 87:1063–6.

128. Allan A, Andrews H, Hilton CJ et al. Segmental colonic resection is an appropriate operation for short skip lesions due to Crohn's disease in the colon. World J Surg 1989; 13:611–14.

129. Makowiec F, Paczulla D, Schmidtke C et al. Crohn's colitis: segmental resection or colectomy. Gastroenterology 1996; 110:A1402.

130. Prabhakar LP, Laramee C, Nelson H et al. Avoiding a stoma: the role of segmental colectomy in Crohn's colitis. Dis Colon Rectum 1997; 40:71–8.

131. Goligher JC. The long-term results of excisional surgery for primary and recurrent Crohn's disease of the large intestine. Dis Colon Rectum 1985; 28:51–5.

132. Keighley MRB, Buchmann P, Lee JR. Assessment of anorectal function in selection of patients for ileorectal anastomosis in Crohn's colitis. Gut 1982; 23:102–7.

133. Chevalier JM, Jones DJ, Ratelle R et al. Colectomy and ileorectal anastomosis in patients with Crohn's disease. Br J Surg 1994; 81:1379–81.

134. Longo WE, Oakley JR, Lavery IC et al. Outcome of ileorectal anastomosis for Crohn's colitis. Dis Colon Rectum 1992; 35:1066–71.

135. Lee ECG, Dowling BL. Perimuscular excision of the rectum for Crohn's disease and ulcerative colitis. Br J Surg 1972; 59:29–32.

136. Elliot MS, Todd IP. Primary suture of the perineal wound using constant suction and irrigation, following rectal excision for inflammatory bowel disease. Ann R Coll Surg Engl 1985; 67:6–7.

137. Scammell BE, Keighley MR. Delayed perineal wound healing after proctectomy for Crohn's colitis. Br J Surg 1986; 73:150–2.

138. Brough WA, Schofield PF. The value of the rectus abdominis myocutaneous flap in the treatment of complex perineal fistula. Dis Colon Rectum 1991; 34:148–50.

139. Reed JB, McLean NR, Griffith CD. Crohn's disease involving a rectus abdominis myocutaneous flap. Br J Surg 1993; 80:1069.

140. Panis P, Poupard B, Neneth J et al. Ileal pouch–anal anastomosis for Crohn's disease. Lancet 1996; 347:854–7.

141. Panis Y. Is there a place for ileal pouch–anal anastomosis in patients with Crohn's colitis? Neth J Med 1998; 53:S47–S51.

142. Phillips RKS. Ileal pouch–anal anastomosis for Crohn's disease. Gut 1998; 43:303–8.

143. Regimbeau JM, Panis Y, Cazaban L et al. Long-term results of faecal diversion for refractory perianal Crohn's disease. Colorectal Dis 2001; 3:232–7.

144. Gillen CD, Walmsley RS, Prior P et al. Ulcerative colitis and Crohn's disease: a comparison of the colorectal cancer risk in extensive colitis. Gut 1994; 35:1590–2.

145. Ribeiro MB, Greenstein AJ, Sachar DB et al. Colorectal adenocarcinoma in Crohn's disease. Ann Surg 1996; 223:186–93.

146. Sigel JE, Petras RE, Lashner BA et al. Intestinal adenocarcinoma in Crohn's disease: a report of 30 cases with a focus on coexisting dysplasia. Am J Surg Pathol 1999; 23:651–5.

147. McKee RF, Keenan RA. Perianal Crohn's disease: is it all bad news. Dis Colon Rectum 1996; 39:136–42.

148. Rankin GB, Watts HD, Melnyk CS et al. National Cooperative Crohn's Disease Study: extraintestinal manifestations and perianal complications. Gastroenterology 1979; 77:914–20.

149. Sangwan YP, Schoetz DJ, Murray JJ et al. Perianal Crohn's disease. Results of local surgical treatment. Dis Colon Rectum 1996; 39:529–35.

150. Pescatori M, Interisano A, Basso L et al. Management of perianal Crohn's disease: results of a multicenter study in Italy. Dis Colon Rectum 1995; 38:121–4.

151. Halme LA, Sainio P. Factors related to frequency, type and outcome of anal fistulas in Crohn's disease. Dis Colon Rectum 1995; 38:55–9.

152. Buchmann P, Keighley MR, Allan RN et al. Natural history of perianal Crohn's disease. Ten year follow-up: a plea for conservatism. Am J Surg 1980; 140:642–4.

153. Scott HJ, Northover MA. Crohn's fistula: the conservative approach. In: Phillips RKS, Luniss PJ (eds)

Anal fistula. Surgical evaluation and managment. London: Chapman & Hall, 1996; pp. 131–41.

154. Sweeney JL, Ritchie JK, Nicholls RJ. Anal fissure in Crohn's disease. Br J Surg 1988; 75:56–7.

155. Buchmann P, Allan RN, Thompson H et al. Carcinoma in rectovaginal fistula in a patient with Crohn's disease. Am J Surg 1980; 140:462–3.

156. Church JM, Fazio VW, Lavery IC et al. The differential diagnosis and comorbidity of hidradenitis suppurativa and perianal Crohn's disease. Int J Colorectal Dis 1993; 8:117–19.

157. Hughes LE, Taylor BA. Perianal lesions in Crohn's disease. In: Allan R, Keighley M, Alexander-Williams J, Hawkins C (eds) Inflammatory bowel disease, 2nd edn. Edinburgh: Churchill Livingstone, 1990; pp. 351–61.

158. Fleshner PR, Schoetz DJ Jr, Roberts PL et al. Anal fissure in Crohn's disease: a plea for aggressive management. Dis Colon Rectum 1995; 38:1137–43.

159. Sonoda T, Hull T, Piedmonte MR et al. Outcomes of primary repair of anorectal and rectovaginal fistulas using the endorectal advancement flap. Dis Colon Rectum 2002; 45:1622–8.

160. Makowiec F, Jehle EC, Becker HD et al. Clinical course after transanal advancement flap repair of perianal fistula in patients with Crohn's disease. Br J Surg 1995; 82:603–6.

161. Ozuner G, Hull TL, Cartmill J et al. Long-term analysis of the use of transanal rectal advancement flaps for complicated anorectal/vaginal fistulas. Dis Colon Rectum 1996; 39:10–14.

162. Williams JG, Rothenberger DA, Nemer FD et al. Fistula-in-ano in Crohn's disease. Results of aggressive surgical treatment. Dis Colon Rectum 1991; 34:378–84.

163. Radcliffe AG, Ritchie JK, Hawley PR et al. Anovaginal and rectovaginal fistulas in Crohn's disease. Dis Colon Rectum 1988; 31:94–9.

164. Giordano P, Drew PJ, Taylor D et al. Vaginography: investigation of choice for clinically suspected vaginal fistulas. Dis Colon Rectum 1996; 39:568–72.

165. Hesterberg R, Schmidt WU, Muller F et al. Treatment of anovaginal fistulas with an anocutaneous flap in patients with Crohn's disease. Int J Colorectal Dis 1993; 8:51–4.

166. Sher ME, Bauer JJ, Gelernt I. Surgical repair of rectovaginal fistulas in patients with Crohn's disease: transvaginal approach. Dis Colon Rectum 1991; 34:641–8.

167. MacRae HM, McLeod RS, Cohen Z et al. Treatment of rectovaginal fistulas that have failed previous repair attempts. Dis Colon Rectum 1995; 38:921–5.

168. Linares L, Moreira LF, Andrews H et al. Natural history and treatment of anorectal strictures complicating Crohn's disease. Br J Surg 1988; 75:653–5.

Asha Senapati

INTRODUCTION

Full-thickness rectal prolapse is a distressing and demoralising condition. Patients are troubled by a protrusion beyond the anal verge that secretes mucus and may bleed. It is frequently associated with incontinence, either because there is an underlying weakness in the sphincter mechanism that allows the prolapse to occur or because the presence of the prolapse protruding through the anal canal leads to poor sphincter function.

Full-thickness rectal prolapse is the complete eversion of the rectum through the anal canal. This chapter deals primarily with its management in adults. Internal rectal prolapse (or intussusception) and rectal prolapse in childhood are considered under separate headings. Although full-thickness rectal prolapse may occur at any age, it is most commonly a condition of elderly women, the mean age of incidence being in the seventh and eighth decades. The sex distribution ranges from 10:1 to 6:1, women to men.

The fact that over 100 different procedures have been described to treat this condition[1] implies that none is entirely satisfactory. Some of these operations are listed in **Box 10.1**.

AETIOLOGY

The cause of rectal prolapse is unknown. The fault may be primarily in the configuration of the rectum and sigmoid colon, with a marked alteration in calibre between the two.[2] Alternatively, the fault may lie in the pelvic floor as many patients are incontinent prior to surgery. It may be a combination of the two. However, it is common to find a lax pelvic floor associated with rectal prolapse and a redundant sigmoid colon. Both these factors are probably responsible for recurrent rectal prolapse no matter what form of treatment is undertaken. Parity is thought to have a limited role in its pathogenesis.[3]

A genetic role has been postulated by the observation that this may occasionally occur in families[4] and in cases of Ehlers–Danlos syndrome type IV.

CLINICAL FEATURES

Patients will usually complain of a lump that prolapses on defecation and which either reduces spontaneously or requires manual reduction. These symptoms are similar to those of prolapsing haemorrhoids and care should be taken during examination to distinguish between the two (see below). Bleeding may also occur as well as discharge of mucus produced by the prolapse.

Incontinence is frequently associated with prolapse, and is often the reason why patients seek advice from the doctor. The presence of a prolapse itself may need to be asked for specifically. Previous surgery for prolapse is not infrequent, occurring in up to 41% of patients in some series.[5] Incontinence associated with rectal prolapse must be assessed carefully if objective measurements are to be made

Box 10.1 • Procedures for the treatment of rectal prolapse

Abdominal procedures

- Ivalon rectopexy
- Ripstein rectopexy
- Anterior resection and rectopexy
- Sigmoid resection and rectopexy
- Extended abdominal rectopexy
- Marlex mesh rectopexy
- Roscoe–Graham repair
- Orr–Loygue rectopexy
- Puborectalis sling
- Rectal plication
- Rectosigmoidectomy
- Hartmann's operation
- Retroperitoneal colopexy
- Absorbable mesh rectopexy
- AP resection
- Presacral suture rectopexy
- Ivalon sling
- Lahaut's operation
- Moschcowitz operation
- Devadhar's operation
- Triple suspension rectopexy
- Ekehorn's rectopexy

Perineal operations

- Thiersch wire
- Silastic sling
- Perineal rectopexy
- Intersphincteric Ivalon rectopexy
- Postanal repair
- Perineal proctectomy
- Transanal fixation
- Modified Thiersch procedure
- Angelchick prosthesis repair
- Graciloplasty
- Alum injection
- Delorme's operation
- Silicone rubber suture
- Cauterisation–plication
- Gant–Miwa operation

about the success of treatment. In particular, many patients complain of incontinence due to the passage of mucus from the prolapse. On questioning, a long history of constipation often predating the prolapse may emerge, and it may be that the weakening of the pelvic floor from the consequent straining results in the prolapse. These patients frequently have hard stools that they find difficult to evacuate, but they are not truly incontinent. Some studies have suggested that many such patients have slow colonic transit underlying their condition.[6,7] Anorectal physiology measuring the pressures preoperatively is a helpful adjunct for assessing the benefit of treatment, as is assessment of colonic function by transit studies.

On examination, full-thickness rectal prolapse has a typical cylindrical appearance which, together with the absence of external skin tags, makes it readily distinguisable from prolapsed haemorrhoids. In addition, on palpating between the two layers of mucosa the prolapsed muscular tube can be clearly felt, and the diagnosis of a full-thickness prolapse is straightforward. However, many patients find it difficult to produce this on demand, particularly in the left lateral position. The diagnosis by a competent observer must be made prior to treatment and effort must be made to see the prolapse. This can be done by asking the patient to squat on the floor and strain. Alternatively, they may sit on the lavatory, a manoeuvre that is usually successful. A modification of this technique using an adapted Leverad toilet seat will facilitate this process.[8] Although undignified, the patient must be examined in this position as sometimes the prolapse reduces on getting up. Occasionally, an examination under anaesthetic is required to make the diagnosis. Rectal examination must also include an assessment of the musculature of the anal canal.

Procidentia of the uterus is frequently associated with a full-thickness rectal prolapse,[9,10] probably because of more complete degeneration of the pelvic floor. Under these circumstances surgery can be fairly debilitating. A combined procedure with a vaginal hysterectomy is often necessary,[10,12] but success with an abdominal approach has been reported.[13] Vaginal hysterectomy with laparoscopic rectopexy has also been reported.[14] Investigation of the pelvic floor by magnetic resonance imaging (MRI) may be helpful prior to surgery.[15,16] Dynamic MRI is currently under evaluation.

COMPLICATIONS

The main complication of rectal prolapse is difficulty in reduction, which may lead to strangulation. Some patients present with a long history of prolapse that has suddenly become irreducible, whereas others present for the first time with an irreducible prolapse. The latter may be managed by reduction of the prolapse and no further treatment and the patient may subsequently have no further episodes. However, the longer any prolapse remains out, the more difficult it is to reduce and the more difficult any surgical manoeuvre becomes. Acute urinary retention may occur.

To treat an irreducible rectal prolapse, elevate the foot of the bed and apply cold compresses to the prolapse in an attempt to reduce the oedema. Application of sugar (sucrose) may assist by causing desiccation.[17] Hyaluronidase has also been used.[18] When the swelling has reduced, gentle manual pressure on the prolapse will nearly always result in reduction, but it may recur almost immediately. If this happens, it must be reduced yet again and urgent surgical treatment planned. If strangulation has occurred, resection must be considered, which may be done via the perineum.[19] Rupture with ileal evisceration has been reported.[20]

TREATMENT

Procedures described to treat full-thickness rectal prolapse can be broadly classified into two groups, abdominal and perineal procedures (see **Box 10.1**).

However, there is little objective evidence or comparative data to support each particular method. As discussed in a Cochrane review, only 324 patients have ever been randomised into 10 different trials of rectal prolapse treatment.[21] The largest of these included 63 patients.[22]

Abdominal procedures

Among abdominal procedures, the most frequently used is some form of posterior rectopexy, which involves mobilisation of the rectum from the sacrum and fixation either directly (suture rectopexy) or by using an artificial material such as Marlex mesh, Ivalon sponge (Well's operation) or an absorbable mesh such as Vicryl. Fascia lata may be used as in the Orr–Loygue operation. A variation to posterior rectopexy is an anterior rectopexy such as Ripstein's operation. Rectopexy may be combined with excision of the sigmoid colon in what is known as resection rectopexy. It has been suggested that the process of rectal mobilisation alone is the main component resulting in the success of abdominal procedures.[23] A summary of the results of these procedures is given in **Table 10.1**.

The recurrence rate after posterior rectopexy is usually low (<5%) but follow-up may not be long and is often incomplete, making the true recurrence rate difficult to determine, although it is likely to be low. However, in one series looking at young patients followed up for many years, the recurrence rate was 20%.[20]

Defecatory disorders after rectopexy are common, intractable constipation being the most distressing. The extent and severity of the problem are not clear. Many patients are not specifically followed up for this problem, which may not be readily apparent, so the true incidence is not known although it can be high (see **Table 10.1**). Madden et al.[4] prospectively studied detailed bowel function in 23 patients and found that incontinence was improved in 82%, 42% became constipated postoperatively, but 36% who were constipated beforehand were relieved, with no deterioration overall in the series. Those who became constipated after surgery could not be predicted on the basis of preoperative questioning and tests.

The mechanism of constipation after rectopexy is not known. Some have suggested that it is due to scarring and rigidity around the rectum from the implant. However, it occurs even without an implant, so some have supposed that the redundant sigmoid may prolapse into the pouch of Douglas, creating a mechanical obstruction by kinking. Alternatively, rectal mobilisation may denervate the rectum by dividing the parasympathetic inflow. In Ripstein's operation, the lateral ligaments are preserved, which may explain the better functional outcome from this operation in some series.[45,46]

In a randomised trial comparing Marlex mesh rectopexy with and without division of the lateral ligaments,[47] there was a higher incidence of constipation (8% vs. 50%) after division of the lateral ligaments, although there was a higher incidence of recurrence in those with lateral ligament preservation, a finding confirmed by others.[48]

Table 10.1 • Results of abdominal rectopexy for rectal prolapse

Reference	Year	Type	N	Morbidity (%)	Mortality (%)	Recurrence (%)	Constipation (%)	Improved continence (%)
Morgan et al.[24]	1972	Ivalon	150	–	2.6	3.2	0	52
Penfold & Hawley[25]	1972	Ivalon	95	6	0	3	23	55
Boulos et al.[26]	1984	Ivalon	25	–	0	20	0	75
Atkinson & Taylor[27]	1984	Ivalon	40	2.5	0	10	–	71
Mann & Hoffman[28]	1988	Ivalon	51	39	0	0	18	38
McCue & Thomson[29]	1991	Ivalon	53	15	0	3.8	15	38
Madden et al.[4]	1992	Ivalon	26	–	0	0	42	82
Keighley et al.[30]	1983	Marlex	86	–	0	0	–	64
Winde et al.[31]	1993	Absorbable mesh	47	28	0	0	–	51
Launer et al.[32]	1982	Ripstein	54	28	0	12	18	–
Holmstrom et al.[33]	1986	Ripstein	97	3.7	2.8	4.1	16	39
Tjandra et al.[34]	1993	Ripstein	142	16	0.6	8	28	48
Watts et al.[35]	1985	Resection	102	–	0	1.9	–	77
Luukkonen et al.[36]	1992	Resection	15	20	6.6	0	0	72
		Absorbable mesh	15	13	0	0	33	83
Madoff et al.[37]	1992	Resection	47	–	–	6.3	6	38
Cirocco & Brown[38]	1993	Resection	41	15	0	7	8	48
Deen et al.[39]	1994	Resection	10	30	0	0	0	90
Huber et al.[40]	1995	Resection	42	7	0	0	0	43
Athanasiadis et al.[41]	1995	Resection	25	–	–	2.6	0	–
McKee et al.[42]	1992	Resection	9	16	0	0	improved 22	0
		Suture	9			0	worsened 25	80
Duthie & Bartolo[43]	1992	Suture	10	–	0	0	improved 60	88
		Ivalon	9				improved 17	40
		Marlex	20	–	0	0	improved 38	67
		Resection	29	–	–	–	improved 44	78
Novell et al.[22]	1994	Ivalon	31	19	0	3	48	40
		Suture	32	9	0	3	31	80
Kim et al.[44]	1999	Resection	161	20	0	5	–	55
Schultz et al.[45]	2000	Ripstein	69	33	0	1.6	improved 37	43

Estimating the prevalence of constipation after surgery is not as helpful as determining whether patients with normal preoperative function have deteriorated. When this was done prospectively by Madden et al.,[4] it was found that 42% of patients who were unaffected before Marlex rectopexy became constipated afterwards. Broden et al.[49] also found that 40% of patients who were not constipated before a Ripstein operation became so after surgery.

Resection rectopexy aims to decrease rectosigmoid kinking by performing sigmoidectomy.[11] Despite concerns that rectosigmoid 'kinking' is not an established cause of constipation and that surgery for constipation alone is rather unpredictable even when much more extensive lengths of colon are removed, the studies that have been performed nevertheless suggest that constipation is improved, particularly in those known preoperatively to be constipated.[35,36,38,40–42,50] The finding has been supported by retained radio-opaque markers that have been demonstrated after rectopexy alone but not after rectopexy with sigmoidectomy.[42]

Comparisons between different types of rectopexy give no clear picture. For example, sponge rectopexy gives similar results to sutured rectopexy.[22]

 In a randomised trial of Ivalon vs. suture rectopexy,[22] the results were similar, leading to the conclusion that it is not necessary to use artificial material in performing a rectopexy.

Duthie and Bartolo[43] compared different methods of rectopexy and found no increase in constipation after rectopexy itself, but emptying after resection was significantly improved. Better results as far as continence is concerned were obtained by avoiding prosthetic material.

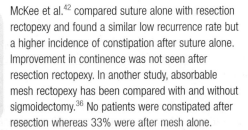 McKee et al.[42] compared suture alone with resection rectopexy and found a similar low recurrence rate but a higher incidence of constipation after suture alone. Improvement in continence was not seen after resection rectopexy. In another study, absorbable mesh rectopexy has been compared with and without sigmoidectomy.[36] No patients were constipated after resection whereas 33% were after mesh alone.

However, one of the concerns with mesh rectopexy is the possibility of infection in the mesh. Although the incidence is low (0–2.6%),[24–26,28,30,33] it is serious when it occurs.

 Absorbable mesh has been used,[31] with good results[51] and no infection of the mesh.[52]

In a series of 59 patients treated by extended abdominal rectopexy[28] (suspension of the uterus and reattachment of the lateral ligaments to the sacral promontory, in addition to conventional mobilisation for an Ivalon rectopexy), there was no mortality and a 12% morbidity. There were no recurrences, but the percentage of patients constipated rose from 29% before surgery to 47% after. Incontinence improved in 38%. Of 151 cases treated by Ivalon rectopexy alone,[24] 3% died and 3% recurred within 3 years. Constipation after surgery was recorded in 27% but it is not clear how many were constipated before. Incontinence improved in 52%. Another study of 40 patients treated by Ivalon rectopexy[27] reported no deaths and 10% recurrence. Constipation was not discussed in detail. Incontinence improved in 71%. In a large series of 101 patients reported from St Mark's Hospital[25] treated by Ivalon rectopexy, there was no mortality, 6% morbidity and 3% recurrence. Continence was improved in 73% but 29% had constipation after surgery, having not been constipated before. Urinary disturbances were also seen in 9%.

Boulos et al.[26] reviewed 40 young patients after Ivalon sponge rectopexy and reported 20% recurrence, three occurring late (5 years). Continence improved in 55% and no patient became constipated who had not been so before surgery. Rogers and Jeffery[53] treated 24 patients with Ivalon rectopexy and an added postanal repair and reported 4% recurrence and 100% improvement in continence. They do not discuss constipation. In 100 patients treated by Marlex mesh rectopexy,[30] there were no recurrences, with 86% of the patients being followed up for over 2 years. Constipation was not discussed. In another study, 47 patients treated by a cross-shaped knitted propylene mesh had no recurrences after 4 years.[54]

Rectopexy combined with anterior resection is popular in the USA, where it is often known as the Frykman–Goldberg operation. In a series of 102 patients[35] (81% followed up for more than 2 years), only 2% developed recurrences, but 20% considered their operation to be unsatisfactory because of either constipation or incontinence. In another study, the Ripstein operation (anterior rectopexy) was performed in 108 patients,[33] with 3% mortality and 4% recurrence. However, defecation disturbances increased from 27 to 43%.

The long-term results of resection rectopexy seem satisfactory,[37] with low recurrence and reasonable bowel function, although no specific mention was made in this study of constipation after surgery. Indeed, anterior resection[35] has also had good results. Rectopexy after resection should not involve non-absorbable mesh as there is a risk of sepsis; either the rectopexy should be sutured or absorbable mesh used.

Absorbable mesh rectopexy has been compared with and without sigmoidectomy,[36] there being increased morbidity with resection but less postoperative constipation. Infection rates without resection were lower than after resection.[55]

Laparoscopic procedures

Laparoscopic rectopexy was first reported in 1993.[56] The technique[57,58] involves mobilising the rectum down to the pelvic floor, facilitated by upward traction of the sigmoid using bowel-holding forceps and/or a tape placed around the colon. A vaginal obturator may help the anterior dissection in females. After fixation, the peritoneum is closed with sutures or staples.

There have now been a few series of mesh rectopexy performed laparoscopically.[59–63] Himpens et al.[64] described 37 patients with a mean age of 62 years, a mean operating time of 130 minutes and a median hospital stay of 7 days. Suture rectopexy without resection in 25 patients was reported, with no recurrence at a mean of 26 months follow-up.[65] Similar results were reported by others[66,76] A large observational study of 124 resection and 26 non-resection rectopexies (85 with a mesh) reported a 5.3% conversion rate.[67] The postoperative morbidity was reasonably low but no long-term outcomes were reported.

A clinically based approach to resection versus mesh rectopexy, both done laparoscopically, was conducted in 24 patients by Madbouly et al.[68] The decision was based on bowel function and incontinence. There were no recurrences after a mean

follow-up of 18 months, and the functional outcomes were good.

A small randomised trial[69] showed no significant differences between a laparoscopic and open Well's rectopexy.

It therefore appears that a similar operation to an open rectopexy can be achieved, so the same arguments for and against abdominal rectopexy can probably be reasonably applied to laparoscopic rectal prolapse surgery, but with the proviso that adhesions may if anything be less dense (and thus recurrence potentially higher) and difficulty/inexperience may lead to collateral injuries (e.g. to the ureters) during the learning curve.[11]

Resection rectopexy has also been performed in a laparoscopically assisted manner since 1992,[70,75,77] again with minimal morbidity and mortality. Recurrence rates were low (0–6%) but follow-up was short.

Studies that have retrospectively compared the results of laparoscopic and conventional surgery[73,74,77] have found that analgesic requirement, postoperative stay and the time to oral intake were reduced with a laparoscopic approach, but the operating time was longer. A case–control study of 53 patients in each group compared laparoscopic with open surgery and found similar outcomes, with a shorter hospital stay after laparoscopy.[78] The functional outcome after laparoscopic rectopexy is considered to be similar to the open procedure.[79] However, not only do retrospective comparisons need to be considered with caution, but it is now also widely appreciated that in the past many patients operated on conventionally were starved for too long and mobilized too slowly. Any difference in hospital stay may in part simply reflect different attitudes to postoperative management rather than real differences in surgical outcomes.

A randomised trial of 40 patients to laparscopic vs. open abdominal rectopexy found that clinical recovery was better in the laparoscopic group.[80]

The conversion rate to open surgery and postoperative morbidity have been low. The longer term issues of recurrent rectal prolapse and function are continuing to be assessed. Overall, it seems as if laparoscopic rectal prolapse surgery holds potential and has a definite place in rectal prolapse surgery. There is little doubt that equivalent operations to their open counterparts can be done. It is now necessary to conduct prospective studies with adequate follow-up to determine whether high rates of recurrence and constipation can be avoided. If it is just the more 'minimal' nature of laparoscopic rectal prolapse surgery that attracts, then the approach may encounter problems. The perineal operations described below are even more minimal. They do not seem to induce constipation, but their Achilles heel is their high recurrence rate. Open abdominal operations can also be adapted to more cosmetic incisions (e.g. Pfannenstiel), so if a resection rectopexy becomes the established norm for an abdominal approach, a laparoscopically assisted operation that may require an incision to remove the specimen may show few advantages.

Perineal procedures

Perineal operations are attractive as they can be applied in sick, elderly or high-risk patients without the use of general anaesthesia. In addition, in young men a pelvic operation, with its associated risks to sexual and bladder function, can be avoided. As with abdominal approaches, there is a wide variety of operations (see **Box 10.1**), of which Delorme's operation and perineal rectosigmoidectomy (originally known as Altemeier's operation) are discussed in more detail.

DELORME'S OPERATION

Technique

The technique is illustrated in **Figs 10.1–10.4**. The rectum is prolapsed to its full extent and a circumferential incision is made in the mucosa 1–2 cm above the dentate line. The mucosa is then dissected off the underlying muscle. This dissection may be facilitated either by repeated submucous injections of dilute adrenaline (epinephrine) or by using diathermy, or both. The mucosa is separated circumferentially. As the dissection proceeds first over the external aspect and then the internal aspect of the prolapse, the surgeon is left holding a cylinder of mucosa in his or her non-dominant hand, which allows traction. The dissection proceeds until no further rectal wall can be prolapsed by traction; the

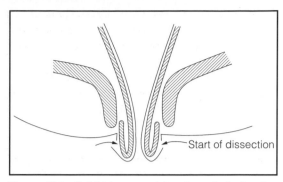

Figure 10.1 • Full-thickness rectal prolapse indicating the start of the dissection.

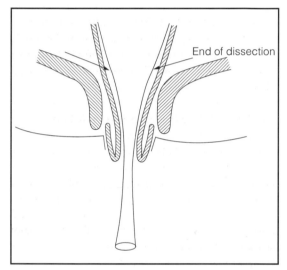

Figure 10.2 • The rectal mucosa has been dissected off the prolapse.

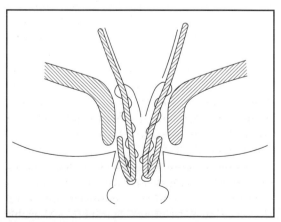

Figure 10.3 • Plication sutures have been inserted.

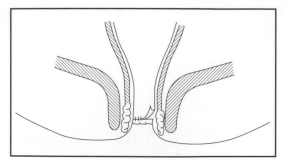

Figure 10.4 • Sutures approximate the cut ends of mucosa.

cylinder of mucosa also becomes narrow and is sometimes up to 40 cm in length. If a full-thickness defect is made in the bowel wall, recognised by seeing fat, it is repaired immediately, but it should not be cause for concern as it will also be taken up in the plication. Several (between four and eight) plicating absorbable (e.g. Vicryl) sutures are then inserted into the muscle starting from the top of the dissection and finishing just above the dentate line but not including the mucosa. These are then tightened, drawing the proximal dissection margin down towards the distal margin. The mucosal cylinder is divided, and mucosa-to-mucosa interrupted sutures inserted to complete the anastomosis. A modification of this procedure[81] is to suture the plicated rectal wall posteriorly in order to tighten the sphincter mechanism.

Discussion

Delorme himself did not describe plication of the muscle.[82] Indeed, he described only three patients, one of whom died of sepsis. Perhaps not surprisingly interest waned in the technique for many years, but since the 1970s there have been a number of publications describing this operation (**Table 10.2**). The mortality is low and the complications are minor. The recurrence rate has varied from 5 to 26% over an average follow-up of 2 years or more. Furthermore, many of these recurrences have been relatively asymptomatic and have not always required treatment. When recurrence has needed to be treated the operation can be repeated, if necessary as many as three times with minimal patient discomfort. There may be some increased bowel frequency after Delorme's operation, presumably due to relative loss of rectal reservoir capacity.

The problem of postoperative constipation after Delorme's operation has seldom been addressed, but when it has the incidence is zero.[5,94] In general, postoperative bowel disturbances are not usually a problem.

PERINEAL RECTOSIGMOIDECTOMY (ALTEMEIER'S OPERATION)

Technique

Perineal rectosigmoidectomy is performed with the patient in either the lithotomy or the prone jack-knife position. After the prolapse has been delivered,[101] a circumferential incision is made through the full thickness of the outer rectal wall 2 cm above the dentate line. The inner tube of rectum and distal sigmoid colon are mobilised, with the blood vessels being ligated close to the bowel wall until the bowel can be prolapsed no further. After transecting the colon and removing the specimen, anastomosis is made either by hand or using staples.[105–107] This procedure may with advantage be combined with a levatoroplasty.[101] Assistance by laparoscopic mobilisation has also been reported.[108,109]

Discussion

In a series of 114 patients,[101] postoperative complications were seen in 12%, recurrent full-thickness rectal prolapse occurred in 10% and improvement in continence was seen in 46%, some of whom had undergone a levatoroplasty. Series outlining this procedure in the elderly have described satisfactory results.[99,102–104] Recurrence varied from 0 to 15.8% and continence improved in 46–88%. A 19-year experience with this technique has been reported with a 15.8% recurrence.[44]

Perineal rectosigmoidectomy has been compared in a small randomised trial of 20 patients with abdominal resection rectopexy, both procedures being combined with a pelvic floor repair.[39] One recurrence was seen after perineal rectosigmoidectomy, no one became constipated postoperatively but continence improved more after the abdominal procedure.

This procedure has been safely done with a less than 24-hour hospital stay in 80% of patients.[104] The results are summarised in **Table 10.2**.

Table 10.2 • Results of perineal operations for rectal prolapse

Reference	Year	Operation	N	Morbidity (%)	Mortality (%)	Recurrence (%)	Constipation (%)	Improved continence (%)
Uhlig & Sullivan[81]	1979	Delorme	44	34	0	6.8	–	–
Christiansen & Kirkgaard[83]	1981	Delorme	12	–	0	17	–	50
Gunderson et al.[84]	1985	Delorme	18	17	0	6	–	–
Houry et al.[85]	1986	Delorme	18	–	0	17	–	44
Monson et al.[86]	1986	Delorme	27	0	0	7.4	–	83
Heaton & Rennie[87]	1988	Delorme	5	0	0	20	–	–
Abulafi et al.[88]	1990	Delorme	22	28	0	5	–	75
Graf et al.[89]	1992	Delorme	14	0	0	21	–	55
Tobin & Scott[90]	1994	Delorme	49	8	0	22	0	50
Oliver et al.[91]	1994	Delorme	41	39	2.4	22	–	68
Senapati et al.[5]	1994	Delorme	32	6	0	12.5	0	46
Lechaux et al.[92]	1995	Delorme	85	14	2.4	13.5	0	69
Plusa et al.[93]	1995	Delorme	19	0	0	–	0	31
Pescatori et al.[94]	1998	Delorme	33	45	0	21	0	30
Watts & Thompson[95]	2000	Delorme	113	–	3.5	26.5	0	40
Watkins et al.[96]	2003	Delorme	52	25	0	10	0	83
Tsunoda et al.[97]	2003	Delorme	31	13	0	13	0	63
Miles[93]	1933	Altemeier	31	0	3.2	3.2	–	–
Prasad et al.[99]	1986	Altemeier	25	0	0	0	–	88
Thorne & Polglase[100]	1992	Altemeier	16	12.5	0	12.5	–	50
Williams et al.[101]	1992	Altemeier	114	12	0	10	–	46
Johansen et al.[102]	1993	Altemeier	20	5	5	0	–	85
Ramanujam et al.[103]	1994	Altemeier	72	10.8	0	5.5	–	67
Deen et al.[39]	1994	Altemeier	10	10	0	0	0	80
Kim et al.[44]	1999	Altemeier	183	14	0.5	15.8	–	53
Kimmins et al.[104]	2001	Altemeier	63	10	0	6.4	0	50

FUNCTIONAL PROBLEMS

Attention to the functional problems associated with rectal prolapse has allowed the potential for a tailored approach to treatment.[7,110]

Constipation

There is increasing awareness of the problem of postoperative constipation after abdominal procedures. As there appears to be a lower incidence of this problem after resection rectopexy, this procedure has been advocated when patients are already constipated before surgery.

Incontinence

Incontinence is common in rectal prolapse and in one series was particularly associated with pudendal neuropathy.[111] Incontinence is improved after all procedures that treat rectal prolapse. Part of the reason may be the cessation of mucus leakage from the prolapse previously interpreted as incontinence. Information is scanty, most studies being retrospective and not classifying or recording incontinence in a systematic way.

A prospective study before and after Delorme's operation[94] showed that although there was improved rectal sensation and lowered compliance, there was no difference in the anal pressures even though continence was improved in 31%. Nevertheless, few would doubt that postoperatively there is a real improvement in continence. Bartolo has proposed that the prolapse itself triggers the recto-anal inhibitory reflex, and thereby leads to incontinence. Certainly, resting anal pressure has been shown to increase after posterior rectopexy[112,113] and after a Ripstein procedure,[114–116] although this increase was not always shown to correlate with continence.[117] However, none of these values rose significantly after surgery despite continence being restored in the majority.

Electrophysiological studies performed preoperatively do not seem to predict continence after rectopexy.[118] In an earlier publication,[119] reductions in basal and squeeze pressures were found only in patients with prolapse and incontinence but not with prolapse alone. There was no significant rise in pressures after surgery and pressures were not related to the clinical results. Pelvic floor repair at the time of prolapse surgery seems to improve continence,[39,103] as does postanal repair,[120] but of course this can be delayed and applied later as a separate operation in those who do not do well.

Biofeedback may be used postoperatively for continuing incontinence but it is only likely to be effective in improving external sphincter function.[121]

Other related conditions

SOLITARY RECTAL ULCER AND INTERNAL INTUSSUSCEPTION

A number of patients with disordered defecation do not have an external prolapse but can be demonstrated on proctography or during rigid sigmoidoscopy to have internal intussusception. It is not known if this is the same disorder.[122] The solitary rectal ulcer syndrome is characterised by chronic, prolonged and multiple visits to the lavatory where the subject sits and strains for periods of upwards of half an hour. Mucus and blood may be passed and the patient, frantic to satisfy an intense urge to defecate, may insert a finger anally in an attempt to extract stool digitally.

The cause of the ulceration seen on rigid sigmoidoscopy is uncertain, some arguing that direct digital trauma is responsible, others that the intussusception allows the apex to become traumatised against a closed anal canal. Not all patients have frank ulceration, some having instead a salmon-pink patch characteristically situated on the anterior rectal wall between 5 and 8 cm from the anal verge. Biopsy reveals diagnostic histological features also seen in other areas in the gastrointestinal tract where there is prolapsing mucosa.

Treatment is difficult. Anterior and posterior Marlex mesh rectopexy has been tried with some early enthusiasm,[123] some patients have undergone an intra-anal Delorme's operation, and indeed some have gone on to proctectomy and either coloanal anastomosis or end colostomy.[124] In a study of 81 patients with solitary rectal ulcer syndrome,[128] only 59% of patients had benefit from rectopexy. The finding of solitary rectal ulcer in either the coloanal segment or the colostomy in some patients and the extremely unpredictable results of surgery make alternatives, such as biofeedback, attractive.

Therapy directed towards improving the defecatory disorder is likely to be more beneficial.[125]

When investigating a patient with a defecatory disorder, a proctogram or rigid sigmoidoscopy may show internal intussusception but without an associated solitary rectal ulcer or other clinical features of the solitary rectal ulcer syndrome. Abdominal rectopexy has been tried in these patients[126] but without clear benefit even though the proctographic appearances may improve.[127] Of note, internal intussusception does not appear to progress to full-thickness prolapse.[129]

PROLAPSE IN CHILDHOOD

Rectal prolapse is not infrequent under the age of 2 years, sometimes being precipitated by a diarrhoeal illness or a prolonged bout of coughing (and even described in association with *Clostridium difficile* infection[130]). It has a strong association with cystic fibrosis, making a sweat test mandatory.[131] The prolapse usually resolves spontaneously, requiring no other treatment than reduction and parental reassurance. Recurrent prolapse also usually resolves spontaneously.

However, there are instances where surgical treatment may be necessary. Injection sclerotherapy has been advocated as the first-line treatment.[131,132] In Ekehorn's rectopexy,[133,134] the rectum is sutured to the lowermost part of the sacrum for 10 days before suture removal; local inflammation causes adhesions between the rectal wall and the perirectal tissue. There were no recurrences and there was no major morbidity in 78 patients. A modification of a Thiersch wire using catgut was used with success in 40 patients with rectal prolapse after acute diarrhoeal illnesses.[135] A posterior approach through the natal cleft dividing the levator muscles and suturing the rectum to the coccyx has also been described,[136] with no recurrence in 14 patients. A minimally invasive technique using sutures to anchor the rectum to the sacrum was used successfully in 42 children.[137]

COLORECTAL CANCER

There is no clear link with colorectal cancer. Some patients with a cancer may be induced to strain sufficiently to produce a prolapse,[138] which may explain the fourfold relative risk for colorectal cancer in one retrospective comparison of 70 prolapse patients with 350 age-matched controls (5.7% vs. 1.5% prevalence of rectosigmoid carcinomas respectively).[139] Clearly, any history of recent change in bowel habit should be investigated fully, regardless of the presence of a rectal prolapse.

THE CHOICE

From a surgeon's perspective, the low morbidity, the apparent absence of constipation and the inherent repeatability of perineal operations makes them attractive. Coupled to this in the young male is the absence of any fear of disturbance of sexual function. On the other hand, recurrence is common and abdominal rectopexy, after a prior Delorme's operation, can be difficult as the concertina makes the anterior plane between rectum and vagina/prostate hard to follow.

There are four groups of patients who suffer rectal prolapse, the first two being particularly rare. The choice of treatment in the four groups is as follows.

1. Babies: reduce the prolapse.
2. Young children: consider injection sclerotherapy or Ekehorn's rectopexy.
3. Young adults: abdominal operations have a more durable outcome, making them more attractive in this group. However, there is a risk of pelvic nerve damage, such that young men may choose a perineal approach.
4. The elderly: here the low morbidity and inherent repeatability make perineal approaches attractive.

The advantages and disadvantages of some procedures are given in **Box 10.2**.

However, there are no clear data to assess which of the various operations are superior to another. Certainly within each approach (abdominal vs. perineal) there is no clarity. An international multicentre randomised controlled trial, PROSPER (PROlapse Surgery PErineal or Rectopexy), is being conducted under the auspices of the Association of Coloproctology of Great Britain and Ireland. The schema is given in **Fig. 10.5**.

Recurrent rectal prolapse

It is difficult to repeat an abdominal procedure, so some believe a perineal operation is best suited to

Box 10.2 • Advantages and disadvantages of abdominal rectopexy and perineal operations

Abdominal rectopexy
Advantage

- Low recurrence rate

Disadvantages

- General anaesthetic
- Abdominal operation
- Risk if anastomosis is performed
- Infection in prosthetic material
- Intractable constipation
- Sexual and urinary disturbance possible

Perineal operations
Advantages

- No abdominal operation
- Can be done under regional anaesthesia
- Short stay in hospital possible
- Minimal postoperative pain
- No constipation

Disadvantages

- Higher recurrence rate
- Risk of anastomosis if performed
- Urgency of defecation

these circumstances.[140] Although perineal operations are easier to repeat, the results of such operations are unknown. Abdominal operations may be more appropriate.[141] The trans-sacral approach has also been used with some success.[142] Pikarsky et al.[143] compared a series of 27 operations for recurrent prolapse with a similar group who had primary prolapse. The outcomes were similar.

SUMMARY

Rectal prolapse is a debilitating benign condition, primarily affecting elderly women, for which there are many choices of operative treatment. The main abdominal ones are mesh rectopexy using either non-absorbable or absorbable mesh, resection rectopexy with sigmoidectomy and sutured rectopexy. Laparoscopic rectal prolapse surgery is certainly feasible but benefits measured against the established objectives of conventional approaches have yet to be demonstrated. The main perineal operations are Delorme's operation and perineal rectosigmoidectomy. The advantage of an abdominal approach is the low recurrence rate, although there is the disadvantage of disordered bowel function postoperatively in up to 50% of cases treated without a resection. The main advantage of the perineal route is its suitability for the elderly and infirm, but the disadvantage is a higher recurrence rate. The evaluation of results from any form of treatment for this condition should be based not only on recurrence rates, complication rates and cosmesis but also on assessment of the effect on bowel function, both incontinence and constipation.

It is probable that different patients will benefit from different treatments.[144] Suture or mesh rectopexy may be appropriate for patients with no preoperative constipation and minimal sigmoid redundancy (although this has yet to be demonstrated, as Madden et al.[4] were not able to predict on the basis of history or physiology testing who would become constipated after surgery). Patients in whom constipation is a prominent feature would certainly seem to be candidates for an abdominal resection rectopexy with suture fixation. The decision in young adults is perhaps the hardest, where the fear in the longer term of recurrence after a perineal approach is balanced by the fear of the huge difficulties of managing lifelong constipation, should it occur, after an abdominal approach. None of this is made any easier in, for example, the young male who is just as concerned about disordered sexual function or the young female disturbed by the prospect of an unsightly abdominal scar. The laparoscopic approach may be used with advantage here. Ultimately the patient should decide, being fully conversant with the advantages and disadvantages of the various approaches.

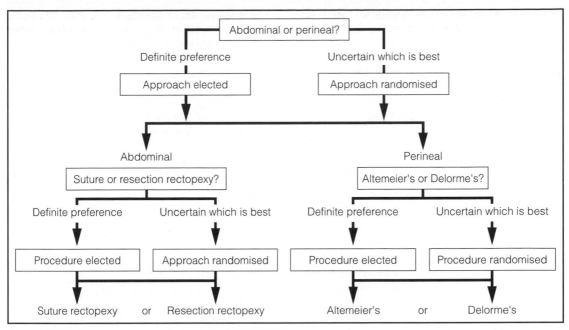

Figure 10.5 • Schema for randomisation in the PROSPER trial.

• Key points

- Symptomatic rectal prolapse requires surgical treatment.
- Several techniques, both abdominal and perineal, have been described.
- Abdominal procedures have a lower recurrence rate but a higher incidence of constipation. This may be improved by doing a resection. These procedures may be done laparoscopically.
- Perineal operations have a higher recurrence rate but satisfactory functional outcome. They have fewer systemic complications than abdominal surgery.
- Few randomised trials have been done to compare different techniques.
- An international multicentre randomised trial (PROSPER) is now comparing abdominal vs. perineal and resection vs. non-resection techniques.

REFERENCES

1. Wassef R, Rothenberger DA, Goldberg SM. Rectal prolapse. Curr Probl Surg 1986; 23:398–451.

2. Stelzner F. Etiology and therapy of rectal prolapse. Experiences with 308 cases 1956–1991. Chirurg 1994; 65:533–45.

3. Karasick S, Spettell CM. Defecography: does parity play a role in the development of rectal prolapse? Eur Radiol 1999; 9:450–3.

4. Madden MV, Kamm MA, Nicholls RJ, Santhanam AN, Cabot R, Speakman CT. Abdominal rectopexy for complete prolapse: prospective study evaluating changes in symptoms and anorectal function. Dis Colon Rectum 1992; 35:48–55.

5. Senapati A, Nicholls RJ, Thomson JP, Phillips RK. Results of Delorme's procedure for rectal prolapse. Dis Colon Rectum 1994; 37:456–60.

6. Brown AJ, Horgan AF, Anderson JH, McKee RF, Finlay IG. Colonic motility is abnormal before surgery for rectal prolapse. Br J Surg 1999; 86:263–6.

7. Eu KW, Seow-Choen F. Functional problems in adult rectal prolapse and controversies in surgical treatment. Br J Surg 1997; 84:904–11.

8. Paice A, Buchanan GN, Murali K, Parker MC. A novel method of demonstrating rectal prolapse. Colorectal Dis 2003; 5:374–5.

9. Barham K, Collopy BT. Posthysterectomy rectal and vaginal prolapse, a commonly overlooked problem. Aust NZ J Obstet Gynaecol 1993; 33:300–3.

10. Bouret JM, De Meeus JB, Kalfon A, Cancel J. Associated rectal and genital prolapse: value of Delorme's operation. A case report. Rev Fr Gynecol Obstet 1992; 87:231–7.

11. Bartolo DC. Rectal prolapse. Br J Surg 1996; 83:3–5.

12. Dekel A, Rabinerson D, Rafael ZB, Kaplan B, Misovaty B, Bayer Y. Concurrent genital and rectal prolapse: two pathologies, one joint operation. Br J Obstet Gynaecol 2000; 107:125–9.

13. Zhioua F, Ferchiou M, Pira JM, Jedoui A, Meriah S. Uterine fixation to the promontory and the Orr-Loygue operation in associated genital and rectal prolapse. Rev Fr Gynecol Obstet 1993; 88:277–81.

14. Kriplani A, Banerjee N, Kriplani AK, Roy KK, Takkar D. Uterovaginal prolapse associated with rectal prolapse. Aust NZ J Obstet Gynaecol 1998; 38:325–6.

15. Pannu HK. Magnetic resonance imaging of pelvic organ prolapse. Abdom Imaging 2002; 27:660–73.

16. Stoker J, Halligan S, Bartram CI. Pelvic floor imaging. Radiology 2001; 218:621–41.

17. Coburn WM III, Russell MA, Hofstetter WL. Sucrose as an aid to manual reduction of incarcerated rectal prolapse. Ann Emerg Med 1997; 30:347–9.

18. Chaudhuri A. Hyaluronidase in the reduction of incarcerated rectal prolapse: a novel use. Int J Colorectal Dis 1999; 14:264.

19. Ramanujam PS, Venkatesh KS. Management of acute incarcerated rectal prolapse. Dis Colon Rectum 1992; 35:1154–6.

20. Hovey MA, Metcalf AM. Incarcerated rectal prolapse–rupture and ileal evisceration after failed reduction: report of a case. Dis Colon Rectum 1997; 40:1254–7.

21.  Brazzelli M, Bachoo P, Grant A. Surgery for complete rectal prolapse in adults (Cochrane review). In: The Cochrane Library, Issue 4, 2003. Chichester: John Wiley & Sons.

22. Novell JR, Osborne MJ, Winslet MC, Lewis AA. Prospective randomized trial of Ivalon sponge versus sutured rectopexy for full-thickness rectal prolapse. Br J Surg 1994; 81:904–6.

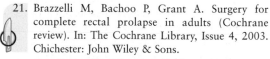
A randomised controlled trial of Ivalon sponge rectopexy vs. suture rectopexy. The results were equivalent.

23. Nelson R, Spitz J, Pearl RK, Abcarian H. What role does full rectal mobilisation alone play in the treatment of rectal prolapse? Tech Coloproctol 2001; 5:33–5.

24. Morgan CN, Porter NH, Klugman DJ. Ivalon (polyvinyl alcohol) sponge in the repair of complete rectal prolapse. Br J Surg 1972; 59:841–6.

25. Penfold JC, Hawley PR. Experiences of Ivalon sponge implant for complete rectal prolapse at St Mark's Hospital 1960–70. Br J Surg 1972; 59:846–8.

26. Boulos PB, Stryker SJ, Nicholls RJ. The long-term results of polyvinyl alcohol (Ivalon) sponge for rectal prolapse in young patients. Br J Surg 1984; 71:213–14.

27. Atkinson KG, Taylor DC. Wells procedure for complete rectal prolapse. Dis Colon Rectum 1984; 27:96–8.

28. Mann CV, Hoffman C. Complete rectal prolapse: the anatomical and functional results of treatment by an extended abdominal rectopexy. Br J Surg 1988; 75:34–7.

29. McCue JL, Thomson JPS. Clinical and functional results of abdominal rectopexy for complete rectal prolapse. Br J Surg 1991; 78:921–3.

30. Keighley MRB, Fielding JWL, Alexander-Williams J. Results of Marlex mesh abdominal rectopexy for rectal prolapse in 100 consecutive patients. Br J Surg 1983; 70:229–32.

31. Winde G, Reers B, Nottberg H, Berns T, Meyer J, Bunte H. Clinical and functional results of abdominal rectopexy with absorbable meshgraft for treatment of complete rectal prolapse. Eur J Surg 1993; 159:301–5.

A randomised trial comparing two different forms of absorbable mesh in abdominal rectopexy: polyglycolic acid and polyglactine. There were no differences between the groups, with no recurrences.

32. Launer DP, Fazio VW, Weakley FL, Turnbull RB, Jagelman DG, Lavery IC. The Ripstein procedure: a 16 year experience. Dis Colon Rectum 1982; 25:41–5.

33. Holstrom B, Broden G, Dolk A. Results of the Ripstein operation in the treatment of rectal prolapse and internal rectal procidentia. Dis Colon Rectum 1986; 29:845–8.

34. Tjandra JJ, Fazio VW, Church JM, Milsom JW, Oakley JR, Lavery IC. Ripstein procedure is an effective treatment for rectal prolapse without constipation. Dis Colon Rectum 1993; 36:501–7.

35. Watts JD, Rothenberger DA, Buls JG, Goldberg SM, Nivatongs S. The management of procidentia. Dis Colon Rectum 1985; 28:96–102.

36. 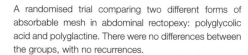 Luukkonen P, Mikkonen U, Jarvinen H. Abdominal rectopexy with sigmoidectomy vs. rectopexy alone for rectal prolapse: a prospective, randomized study. Int J Colorectal Dis 1992; 7:219–22.

A randomised trial comparing polyglycolic acid mesh rectopexy with suture rectopexy and sigmoidectomy. Constipation was lower after resection rectopexy.

37. Madoff RD, Williams JG, Wong WD, Rothenberger DA, Goldberg SM. Long-term functional results of colon resection and rectopexy for overt rectal prolapse. Am J Gastroenterol 1992; 87:101–4.

38. Cirocco WC, Brown AC. Anterior resection for the treatment of rectal prolapse: a 20-year experience. Am Surg 1993; 59:265–9.

39. Deen KI, Grant E, Billingham C, Keighley MR. Abdominal resection rectopexy with pelvic floor repair versus perineal rectosigmoidectomy and pelvic floor repair for full-thickness rectal prolapse. Br J Surg 1994; 81:302–4.

 A randomised trial comparing abdominal resection rectopexy and perineal rectosigmoidectomy, both with pelvic floor repair. Abdominal resection rectopexy gave a better functional outcome than perineal rectosigmoidectomy.

40. Huber FT, Stein H, Siewert JR. Functional results after treatment of rectal prolapse with rectopexy and sigmoid resection. World J Surg 1995; 19:138–43.

41. Athanasiadis S, Heiligers J, Kuprian A, Heumuller L. Surgical therapy of rectal prolapse using rectopexy and resection. Effect of resection treatment on postoperative constipation and sphincter muscle function: a follow-up study of 112 patients. Chirurg 1995; 66:27–33.

42. McKee RF, Lauder JC, Poon FW, Aitchison MA, Finlay IG. A prospective randomized study of abdominal rectopexy with and without sigmoidectomy in rectal prolapse. Surg Gynecol Obstet 1992; 174:145–8.

 A randomised trial comparing suture rectopexy to sigmoid resection with rectopexy. Constipation in the suture rectopexy group was significantly higher compared with the resection rectopexy. There were no recurrences.

43. Duthie GS, Bartolo DC. Abdominal rectopexy for rectal prolapse: a comparison of techniques. Br J Surg 1992; 79:107–13.

44. Kim DS, Tsang CB, Wong WD, Lowry AC, Goldberg SM, Madoff RD. Complete rectal prolapse: evolution of management and results. Dis Colon Rectum 1999; 42:460–6.

45. Schultz I, Mellgren A, Dolk A, Johansson C, Holmstrom B. Long-term results and functional outcome after Ripstein rectopexy. Dis Colon Rectum 2000; 43:35–43.

46. Scaglia M, Fasth S, Hallgren T, Nordgren S, Oresland T, Hulten L. Abdominal rectopexy for rectal prolapse. Influence of surgical technique on functional outcome. Dis Colon Rectum 1994; 37:805–13.

47. Speakman CTM, Madden MV, Nicholls RJ, Kamm MA. Lateral ligament division during rectopexy causes constipation but prevents recurrence: results of a prospective randomised study. Br J Surg 1991; 78:1431–3.

 A randomised controlled trial of rectopexy with and without division of the lateral ligaments. Division of the lateral ligaments resulted in significantly higher incidence of constipation. There was a higher incidence of recurrence in those who did not undergo division of the lateral ligaments.

48. Scaglia M, Comotti F, Fornari M et al. The functional and manometric–volumetric results following abdominal rectopexy for total rectal prolapse. Chir Ital 1992; 44:257–72.

49. Broden G, Dolk A, Holmstrom B. Evacuation difficulties and other characteristics of rectal function associated with procidentia and the Ripstein operation. Dis Colon Rectum 1988; 31:283–6.

50. Benoist S, Taffinder N, Gould S, Chang A, Darzi A. Functional results two years after laparoscopic rectopexy. Am J Surg 2001; 182:168–73.

51. Galili Y, Rabau M. Comparison of polyglycolic acid and polypropylene mesh for rectopexy in the treatment of rectal prolapse. Eur J Surg 1997; 163:445–8.

 Comparison of a non-absorbable mesh and an absorbable mesh in abdominal rectopexy. There was no difference in outcome.

52. Arndt M, Pelster FW, Bunte H. [10 years' experiences used resorbable synthetic mesh in treatment of rectal prolapse.] Helv Chir Acta 1993; 59:707–11.

53. Rogers J, Jeffery PJ. Postnatal repair and intersphincteric Ivalon sponge rectopexy for the treatment of rectal prolapse. Br J Surg 1987; 74:384–6.

54. Bakshi G, Ranka S, Agarwal S, Shetty SV. Modified mesh rectopexy: a study. J Postgrad Med 2000; 46:256–7.

55. Athanasiadis S, Weyand G, Heiligers J, Heumuller L, Barthelmes L. The risk of infection of three synthetic materials used in rectopexy with or without colonic resection for rectal prolapse. Int J Colorectal Dis 1996; 11:42–4.

56. Munro W, Avramovic J, Roney W. Laparoscopic rectopexy. J Laparoendosc Surg 1993; 3:55–8.

57. Berman IR. Sutureless laparoscopic rectopexy for procidentia. Technique and implications. Dis Colon Rectum 1992; 35:689–93.

58. Kwok SP, Carey DP, Lau WY, Li AK. Laparoscopic rectopexy. Dis Colon Rectum 1994; 37:947–8.

59. Cuesta MA, Borgstein PJ, de Jong D, Meijer S. Laparoscopic rectopexy. Surg Laparosc Endosc 1993; 3:456–8.

60. Henry LG, Cattey RP. Rectal prolapse. Surg Laparosc Endosc 1994; 4:357–60.

61. Cuschieri A, Shimi SM, Vander Velpen G, Banting S, Wood RA. Laparoscopic prosthesis fixation rectopexy for complete rectal prolapse. Br J Surg 1994; 81:138–9.

62. Darzi A, Henry MM, Guillou PJ, Shorvon P, Monson JR. Stapled laparoscopic rectopexy for rectal prolapse. Surg Endosc 1995; 9:301–3.

63. Graf W, Stefansson T, Arvidsson D, Pahlman L. Laparoscopic suture rectopexy. Dis Colon Rectum 1995; 38:211–12.

64. Himpens J, Cadiere GB, Bruyns J, Vertruyen M. Laparoscopic rectopexy according to Wells. Surg Endosc 1999; 13:139–41.

65. Heah SM, Hartley JE, Hurley J, Duthie GS, Monson JR. Laparoscopic suture rectopexy without resection is effective treatment for full-thickness rectal prolapse. Dis Colon Rectum 2000; 43:638–43.

66. Kellokumpu IH, Vironen J, Scheinin T. Laparoscopic repair of rectal prolapse: a prospective study evaluating surgical outcome and changes in symptoms and bowel function. Surg Endosc 2000; 14:634–40.

67. Rose J, Schneider C, Scheidbach H et al. Laparoscopic treatment of rectal prolapse: experience gained in a prospective multicenter study. Langenbecks Arch Surg 2002; 387:130–7.

68. Madbouly KM, Senagore AJ, Delaney CP, Duepree HJ, Brady KM, Fazio VW. Clinically based management of rectal prolapse. Surg Endosc 2003; 17:99–103.

69. Boccasanta P, Rosati R, Venturi M et al. Comparison of laparoscopic rectopexy with open technique in the treatment of complete rectal prolapse: clinical and functional results. Surg Laparosc Endosc 1998; 8:460–5.

    A randomised trial between open and laparoscopic rectopexy using polypropylene mesh. The outcomes were the same. The laparoscopic technique was cheaper due to a reduced hospital stay.

70. Ballantyne GH. Laparoscopically assisted anterior resection for rectal prolapse. Surg Laparosc Endosc 1992; 2:230–6.

71. Senagore AJ, Luchtefeld MA, MacKeigan JM. Rectopexy. J Laparoendosc Surg 1993; 3:339–43.

72. Reissman P, Weiss E, Teoh TA, Cohen SM, Wexner SD. Laparoscopic-assisted perineal rectosigmoidectomy for rectal prolapse. Surg Laparosc Endosc 1995; 5:217–18.

73. Ratelle R, Vollant S, Peloquin AB, Gravel D. Abdominal rectopexy (Orr–Loygue) in rectal prolapse: celioscopic approach or conventional surgery? Ann Chir 1994; 48:679–84.

74. Baker R, Senagore AJ, Luchtefeld MA. Laparoscopic-assisted vs. open resection. Rectopexy offers excellent results. Dis Colon Rectum 1995; 38:199–201.

75. Stevenson AR, Stitz RW, Lumley JW. Laparoscopic-assisted resection-rectopexy for rectal prolapse: early and median follow-up. Dis Colon Rectum 1998; 41:46–54.

76. Kessler H, Jerby BL, Milsom JW. Successful treatment of rectal prolapse by laparoscopic suture rectopexy. Surg Endosc 1999; 13:858–61.

77. Xynos E, Chrysos E, Tsiaoussis J, Epanomeritakis E, Vassilakis JS. Resection rectopexy for rectal prolapse. The laparoscopic approach. Surg Endosc 1999; 13:862–4.

78. Kairaluoma MV, Viljakka MT, Kellokumpu IH. Open vs. laparoscopic surgery for rectal prolapse. A case–controlled study assessing short term outcome. Dis Colon Rectum 2003; 46:353–60.

79. Zittel TT, Manncke K, Haug S et al. Functional results after laparoscopic rectopexy for rectal prolapse. J Gastrointest Surg 2000; 4:632–41.

80. Solomon MJ, Young CJ, Eyers AA, Roberts RA. Randomised clinical trial of laparoscopic versus open abdominal rectopexy for rectal prolapse. Br J Surg 2002; 89:35–9.

    A randomised trial of laparoscopic vs. open mesh rectopexy. The recovery after laparoscopic technique was improved with no long-term adverse effects.

81. Uhlig BE, Sullivan ES. The modified Delorme operation. Dis Colon Rectum 1979; 22:513–21.

82. Delorme E. On the treatment of total prolapse of the rectum by excision of the rectal mucous membranes. Bull Mem Soc Chir Paris 1900; 26:499–518.

83. Christiansen J, Kirkgaard P. Delorme's operation for complete rectal prolapse. Br J Surg 1981; 68:537–8.

84. Gunderson AL, Cogbill TH, Landercasper J. Reappraisal of Delorme's procedure for rectal prolapse. Dis Colon Rectum 1985; 28:721–4.

85. Houry S, Lechaux JP, Huguier M, Molkhou JM. Treatment of rectal prolapse by Delorme's operation. Int J Colorectal Dis 1987; 2:149–52.

86. Monson JRT, Jones NAG, Vowden P, Brennan TG. Delorme's operation: the first choice in complete rectal prolapse. Ann R Coll Surg Engl 1986; 68:143–6.

87. Heaton ND, Rennie JA. Extended abdominal rectopexy. Br J Surg 1988; 75:828.

88. Abulafi AM, Sherman IW, Fiddian RV, Rothwell-Jackson RL. Delorme's operation for rectal prolapse. Ann R Coll Surg Engl 1990; 72:382–5.

89. Graf W, Ejerblad S, Krog M, Pahlman L, Gerdin B. Delorme's operation for rectal prolapse in elderly or unfit patients. Eur J Surg 1992; 158:555–7.

90. Tobin SA, Scott IH. Delorme operation for rectal prolapse. Br J Surg 1994; 81:1681–4.

91. Oliver GC, Vachon D, Eisenstat TE, Rubin RJ, Salvati EP. Delorme's procedure for complete rectal

prolapse in severely debilitated patients. Dis Colon Rectum 1994; 37:461–7.

92. Lechaux JP, Lechaux D, Perez M. Results of Delorme's procedure for rectal prolapse. Advantages of a modified technique. Dis Colon Rectum 1995; 38:301–7.

93. Plusa SM, Charig JA, Balaji V, Watts A, Thompson MR. Physiological changes after Delorme's procedure for full-thickness rectal prolapse. Br J Surg 1995; 82:1475–8.

94. Pescatori M, Interisano A, Stolfi VM, Zoffoli M. Delormes operation and sphincteroplasty for rectal prolapse and fecal incontinence. Int J Colorectal Dis 1998; 13:223–7.

95. Watts AMI, Thompson MR. Evaluation of the Delorme's procedure as a treatment for full thickness rectal prolapse. Br J Surg 2000; 87:218–22.

96. Watkins BP, Landercasper J, Belzer E et al. Long term follow-up of the modified Delorme procedure for rectal prolapse. Arch Surg 2003; 138:498–503.

97. Tsunoda A, Yaduda N, Yokoyama N, Kamiyama G, Kusano M. Delorme's procedure for rectal prolapse: clinical and physiological analysis. Dis Colon Rectum 2003; 46:1260–5.

98. Miles WE. Rectosigmoidectomy as a method of treatment for procedentia recti. Proc R Soc Med 1933; 1445–52.

99. Prasad ML, Pearl RK, Abcarian H, Orsay CP, Nelson RL. Perineal proctectomy, posterior rectopexy and postanal levator repair for the treatment of rectal prolapse. Dis Colon Rectum 1986; 29:547–52.

100. Thorne MC, Polglase AL. Perineal proctectomy for rectal prolapse in elderly and debilitated patients. Aust NZ J Surg 1992; 62:791–4.

101. Williams JG, Rothenberger DA, Madoff RD, Goldberg SM. Treatment of rectal prolapse in the elderly by perineal rectosigmoidectomy. Dis Colon Rectum 1992; 35:830–4.

102. Johansen OB, Wexner SD, Daniel N, Nogueras JJ, Jagelman DG. Perineal rectosigmoidectomy in the elderly. Dis Colon Rectum 1993; 36:767–72.

103. Ramanujam PS, Venkatesh KS, Fietz MJ. Perineal excision of rectal procidentia in elderly high-risk patients. A ten-year experience. Dis Colon Rectum 1994; 37:1027–30.

104. Kimmins MH, Evetts BK, Isler J, Billingham R. The Altemeier repair: outpatient treatment of rectal prolapse. Dis Colon Rectum 2001; 44:565–70.

105. Vermeulen FD, Nivatongs S, Fang DT, Balcos EG, Goldberg SM. A technique for perineal rectosigmoidectomy using autosuture devices. Surg Gynecol Obstet 1983; 156:85–6.

106. Hida J, Yasutomi M, Maruyama T et al. Coloanal anastomosis using a circular stapling device follow-ing perineal rectosigmoidectomy for rectal prolapse. Surg Today 1999; 29:93–4.

107. Schutz G. Extracorporal resection of the rectum in the treatment of complete rectal prolapse using a circular stapling device. Dig Surg 2001; 18:274–7; discussion 277–8.

108. Reissman P, Weiss E, Teoh TA, Cohen SM, Wexner SDS. Laparoscopic-assisted perineal rectosigmoidectomy for rectal prolapse. Surg Laparosc Endosc 1995; 5:217–18.

109. Allam M, Piskun G, Fogler R. Laparoscopic-assisted abdominoperineal proctosigmoidectomy for rectal prolapse. A new technique. Surg Endosc 1997; 11:150–1.

110. Farouk R, Duthie GS. The evaluation and treatment of patients with rectal prolapse. Ann Chir Gynaecol 1997; 86:279–84.

111. Roig JV, Buch E, Alos R et al. Anorectal function in patients with complete rectal prolapse. Differences between continent and incontinent individuals. Rev Esp Enferm Dig Nove 1998; 90:794–805.

112. Farouk R, Duthie GS, Bartolo DC, MacGregor AB. Restoration of continence following rectopexy for rectal prolapse and recovery of the internal anal sphincter electromyogram. Br J Surg 1992; 79:439–40.

113. Aitola PT, Hiltunen KM, Matikainen MJ. Functional results of operative treatment of rectal prolapse over an 11-year period: emphasis on transabdominal approach. Dis Colon Rectum 1999; 42:655–60.

114. Holmstrom B, Broden G, Dolk A, Frenckner B. Increased resting anal pressure following the Ripstein operation. Dis Colon Rectum 1986; 29:485–7.

115. Broden G, Dolk A, Holmstrom B. Recovery of the internal anal sphincter following rectopexy: a possible explanation for continence improvement. Int J Colorectal Dis 1988; 3:23–8.

116. Schultz I, Mellgren A, Dolk A, Johansson C, Holmstrom B. Continence is improved after the Ripstein rectopexy. Different mechanisms in rectal prolapse. Dis Colon Rectum 1996; 39:300–6.

117. Yoshioka K, Hyland G, Keighley MR. Anorectal function after abdominal rectopexy: parameters of predictive value in identifying return of continence. Br J Surg 1989; 76:64–8.

118. Schultz I, Mellgren A, Nilsson BY, Dolk A, Holmstrom B. Preoperative electrophysiologic assessment cannot predict continence after rectopexy. Dis Colon Rectum 1998; 41:1392–8.

119. Keighley MR, Makuria T, Alexander-Williams J, Arabi Y. Clinical and manometric evaluation of rectal prolapse and incontinence. Br J Surg 1980; 67:54–6.

120. Seti Carraro P, Nicholls RJ. Postanal repair for faecal incontinence persisting after rectopexy. Br J Surg 1994; 81:305–7.

121. Hamalainen KJ, Raivio P, Antila S, Palmu A, Mecklin JP. Biofeedback therapy in rectal prolapse patients. Dis Colon Rectum 1996; 39:262–5.

122. Kang YS, Kamm MA, Nicholls RJ. Solitary rectal ulcer and complete rectal prolapse: one condition or two? Int J Colorectal Dis 1995; 10:87–90.

123. Nicholls RJ, Simson JNL. Anteroposterior rectopexy in the treatment of solitary rectal ulcer syndrome without overt rectal prolapse. Br J Surg 1986; 73:222–4.

124. Nicholls RJ. Rectal prolapse and the solitary ulcer syndrome. In: Kamm MA, Lennard-Jones JE (eds) Constipation. Peterfield, UK: Wrightson Biomedical, 1994; pp. 289–97.

125. Felt-Bersma RJ, Cuesta MA. Rectal prolapse, rectal intussusception, rectocele, and solitary rectal ulcer syndrome. Gastroenterol Clin North Am 2001; 30:199–222.

126. McCue JL, Thomson JPS. Rectopexy for internal intussusception. Br J Surg 1990; 70:632–4.

127. Halligan S, Nicholls RJ, Bartram CI. Proctographic changes after rectopexy for solitary ulcer syndrome and preoperative predictive factors for a successful outcome. Br J Surg 1995; 82:314–17.

128. Sitzler PJ, Kamm MA, Nicholls RJ, McKee RF. Long-term clinical outcome of surgery for solitary rectal ulcer syndrome. Br J Surg 1998; 85:1246–50.

129. Mellgren A, Schultz I, Johansson C, Dolk A. Internal rectal intussusception seldom develops into total rectal prolapse. Dis Colon Rectum 1997; 40:817–20.

130. Harris PR, Figueroa R. Rectal prolapse in children associated with Clostridium difficile infection. Pediatr Infect Dis J 1995; 14:78–80.

131. Siafakas C, Vottler TP, Andersen JM. Rectal prolapse in pediatrics. Clin Pediatr 1999; 38:63–72.

132. Chan WK, Kay SM, Laberge JM, Gallucci JG, Bensoussan AL, Yazbeck S. Injection sclerotherapy in the treatment of rectal prolapse in infants and children. J Pediatr Surg 1998; 33:255–8.

133. Schepens MA, Verhelst AA. Reappraisal of Ekehorn's rectopexy in the management of rectal prolapse in children. J Pediatr Surg 1993; 28:1494–7.

134. Sander S, Vural O, Unal M. Management of rectal prolapse in children: Ekehorn's rectosacropexy. Pediatr Surg Int 1999; 15:111–14.

135. Chaloner EJ, Duckett J, Lewin J. Paediatric rectal prolapse in Rwanda. J R Soc Med 1996; 89:688–9.

136. Tsugawa C, Matsumoto Y, Nishijima E, Muraji T, Higashimoto Y. Posterior plication of the rectum for rectal prolapse in children. J Pediatr Surg 1995; 30:692–3.

137. Lasheen AE. Closed rectosacropexy for rectal prolapse in children. Surg Today 2003; 33:642–4.

138. Yamazaki T, Sakai Y, Sekine Y, Nihei K, Hatakeyama K. Sigmoid colon cancer presenting as complete rectal prolapse: report of a case. Surg Today 1999; 29:266–7.

139. Rashid Z, Basson MD. Association of rectal prolapse with colorectal cancer. Surgery 1996; 119:51–5.

140. Fengler SA, Pearl RK, Prasad ML et al. Management of recurrent rectal prolapse. Dis Colon Rectum 1997; 40:832–4.

141. Hool GR, Hull TL, Fazio VW. Surgical treatment of recurrent complete rectal prolapse: a thirty-year experience. Dis Colon Rectum 1997; 40:270–2.

142. Araki Y, Isomoto H, Tsuzi Y et al. Transsacral rectopexy for recurrent complete rectal prolapse. Surg Today 1999; 29:970–2.

143. Pikarsky AJ, Joo JS, Wexner SD et al. Recurrent rectal prolapse: what is the next good option? Dis Colon Rectum 2000; 43:1273–6.

144. Berman IR. Different strokes for different folks in repair of rectal prolapse. Dis Colon Rectum 1995; 38:330.

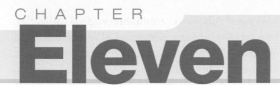

CHAPTER Eleven
Incontinence

Paul Durdey

INTRODUCTION

Faecal incontinence is socially disabling. The true incidence in the general population is grossly underestimated but may be up to 1–2%. This is largely due to embarrassment, with patients maybe unwilling to discuss the problem with their family or their doctor. Urinary incontinence appears to carry less of a social stigma, with women in particular more willing to discuss their problems. Awareness is improving among both patients and the medical profession, and therefore the number of patients who seek treatment for this condition is likely to increase in the future. Faecal incontinence is more common in women and the peak incidence occurs in the elderly.

AETIOLOGY

The aetiology of faecal incontinence is multi-factorial. The ability to retain faeces within the rectum depends on a number of factors, including stool consistency, the capacity and compliance of the rectum, a normal rectoanal inhibitory reflex, normal internal and external sphincter function and normal sensation in the anal canal. Failure in any component can lead to incontinence. The major aetiological factors in faecal incontinence are listed in **Box 11.1**. The majority of patients with the condition who present in surgical practice have an

Box 11.1 • Aetiology of faecal incontinence

Trauma

- Obstetric
- Surgical
- Accidental/war injury

Colorectal disease

- Haemorrhoids
- Rectal prolapse
- Inflammatory bowel disease
- Tumours

Congenital

- Spina bifida
- Operations for imperforate anus
- Hirschsprung's disease

Neurological

- Cerebral
- Spinal
- Peripheral

Miscellaneous

- Behavioural
- Impaction
- Encopresis

obstetric injury, damage to the pudendal nerves (neuropathic or idiopathic faecal incontinence) or iatrogenic injuries due to previous injudicious anal surgery: iatrogenic incontinence following anal surgery is underestimated. Surgery for fistula in ano accounts for the majority of cases. Patients likely to present with incontinence after fistula surgery are those treated for high fistulas or individuals who have undergone multiple operations for recurrent or persistent fistula. A surprising number of patients after haemorrhoidectomy present with minor degrees of soiling. This may be due to loss of the normal anal cushions associated with a degree of sensory impairment in the anal canal. The majority of these patients do not require surgical intervention.

Treatment for anal fissure has been associated with faecal incontinence. Manual dilatation of the anus, which was a popular treatment for a variety of anorectal conditions, can lead to incontinence in up to 20% of patients.[1] The more recent procedure of sphincterotomy has a much lower incidence of incontinence postoperatively; however, this is argued to be the case only if the sphincterotomy is performed in the lateral position and not through the base of the fissure. The latter procedure is claimed to be worse through formation of a keyhole deformity.

Minor degrees of incontinence can follow rectal resection such as low anterior resection and coloanal anastomoses. The aetiology of this is probably twofold. First, there is a reduction in the reservoir capacity of the neorectum, which can be addressed by the formation of a small J-shaped colonic pouch. The second factor probably relates to interference with the intramural nerve pathways to the internal anal sphincter.

Traumatic damage to the perineum can result from accidental injuries such as impalement or from acts of aggression, for example war injury or gunshot wounds. Occasionally, socially acquired injuries will present to the surgeon. The majority of patients who present with severe sphincter injury are those who suffer major pelvic trauma following road traffic accidents. These injuries are often associated with damage to the urinary tract.

The vast majority of patients who present to the surgeon with faecal incontinence are women who have suffered an obstetric injury. Many women presenting with faecal incontinence give a history of prolonged labour or traumatic vaginal deliveries. In a series of studies, Snooks et al.[2,3] demonstrated objective damage to the anal sphincter mechanism in women who had undergone a vaginal delivery, including a fall in resting and squeeze pressures associated with increase in perineal descent and prolonged pudendal nerve terminal motor latencies. Although many of these parameters improved by 6 months after delivery, patients who had undergone a forceps delivery developed a persistent conduction defect of the pudendal nerves.

The risk of faecal incontinence increases with the number of vaginal deliveries, delivery of large babies, prolonged second stage of labour and use of forceps. Severe injuries to the perineum, such as a third-degree tear, can lead to immediate problems with continence. A third-degree tear occurs in 0.5–2% of vaginal deliveries, and although obvious disruption of the sphincter mechanism sustained in a tear is usually repaired immediately by the obstetrician, there is evidence that many women (up to 85%) following such a repair have a persistent defect of the sphincter that can be defined on anal endosonography. Many of these women remain symptomatic.[4,5] Occult sphincter injuries may occur in up to one-third of women who undergo vaginal delivery[6] and in up to 80% following forceps delivery.[4]

In elderly women who present with faecal incontinence the precise aetiology is often unclear. In many cases there is a history of multiparity and prolonged or difficult vaginal delivery. Histochemical analysis of the pelvic floor muscles demonstrates abnormalities compatible with neuropathic damage to the sphincter with subsequent reinnervation. These changes can be seen in the external anal sphincter, puborectalis and levator ani.[7,8] The changes of denervation and reinnervation can be confirmed by electromyography of the pelvic floor striated muscles.

Pudendal neuropathy is present in the majority of patients with idiopathic faecal incontinence.[9–11] Damage to the pudendal nerves leads to low squeeze pressures in the anal canal, evidence of delayed pudendal nerve terminal motor latency, an increase in mean fibre density and decreased anal canal sensation. Further damage to the pudendal nerves may result from chronic straining and perineal descent.

Abnormal descent of the perineum was first described by Parks et al. in 1966.[12] The anorectal junction normally lies above a line drawn between the lower margin of the symphysis pubis and the tip of the coccyx defined on a lateral pelvic radiograph. In patients with the descending perineum syndrome the anorectal junction lies below this and on straining there is further descent of the perineum. Perineal descent also appears to be related to the number of vaginal deliveries and in itself may lead to further trauma to the pudendal nerves. However, the precise relationship between perineal descent and neuropathic damage to the pelvic floor is unclear and recent studies have failed to demonstrate a direct link.[13] It would therefore appear that the majority of cases of faecal incontinence secondary to obstetric damage are due to a combination of traumatic injury to the pelvic floor during delivery associated with trauma to its nerve supply.

sensation demonstrate seepage of faeces due to sensory inattention. Specific features in the history may point to the underlying aetiology. Data from our unit in Bristol have suggested that patients in whom the primary presenting complaint is one of urgency of defecation – in other words they are aware of the need to defecate but are unable to retain stool for more than a few moments – will have deficiency of external anal sphincter function.[14] However, a history of coexisting urinary incontinence would suggest a neuropathic aetiology. Many older patients who present with neurogenic incontinence give a history of insensible faecal loss.

A general history should be taken with particular reference to anorectal surgery or trauma. Specifically, the patient should be asked about any neurological problems and a careful obstetric history is essential. In order to quantify the degree of incontinence it is helpful to use some type of standardised scoring system, of which there are many. My personal preference is the Cleveland Clinic scoring system[15] (Table 11.1).

PRESENTATION

History

It is essential to take an accurate history from patients who present with faecal incontinence. Frequency and severity of incontinence should be documented. It is important to know whether the patient is incontinent to liquids, solids, flatus or all three. Often the history will give some indication as to whether the problem lies primarily within the rectum or sphincter apparatus. A proportion of patients with abnormalities purely of anal canal

Examination

A full examination of the patient's abdomen should be undertaken and neurological assessment made. On inspection of the perineum the patient should be asked to strain in order to assess perineal descent and also to exclude rectal prolapse. The perianal area should be inspected for evidence of previous surgery or the presence of minor anorectal conditions. The anus itself should be assessed at rest to see whether it is closed or patulous.

Table 11.1 • Cleveland Clinic scoring system for assessment of faecal incontinence

	Never	Rarely	Sometimes	Usually	Always
Solids	0	1	2	3	4
Liquids	0	1	2	3	4
Flatus	0	1	2	3	4
Use of pad	0	1	2	3	4
Lifestyle alteration	0	1	2	3	4

Definitions
Rarely: less than once a month. Sometimes: more than once a month but less than once a week. Usually: more than once a week but less than once a day. Always: more than once a day.

Digital rectal examination can provide some information. An assessment can be made of resting anal tone, although the correlation between clinical examination and physiological evaluation is controversial. The patient should be asked to contract the external anal sphincter voluntarily. It is possible to assess movement of the external sphincter and puborectalis separately. Patients who have a deficiency in the anterior part of the sphincter can be recognised. An assessment should be made for the presence or absence of a rectocele, and proctoscopy and sigmoidoscopy are mandatory to exclude other significant pathology.

Special investigations

Physiological assessment of the anorectum has been comprehensively addressed in Chapter 1. My practice is to assess all patients who present with symptomatic incontinence in the anorectal physiology laboratory. The tests that are performed routinely include three-dimensional manometry examining resting and squeeze pressures. This method allows a pressure profile of the anal sphincter mechanism to be constructed, which is particularly useful when searching for defects in the sphincter mechanism and can be correlated with the anatomical appearances on anorectal ultrasound. Assessment of the sphincters by endoanal ultrasound is an extremely useful method of identifying specific anatomic defects in the internal and external anal sphincter and for monitoring the results of surgery. Patients also undergo assessment of anal mucosal electrosensitivity, pudendal nerve latency and rectal compliance. Not all patients require assessment by measurement of mean fibre density or neuromuscular jitter, but the latter has been found to be helpful in our unit in identifying those patients with neurogenic incontinence who are likely to benefit least from surgical intervention.

It is not my practice to perform invasive electromyography on every patient; future developments in improving acquisition of data from surface electrodes may obviate the need for such techniques. We also do not routinely use defecography in the assessment of faecally incontinent patients unless an overt rectal prolapse that is not apparent clinically or an intrarectal intussusception is suspected.

TREATMENT OF FAECAL INCONTINENCE

The treatment of faecal incontinence depends on its aetiology. Minor degrees of perianal soiling may require nothing more than careful perianal hygiene, but for patients with established and troublesome faecal incontinence the choice lies between conservative measures or surgical repair of the sphincter apparatus. The majority of patients who have a specific sphincter defect following obstetric or direct injury identified by three-dimensional manometry or endoanal ultrasound are best served by surgical repair. However, those in whom the incontinence is thought to be neurological in origin may benefit from a conservative approach, at least initially.

Conservative treatment

There is a proportion of patients in whom incontinence is related to fluidity of the bowel action. These patients may be continent if their stool remains solid. In such patients it is appropriate to try antidiarrhoeal medication and sometimes even bulking agents in order to improve stool consistency. A simple regimen of bulking agents and loperamide may succeed in controlling diarrhoea and avoid the necessity of invasive treatment, as may an opposite approach of avoiding fibre in the diet.

Similarly, many patients report troublesome faecal leakage after defecation. This can be improved if the rectum can be fully evacuated. Glycerin or bisacodyl suppositories may be helpful, or alternatively the patient may require a daily phosphate enema. Isolated internal sphincter dysfunction may respond to topical application of 10% phenylephrine gel.[16]

Physiotherapy and pelvic floor retraining (biofeedback) can be helpful in a proportion of patients with incontinence. Biofeedback is particularly useful in patients who have primarily a sensory problem in the anal canal leading to insensible loss of faeces. Patients can be trained using either electromyographic or manometric feedback to improve the strength of their anal sphincters and, if coupled with an intrarectal balloon, may improve their rectal sensory awareness. Biofeedback training can be undertaken as an inpatient; however, the best results are often obtained when patients are allowed to take the biofeedback apparatus home and practise for 2–3 months.

Simple pelvic floor exercises, such as those recommended after delivery, can be beneficial in some patients. However, I have found that more specific physiotherapy using either interferential treatment of the pelvic floor and, in particular, trophic stimulation via an anal plug electrode can be extremely successful. The latter technique uses electrical impulses designed to mimic the train of signals along the pudendal nerve. The precise role of electrical stimulation of the pelvic floor is unclear.[17,18] In our hands the results of intensive physiotherapy are almost equivalent to those obtained by postanal repair in patients with neurogenic incontinence. Enthusiasts of biofeedback training have reported improvement in up to 70% of patients.[19] Biofeedback can certainly improve patients with structural defects of the anal sphincter, although long-term results are unclear.[20] There are few randomised trials.[21,22]

 A recent review of published series confirms the benefit of biofeedback.[22]

Surgical treatment

Surgical treatment of faecal incontinence can be divided into procedures designed to repair sphincter defects, such as have occurred after direct injury or obstetric trauma, and plication procedures, where the primary problem appears to be of neurogenic origin. In cases where the sphincter cannot be repaired further or where direct repair of the sphincter has failed, there are various techniques for augmenting or replacing the anal musculature. Such methods include gracilis muscle transposition, placement of a silastic sling around the anus, the use of an artificial anal sphincter, and sacral nerve stimulation.

The choice of operation is largely determined by the preoperative physiological and radiological findings. If the primary problem appears to be a specific sphincter defect identified manometrically or ultrasonographically, then this should be repaired directly. For patients in whom an anterior sphincter deficit is apparent clinically or on investigation, and usually following an obstetric injury, my preference is to perform an anterior sphincter repair with

levatorplasty. Many of these patients will have a degree of coexisting neuropathic damage to the pelvic floor, particularly if they have undergone multiple vaginal deliveries. Such patients are still suitable for an anterior repair.[23]

For patients in whom the primary aetiology appears to be neurogenic and in whom preoperative investigations have failed to reveal a sphincter defect, the choice lies between a postanal repair, anterior repair or total pelvic floor repair.

SPHINCTER REPAIR PROCEDURES

Preoperative preparation

In the early days of sphincter reconstruction many patients routinely underwent a defunctioning stoma. Few surgeons now use a stoma as an adjunct to sphincter repair in the elective case. However, complex sphincter reconstruction may still require protection, for example in a patient with Crohn's disease, for a cloacal defect or when there is an associated anovaginal or rectovaginal fistula.

Many surgeons use full mechanical bowel preparation prior to sphincter repair. My preference is to use two phosphate enemas, one the evening before and one the morning of surgery. The rationale for this is that a failed full mechanical bowel preparation may be worse than no bowel preparation at all, with liquid faeces running over the operation site.

All patients undergoing sphincter repair are routinely administered three perioperative doses of antibiotics, such as cefuroxime and metronidazole.

Anterior sphincter repair and levatorplasty

This is the operation of choice for patients with an anterior injury. Classically, the majority of surgeons in the UK perform this operation with the patient in the lithotomy position. My practice for a number of years has been to use the prone jack-knife position, as used by the majority of surgeons in the USA. The patients are not routinely catheterised.

The intersphincteric plane is approached through a curvilinear incision close to the vaginal introitus and extending laterally around the anal margin. In a small number of women with severe obstetric injuries there may be little skin between the vagina and anal orifice, with mucosa-to-mucosa apposition. In such cases a Z-plasty is required (**Fig. 11.1**). The skin flap is dissected towards the anal margin to

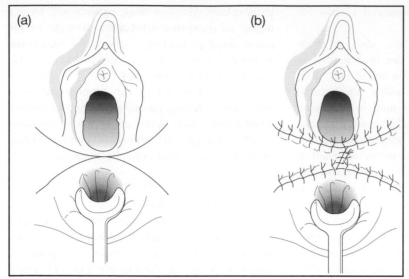

Figure 11.1 • Double Z-plasty for sphincter repair: **(a)** a cruciate incision is made over the perineal body, which is grossly deficient; **(b)** the completed operation with elongation of the skin over the perineal body. From Keighley MRB, Williams NS. Surgery of the anus, rectum and colon. Philadelphia: WB Saunders, 1993, with permission.

expose the fibres of the external sphincter. In severe cases of obstetric injury the external sphincter may be completely divided and replaced by scar tissue.

The intersphincteric plane between internal and external sphincter is dissected. This is a relatively avascular plane. The anterior border of the external sphincter is identified by sharp dissection close to the vaginal wall. The external sphincter may be tethered by surrounding fibrosis. This dissection can be technically demanding. By dissecting laterally, normal external anal sphincter is identified. Great care must be taken in not extending the exploration too far laterally as there is a danger of damaging the neurovascular bundles to the external sphincter, which may result in a poor postoperative result.

Once the external sphincter has been mobilised from surrounding fibrosis, it is retracted caudally and dissection continued in the rectovaginal septum. The septum, particularly in young women, can be vascular and troublesome bleeding may be encountered. Great care must be taken not to enter the rectum. The vagina is carefully separated through its entire length from the anterior rectal wall. The levator muscles can then be identified in the base of the wound running anteriorly and superiorly.

An anterior levatorplasty is performed by suturing together the two sides of the levator using two or three interrupted sutures (**Fig. 11.2**). Many authorities prefer to use a non-absorbable suture such as prolene for this; however, my preference is to use 2/0 PDS (polydioxanone suture; Ethicon

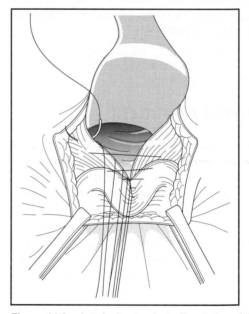

Figure 11.2 • Anterior levatorplasty. By rotation of the anterior retractor the anterior fibres of the puborectalis can be identified and then plicated so as to oppose the pelvic floor in the midline anteriorly. From Keighley MRB, Williams NS. Surgery of the anus, rectum and colon. Philadelphia: WB Saunders, 1993, with permission.

Limited UK). If the external sphincter has been completely divided and continuity maintained by scar tissue, the external sphincter is divided through the scar tissue. An overlapping repair is performed (**Fig. 11.3**) using two layers of horizontal mattress

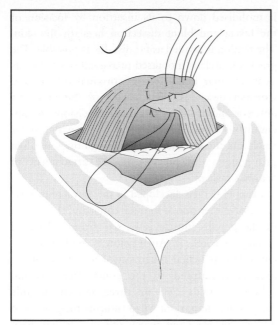

Figure 11.3 • A two-layer flap-over repair is formed. From Keighley MRB, Williams NS. Surgery of the anus, rectum and colon. Philadelphia: WB Saunders, 1993, with permission.

sutures of 2/0 PDS. For each layer all the sutures should be placed prior to tying them. Some surgeons prefer not to overlap the muscle but perform an end-to-end apposition. Results appear similar.

Obstetric injuries are often associated with damage to the perineal body and distal rectovaginal septum, but attempts to correct these defects by imbrication of the rectal wall above the sphincter and internal sphincter imbrication appear to confer little benefit over simple overlapping repair of the external anal sphincter, and they are associated with more complications.[24]

It is often the case that after anterior sphincter repair and levatorplasty the skin wound, which was semicircular, has now become almost longitudinal. The skin is closed using an absorbable suture such as Vicryl. A small defect is left in the wound to facilitate drainage of any haematoma.

Postoperatively, some surgeons place the patient on fluids only and constipating agents for 48–72 hours, whereas others use laxatives and a normal diet and encourage early defecation.

Recent evidence suggests that bowel confinement may be unnecessary.[25]

In our unit, postoperative physiotherapy after wound healing at approximately 6–8 weeks using trophic stimulation has been found to be a useful adjunct to all types of sphincter repair.

A similar technique is used for patients in whom a traumatic injury to the external sphincter apparatus has been sustained. Having identified the site of injury, the tissues are dissected back to healthy muscle. The sphincter is divided through the scar tissue and an overlapping repair performed. Often the wound is left open to granulate.

Postanal repair

Postanal repair was developed in 1975 by Parks.[26] The operation was devised to restore the normal anorectal angle, which Parks had discovered was obtuse in many patients with idiopathic faecal incontinence. Parks concluded that the puborectalis muscle was responsible for maintaining this angle and postanal repair was designed to restore the normal anatomy. It is my view that this procedure is now indicated in very few patients.

Total pelvic floor repair

The operation of total pelvic floor repair was devised in response to disappointing long-term results following postanal repair for neurogenic incontinence, and in response to the fact that many such patients have anatomical defects such as rectocele and abnormal perineal descent.[27] It combines postanal repair with anterior sphincter plication and levatorplasty. The postanal repair is performed first using a standard technique including suture of ischiococcygeus and iliococcygeus. An anterior perineal incision is then made and an anterior levatorplasty and plication of the anterior sphincter performed. The skin wounds are closed and suction drains placed into both spaces. Postoperative management is similar to that described above for anterior sphincter repair. In our unit, postoperative physiotherapy commences 6–8 weeks after the operation as a routine. This procedure has not been widely adopted and its use in the future will decline.

The question of whether to plicate the internal anal sphincter is conjectural, evidence from a recent randomised trial suggesting that it adds nothing to a standard pelvic floor repair.[28]

Isolated injuries to the internal anal sphincter can be treated by injection of silicone. Results are variable and appear short term.

Plication procedures

Simple reefing procedures for the anal sphincter have been described in the literature for over 100 years. However, in my opinion the role for simple reefing of the external sphincter is limited. Occasionally, in patients who appear to have an anterior deficit secondary to obstetric trauma, the external sphincter is not divided but merely thinned, sitting loosely around the anal canal. Simple plication without division of the muscle can be combined with a formal reconstruction of the perineal body via levatorplasty. I think there are few indications for simple reefing of the external sphincter posteriorly, but there are isolated cases of unexplained male incontinence where the procedure can be surprisingly effective.

SPHINCTER AUGMENTATION PROCEDURES

In a minority of patients direct sphincter repair is not possible due to insufficient residual sphincter, major neurological deficit or previous failed repairs. In such patients, consideration should be given to some form of sphincter augmentation. Various muscles have been used, including gluteus maximus, sartorius, adductor longus and, most commonly, gracilis.

Gracilis muscle transposition

The gracilis muscle has been used for anal sphincter supplementation since 1952; however, it was Corman[29] in 1978 who popularised the technique. However, Corman stressed that this approach should be used only for young patients and only under limited circumstances. The advantage of the gracilis muscle is that it is the most superficial muscle in the medial aspect of the thigh. It is approximately the right size and the blood and nerve supply enter proximally. Thus distal division of the muscle does not necessarily compromise the blood supply.

The technique of gracilis transposition is best carried out with the patient in the Lloyd-Davies position, which allows access to the medial aspect of the thigh over which three incisions are recommended in order to mobilise and divide the distal tendon of the gracilis (**Fig. 11.4**). The muscle is mobilised down to its insertion by incision of the fascia and blunt dissection beneath the skin. The tendon is divided as far distally as possible. The gracilis muscle is mobilised proximally as far as its neurovascular bundle. In his original description, Corman describes encirclement of the anus via anterior and posterior circumanal incisions. A subcutaneous tunnel is developed between the upper thigh and the perianal area, although this can often prove quite difficult due to the attachment of Scarpa's fascia.

A tunnel is then developed in the extrasphincteric space on either side of the anal canal and the tendon of the gracilis muscle is passed around the anal canal to encircle it. An incision is made over the contralateral ischial tuberosity. The tendon of the gracilis is sutured to the contralateral ischial tuberosity with two or three non-absorbable sutures. It is important when suturing the gracilis to adduct the leg from which the muscle has been taken in order that the tension can be adjusted accordingly. Postoperatively, it is recommended that the bowels are confined for a period of 1 week.

It is possible to use both gracilis muscles to form a bilateral wrap.

Electrically stimulated gracilis neosphincter

One problem with transposition of muscles around the anal canal is the difference in physiology between the external anal sphincter and other adjacent skeletal muscles. The external sphincter has resting tone and a preponderance of slow twitch fibres. None of the other skeletal muscles used to augment the sphincter has these properties. This led several groups to explore the possibility of electrical stimulation of the gracilis muscle to determine whether this provided a better physiological replacement for the external sphincter.[30–32] The principle of the procedure is to provide continuous electrical stimulation to the gracilis via its nerve supply or directly into the muscle. Stimulation is achieved via an implanted stimulator. This technique has been used not only to augment an existing anal sphincter but also in patients with anorectal agenesis. The method has also been applied to patients who have undergone abdominoperineal excision of the rectum who cannot tolerate a permanent stoma for religious or social reasons. The procedure is contraindicated in patients in whom the gracilis muscle is

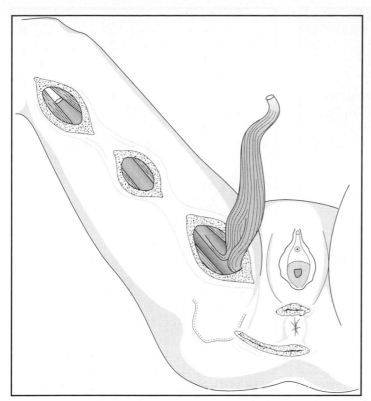

Figure 11.4 • Graciloplasty. A series of thigh incisions is used to identify and mobilise the gracilis muscle. Care is taken not to damage the neurovascular bundle. The tendon's insertion to the medial aspect of the tibia is divided. From Keighley MRB, Williams NS. Surgery of the anus, rectum and colon. Philadelphia: WB Saunders, 1993, with permission.

damaged for any reason or where perineal sepsis is likely to be problematic.

The technique is not suitable for elderly or infirm patients nor for those who cannot manage control of the stimulator. Due to the complexity of the procedure, initial studies included a covering stoma, to be fashioned before embarking on the transposition and sited on the opposite side to the proposed gracilis muscle transfer. However, more recent series have suggested that a stoma is not always necessary, that it may not prevent perineal sepsis and that it has a morbidity of its own.[33,34]

Initial results of this operation were marred by a high incidence of necrosis of the distal half of the gracilis. In the original studies, in order to prevent ischaemic necrosis the first stage of the operation consisted of mobilisation of the distal half of the gracilis. This was performed by a longitudinal incision over the innermost aspect of the thigh. The gracilis was mobilised by division and ligation of small vessels that supply the lateral aspect of the muscle in its distal half. The tendon was not divided and the wound was closed. Again, recent studies

suggest that this prior mobilisation may not be necessary.[33]

Approximately 4–6 weeks after the initial mobilisation the previous incision in the thigh is extended proximally and the tendon of the gracilis muscle traced to its insertion where it is divided. The muscle is then mobilised proximally towards the neurovascular bundle. The main nerve to the gracilis muscle lies above the main vascular pedicle and this is identified using a nerve stimulator. The main branch of the nerve lies on the adductor brevis muscle.

There are two techniques for muscle stimulation. In the procedure devised by Williams et al.,[30] the electrodes are placed directly over the nerve to gracilis. Having identified the nerve, the stimulator and electrodes are attached. The stimulator lies in a pocket overlying the lower ribs. The lead is tunnelled subcutaneously via a small incision in the suprainguinal region and the electrode brought down to the appropriate nerve. The electrode plate is sutured over the main nerve bundle in a longitudinal fashion (**Fig. 11.5**). The electrode plate is

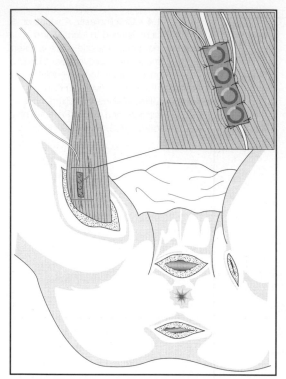
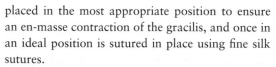

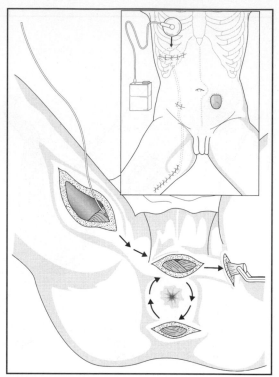

Figure 11.5 • Continuous electrical stimulation of the gracilis. An electrode for electrical stimulation is sutured to the proximal gracilis muscle near the neurovascular bundle. From Keighley MRB, Williams NS. Surgery of the anus, rectum and colon. Philadelphia: WB Saunders, 1993, with permission.

Figure 11.6 • The gracilis muscle is rerouted around the anal canal. Stimulation is triggered by an external pulse generator, which activates a receiving device under the costal margin. From Keighley MRB, Williams NS. Surgery of the anus, rectum and colon. Philadelphia: WB Saunders, 1993, with permission.

placed in the most appropriate position to ensure an en-masse contraction of the gracilis, and once in an ideal position is sutured in place using fine silk sutures.

The alternative technique[31] utilises insertion of electrodes into the gracilis muscle adjacent to the supplying nerve (Medtronic, Minneapolis, USA). This technique has become more widely adopted due to complications associated with applying the electrode directly on to the nerve.

The connection to the stimulator can be assessed using an external telemetry programmer. The gracilis muscle is then transposed around the anal canal in a tunnel in the extrasphincteric plane. Two lateral incisions placed well away from the anal canal are recommended in order to achieve this. It is also recommended that the muscle is taken around the anal canal in a gamma configuration (**Fig. 11.6**) and sutured to the periosteum of the contralateral ischial tuberosity. It is essential that the anal canal

is surrounded by the muscle and not its tendon for optimal function.

Postoperatively, the patient is nursed with legs bandaged loosely together. Electrical stimulation of the muscle commences at day 10, provided the wounds are healed satisfactorily. The stimulator is programmed using a standard training protocol. Once the muscle is trained, the patient can be admitted for closure of the covering stoma. The stimulator can be switched on or off by passing a magnet over it.

Gluteus maximus transposition

In many respects the gluteus maximus muscle is in an ideal position to augment anal sphincter function, and recent reports of this technique have proved encouraging.[35,36] It involves formation of a defunctioning stoma as a preliminary procedure. The patient is positioned in the prone jack-knife position. Two mirror-image cutaneous incisions are

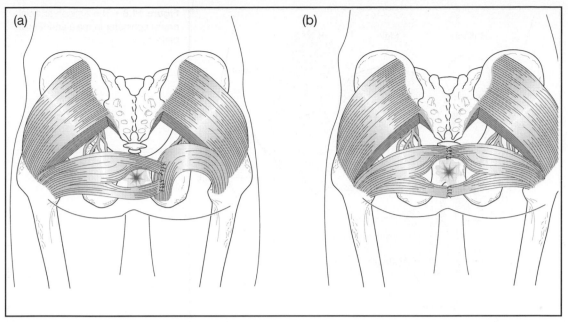

Figure 11.7 • Gluteus maximus transposition: **(a)** reconstruction with one muscle split to attach to the opposite side; **(b)** alternative reconstruction. From Keighley MRB, Williams NS. Surgery of the anus, rectum and colon. Philadelphia: WB Saunders, 1993, with permission.

made on each side from the border of the mid-sacrum towards the acetabulum. The sacrococcygeal origin of the gluteus maximus is detached with its aponeurosis. A 5-cm wide strip of muscle is divided parallel with the fascia up to the point where the neurovascular pedicle enters the deep surface. Blunt dissection of the muscle is continued until it is sufficiently mobilised to allow transposition around the anal orifice. Two lateral incisions are made parallel to the anal margin 2 cm from the anal orifice. The detached inferior halves of the gluteus maximus muscles are then wrapped around the anal canal (**Fig. 11.7**). Various techniques for achieving this have been described. The muscles are usually sutured using PDS. The incisions are drained. It is also possible to use a stimulator for gluteal transposition.[36] This procedure is now uncommon and may become obsolete.

Implants and artificial anal sphincters

DACRON-IMPREGNATED SILASTIC SLING

The use of an artificial sling to encircle the anal canal as an adjunct to continence has gained little popularity in the UK, but in the USA is used more frequently.[37] Two incisions are made 3 cm lateral to either side of the anal verge. The ischiorectal fossae are then entered and a tunnel developed around the anal canal. A 1.5-cm strip of silastic sheet is cut. The strip is placed around the anal canal using two clamps and the adequacy of the anal lumen assessed. Once the position of the mesh is correctly identified, the ends are secured using a 30-mm linear stapler. The suture line can be reinforced with interrupted non-absorbable suture if required.

ARTIFICIAL SPHINCTER FOR FAECAL INCONTINENCE

The artificial bowel sphincter for faecal incontinence (**Fig. 11.8**) has not proved as successful as artificial sphincters for urinary incontinence, although in 1989 Christiansen and Lorentzem reported five cases using an AMS 800 artificial urinary sphincter.[38] The cuff of the sphincter was inserted around the anal canal and the pump placed in the left side of the scrotum or the left labium majus. The pressure-regulating balloon was placed extraperitoneally to the left of the bladder.

A modified artificial bowel sphincter has now been evaluated.[39,40] Indications for use of an artificial

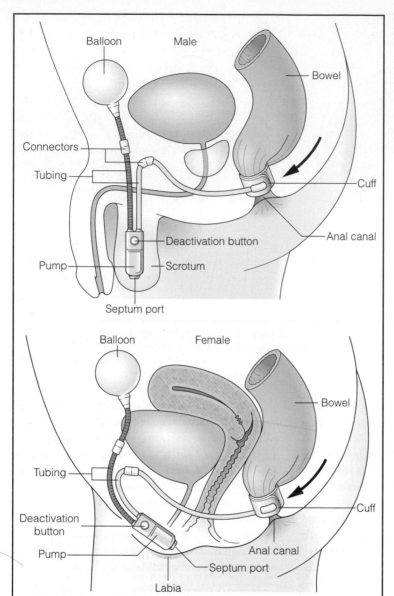

Figure 11.8 • The Acticon artificial bowel sphincter in male and female patients.

bowel sphincter include congenital anorectal abnormalities, traumatic injuries, neurological dysfunction or failure of previous sphincter repair. This device is specifically designed with different-sized cuffs to encircle the anal canal. Similar to the urinary sphincter the device has a reservoir implanted in the abdominal wall with a control pump placed in the scrotum or labium. The occlusive cuff containing a fluid-filled inflatable shell is implanted around a segment of the anal canal using multiple incisions. A tunnel is created around the anal canal by blunt dissection, with care taken to avoid injury to the rectal wall of the vagina. It is important to ensure that the cuff is inserted deeply into the tissues to avoid postoperative skin erosion. The pressure-regulating balloon is implanted in the prevesical space using a Pfannenstiel incision. The control pump is implanted into the soft tissue of the labium or scrotum. The control pump is a soft bulb that the patient squeezes and releases to transfer fluid into or out of the cuff. The technique is associated with considerable morbidity. Results of a multicentre trial suggest that the majority of patients who underwent the procedure had a device-related complication. The commonest complications reported are infection, erosion of the device, malfunction and migration. Over one-third of the patients required explant of the device due to postoperative complications. Data from a multicentre study in the USA revealed that in 1 year two-thirds of patients retained a functioning device. Lessons from the larger studies suggest that a single perianal incision is preferable and that the cuff should be placed at least 3 cm deep at its lower border. Selection of the pressure-regulating balloon appears to be important. It is not considered that a diverting stoma is necessary in the majority of patients.

Alternative procedures

SACRAL NERVE STIMULATION

Sacral nerve stimulation (**Fig. 11.9**) has been used in the treatment of urinary incontinence. A similar technique has been utilised for faecal incontinence with promising initial results.[41,42] An initial trial stimulation is undertaken. A percutaneous wire is inserted under general or local anaesthesia into the second, third or fourth sacral foramen. Successful position is indicated by ballooning of the pelvic

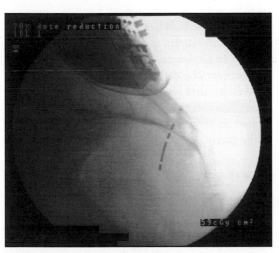

Figure 11.9 • Sacral nerve stimulation: radiograph of a percutaneously introduced tined permanent electrode with implanted stimulator.

floor and flexion of the ipsilateral great toe. The wire is connected to an external stimulator and the results monitored for a period of 2–3 weeks. If successful, a permanent indwelling stimulator can be inserted. A permanent electrode is implanted via an operative approach. More recently, a percutaneous system for introducing the permanent electrode has been developed. The technique appears to benefit patients who have an intact anal sphincter on ultrasound and some preservation of pudendal nerve function. In selected patients, improvement in continence occurs in approximately 70%.[41,42]

ANAL PLUG

One simple technique suggested for control of faecal incontinence is the anal continence plug.[43] This may have a role to play in some patients' treatment.

STOMA FORMATION

When all else fails, consideration should be given to a defunctioning stoma, which can be performed laparoscopically. Generally, an end-colostomy is preferable to a loop. However, if the rectal stump remains, patients can be troubled by incontinence of mucus, and on occasions this will require a formal proctectomy. An alternative procedure is to form a continent colonic conduit in sigmoid or transverse colon to allow antegrade colonic lavage.[44]

RESULTS OF TREATMENT

Direct sphincter repair

Direct repair of the anal sphincter following anorectal trauma or iatrogenic injuries has achieved good results. Browning and Motson[45] reported on 97 patients who had undergone direct sphincter repair, the vast majority of whom were in one of the above two categories. These authors reported a 78% success rate, with patients being rendered completely continent of liquids and solids. (It is noteworthy, though, that the results of the minority of patients in this series with obstetric damage were poor when treated by this approach.) Similar results of direct repair have been obtained by other authors (**Table 11.2**).

Table 11.2 • Results of direct sphincter repair

Reference	N	Patients with complete continence (%)
Manning & Pratt[46]	102	74
Fang et al.[47]	79	58
Corman[48]	28	100
Cterceko et al.[49]	44	54

ANTERIOR SPHINCTER REPAIR

The results for anterior sphincter repair with or without levatorplasty are shown in **Table 11.3**, and overall can be expected to be good in approximately three-quarters of patients. It would appear that the patients who fail to derive benefit from the operation are those in whom there is coexisting pudendal neuropathy.[54,55] A proportion of patients who have poor postoperative function have persistent defects in the anal sphincter, demonstrable on postoperative anal endosonography.[54] It is of note that age in itself does not adversely influence outcome.[53] Physiological changes seen after anterior sphincter repair include restoration of mean resting pressure and increased length of the anal canal. However, the most important improved physiological parameter appears to be an increase in the maximum squeeze pressure.[56] However, not all authors report such a direct correlation between improvement in function and measurable parameters.[54]

On longer term follow-up, initial studies suggested that the success rate is maintained.[57]

Table 11.3 • Results of published series of anterior sphincteroplasty

Reference	N	Good/excellent results (%)
Laurberg et al.[50]	19	47
Yoshioka & Keighley[51]	27	74
Orrom et al.[23]	16	62
Wexner et al.[52]	16	74
Fleshman et al.[53]	28	75
Engel et al.[54]	55	76
Oliveira et al.[55]	55	71

Unfortunately, more recent studies have demonstrated that the long-term success rates of anterior sphincter repair after obstetric trauma may not be maintained. In the long term, only about 40% of patients remain satisfactorily continent.[58,59]

POSTANAL REPAIR

The early results of postanal repair were encouraging (**Table 11.4**). Unfortunately, long-term follow-up of patients has revealed that postoperative function deteriorates over time. A frank appraisal of data from patients who had undergone postanal repair from the Birmingham group demonstrated that 3 years after surgery only 34% were completely continent of liquids, solids and flatus.[60–62]

SUMMARY

Physiological changes after sphincter repair are difficult to document. The Birmingham series of postanal repair reported no significant improvement in resting or squeeze pressures within the anal canal and, significantly, no improvement in the anorectal angle, the parameter which Sir Alan Parks designed the operation to correct. Preoperative physiological factors that correlate with a failure to improve after postanal repair include low resting and squeeze anal canal pressures, severe neuropathy of the pelvic floor, perineal descent and the presence of rectal prolapse. Electrophysiological investigations surprisingly reveal increased neurogenic damage to striated sphincteric muscle after postanal repair, even in some patients whose function improves postoperatively.[63] When patients deteriorate after surgery, a significant increase in neurogenic abnormality can be demonstrated. Thus it would appear that patients who do badly after postanal repair have progressive denervation. Further evidence for this comes from our own studies, which have demonstrated an abnormal degree of neuromuscular jitter in the external anal sphincter of patients who have

Table 11.4 • Results of major series of postanal repair

Reference	N	Good/excellent results (%)
Browning & Parks[60]	140	86
Henry & Simson[61]	129	70
Yoshioka & Keighley[62]	116	57

poor functional results after postanal repair for faecal incontinence. The aetiology of this progressive denervation remains conjectural.

Results from total pelvic floor repair were initially encouraging, with 90% of patients either being fully continent or with improved continence. However, long-term follow-up of a group of 57 patients revealed that only 14% were rendered completely continent and social activity remained compromised in 76%.[64] Careful clinical and physiological evaluation of the pelvic floor can identify patients with a specific sphincter defect in the absence of neuropathic damage, or who have primarily a neuropathic sphincter injury with no obvious anatomical defect, or in whom the injuries are combined.

The optimum treatment we can offer patients at the moment is to repair the sphincter directly by anterior sphincteroplasty, or by overlapping repair of a traumatic sphincter defect in those in whom such a defect is demonstrated. The presence of neuropathic change does not alter the surgical management, but has prognostic significance.

Patients with severe neuropathic incontinence are best treated by intensive conservative management with control of stool consistency. Surgical options are limited. As many of these patients do have an anterior defect on ultrasonography it is often preferable to repair this, possibly with an adjunctive postanal repair as a secondary procedure.

In young patients with severe sphincter injuries or in those in whom previous repairs have failed, consideration should be given to some form of sphincter augmentation. In the elderly with poor prognostic factors, one must be realistic in advising patients what can be achieved. It may be in the patient's best interest not to attempt sphincter reconstruction but rather to offer a permanent colostomy, which may well restore quality of life in the least traumatic way.

Sphincter augmentation

DYNAMIC GRACILOPLASTY

Unstimulated gracilis transposition has proved disappointing in the long term. There have been studies on bilateral unstimulated gracilis muscle transposition; however, the majority of data now available are on the results of the electrically stimulated gracilis neosphincter over the medium to long term.[65]

The technique has evolved, with most authorities now using intramuscular electrodes rather than direct stimulation of the nerve to gracilis. The latter is associated with significantly greater mechanical problems, particularly perineural fibrosis and electrode migration, which require revisional surgery.[33,35]

Results of recent studies including multicentre trials have demonstrated a success rate for graciloplasty of 60–80%. There remains significant morbidity, with approximately one-third of patients developing wound complications.[35,66,67]

ARTIFICIAL BOWEL SPHINCTER

There are few units in this country with extensive experience of the artificial bowel sphincter. There have been two recent reports of large series giving detailed results.[40,67] The procedure is associated with significant complications, as outlined previously. Short-term follow-up would indicate that over two-thirds of patients retain a functioning artificial sphincter, and in these patients the results are good with approximately 80% of patients achieving improvement of incontinence, particularly to solid stool. A longer term study with immediate follow-up of 7 years in a small group of patients would suggest that these results are not maintained, with less than 50% of patients retaining a functioning neosphincter at the end of follow-up, with an overall clinical success rate of 47%.[68]

A report of a multicentre cohort study[69] demonstrated that this procedure is associated with significant complications: 45% of patients required revisional surgery and 37% required removal of the device. In those patients who retained their device, continence was satisfactory in over 80%. A recent systematic review has queried the use of the device due to complications and limited efficacy.[70]

Experience of the anterior bowel sphincter is limited in this country.

Failed sphincter repair

A patient in whom a previous repair has failed can be a dilemma for the treating surgeon. There is evidence that patients in whom previous anterior repairs failed can undergo a repeat sphincter repair, with a good outcome in 50–60% of patients.[71,72]

Patients unsuitable for a repeat sphincter repair could be considered for dynamic graciloplasty, artificial bowel sphincter or sacral nerve stimulation.

Sacral nerve stimulation

Several studies have now reported on the safety and efficacy of sacral nerve stimulation.[41,42,73] A recent review of sacral nerve stimulation for the treatment of faecal incontinence[74] has demonstrated that the trial stimulation is associated with a very low level of complications, and a complication rate of 5–10% for insertion of a permanent implant. Overall, sacral nerve stimulation appears to improve continence in approximately 80% of patients who are permanently implanted. The mechanism of action of sacral nerve stimulation remains unknown. Sacral nerve stimulation is an exciting new therapy for the treatment of faecal incontinence and may supersede many of the more traditional methods and management.

THE FUTURE

Increased awareness among patients and doctors that faecal incontinence can be successfully treated in the majority will lead to an increase in referrals. Similarly, greater awareness of injury at the time of vaginal delivery may improve obstetric practice and obviate the necessity for many of the surgical procedures listed. However, prevention of obstetric trauma altogether is unlikely, although obstetricians are becoming aware of the need to recognise injuries at the time of delivery and of the requirement that these injuries be repaired by appropriately skilled personnel.

It is well recognised that even a normal vaginal delivery is associated with a degree of damage to the nerve supply to the pelvic floor. There has been considerable interest recently in the field of nerve growth factors. It is possible in the future that use of such growth factors in the immediate postnatal period may optimise the reinnervation process in the pelvic floor. Similarly, newer electrophysiological tests and improvement in endoanal imaging could improve the selection of patients and the overall long-term outlook.

The indications for stimulated neosphincter formation are expanding and the number of patients suitable for this procedure will undoubtedly increase. The use of the artificial bowel sphincter remains controversial. Its use in the future is speculative. Sacral nerve stimulation is an exciting new procedure that appears to benefit the majority of patients with faecal incontinence, particularly those with neuropathic damage of the pelvic floor. It is likely that the use of sacral nerve stimulation will increase in the future.

• Key points

- Faecal incontinence is a relatively common condition.
- The commonest cause for faecal incontinence in women is obstetric trauma.
- Following careful assessment and investigation, the majority of patients may benefit from conservative treatment.
- The majority of patients with obstetric trauma who have an identified defect on anal ultrasound will benefit from anterior sphincter repair in the short term.
- The long-term results of anterior sphincter repair suggest that only 40% of women will remain fully continent.
- Sphincter augmentation procedures are becoming increasingly used for patients who are not suitable for direct repair or in whom a previous repair has failed.
- Sacral nerve stimulation appears to be a promising innovation in the treatment of faecal incontinence.

REFERENCES

1. MacIntyre IMC, Balfour TW. Results of the Lord non-operative treatment for haemorrhoids. Lancet 1977; i:1094.

2. Snooks SJ, Swash M, Henry MM, Setchell MM. Risk factors in childbirth causing damage to the pelvic floor innervation. Int J Colorectal Dis 1986; 1:20–4.

3. Snooks SJ, Swash M, Mathers SE, Henry MM. Effect of vaginal delivery on the pelvic floor: a 5 year follow-up. Br J Surg 1990; 77:1358–60.

4. Sultan AH, Kamm MA, Bartram CI, Hudson CN. Third degree obstetric anal sphincter tears: risk factors and outcome of primary repair. Br Med J 1994; 308:887–91.

5. Gjessing H, Backe B, Sahlin Y. Third degree obstetric tears: outcome after primary repair. Acta Obstet Gynaecol Scand 1998; 77:736–40.

6. Cook TA, Mortensen NJ. Management of faecal incontinence following obstetric injury. Br J Surg 1998; 85:293–9.

7. Perry RE, Blatchford GJ, Christensen MA et al. Manometric diagnosis of anal sphincter injuries. Am J Surg 1990; 159:112.

8. Parks AG, Swash M. Denervation of the anal sphincter causing idiopathic anorectal incontinence. J R Coll Surg Edinb 1979; 24:94–6.

9. Neill ME, Parks AG, Swash M. Physiological studies of the pelvic floor in idiopathic faecal incontinence and rectal prolapse. Br J Surg 1981; 68:531–6.

10. Kiff ES, Swash M. Slowed conduction in the pudendal nerves in idiopathic (neurogenic) faecal incontinence. Br J Surg 1984; 71:614–16.

11. Rogers J, Henry MM, Misiewicz JJ. Combined sensory and motor deficit in primary neuropathic faecal incontinence. Gut 1988; 29:5–9.

12. Parks AG, Porter NH, Hardcastle JD. The syndrome of the descending perineum. Proc R Soc Med 1966; 59:477–82.

13. Jorge JMN, Wexner SD, Ehrenpreis E et al. Does perianal descent correlate with pudendal neuropathy? Dis Colon Rectum 1992; 35:11–12.

14. Gee AS, Durdey P. Urge incontinence of faeces is a mark of severe anal sphincter dysfunction. Br J Surg 1995; 82:1179–82.

15. Jorge JM, Wexner SD. Etiology and management of fecal incontinence. Dis Colon Rectum 1993; 36:77–97.

16. Carapeti EA, Kamm MA, Evans BK, Phillips RKS. Topical phenylephrine increases anal sphincter resting pressure. Br J Surg 1999; 86:267–70.

17. Fynes MM, Marshall K, Cassidy M et al. A prospective randomized study comparing the effect of augmented biofeedback with sensory biofeedback alone on faecal incontinence after obstetric trauma. Dis Colon Rectum 1999; 42:753–61.

18. Osterberg A, Graf W, Eeg-Olofsson K, Hallden M, Pahlman L. Is electrostimulation of the pelvic floor an effective treatment for neurogenic faecal incontinence? Scand J Gastroenterol 1999; 34:319–24.

19. Norton C, Kamm MA. Outcome of biofeedback for incontinence training. Br J Surg 1999; 86:1159–63.

20. Macleod JH. Biofeedback in the management of partial anal incontinence. Dis Colon Rectum 1983; 26:244–6.

21. Heyman S, Jones KR, Ringel Y, Scarlett Y, Whitehead WE. Biofeedback treatment of fecal incontinence. Dis Colon Rectum 2001; 44:728–36.

A review of 35 studies of biofeedback in faecal incontinence. Most studies demonstrate efficacy of biofeedback.

22. Norton C, Chelvanayagam S, Wilson-Barnet J, Refern S, Kamm MA. Randomised controlled trial of biofeedback for fecal incontinence. Gastroenterology 2003; 125:1320–9.

23. Orrom WJ, Miller R, Cornes H et al. Comparison of anterior sphincteroplasty and postanal repair in the treatment of idiopathic fecal incontinence. Dis Colon Rectum 1991; 34:305–10.

24. Briel JW, De Boer LM, Hop CJ, Schouten WR. Clinical outcome of anterior overlapping external anal sphincter repair with internal sphincter imbrication. Dis Colon Rectum 1998; 41:209–14.

25. Nessim A, Wexner SD, Agachan F et al. Is bowel confinement necessary after anorectal reconstructive surgery? A prospective randomized surgeon trial. Dis Colon Rectum 1999; 42:16–23.

This trial has demonstrated that it is unncessary to restrict oral intake following reconstructive surgery of the anorectum.

26. Parks AG. Anorectal incontinence. Proc R Soc Med 1975; 68:681–90.

27. Pinho M, Ortiz J, Oya M et al. Total pelvic floor repair for the treatment of neuropathic fecal incontinence. Am J Surg 1992; 163:340–3.

28. Deen KI, Kumar D, Williams JG et al. Randomised trial of internal anal sphincter plication with pelvic floor repair for neuropathic fecal incontinence. Dis Colon Rectum 1995; 38:14–18.

This trial demonstrated that there is no value in plicating the internal sphincter during pelvic floor repair. In this study, however, the internal sphincter was plicated longitudinally.

29. Corman ML. Gracilis muscle transposition. Contemp Surg 1978; 13:9–16.

30. Williams NS, Patel J, George BD et al. Development of an electrically stimulated neoanal sphincter. Lancet 1991; 338:1166–9.

31. Baeten CGMI, Konsten J, Spaans F et al. Dynamic graciloplasty for treatment of faecal incontinence. Lancet 1991; 338:1163–5.

32. Sielezneff I, Malouf AJ, Bartolo DCC, Pryde A, Douglas S. Dynamic graciloplasty in the treatment of patients with faecal incontinence. Br J Surg 1999; 86:61–5.

33. Navrantonis C, Wexner SD. Stimulated graciloplasty for treatment of intractable fecal incontinence. Dis Colon Rectum 1999; 42:497–504.

34. Cavina E, Seccia M, Evangelista G et al. Perineal colostomy and electrostimulated gracilis neosphincter after abdominoperineal resection of the colon and anorectum: a surgical experience and follow-up study in 47 cases. Int J Colorectal Dis 1990; 5:6–11.

35. Madoff RD, Rosen HR, Baeten CG et al. Safety and efficacy of dynamic muscle plasty for anal incontinence: lessons from a prospective multicenter trial. Gastroenterology 1999; 116:549–56.

36. Devesa JM, Vincente E, Enriquez JM et al. Total fecal incontinence. A new method of gluteus maximus transposition: preliminary results and report of previous experience. Dis Colon Rectum 1992; 35:339–49.

37. Corman ML. The management of anal incontinence. Surg Clin North Am 1983; 63:177–92.

38. Christiansen J, Lorentzem M. Implantation of artificial sphincter for anal incontinence. Report of five cases. Dis Colon Rectum 1989; 32:432–6.

39. Wong WD, Jensen LL, Bartolo DCC, Rotherberger DA. Artificial anal sphincter. Dis Colon Rectum 1996; 39:1345–51.

40. Christiansen J, Rasmussen OO, Lindorf-Larsen K. Long term results of artificial anal sphincter implantation for severe anal incontinence. Ann Surg 1999; 230:45–8.

41. Ganio E, Lue AR, Clerico G, Trumpetts M. Sacral nerve stimulation for treatment of fecal incontinence. A novel approach for intractable fecal incontinence. Dis Colon Rectum 2001; 44:619–31.

42. Matzel KE, Stadelmaier U, Hohenfellner M, Gall FP. Electrical stimulation of sacral spinal nerves for treatment of faecal incontinence. Lancet 1995; 346:1124–7.

43. Mortensen N, Smilgin Humphreys M. The anal continence plug: a disposable device for patients with anorectal incontinence. Lancet 1991; 338:295–7.

44. Hughes SF, Williams NS. Continent conduit for the treatment of faecal incontinence associated with disordered evacuation. Br J Surg 1995; 82:1318–20.

45. Browning GGP, Motson RW. Anal sphincter injury. Management and results of Parks sphincter repair. Ann Surg 1984; 199:351–6.

46. Manning PC, Pratt JH. Faecal incontinence caused by laceration of the perineum. Arch Surg 1964; 88:569–76.

47. Fang DT, Nivatvongs S, Vermeulen FD et al. Overlapping sphincteroplasty for acquired anal incontinence. Dis Colon Rectum 1984; 27:720–2.

48. Corman ML. Anal incontinence following obstetric injury. Dis Colon Rectum 1985; 28:86–9.

49. Cterceko GC, Fazio VW, Jagelman DG et al. Anal sphincter repair: a report of 66 cases and review of the literature. Aust NZ J Surg 1988; 58:703–10.

50. Laurberg S, Swash M, Henry MM. Delayed external sphincter repair for obstetric tear. Br J Surg 1988; 75:786–8.

51. Yoshioka K, Keighley MRB. Sphincter repair for faecal incontinence. Dis Colon Rectum 1989; 32:39–42.

52. Wexner SD, Marchetti F, Jagelman JD. The role of sphincteroplasty for faecal incontinence re-evaluated. A prospective physiologic and functional review. Dis Colon Rectum 1991; 34:22–30.

53. Fleshman JW, Dreznik Z, Fry RD et al. Anal sphincter repair for obstetric injury: manometric evaluation of functional results. Dis Colon Rectum 1991; 34:1061–7.

54. Engel AF, Kamm MA, Sultan AH et al. Anterior anal sphincter repair in patients with obstetric trauma. Br J Surg 1994; 81:1231–4.

55. Oliveira L, Pfeifer J, Wexner SD. Physiological and clinical outcome of anterior sphincteroplasty. Br J Surg 1996; 83:502–5.

56. Simmans C, Birnbaum EH, Kodner IJ et al. Anal sphincter reconstruction in the elderly: does advancing age affect outcome? Dis Colon Rectum 1994; 37:1065–9.

57. Engel AF, van Baal SJ, Brummeckamp WH. Late results of anterior sphincter plication for traumatic faecal incontinence. Eur J Surg 1994; 160:633–6.

58. Malouf AJ, Norton CS, Engel AF, Nicholls RJ, Kamm MA. Long term results of overlapping anterior anal sphincter repair for obstetric trauma. Lancet 2000; 355:260–5.

This study has confirmed that the long-term results of anterior sphincter repair are not as good as expected. Only 40% of patients following a secondary repair can expect to be continent.

59. Halverson AL, Hull TL. Long term outcome of overlapping anal sphincter repair. Dis Colon Rectum 2002; 45:345–8.

60. Browning GGP, Parks AG. Postanal repair for neuropathic faecal incontinence: correlation of clinical results and anal cancer pressures. Br J Surg 1983; 70:101–4.

61. Henry MM, Simson JNL. Results of postanal repair: a retrospective study. Br J Surg 1985; 72(suppl.): 517–19.

62. Yoshioka K, Keighley MRB. Critical assessment of quality of continence after postanal repair for faecal incontinence. Br J Surg 1989; 76:1054–7.

63. Laurberg S, Swash M, Henry MM. Effect of postanal repair on the progress of neurogenic damage to the pelvic floor. Br J Surg 1990; 77:519–22.

64. Pinho M, Keighley MRB. Results of surgery in idiopathic faecal incontinence. Ann Med 1990; 22:425–33.

65. Keighley MRB, Korsgen S. Long term results and predictive parameters of outcome following total pelvic floor repair. Dis Colon Rectum 1996; 39:A15.

66. Wexner SD, Baeten C, Bailey R et al. Long term efficacy of dynamic graciloplasty for fecal incontinence. Dis Colon Rectum 2002; 45:809–18.

67. Rongen MGM, Uludas O, El Naggar K et al. Long term follow up of dynamic graciloplasty for fecal incontinence. Dis Colon Rectum 2003; 46:716–21.

These studies (65–67) have now demonstrated the long-term follow-up of dynamic graciloplasty. They confirm that the procedure has significant morbidity, although the long-term success rates appear good.

68. Devesa JM, Rey A, Hervas PL et al. Artificial anal sphincters: complications and functional results of a large personal series. Dis Colon Rectum 2002; 45:1154–63.

69. Wong WD, Congliosi SM, Spencer MP et al. The safety and efficacy of the artificial bowel sphincter for faecal incontinence: the results from a multi-centre cohort study. Dis Colon Rectum 2002; 45:1139–53.

70. Mundy L, Merlin TL, Maddern GJ, Hiller JE. Systematic review of safety and effectiveness of an artificial bowel sphincter for faecal incontinence. Br J Surg 2004; 91:665–72.

This trial has demonstrated that in selected patients the artificial bowel sphincter may be a viable alternative. It is still associated with considerable morbidity.

71. Pinedo G, Vaizey CJ, Nicholls RJ et al Results of repeat anal sphincter repair. Br J Surg 1999; 86:66–9.

72. Giordano P, Renzi A, Efron J et al Previous sphincter repair does not affect the outcome of a previous repair. Dis Colon Rectum 2002; 45:635–40.

73. Malouf AJ, Vaizey CJ, Nicholls RJ, Kamm MA. Permanent sacral nerve stimulation for fecal incontinence. Ann Surg 2000; 232:143–8.

74. Kenefick NJ, Christiansen J. A review of sacral nerve stimulation for the treatment of faecal incontinence. Colorectal Dis 2004; 6:75–80.

Twelve

Functional problems and their management

Anton V. Emmanuel

INTRODUCTION

Symptoms related to functional gastrointestinal disorders (FGIDs) are highly prevalent. In community-based studies, up to 22% of 'normal' UK subjects can be diagnosed as having irritable bowel syndrome (IBS)[1] and up to 28% have functional constipation.[1,2] These disorders are constellations of symptoms – they are not diseases. As such, the emphasis of management of these patients should be based on simple principles: the exclusion of organic disease, alteration of lifestyle where appropriate, addressing any relevant psychological and social factors, simple pharmacological therapy and avoidance of surgery. This chapter deals primarily with IBS and functional constipation, leaving the treatment of faecal incontinence to Chapter 11. Similarly, rectal prolapse, which is a frequent comorbidity of chronic constipation, is dealt with in Chapter 10.

The prevalence of functional disorders relates to the nature of the diagnostic criteria used; the current standard for diagnosis of FGIDs is the Rome II criteria.[3] The diagnostic requirements for IBS include the presence of abdominal pain related to bowel function in association with altered stool form or frequency. The definition of functional constipation requires the presence of at least two of the following: less than three bowel actions a week, need to strain or manually assist evacuation on more than 25% of occasions, passage of hard stools on more than 25% of occasions or a sensation of abnormal evacuation on more than 25% of occasions. These symptoms need only be present for 12 weeks (not necessarily consecutive) of the preceding 12 months. Although these criteria can be criticised for being over-inclusive, what is clear is that FGIDs represent a major burden in secondary and tertiary outpatient clinics and that IBS is the commonest diagnosis in gastrointestinal clinics.[4] An important confounding factor to be borne in mind when reviewing the literature on FGIDs is that the overwhelming majority of studies originate from tertiary centres. Patients attending such institutions are known to have disproportionately high scores on scales of depression, health-related anxiety and somatisation.[5,6] One further compounding variable in assessing studies of FGIDs is that there is a notoriously high placebo response, ranging from 30 to 80%.[7]

IRRITABLE BOWEL SYNDROME

The key to successful management of IBS is strong, empathic reassurance. This will need to be individually directed according to the particular patient's symptoms, beliefs and anxieties.[8] A central component of the reassurance is provision of a simple explanation of the benign nature and prognosis of the condition. Patients should be advised that no more than 2% of patients need their diagnosis of IBS to be revised at 30 years of follow-up.[9] The less good news is that 88% of patients have recurring episodes of gastrointestinal symptoms, and so reassurance should be tempered by the fact that IBS is frequently a chronic and recurrent disorder.[9]

Investigation

The presence of alarm features, such as symptom onset after age 50, rectal bleeding, significant weight loss or abdominal mass, mandates serological and luminal investigation to exclude organic disease. Investigations of these frequently young patients (the majority are aged less than 35 years at presentation[2]) should otherwise be avoided since they may both exacerbate the patient's anxieties and undermine confidence in the clinician.

An important diagnosis to consider, especially in the presence of low-grade anaemia, is coeliac disease.

Approximately 5% of patients fulfilling Rome II criteria will have histological evidence of coeliac disease compared with 0.5% of controls without IBS symptoms.[10]

Treatment

LIFESTYLE MODIFICATION

No strong, reproducible, clinical trial evidence exists in favour of any particular lifestyle modification or dietary intervention in IBS.

Behavioural training to encourage patients to alter patterns of phobic avoidance of public toilets is a central component of biofeedback, and is of undoubted value in some patients.[8,11]

True food allergies are much rarer than lay perception would predict,[12] and food fads and avoidances should be discouraged. The one helpful dietary intervention worth bearing in mind in IBS patients with a tendency to frequent stool passage is that excess caffeine and sorbitol (found in chewing gum and sweeteners) can further irritate an irritable bowel.[13]

A small number of studies have reported the effect of dietary fibre augmentation in IBS patients.[14–17] Two early placebo-controlled crossover studies showed some acceleration of transit but no significant effect on symptoms.[14,15] Two later studies have corroborated the absence of beneficial effect on symptoms and suggested that there is an increase in abdominal bloating, discomfort and flatulence during dietary fibre supplementation.[16,17] In summary, the effect of dietary fibre in IBS is not significantly beneficial, and the diet is frequently difficult to adhere to in the long term.[18]

PHARMACOLOGICAL TREATMENTS

Most patients with FGIDs do not need drug therapy. The strongest evidence for a single agent in patients with IBS is in those with loose or frequent stools, where loperamide is a well-tolerated and effective treatment of diarrhoea and urgency.[19]

The popular aetiological theory that IBS symptoms relate to gut spasm has led to a huge number of uniformly low-quality studies of antispasmodics in IBS patients. These have been subject to recent meta-analyses.[7,20] In essence what can be concluded is that, even allowing for publication bias in favour of positive studies, there is no evidence that anticholinergics (e.g. dicycloverine, hyoscine) or antispasmodics (mebeverine, peppermint) have any advantage over placebo in treating the symptoms of IBS. In contrast, the data for the efficacy of tricyclic antidepressants show unequivocal benefit in favour of low-dose usage of these agents.[21] Doses of amitriptyline or nortriptyline of 10–50 mg seem to be effective at both central (anxiety and depression) and peripheral (neuromodulatory) level, improving symptoms with an impressively low 'number needed to treat' of 3.

One putative mechanism of action of tricyclic agents is through an effect at gut serotonin receptors. A number of drugs that activate or inhibit these receptors have been developed, although the effect of all these drugs seems at best to be modest, amounting to no more than a 10–20% advantage over placebo.[9] None of these agents is licensed for use in the UK at present. Finally, preliminary evidence suggests the possibility that some probiotic strains may have a beneficial influence in patients with IBS.

PSYCHOLOGICAL TREATMENTS

A landmark study by Creed et al.[22] showed that cognitive behavioural therapy directed towards bowel symptoms is effective in treating women with IBS, with a 'number needed to treat' of 3.

The essence of such treatment is that it is gut focused, since general cognitive behavioural and relaxation therapies are no more effective than standard care.[23] A frequent criticism of psychotherapeutic approaches towards patients with FGIDs is that such treatment is neither cost-effective nor beneficial in the long term. The study of Creed et al. showed unequivocal benefit at follow-up 1 year after the cessation of therapy, and demonstrated that health-care costs at that time amounted to £610 compared with £1040 for standard care.[22] In summary, anecdotal and trial evidence favours the provision of psychological services to complement standard care for patients with FGIDs.[8,22]

A number of studies in the literature show the benefit of hypnotherapy in IBS, including in the long-term setting, at up to 6 years following cessation of therapy.[24,25]

In brief, three-quarters of patients report symptom alleviation after hypnotherapy, and over 80% of these responders remain well at a median follow-up of 5 years.[25]

SURGERY

Patients with IBS are disproportionately more likely to undergo abdominal and pelvic surgery than age- and sex-matched controls.[26,27] Patients with IBS have a prevalence of cholecystectomy of 4.6% compared with 2.4% in controls, and a prevalence of hysterectomy of 18% compared with 12% in controls. There is also evidence that IBS patients are more likely to undergo appendicectomy (35% prevalence compared with 8% in control patients with ulcerative colitis).[28] Furthermore, in IBS patients these examinations are more likely to yield normal findings macroscopically and histologically.[29]

The factors resulting in this increased rate of frequently unnecessary surgery have not been addressed in the available studies. One hypothesis is that abdominal or pelvic surgery predisposes to the development of functional symptoms through mechanical, neural or hormonal impairments. Heaton et al.[30] reported that 44% of subjects develop new symptoms of urgency after cholecystectomy and 27% report constipation symptoms beginning after hysterectomy. An alternative hypothesis is suggested by the high prevalence of normal histological material obtained from surgery in IBS patients. This would suggest that the preoperative diagnoses may be erroneous, contributed to in part by the considerable overlap between the symptoms of functional and organic disorders. In the face of this controversy, what these studies do highlight is the key importance of trying to minimise surgery in patients with FGIDs. In those patients who do undergo an operation it is implicit that there is complete explanation of the possibility of developing new symptoms postoperatively. The corollary of this is that patients in whom there is a high suspicion of FGID (based on symptoms and normal investigations) should be dissuaded from undergoing diagnostic laparoscopy, which is not usually revealing and which may result in new complaints.

FUNCTIONAL CONSTIPATION

Estimates from the USA suggest that 1.2% of the population consult a physician every year with the complaint of constipation.[31] Since 85% of these consultations result in the prescription of a laxative,[31] it should come as no surprise that the estimated annual expenditure on prescription laxatives in the UK is £48 million,[32] more than is spent on treating hypertension. This figure does not include the cost of over-the-counter laxatives. It also does not include the costs of specialist investigation and work absenteeism resulting from constipation. What these figures reflect is the importance of the role of the hospital specialist in identifying appropriate patients for further investigation and specific treatments.

In terms of pathophysiology, functional constipation is considered as being due to slow whole-gut transit ('colonic inertia') or rectal evacuatory dysfunction, or a combination of both these abnormalities. The commonest cause of slow transit in general practice is as an adverse effect of drug therapy for other reasons. The commonest culprit drugs are opiates, anticholinergics, antihypertensives, iron supplements, antacids and non-steroidal anti-inflammatory drugs.[33]

Investigation

As with the case of patients with IBS, luminal investigation is reserved for patients with alarm symptoms in whom there is the need to exclude colorectal cancer. In addition to the drug causes listed above, which can be identified from a careful history, the other common associations are with neurological disease (multiple sclerosis, Parkinson's disease, diabetic autonomic neuropathy). Causes of constipation that can be identified from simple serological testing include hypothyroidism, hypercalcaemia and hypokalaemia.

Whereas the diagnosis of IBS is one of exclusion, there are investigations available that both define the pathophysiological abnormality and confirm the presence of constipation. Colonic transit can be simply measured by use of radio-opaque markers followed by plain abdominal radiography. One well-described assessment comprises ingestion of three sets of radiologically distinct markers at 24-hour intervals and an abdominal radiograph taken at 120 hours; retention of more than the normal range for any one of the three sets of markers reflects slow transit.[34] The test is cheap, sensitive and reproducible and provides clinically helpful information in the management of patients with constipation.[35]

Defecating proctography and the balloon expulsion test are means of quantifying the anatomical and physiological disturbances of rectal evacuation in patients with functional constipation. Supposed abnormalities, such as paradoxical anal sphincter contraction, impaired pelvic floor relaxation, anal intusussception and rectal prolapse, can be demonstrated by these techniques.[36] No firm evidence exists of the value of demonstrating these abnormalities in the management of patients with constipation.[37] The place of anorectal manometry in patients with chronic constipation is primarily in the exclusion of Hirschsprung's disease.[37]

Treatment

DIETARY FIBRE SUPPLEMENTATION

This is the traditional first-line therapy of chronic constipation and by the time of specialist referral most patients would have already undertaken trials of such therapy. Fibre supplementation increases gut transit and stool bulk by a fraction of the starting value, and as such is only effective in patients with mild constipation.[38] In those small number of patients seen in hospital who have not tried fibre supplementation, advice needs to be offered about a gradual stepwise increase in fibre intake. Patients need to be counselled that the effect is not apparent until therapy has been established for several weeks. Patients need to continue with the diet in the long term,[36] and there is evidence that this can be difficult in a significant proportion.[18] Increasing liquid intake and attempting to maintain regular meal-time patterns seem also to have a place in improving symptoms, although the evidence is strongest in the elderly.[39]

LAXATIVES, SUPPOSITORIES, ENEMAS AND NOVEL PROKINETICS

There are widely held misconceptions of the danger of 'self-poisoning' without a daily bowel action. Given the limited evidence base for the use of laxatives, the first step in the management of constipation is to discourage laxative abuse.[40] The effect of laxatives in chronic constipation is modest at best. Only a very small number of trials have compared a laxative regimen with placebo, and meta-analysis would not be statistically or clinically meaningful.[32] Compared with the dearth of placebo-controlled studies, there are a number of open and blinded comparisons between different laxatives. These have been systematically reviewed recently[32,41] and, as might be predicted, the opinion of the reviewers is that methodological flaws and inconsistencies prevent meaningful conclusions being drawn. The conclusions that can be drawn are listed below. Overall, the review by Tramonte et al.[41] suggested an increase in stool frequency with bulking agents of 1.4 bowel movements per week, and with other laxative classes of 1.5 bowel movements per week.

Bulk laxatives

Bulk laxatives have a limited role in chronic constipation. They should be reserved for patients who are unable to consume adequate dietary fibre. They have no role in either patients with severe constipation or those who need rapid relief of symptoms.

Osmotic agents

Osmotic agents comprise either poorly absorbed ionic salts or non-absorbed sugars and alcohols.

 Dose titration is possible with osmotic laxatives, which have a particular place in the management of megacolon and megarectum once the patient has been disimpacted.

Stimulant laxatives

Stimulant laxatives (anthranoid compounds such as senna, or polyphenolic compounds such as bisacodyl) usually have an effect on stool output within 24 hours of ingestion, and are most suitable for occasional rather than regular use. The effect of these drugs is unpredictable, and dose escalation is often required. Nevertheless, they appear to be harmless and are frequently used in chronic severe constipation. What is clear is that the previous fears that chronic use of anthranoid laxatives may result in enteric nerve damage is highly unlikely.[42] Stool softeners and compound mixtures of the above classes of laxative are also commonly used, although their efficacy has not been rigorously demonstrated.

Suppositories and enemas

Suppositories induce a chemically induced reflex rectal contraction. Enemas act by either inducing rectal contraction or softening hard stool. Suppositories and enemas can be effective in alleviating the symptoms of evacuation difficulty if dietary modification and behavioural therapy have been unsuccessful. Used on an as-required basis, enemas have a particular place in managing rectal impaction.

Prokinetics

Cisapride was the first prokinetic to be studied in chronic functional constipation, showing a limited short-lived effect. Prucalopride and tegaserod are agonists at the serotonin-4 receptor and seem to accelerate both upper and lower gut transit.[43,44] Both drugs rapidly improve symptoms, although the optimal duration of treatment remains uncertain.

BEHAVIOURAL THERAPY (BIOFEEDBACK)

Gut-directed behavioural therapy, biofeedback, is now an established therapy for functional constipation, and in a number of specialist centres is first-line therapy for new referrals.[45,46] Biofeedback is a learning strategy based on operant conditioning. Although the main focus is on abdominal and pelvic coordination, patients with slow transit respond as frequently as those with evacuation dysfunction.[11,46]

 Short- and long-term benefit is evident in over 60% of unselected patients in specialist centres.[11,45–47]

The effect of treatment is seen not only in symptoms (improved bowel frequency, reduced need to strain) but also in terms of reduced laxative use and improved quality-of-life scores.[11]

Biofeedback seems to have its effect through alteration of a variety of pathophysiological disturbances. There is evidence that successful outcome with biofeedback is associated with specifically improved autonomic innervation to the colon, and improved transit time for patients with slow and normal transit.[11] Additionally, treatment may improve pelvic floor coordination, thereby allowing antegrade peristalsis and preventing retrograde movement of colonic content. What is important is that biofeedback is successful not just in patients with mild symptoms but also in those with intractable symptoms being considered for surgery.[46,48]

SURGICAL TREATMENT

In those patients with proven slow transit who have failed to respond to dietary modification, biofeedback and long-term trials of laxatives and prokinetics, the traditional algorithm dictates consideration of a surgical approach. The standard surgical procedure has been total colectomy (performed to the level of the sacral promontory) and ileorectal anastomosis.[49] Ileorectostomy is reported as being more successful than ileosigmoidostomy in terms of successful relief of constipation and, providing greater than 7–10 cm of rectum is left intact, bowel frequency and urgency are not unduly frequent.[50]

 Almost every major colorectal institution and a huge number of other centres have published their experience of subtotal colectomy for slow transit constipation. Results vary widely, with satisfaction rates ranging from 39 to 100%.[51–54]

While median scores of bowel frequency tend to show statistically significant improvements, what these composite figures mask are the facts that, firstly, approximately one in three patients do not improve at all and, secondly, that some patients develop diarrhoea. The strongest argument against colectomy for slow transit constipation is that the disorder is a pan-enteric one, and so mere removal of the colon is unlikely to yield sustained benefit.[55]

There are two unequivocal conclusions that emerge from the welter of small studies in the literature. Firstly, adverse effects occur in over half of all patients. Most common is episodic subacute small bowel obstruction (occurring in up to two-thirds of patients in some series), followed by the need for further abdominal surgery (in up to one-third of patients), persisting constipation (in up to one-quarter), diarrhoea (in up to one-quarter) and faecal incontinence (in up to 10%). The second conclusion, related to the incidence of adverse events, is the importance of careful patient selection. Thus, of the many patients complaining of constipation in the community, only a tiny proportion (approximately 1%) are referred for tertiary care, of whom only a small fraction (<5%) might benefit from surgical treatment.[49,54] Patient selection must initially be on clinical grounds (including careful consideration of potential psychiatric disorders) and the physiological demonstration of slow transit. Some authors have recommended extensive anorectal sensory and motor physiological testing, defecating proctography and upper gut motility studies to aid identification of subgroups in whom surgery may be more successful.[56,57] In contrast, Rantis et al.[58] identified only 23% of patients in whom such extensive testing altered clinical management; additionally, the cost of this testing was great (US$140 000 in 1997).

In view of the controversy about subtotal colectomy, a vogue for alternative surgical therapies arose. Two particular surgical approaches have received sustained study: stoma formation and segmental colonic resection.

However, the data on efficacy and morbidity of these techniques are little different and no less controversial than those for subtotal colectomy.[36,59,60] There is unequivocally no place for division of puborectalis in an attempt to treat rectal evacuatory dysfunction.[61]

A less invasive surgical approach to functional constipation has been the antegrade continence enema (Malone procedure). Initially used in patients with constipation secondary to neurological disease, the technique has been widely reported in functional constipation.[62,63] Patients intubate their stoma (appendix or plastic conduit) and irrigate with either water or a stimulant or osmotic laxative.

Although there are stomal complications in over 50% of patients (stenosis, mucus leak, pain), three-quarters of patients report 'high' or 'very high' satisfaction with the procedure.[62,63]

Current-day trials of medical therapy for FGIDs require quality-of-life data to complement conventional efficacy data. There is only one such paper in the surgical literature to date, and tellingly this shows that although stool frequency improves, gut-specific quality of life does not.[64]

PUTATIVE TREATMENTS OF CONSTIPATION

The future of medical therapy for functional constipation seems to relate to the development of novel prokinetic drugs.[44,65] The major recent development with regard to surgical therapy for constipation has been sacral nerve stimulation.[66] In the single publication to date, two patients were studied in a double-blind crossover fashion with their sacral nerve stimulator turned either on or off. There was a clear improvement in both symptoms and quality of life with the stimulator turned on, potentially extending the role of sacral nerve stimulation from its existing licence for the treatment of faecal incontinence.

IDIOPATHIC MEGARECTUM AND MEGACOLON

Megarectum and megacolon are uncommon clinical conditions of unknown aetiology that present typically, but not exclusively, with intractable constipation in the first two decades of life.[67] Other conditions presenting with constipation in the context of gut dilatation (e.g. Hirschsprung's disease, chronic intestinal pseudo-obstruction) are not included since the aetiology of these disorders is known. Patients with idiopathic megarectum tend to present with faecal incontinence in the context of recurrent faecal impaction frequently requiring surgical disimpaction. In contrast, patients with idiopathic megacolon more frequently present with abdominal pain and distension in the context of chronic constipation.[67]

The majority of patients with idiopathic megarectum and megacolon can be successfully managed by disimpaction followed by the use of osmotic laxatives. The osmotic agent needs titration in order that the patient obtains a semiformed ('porridgey') stool that is passed three times a day. Occasionally, rectal evacuation techniques (such as suppository use or biofeedback therapy) are required to empty the rectum of the semiformed stool.[68]

When medical therapy fails (due to compliance failure or lack of success in avoiding recurrent impaction), surgical therapy is warranted. A number of surgical procedures have been performed, with variable reports of success. As with reports of surgery for idiopathic constipation, the longer the duration of follow-up, the worse the documented outcome. Anorectal physiology, whole-gut transit studies and evacuation proctography neither help identify patients who may benefit nor help with the choice of surgical procedure.[69] Anorectal physiology testing does have a role in identifying the presence of a rectoanal inhibitory reflex, which when present excludes the differential diagnosis of Hirschsprung's disease.

With regard to resectional surgery, colectomy offers good results in the majority of patients (80%), with ileorectal anastomosis yielding the highest levels of patient satisfaction.[70] Outcomes with the Duhamel procedure, anal myomectomy and restorative proctocolectomy are also favourable in the majority of cases, approaching 70% in the majority of series.[70] In situations where initial surgery has failed, formation of a stoma (colostomy or ileostomy) is associated with excellent results.[71] Stoma formation as a primary procedure is also successful in the vast majority of cases.[71] The ultimate choice of surgical procedure will depend on available expertise, patient physical and psychological factors and the patient's choice.

• Key points

- Dietary manipulation is rarely helpful in managing symptoms in hospital-referred patients with functional disorders.
- Drug therapy is rarely needed in treating patients with IBS.
- Loperamide is unequivocally beneficial in patients with loose stools and urgency.
- Low-dose tricyclic antidepressants are effective in relieving functional abdominal pain.
- A comprehensive approach to therapy of functional disorders requires close liaison with psychological services.
- The effect of laxatives in chronic constipation is minimally superior to placebo.
- Biofeedback is effective in almost two-thirds of patients with constipation, whether due to slow transit or evacuatory dysfunction.
- Subtotal colectomy and ileorectal anastomosis are beneficial in a small number of highly selected patients, although surgical morbidity is frequently high.
- The majority of patients with idiopathic megarectum and megacolon can be managed by disimpaction and initiation of osmotic laxatives.

REFERENCES

1. Jones R, Lydiard S. Irritable bowel syndrome in the general population. Br Med J 1991; 304:87–90.

2. Heaton KW, O'Donnell LJ, Braddon FEM et al. Symptoms of irritable bowel syndrome in a British urban community: consulters and non-consulters. Gastroenterology 1992; 102:1962–7.

3. Thompson WG, Longstreth GF, Drossman DA et al. Functional bowel disorders and functional abdominal pain. Gut 1999; 45(suppl. II):I143–I147.

4. Drossman DA, Whitehead WE, Camilleri M. Irritable bowel syndrome: a technical review for practice guideline development. Gastroenterology 1997; 112:2120–37.

5. Drossman DA, Sandler RS, McKee DC et al. Bowel patterns among subjects not seeking health care: use of a questionnaire to identify a population with bowel dysfunction. Gastroenterology 1982; 83:529–34.

6. Emmanuel AV, Mason HJ, Kamm MA. Relationship between psychological state and level of

activity of extrinsic gut innervation in patients with a functional gastrointestinal disorder. Gut 2001; 49:214–19.

7. Akehurst R, Kaltenthaler E. Treatment of irritable bowel syndrome: a review of randomised controlled trials. Gut 2001; 48:272–82.

8. Stern JM. Review article: psychiatry, psychotherapy and gastroenterology: bringing it all together. Aliment Pharmacol Ther 2003; 17:175–84.

9. Thompson WG. Review article: the treatment of the irritable bowel syndrome. Aliment Pharmacol Ther 2002; 16:1395–406.

10. Sanders DS, Carter MJ, Hurlstone DP et al. Association of adult coeliac disease with irritable bowel syndrome: a case control study in patients fulfilling the Rome II criteria referred to secondary care. Lancet 2001; 358:1504–8.

11. Emmanuel AV, Mason HJ, Kamm MA. Response to a behavioural treatment, biofeedback, in constipated patients is associated with improved gut transit and autonomic innervation. Gut 2001; 49:209–13.

12. Pearson DJ. Pseudo food allergy. Br Med J 1986; 292:221–2.

13. Hyams JS. Sorbitol intolerance: an unappreciated cause of functional gastrointestinal complaints. Gastroenterology 1983: 84:30–3.

14. Arffmann S, Andersen JR, Hegnhoj J et al. The effect of coarse wheat bran in the irritable bowel syndrome: a double-blind cross-over study. Scand J Gastroenterol 1985; 20:295–8.

15. Lucey MR, Clark ML, Lowndes J et al. Is bran efficacious in irritable bowel syndrome? A double blind placebo-controlled crossover study. Gut 1987; 28:221–5.

16. Snook J, Shepherd HA. Bran supplementation in the treatment of irritable bowel syndrome. Aliment Pharmacol Ther 1994; 8:511–14.

While some patients can expect improvement in stool output with bran, the majority of patients experience an increase in abdominal distension and discomfort.

17. Francis CY, Whorwell PJ. Bran and irritable bowel syndrome: time for reappraisal. Lancet 1994; 344:39–40.

18. Hillman LC, Stace NH, Pomare EW. Irritable bowel patients and their long-term response to a high fibre diet. Am J Gastroenterol 1984; 79:1–7.

19. Cann PA, Read NW, Holdsworth CD et al. Role of loperamide and placebo in management of irritable bowel syndrome. Dig Dis Sci 1984; 29:239–47.

Loperamide is effective in slowing gut transit, reducing stool frequency and urgency in patients with IBS.

20. Poynard T, Regimgeau C, Benhamou Y. Meta-analysis of smooth muscle relaxants in the treatment of irritable bowel syndrome. Aliment Pharmacol Ther 2001; 15:355–61.

21. Jackson AL, O'Malley PG, Tomkins G et al. Treatment of functional gastrointestinal disorders with antidepressant medications. Am J Med 2000; 108:65–72.

Meta-analysis of studies using a variety of tricyclic antidepressants in varying doses in patients with FGIDs, showing clear benefit for low-dose tricyclics over placebo.

22. Creed F, Fernandes L, Guthrie E et al. The cost-effectiveness of psychotherapy and paroxetine for severe irritable bowel syndrome. Gastroenterology 2003; 124:303–17.

23. Boyce PM, Talley NJ, Balaam B et al. A randomised controlled trial of cognitive behavioural therapy, relaxation training and routine clinical care for the irritable bowel syndrome. Am J Gastroenterol 2003; 98:2209–18.

24. Whorwell PJ, Prior A, Faragher EB. Controlled trial of hypnotherapy in the treatment of severe refractory irritable bowel syndrome. Lancet 1984; ii:1232–4.

25. Gonsalkorale WM, Miller V, Afzal A et al. Long term benefits of hypnotherapy for irritable bowel syndrome. Gut 2003; 52:1623–9.

26. Kennedy TM, Jones RH. Epidemiology of cholecystectomy and irritable bowel syndrome in a UK population. Br J Surg 2000; 87:1658–63.

27. Kennedy TM, Jones RH. The epidemiology of hysterectomy and irritable bowel syndrome in a UK population. Int J Clin Pract 2000; 54:647–50.

28. Burns DG. The risk of abdominal surgery in irritable bowel syndrome. S Afr Med J 1986; 70:91–3.

29. Longstreth GF, Preskill DB, Youkeles L. Irritable bowel syndrome in women having diagnostic laparoscopy or hysterectomy: relation to gynaecologic features and outcome. Dig Dis Sci 1990; 35:1285–90.

30. Heaton KW, Parker D, Cripps H. Bowel function and irritable bowel symptoms after hysterectomy and cholecystectomy: a population based study. Gut 1993; 34:1108–11.

31. Sonnenberg A, Koch TR. Physician visits in the United States for constipation: 1958–1986. Dig Dis Sci 1989; 34:606–11.

32. Petticrew M, Watt I, Brand M. What's the 'best buy' for treatment of constipation? Results of a systematic review of the efficacy and comparative efficacy of laxatives in the elderly. Br J Gen Pract 1999; 49:387–93.

33. Emmanuel AV. The use and abuse of laxatives in the elderly. In: Potter J, Norton C, Cottenden AM (eds) Bowel care in frail older people. London: Royal College of Physicians, 2002; chapter 6.

34. Evans RC, Kamm MA, Hinton JM et al. The normal range and a simple diagram for recording whole gut transit. Int J Colorectal Dis 1992; 7:15–17.

35. Degen LP, Phillips SF. Variability of gastrointestinal transit in healthy men and women. Gut 1996; 39:299–305.

36. Locke GR, Pemberton JH, Phillips SF. AGA technical review of constipation. Gastroenterology 2000; 119:1766–78.

37. Diamant NE, Kamm MA, Wald A et al. AGA technical review on anorectal testing techniques. Gastroenterology 1999; 116:735–54.

38. Kamm MA. Constipation. Br J Hosp Med 1989; 41:244–50.

39. Harari D, Gurwitz JH, Minaker KL. Constipation in the elderly. J Am Geriatr Soc 1993; 41:1130–40.

40. Jones MP, Talley NJ, Nuyts G et al. Lack of objective evidence of efficacy of laxatives in chronic constipation. Dig Dis Sci 2002; 47:2222–30.

41. Tramonte SM, Brand MB, Mulrow CD et al. The treatment of chronic constipation in adults. J Gen Intern Med 1997; 12:15–24.

Systematic review of the placebo-controlled laxative studies and those comparing different laxative classes. The limited benefit of these drugs over placebo is highlighted.

42. Kieman JA, Heinicke EA. Sennosides do not kill myenteric neurons in the colon of the rat or mouse. Neuroscience 1989; 30:837–42.

43. Emmanuel AV, Roy AJ, Nicholls TJ. Prucalopride, a systemic enterokinetic, for the treatment of constipation. Aliment Pharmacol Ther 2002; 16:1347–56.

Large single-centre study of the effect of a serotonin agonist on gut physiology and symptoms in patients with functional constipation.

44. Callaghan MJ. Irritable bowel syndrome neuropharmacology: a review of approved and investigational compounds. J Clin Gastroenterol 2002; 35(suppl. 1):S58–S67.

45. Enck P. Biofeedback training in disordered defaecation: a critical review. Dig Dis Sci 1993; 38:1953–60.

46. Chiotakakou-Faliakou E, Kamm MA, Roy AJ et al. Biofeedback provides long term benefit for patients with intractable slow and normal transit constipation. Gut 1998; 42:517–21.

Demonstration of long-term efficacy of biofeedback in patients who have an initially good response to treatment.

47. Bassotti G, Whitehead WE. Biofeedback as a treatment approach to gastrointestinal tract disorders. Am J Gastroenterol 1994; 89:159–64.

48. Brown SR, Donati D, Seow-Chen F et al. Biofeedback avoids surgery in patients with slow transit constipation: report of four cases. Dis Colon Rectum 2001; 44:737–9.

49. Nyam DC, Pemberton JH, Ilstrupp DM et al. Long term results of surgery for chronic constipation. Dis Colon Rectum 1997; 40:273–9.

50. Vasilevsky CA, Nemer FD, Balcos EG et al. Is subtotal colectomy a viable option in the management of chronic constipation? Dis Colon Rectum 1988; 31:679–81.

51. Kamm MA, Hawley PR, Lennard-Jones JE. Outcome of colectomy for severe idiopathic constipation. Gut 1988; 29:969–73.

52. Pfeifer J, Agachan F, Wexner SD. Surgery for constipation: a review. Dis Colon Rectum 1996; 39:444–60.

53. Lubowski DZ, Chen FC, Kennedy ML et al. Results of colectomy for severe slow transit constipation. Dis Colon Rectum 1996; 39:23–9.

54. Knowles CH, Scott M, Lunniss PJ. Outcome of colectomy for slow transit constipation. Ann Surg 1999; 230:627–38.

Systematic review of most of the small reports of subtotal colectomy showing that efficacy is inversely related to duration of follow-up. A rationale for patient selection is presented.

55. Altomare DF, Portincasa P, Rinaldi M et al. Slow transit constipation: solitary symptom of a systemic gastrointestinal disease. Dis Colon Rectum 1999; 42:231–40.

56. Rex DK, Lappas JC, Goulet RC et al. Selection of constipated patients as subtotal colectomy candidates. J Clin Gastroenterol 1992; 15:212–17.

57. Redmond JM, Smith GW, Barofsky I et al. Physiologic tests to predict long-term outcome of total abdominal colectomy for intractable constipation. Am J Gastroenterol 1995; 90:748–53.

58. Rantis PC, Vernava AM, Daniel GL et al. Chronic constipation: is the work-up worth the cost? Dis Colon Rectum 1997; 40:280–6.

59. Kamm MA, van der Sijp JR, Hawley PR et al. Left hemicolectomy with rectal excision for severe idiopathic constipation. Int J Colorectal Dis 1991; 6:49–51.

60. Lundin E, Karlbom U, Pahlman L et al. Outcome of segmental colonic resection for slow-transit constipation. Br J Surg 2002; 89:1270–4.

61. Kamm MA, Hawley PR, Lennard-Jones JE. Lateral division of puborectalis in the management of severe constipation. Br J Surg 1988; 75:661–3.

62. Krogh K, Laurberg S. Malon antegrade continence enema for faecal incontinence and constipation in adults. Br J Surg 1998; 85:974–7.

63. Marshall J, Hutson JM, Anticich N et al. Antegrade continence enemas in the treatment of slow-transit constipation. J Pediatr Surg 2001; 36:1227–30.

64. FitzHarris GP, Garcia-Aguilar J, Parker SC et al. Quality of life after subtotal colectomy for slow-transit constipation: both quality and quantity count. Dis Colon Rectum 2003; 46:433–40.

65. Coulie B, Szarka LA, Camilleri M et al. Recombinant human neuropathic factors accelerate colonic transit and relieve constipation in humans. Gastroenterology 2000; 119:41–50.

66. Kenefick NJ, Vaizey CJ, Cohen CR et al. Double-blind placebo-controlled crossover study of sacral nerve stimulation for idiopathic constipation. Br J Surg 2002; 89:1570–1.

67. Gattuso JM, Kamm MA. Clinical features of idiopathic megarectum and idiopathic megacolon. Gut 1997; 41:93–9.

> The only true prospective comparison of symptoms, pathophysiology and management between patients with idiopathic megarectum and megacolon.

68. Mimura T, Nicholls T, Storrie JB et al. Treatment of constipation in adults associated with idiopathic megarectum by behavioural retraining including biofeedback. Colorectal Dis 2002; 4:477–82.

69. O'Suillbhain CB, Anderson JH, McKee RF et al. Strategy for the surgical management of patients with idiopathic megarectum and megacolon. Br J Surg 2001; 88:1392–6.

70. Stabile G, Kamm MA, Hawley PR et al. Colectomy for idiopathic megarectum and megacolon. Gut 1991; 32:1538–40.

71. Stabile G, Kamm MA, Hawley PR et al. Results of stoma formation for idiopathic megarectum and megacolon. Int J Colorectal Dis 1992; 7:82–4.

Thirteen

Anal fistula: evaluation and management

Peter J. Lunniss and
Robin K.S. Phillips

INTRODUCTION

Anorectal sepsis is common, presenting as either an acute abscess or a chronic anal fistula. The majority of cases can be dealt with avoiding complication, but a small minority can present a major challenge to both sufferer and surgeon.

Although fistula in ano may be found in association with a variety of specific conditions, the majority seen in the UK today are classified as non-specific, idiopathic or cryptoglandular, their exact aetiology having not been fully proven, although the diseased anal gland in the intersphincteric space is considered central. Fistulas may be seen in association with Crohn's disease,[1] tuberculosis,[2] pilonidal disease, hidradenitis suppurativa,[3] lymphogranuloma venereum,[4] presacral dermoids,[5] rectal duplication,[6] actinomycosis,[7] trauma and foreign bodies.[8] An important association is malignancy,[9] which may manifest itself as a discharging opening on the perineum from a pelvic source, but which may also arise in long-standing fistulas, either cryptoglandular, as part of perianal Crohn's disease, or even in hidradenitis suppurativa.

There is only scant information about the exact incidence of idiopathic anal fistula in the general population, as most data come from hospital analysis in tertiary referral centres, which attract only the more difficult cases. Perhaps the most accurate information about incidence comes from

Scandinavia. In the County of Stockholm, the incidence is about 1 per 10 000.[10] Sainio[11] reported a mean incidence of 8.6 per 100 000 population in Helsinki.

All reported series have demonstrated a male predominance. Most report a male to female ratio of between 2:1 and 4:1; the much higher ratios reported from the Indian subcontinent[12–14] may reflect different cultural attitudes of women towards attending often male doctors. Otherwise, the gender difference in incidence is unexplained. McColl[15] found no sex differences in histology or distribution of anal glands in 50 normal human anal canals, and we have found no differences in circulating sex hormone concentrations between sufferers of either sex and healthy controls.[16] Furthermore, the sex difference is not limited to humans. The German Shepherd dog is a breed particularly prone to the development of anal fistula compared with other breeds, and this is not due to any differences in anal crypt or gland anatomy.[17] Vasseur[18] reported a 3:1 male to female ratio of the incidence of canine fistulas, compared to a 1:1 ratio for the whole dog population; the incidence of fistula is much lower in neutered dogs and bitches compared with those that are sexually intact.[19]

Anal fistulas most commonly afflict people in their third, fourth or fifth decades.[20–22] There is little information on racial differences in incidence, although the peak incidence has been reported at a lower age in Nigerians[23] and in black Americans.[24] Sedentary occupations cannot be implicated.[13,21] Whether bowel habit may be influential is unclear. Some authors take the view that diarrhoea may allow easier access of bacteria to the anal glands, especially in infants;[25] others feel that hard stools are implicated by their abrasive passage through the anal canal.[26]

The overall morbidity from fistula is difficult to assess in either individual or economic terms. For the majority of patients with simple fistulas, the time spent off work with the parent abscess and subsequent fistula management may be relatively short. However, it is not that uncommon for a patient with a complex fistula to have had multiple hospital admissions for attempted cure over several years, only to end up incontinent and permanently incapacitated. For these patients in particular, tertiary referral centres that have gained the necessary expertise are essential, expertise lying in the hands of not only the surgeons but also the nurses, radiologists, physiologists and psychologists who all play an important part in management.

AETIOLOGY

Anal glands and their link with anal fistulas have been historically attributed to Chiari[27] and to Herrmann and Desfosses.[28] The function of the anal glands is uncertain. They have been shown to secrete mucin,[29] but this has a different composition from that secreted by rectal mucosa.[30] From comparative anatomical studies, McColl[15] showed that the anal glands are not vestigial remnants of sexual scent glands; and Shafik's[31] suggestion that they are not true glands at all but rather vestigial epithelial remnants left after proctodeal invagination into the hindgut has not been substantiated.[32]

Current thinking lays the blame at those anal glands situated in the intersphincteric space; these may constitute one-third to two-thirds of the total number of anal glands found in an anal canal.[15,33]

Eisenhammer[34] considered all non-specific abscesses and fistulas to be the result of extension of sepsis from an intramuscular anal gland, the sepsis being unable to drain spontaneously into the anal lumen because of infective obstruction of its connecting duct across the internal sphincter.

Parks[29] proposed that should the initial abscess in relation to the intersphincteric anal gland subside, the diseased gland might become the seat of chronic infection with subsequent fistula formation. The fistula is thus a granulation tissue-lined track kept open by the infective source, which is the abscess around a diseased anal gland deep to the internal sphincter. Parks[29] studied 30 consecutive cases of anal fistula and found cystic dilatation of anal glands in eight, which he attributed to acquired duct dilatation or more probably a congenital abnormality, a precursor to infection within a mucin-filled cavity.

There have been few studies which have examined the cryptoglandular hypothesis. Goligher et al.[35] found intersphincteric space sepsis in only 8 of 28 cases of acute anorectal sepsis; of 32 cases of anal fistula, only 14 had evidence of either intersphincteric sepsis or the track travelling within (rather than simply across) the intersphincteric space. However, Goligher failed to acknowledge that a proportion of cases of acute sepsis have nothing to do with fistula and that some common fistulas (e.g. superficial fistulas and those arising from a chronic anal fissure) have an aetiology separate from that postulated by Parks.

Another question arises from studies of the microbiology of fistula tissue. Although infection and its effective drainage are the primary problems in the acute stage, and although failure to treat secondary extensions and abscesses adequately will inevitably lead to recurrence, the possibility that the anal gland becomes the seat of chronic infection in the established fistula has found little support in the only two studies directed at this aspect of the hypothesis.[36,37] A more attractive theory as to why idiopathic fistulas persist is that they become (at least partly) epithelialised, a factor responsible for failure of healing of fistulas at other sites in the body. A histological study of the intersphincteric component of 18 consecutive idiopathic anal fistulas showed that although an association between anal gland and fistula may be demonstrated (as had been suggested by Gordon-Watson and Dodd[38] in 1935) in a minority of cases, epithelialisation from either or both ends of the fistula track is a more common finding.[39]

Spread of sepsis from an acutely infected anal gland may occur in any of the three planes, vertical, horizontal or circumferential. Caudal spread is the simplest and most usual way by which infection is thought to disseminate[40] to present acutely as a perianal abscess (labelled **a** in **Fig. 13.1**). Cephalad extension in the same space will result in a high intermuscular abscess (**b** in **Fig. 13.1**)[41] or a supra-levator pararectal (syn. pelvirectal) abscess (**c** in **Fig. 13.1**), depending on the relation of the sepsis to the longitudinal muscle layer. Lateral spread across the external sphincter will reach the ischiorectal fossa (**d** in **Fig. 13.1**), where further caudal spread will result in the abscess pointing at the skin as an ischiorectal abscess; and upward spread may penetrate the levators to reach the supralevator pararectal space. Circumferential spread (**Fig. 13.2**) may occur in any of the three planes, intermuscular (synonymous with intramuscular and equivalent to intersphincteric but with no restriction to a level beneath the anorectal ring), ischiorectal or supra-levator. All those conditions which Eisenhammer[42] considered not to be of cryptoglandular origin he placed into the miscellaneous group of acute ano-rectal non-cryptoglandular non-fistulous abscesses (**Fig. 13.3**). These included the submucous abscess (arising from an infected haemorrhoid, sclero-therapy or trauma), the mucocutaneous or marginal abscess (infected haematoma), the perianal abscess (follicular skin infection), some ischiorectal abscesses (primary infection or foreign body) and the pelvirectal supralevator abscess originating in pelvic disease.

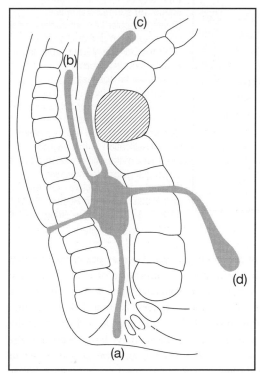

Figure 13.1 • The possible courses of spread of sepsis from the diseased anal gland in the intersphincteric space. See text for explanation. With permission from Parks AG. The pathogenesis and treatment of fistula-in-ano. Br Med J 1961; i:463–9.

MANAGEMENT OF ACUTE SEPSIS

The majority of chronic anal fistulas are preceded by an episode of acute anorectal sepsis, although

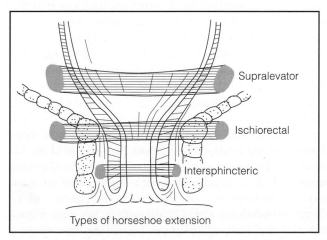

Figure 13.2 • The three planes in which sepsis may spread circumferentially. With permission from Parks AG, Gordon PH, Hardcastle JD. A classification of fistula-in-ano. Br J Surg 1976; 63:1–12.

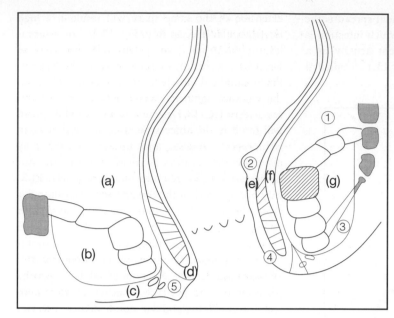

Figure 13.3 • The acute anorectal non-cryptoglandular non-fistulous abscesses of Eisenhammer.
(a) Pelvirectal supralevator space; **(b)** ischiorectal space; **(c)** perianal or superficial ischiorectal space; **(d)** marginal or mucocutaneous space; **(e)** submucous space; **(f)** intermuscular (syn. intersphincteric) space; (g) deep postanal space. 1, Pelvirectal supralevator abscess; 2, submucous abscess; 3, ischiorectal abscess; 4, mucocutaneous or marginal abscess; 5, perianal or subcutaneous abscess. With permission from Eisenhammer S. The final evaluation and classification of the surgical treatment of the primary anorectal cryptoglandular intermuscular (intersphincteric) fistulous abscess and fistula. Dis Colon Rectum 1978; 21:237–54. © Springer-Verlag.

acute sepsis does not inevitably lead to fistula formation. The reported rates of recurrent abscess or fistula development following simple incision and drainage range from 17 to 87%.[43,44] The optimal management of acute sepsis should reside in an understanding of aetiology. Pilonidal infection, hidradenitis and perianal Crohn's disease are usually fairly easy to recognise by history and examination. Pus in the perianal space may result from caudal spread of intersphincteric (cryptoglandular) infection or from simple skin appendage infection. Similarly, pus in the ischiorectal space may or may not be related to presumed anal gland disease.

Patients with acute anorectal sepsis usually present via the accident and emergency department rather than the outpatient clinic. Those with perianal sepsis tend to present early, 2 or 3 days after onset of symptoms, with pain and a palpable tender lump close to the anal margin, and usually with no constitutional symptoms. Patients with ischiorectal abscesses tend to present later with more vague discomfort, but because much more pus may accumulate in the large relatively avascular loose areolar tissue of the ischiorectal fossa, they often have fever and constitutional upset. Examination may reveal tender induration over the abscess rather than an exquisitely tender well-defined lump as found when the sepsis is perianal. Sepsis higher

up in the sphincter complex may present with rectal pain, and possibly disturbance of micturition, and there may be no external signs of pathology. The rare submucosal abscess is revealed on digital examination of the anal canal as a distinct tender bulge, and the patient may have reported the passage of pus from the anal canal with relief of symptoms.

Clues as to the aetiology of perineal sepsis may be gleaned from microbiology of the drained pus:[45] if skin organisms alone are cultured and the acute abscess adequately drained, the patient may be told with confidence that recurrence should not occur and that a fistula will not result. If gut organisms are cultured, however, it is probable but not inevitable that there is an underlying fistula. The results of microbiology are therefore sensitive (100%) but not totally specific (60–80%), and of course are not available at the time of initial surgery.

Determination of the presence or absence of sepsis in the intersphincteric space (irrespective of the site of the main abscess or whether an internal opening is demonstrable) has been shown to be the most accurate way of determining the presence of an underlying fistula,[46] although it has been argued that such exploration is beyond the expertise of a general surgical trainee untrained in proctology for whom simple incision and drainage represents the safest option in the acute stage.

Those who advocate a more aggressive approach to acute sepsis do so on the basis that incision and drainage can only be effective if the abscess is not cryptoglandular,[42] that definitive treatment in the initial stage obviates further surgery, and that such a policy reduces the incidence of complex fistulas arising through incompletely drained sepsis. Certainly, the reported recurrence/fistula rate following primary fistulotomy (0–7%) would support this.[47–49] There are drawbacks however: internal openings are evident in only about one-third of cases; the acute situation lends itself to the creation of false tracks and internal openings; and the unknown proportion of patients with crypto-glandular sepsis who might be cured by incision and drainage alone would not be well served by a procedure associated with a greater risk of flatus incontinence and soiling.[50]

A recent prospective randomised trial involving 200 patients presenting with anal sepsis compared simple drainage to drainage plus primary fistulotomy, when the fistula was deemed low (subcutaneous, intersphincteric or low trans-sphincteric). This yielded recurrence rates of 36.7% in the drainage-alone group and 5% in those in whom the underlying fistula was laid open.[51] There was no reported incontinence following simple drainage, compared with 2.8% in the fistulotomy group.

A policy (in experienced hands) of simple incision when a fistula is not evident, and primary fistulotomy when a fistula is evident and low (or a draining loose seton placed if there is any doubt about the level, or concern about continence) is sensible, as long as the patient has been adequately counselled.

Patients with an established fistula usually give a history of intermittent pain and purulent discharge from an opening on the perineum, the pain building up until relief is felt when the pus escapes. Patients in whom the internal opening is rectal, and those with large internal openings irrespective of site, may pass flatus and stool through the external opening(s).

CLASSIFICATION OF ANAL FISTULA

Successful surgical management of anal fistula depends upon accurate knowledge of anal sphincter anatomy and the fistula's course through it. Failure to understand either may result in fistula recurrence or incontinence. To this end, classification of pathology is extremely important.

The most comprehensive and practical classification, and the one most widely used presently, is that devised at St Mark's, based on a study of 400 fistulas treated there.[52]

The cryptoglandular hypothesis is central to this classification, which holds firstly that the majority of fistulas arise from an abscess in the inter-sphincteric plane and, secondly, that the relation of the primary track to the external sphincter is para-mount in surgical management. Four main groups exist: intersphincteric, trans-sphincteric, supra-sphincteric and extrasphincteric. These groups can be further subdivided according to the presence and course of any extensions or secondary tracks.

Intersphincteric fistulas (**Fig. 13.4**), constituting 45% of cases in the original St Mark's series, are

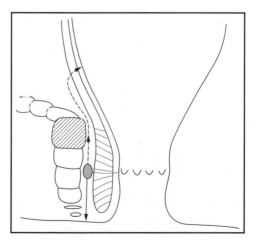

Figure 13.4 • The possible courses of an intersphincteric fistula. With permission from Marks CG, Ritchie JR. Anal fistulas at St Mark's Hospital. Br J Surg 1977; 64:84–91. Copyright British Journal of Surgery Society Ltd. Reproduced with permission. Permission is granted by John Wiley & Sons Ltd on behalf on the BJSS Ltd.

usually simple; however, others have a high blind track, or a high opening into the rectum or no perineal opening, or even have pelvic extension, or arise from pelvic disease. Trans-sphincteric fistulas (**Fig. 13.5**) (29%) have a primary track that passes through the external sphincter at varying levels into the ischiorectal fossa. Such fistulas may be uncomplicated, consisting only of the primary track, or can have a high blind track that may terminate below or above the levator ani muscles.

Suprasphincteric fistulas (**Fig. 13.6**) (20% in the 1976 series[52]) run up to a level above puborectalis and then curl down through the levators and ischiorectal fossa to reach the skin. Extrasphincteric fistulas (**Fig. 13.7**) (5%) run without relation to the sphincters and are classified according to their pathogenesis. In addition to horizontal and vertical spread, sepsis may spread circumferentially in any of the three spaces: intersphincteric, ischiorectal or pararectal.

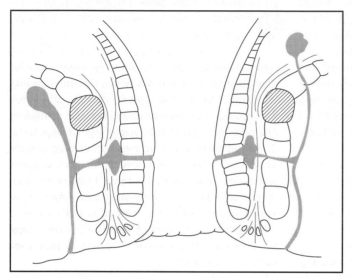

Figure 13.5 • A trans-sphincteric fistula with blind infralevator ischiorectal extension (left) and supralevator pararectal extension (right). With permission from Parks AG, Gordon PH, Hardcastle JD. A classification of fistula-in-ano. Br J Surg 1976; 63:1–12.

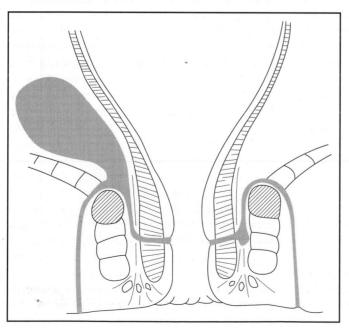

Figure 13.6 • Simple suprasphincteric fistula (right) and more complex form with associated secondary pelvic abscess (left). With permission from Parks AG, Gordon PH, Hardcastle JD. A classification of fistula-in-ano. Br J Surg 1976; 63:1–12.

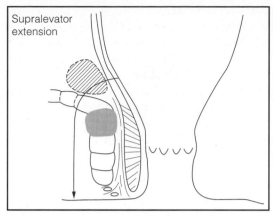

Figure 13.7 • Extrasphincteric fistula running without relation to the sphincter complex. With permission from Marks CG, Ritchie JK. Anal fistulas at St Mark's Hospital. Br J Surg 1977; 64:84–91. Copyright British Journal of Surgery Society Ltd. Reproduced with permission. Permission is granted by John Wiley & Sons Ltd on behalf on the BJSS Ltd.

The St Mark's classification does have a few drawbacks,[53] but these are of little clinical significance. Superficial fistulas, and those associated with bridged fissures (commonly seen outside tertiary referral centres), are not acknowledged by a classification whose emphasis is the intersphincteric space. There can be clinical difficulty in differentiating between a simple intersphincteric fistula and a very low trans-sphincteric fistula that crosses the lowermost fibres of the subcutaneous portion of the external sphincter. And some argue whether suprasphincteric tracks can be part of a classification based on cryptoglandular pathology (arguing indeed that many are iatrogenic). The extreme rarity of suprasphincteric fistulas and the difficulty of distinguishing them from high trans-sphincteric tracks even raise doubts about their very existence. However, clinical differentiation from high trans-sphincteric fistulas is in most cases immaterial since the same methods of treatment would be employed.

ASSESSMENT

Clinical

A full history and examination including proctosigmoidoscopy are essential in all cases to exclude any associated conditions. Clinical assessment involves five essential points, enumerated by Goodsall and Miles[54] at the end of the nineteenth century:

1. location of the internal opening;
2. location of the external opening;
3. course of the primary track;
4. presence of secondary extensions;
5. presence of other diseases complicating the fistula.

The relative positions of the external and internal openings will indicate the likely course of the primary track, and the presence of any palpable induration, especially supralevator, should alert the surgeon to a secondary track.[55] The distance of the external opening from the anal verge may assist in differentiating an intersphincteric from a trans-sphincteric fistula; the greater the distance, the greater the likelihood of a complex cephalad extension.[21,56] Goodsall's rule generally applies in that the likely site of the internal opening can be predicted by the position around the anal circumference of the external opening. Exceptions to this rule include anteriorly located openings more than 3 cm from the anal verge (which may be anterior extensions of posterior horseshoe fistulas) and fistulas associated with other diseases, especially Crohn's and malignancy.

Thus, the first step in examining the anus is to identify the position of the external opening (or openings). Next, the perianal area should be carefully palpated with a well-lubricated finger to feel for the presence and direction of induration, which will indicate the course of the primary track (**Fig. 13.8**). If the track is not palpable, it is probable that the fistula is not intersphincteric or low trans-sphincteric. Digital examination within the anorectal lumen is then performed with the specific intention of feeling for any indentation/induration as the sign marking the site of the internal opening. Asking the patient to contract the anal sphincters allows an assessment of the position of the primary track in relation to the puborectalis sling (if posterior) or upper border of the external anal sphincter (if anterior), although it must be remembered that in trans-sphincteric fistulas the level of the internal opening may not be the same as that at which the primary track crosses the external sphincter (it may be higher, especially if the internal opening is above the dentate line). The finger is then

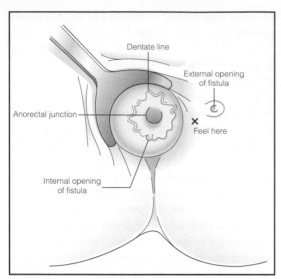

Figure 13.8 • Palpating for the direction and depth of the primary tract. With permission from Phillips RKS. Operative management of low cryptoglandular fistula-in-ano. Operat Tech Gen Surg 2001; 3(3):134–141.

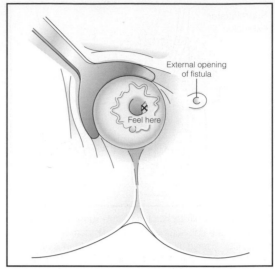

Figure 13.9 • Palpating for the presence of induration, indicating either a high primary tract or secondary extension in the roof of the ischiorectal fossa or supralevator space. With permission from Phillips RKS. Operative management of low cryptoglandular fistula-in-ano. Operat Tech Gen Surg 2001; 3(3):134–141.

advanced into the rectum and any supralevator induration is sought (it feels like bone and is easier to notice when it is unilateral as there will be asymmetry) (**Fig. 13.9**). Digital assessment of the primary track by an experienced coloproctologist has been shown to be 85% accurate.[57]

Examination under anaesthesia complements examination in the awake patient. The internal opening may be easily seen at proctoscopy, aided if necessary by gentle downward retraction of the dentate line, which may expose openings concealed by prominent valves or papillae.[58] Lateral traction of an opened Eisenhammer proctoscope may reveal dimpling at the internal opening through its underlying fibrous inelasticity. Sometimes, the site of the responsible crypt may be seen only as scar tissue if the internal opening is not patent.[59] Digital massage of the track may reveal the site of the internal opening as a bead of pus. If the track is simple, a probe may traverse its entire length, but if the probe comes to lie above or remote from the dentate line, a direct association between the track and the adjacent anoderm cannot be assumed.[58] The instillation of various agents along the track via the external opening has also been advocated, including saline,[60] hydrogen peroxide[61] and dyes such as methylene blue and indigo carmine.[42,58] In practical terms, instillation of dilute hydrogen peroxide is the easiest way of locating the internal opening, as staining is avoided.[58,62]

Careful probing can delineate primary and secondary tracks. If the internal and external openings are easily detected but the probe cannot easily traverse the path of the track, it is possible that there is a high extension, and a probe passed via each opening may then delineate the primary track. Failure to negotiate probes around a horse-shoe posterior trans-sphincteric fistula suggests at least one acute bend in the track, within the intersphincteric space and crossing the external sphincter, or in the roof of the ischiorectal fossa, in which case anatomy will only be defined once surgery is under way (**Fig. 13.10**). Persistence of granulation tissue after curettage during the operation is an indication of a secondary extension.[62]

Imaging

Careful examination of a fistula under anaesthesia has been considered the most important part of any assessment.[57] However, previous surgery leads to scarring and deformity, as well as the creation of

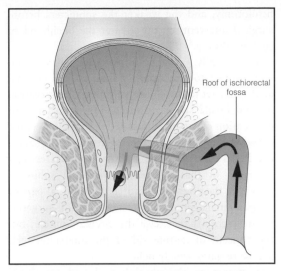

Figure 13.10 • Trans-sphincteric horseshoe fistulas may have several sharp bends along their course, preventing exact delineation unless the ischiorectal fossa is opened widely (to reach the acute bend in the roof of the ischiorectal fossa), and often necessitating dislocation of the posterior sphincter from its ligamentous attachments (to ascertain the site at which the tract crosses the external sphincter). With permission from Phillips RKS. Operative management of low cryptoglandular fistula-in-ano. Operat Tech Gen Surg 2001; 3(3):134–141.

unusual primary tracks, which can make clinical assessment extremely difficult. Until recently, techniques aimed at helping in fistula assessment have proved disappointing.

The accuracy of fistulography has been variously reported. Some have found it useful in recurrent cases,[63,64] but its low sensitivity in identifying internal openings and their positions, its low sensitivity combined with significant false positivity in determining high extensions,[59,65] the discomfort of the technique and potential for dissemination of sepsis,[66] and the introduction of more accurate methods have rendered it almost obsolete. Fistulography is necessary to outline an extra-sphincteric track, so the method should not be completely ruled out. However, extrasphincteric tracks are rare, and in other circumstances fistulography does not seem worthwhile. Computed tomography suffers other disadvantages,[67,68] and is indicated only when there is suspicion that the fistula arises from an intra-abdominal or pelvic source.

Anal endosonography (AES) using a 7-MHz rotating endoprobe encased within a hard sonolucent cone

in the evaluation of intersphincteric and trans-sphincteric tracks produced results that were initially promising.[69] Unfortunately, the limited focal range of the probe made evaluation of pathology beyond the sphincters (either lateral to or above) difficult to assess, and it is in these areas that difficulty in clinical assessment often arises. Sepsis and scarring can confuse fistula assessment in those who have undergone previous surgery[70] and although the method is cheap and is currently the gold standard in determining internal and external sphincter integrity, its low positive predictive value, especially in the demonstration of extensions,[70] limits its usefulness when dealing with difficult fistulas. More recent studies have shown better concordance rates between AES and operative findings,[71] that hydrogen peroxide may improve resolution and help localize the internal opening,[72] and that AES has been shown to be superior to clinical evaluation.[73] The results of prospective studies assessing three-dimensional ultrasound assessment of anal fistulas are awaited.

The potential advantages of magnetic resonance imaging (MRI) include the lack of ionising radiation, the ability to image in any plane and the high soft-tissue resolution.[74,75]

 Short tau inversion recovery (STIR) sequencing (a fat-suppression technique) to highlight the presence of pus and granulation tissue without the need for any contrast media[76] was used in a prospective study involving 35 patients at St Mark's Hospital that favourably compared MRI interpretations with the independently documented operative findings.[70]

Concordance between MRI and operative findings was 86% for the presence and course of the primary track, 86% for the presence and site of secondary extensions and abscesses, and 97% for the presence of horseshoeing. The positive predictive value of MRI in demonstrating secondary extensions and abscesses was 100%. More importantly, in five patients (14%) failure of healing was related to pathology missed at surgery that had been demonstrated on preoperative MRI. Further prospective studies[77] have confirmed that the technique certainly challenges operative assessment by an experienced coloproctologist as the 'gold standard'. A recent prospective study has demonstrated a therapeutic impact of MRI in the management of 10% of patients treated for primary anal fistulas,[78] although the therapeutic impact is much greater when used to assess recurrent fistulas.[79]

Perhaps a logical approach is that patients with (suspected) primary anal fistulas undergo AES, and those in whom there is clinical or sonographic suspicion of complexity go on to MRI. There is strong evidence that all recurrent fistulas should be examined using MRI preoperatively, and that the surgeon uses the scans to aid surgery. It is unlikely that imaging with an endoanal coil[80,81] will have a great impact in fistula surgery. The accuracy of MRI also means that we are now able to refute or confirm the presence of sepsis in those patients with symptoms but in whom clinical examination is unrevealing, and in the prospective assessment of newer methods of attempted fistula eradication.

Physiological

The correlation between subjective assessment of an individual's continence and physiological static measurements recorded in a laboratory may be debatable, but the argument for physiological assessment (anal canal length, pressures along it, anorectal sensitivity, sphincter integrity and pudendal nerve conduction studies) in the clinical context of a patient with a complex fistula (or one deemed to have, or be at risk of, compromise in function) is nowadays strong. Continence may be regarded as a balance between rectal pressure and the power of the sphincters to overcome this, orchestrated by anorectal sensation.

Milligan and Morgan[82] stressed the importance of the anorectal ring in fistula surgery: 'if this ring be cut, loss of control surely results, yet as long as the narrowest complete ring of muscle remains, control is preserved. All the anal sphincter muscles below this ring may be divided in any manner without harmful loss of control'.

Certainly, complete division of the puborectalis sling in suprasphincteric and extrasphincteric fistulas results in total incontinence to all rectal contents, but division of muscles below the ring may result in equally devastating consequences. It is reasonable to suppose that the higher the level at which the primary track crosses the sphincter complex, the greater the possibility of impaired function after

fistulotomy; and the weaker the sphincters before surgical intervention, the greater the likelihood of such morbidity.[83]

Traditionally, more importance has been apportioned to the external than to the internal anal sphincter in the context of muscle preservation in anal fistula surgery. Indeed, the importance of eradication of the presumed aetiological source, the diseased anal gland in the intersphincteric space, led Parks[29] to advocate internal sphincterectomy (excision of that segment of internal sphincter overlying the diseased gland) as an essential part of surgical management. Nowadays, most surgeons divide rather than excise the circular muscle, but the concept of getting rid of the intersphincteric source remains widely held.

To determine the physiological and functional effects of fistula surgery, we conducted a prospective study[84] of 37 patients successfully treated for either intersphincteric (15 patients) or trans-sphincteric fistulas. All patients underwent division of the internal anal sphincter and anoderm below the level of the primary track; 15 of the 22 patients with trans-sphincteric fistulas also underwent division of the external sphincter, at least to the level of the dentate line, whereas the remaining seven patients with trans-sphincteric fistulas were successfully treated without recourse to external sphincter division. As might be predicted, distal anal canal and maximum resting pressures were reduced in all patients after surgery, external sphincter division resulting in no greater reduction of maximum resting pressure than occurred after internal sphincter division alone. Squeeze pressures were unaffected in those in whom the external sphincter had been preserved, but division in the 15 patients who underwent fistulotomy of trans-sphincteric tracks resulted in significant reductions in distal anal canal squeeze pressures and maximum squeeze pressure.

However, functional outcome was not related to division of the external sphincter, with equal incidence of minor disturbances of continence reported by those in whom it had been preserved (53% vs. 50% respectively). Furthermore, the severity of postoperative symptoms was no different between the two groups, being related to reduced postoperative resting pressures, reduced maximum resting pressure and higher thresholds of anal electrosensitivity in the sector of surgery, rather than to postoperative squeeze pressures.

It appears that total sphincter conservation would be optimal in terms of functional outcome, but the drawback is that no sphincter-preserving method heals the underlying fistula as surely as lay open. This is important, because although this study revealed a relatively high incidence of functional disturbance, the vast majority of patients were satisfied with their management and tolerated a reduction in function as a reasonable price to pay in order to be rid of chronic anal sepsis. Nevertheless, there is a functional price to pay, even for curing the more minor forms of fistula, and this justifies continued attempts at methods that preserve sphincter integrity and function when appropriate.

PRINCIPLES OF FISTULA SURGERY

Acute sepsis is an indication for early surgical intervention and drainage. However, in cases where a more complex procedure than lay open is contemplated, acute sepsis should have been eradicated long before, leaving well-established chronic tracks. A loose seton may be required to achieve adequate drainage of the primary track. Secondary tracks should be either laid open, curetted or drained, according to their position in relation to the levators. Some authors advise bowel preparation before fistula surgery, although laid-open wounds in the perineum heal remarkably well despite the continual bacterial load. Most authors recommend parenteral antibiotics peroperatively and postoperatively for any of the more complex procedures.

In the UK, fistula surgery is usually performed under general anaesthesia, but in North America local or regional anaesthesia is more widely employed. Similarly, in the UK most anal fistula surgery is performed with the patient in the lithotomy position, although the prone jack-knife position is gaining in popularity, at least among some surgeons. Prophylaxis against development of venous thrombosis is advised, and in the UK is usually achieved with a combination of low-dose subcutaneous heparin and elasticated stockings. Finally, the operative findings and treatment should be recorded. The St Mark's Hospital fistula operation sheet (**Fig. 13.11**) based on Parks' classifi-

cation provides an excellent standardised format for documentation both by description and by illustration.

SURGICAL TREATMENT

Lay open remains the surest way of eliminating an anal fistula. The multiplicity of techniques designed to preserve sphincter function and at the same time eradicate fistula pathology reflects their relative lack of success. A degree of caution and scepticism may be appropriately apportioned when assessing reported results of the various approaches towards complex fistula, since:

1. patient populations may be markedly different;
2. fistula classification may be variable;
3. reports of successes may not be tempered by honest reporting of failures;
4. reports of success in terms of fistula cure have historically not always been accompanied by reports of changes in continence;
5. despite the increasing drive for evidence-based medicine, the use of prospective randomised trials is probably unachievable, because of individual fistula (and sphincter) variability and individual surgeon preference and skill;
6. follow-up may be inadequate.

Fistulotomy

Fistulotomy means laying open and allowing to heal by secondary intention. Its application should, in the first instance, be restricted to situations where a significant degree of incontinence would not result. In principle, high trans-sphincteric (especially anterior tracks in women) and suprasphincteric tracks should not be treated by one-stage fistulotomy. Intersphincteric and low trans-sphincteric tracks are probably best treated by this method, but the decision whether to lay open rests on the skill and experience of the surgeon after informed advice to the patient.

Abcarian[85] recommends the following technique: after initial assessment of the track, a crypt hook is placed into the internal opening which is laid open by diathermy cautery, the latter maintaining a dry operative field and thus allowing easy identification of granulation tissue. If examination with the

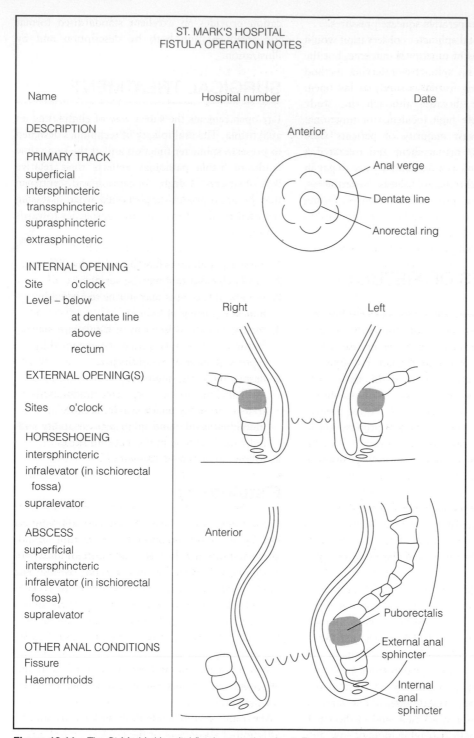

ST. MARK'S HOSPITAL
FISTULA OPERATION NOTES

Name   Hospital number   Date

DESCRIPTION

Anterior

PRIMARY TRACK
superficial
intersphincteric
transsphincteric
suprasphincteric
extrasphincteric

Anal verge

Dentate line

Anorectal ring

INTERNAL OPENING
Site   o'clock
Level – below
        at dentate line
        above
        rectum

Right   Left

EXTERNAL OPENING(S)

Sites   o'clock

HORSESHOEING
intersphincteric
infralevator (in ischiorectal
    fossa)
supralevator

ABSCESS
superficial
intersphincteric
infralevator (in ischiorectal
    fossa)
supralevator

Anterior

Puborectalis

External anal
sphincter

OTHER ANAL CONDITIONS
Fissure
Haemorrhoids

Internal
anal
sphincter

Figure 13.11 • The St Mark's Hospital fistula operation sheet. Reproduced with thanks to Mr James P.S. Thompson.

crypt hook reveals the primary track to be inter-sphincteric or to involve only the lowermost fibres of the external anal sphincter, the tissue overlying the probe is divided along its length. If, however, the probe enters the depths outside the external sphincter, it is left in place and a second probe gently passed via the external opening, and the two probes manipulated until they can be felt or heard to touch. That portion of the track outside the external sphincter is laid open, and the internal sphincter divided over the crypt hook. An assessment is then made as to how much voluntary muscle lies below the track and the decision is made either to lay the track open or to resort to a sphincter-saving procedure. Marsupialisation, i.e. suturing the divided wound edge to the edges of the curetted fibrous track, results in a smaller wound and faster healing.

Secondary extensions from the primary track can be dealt with in two ways. The traditional method in the UK is to lay these open widely to allow maximal drainage, which is followed by healing by secondary intention. As long as the external sphincter is intact, the residual scarring after healing is remarkably little. In the USA, the use of incisions, counter-incisions and the placement of encircling drains is sometimes preferred; these drains are left in for 2–4 weeks, with more rapid healing and less deformity claimed.[86,87]

Fistulotomy and immediate reconstitution

Parkash et al.[88] reported a series of 120 patients treated by fistulotomy and immediate reconstruction of the divided musculature, and with primary wound closure. The reported results were impressive: 88% of wounds had healed by 2 weeks, there was a 4% recurrence rate, and all patients were satisfied with the functional outcome. However, 118 of the 120 fistulas were classified as low intersphincteric or simple trans-sphincteric, and the authors admitted that similar success would not be expected with more complex fistulas. Sood[89] had earlier obtained equally impressive results in 136 patients with low fistulas treated by the same method, and reported shorter healing time and less postoperative pain than in 100 patients treated by conventional fistulotomy. There is no literature addressing the technique in patients in whom fistulotomy is not indicated.

Fistulectomy

The technique of fistulectomy, which excises rather than incises the fistula track, has been criticised on the basis that the greater tissue loss leads to delayed healing.[90]

However, Lewis[91] advocates fistulectomy, but by a core-out technique rather than excision of the track, because he claims that:

1. the precise course of the track is more accurately determined by core-out under direct vision, and does not involve the passage of probes along the track and thus creation of false tracks – a probe is used only to open the external opening and assist in inserting a stay suture around it;
2. coring out the primary track reduces the risk of missing secondary tracks, which are seen as transected granulation tissue and which may be followed by the same technique;
3. the relation of the primary track to the external anal sphincter may be correctly ascertained before any sphincter muscle is divided;
4. a complete specimen is available for histology.

Once the track has been cored out, from the external towards the internal opening using either scissors or cautery dissection, the decision as to whether the tunnel left after the core-out can be safely laid open is made. For a non-recurrent single trans-sphincteric track, Lewis recommends simple anatomical closure of the cored-out tunnel, with mucosal closure and closure of the holes in the muscles. The wound outside the sphincters is lightly packed.

Of 67 low fistulas treated by Lewis[92] between 1985 and 1992 by coring out and laying open the resultant tunnel, there has been one recurrence. Of 32 patients with high trans-sphincteric or supra-sphincteric fistulas treated between 1972 and 1992 by core-out and simple anatomical closure, a temporary colostomy was raised in four and there have been three recurrences.[80] In the case of recurrent or more complex fistulas, Lewis recommends the adoption of other sphincter-conserving methods, since excessive scarring and the larger defect created by coring out this tissue makes simple anatomical closure inappropriate.

Setons

THE LOOSE SETON

Setons may be classified as loose, tight or chemical according to their different properties and modes of action. A thread, loosely tied, is often used as a marker of a fistula track when its exact position and level in relation to the external sphincter is unclear at surgery, perhaps because of scarring from previous surgery or because of the depth of sphincter muscle relaxation under anaesthesia. In such circumstances, the proportions of muscle above and below the fistula may be more accurately determined when the patient is awake and with the track palpably delineated by the thread. Similarly, a loosely tied thread can be used as a drain of acute sepsis, to allow subsidence of acute inflammatory changes and safer definitive fistula surgery.

More specifically in the field of sphincter and continence preservation, the loose seton can be used in three ways: to preserve the entire external sphincter; to preserve part of the voluntary muscle; or as part of a staged fistulotomy in order to reduce the consequences of division of large amounts of muscle in one procedure.

The key points of a staged fistulotomy are the amount of muscle divided at each stage and the time allowed for fibrosis to develop between the divided muscle edges before a further length of sphincter is divided. Ramanujan et al.[93] reported a series of 45 patients with suprasphincteric fistulas in whom the first stage involved laying open the upper sphincter while preserving the distal sphincter within a seton; the seton-enclosed muscle was divided about 2 months later. There was just one recurrence and in only one patient did any disturbance of continence (intermittent leakage of flatus) result. Others have preserved the upper sphincter within a seton while laying open the lower portion. Kuypers[94] described this technique in 10 patients with trans-sphincteric fistulas with supralevator extensions opening into the rectum. The seton-enclosed muscle was divided 3 months after the first stage. There were no recurrences, one

patient was incontinent and six reported minor soiling.

Parks and Stitz[95] reported a series of 80 patients from St Mark's Hospital with trans-sphincteric and suprasphincteric fistulas in whom, at the first stage, the lower one-third to one-half of the sphincter was divided and at the second stage a few months later either the seton removed (if all had healed) or the seton-enclosed muscle divided (if there were high tracks or cavities that had failed to close in). About 38% of patients required division of the upper sphincter to achieve healing; unfortunately, the functional outcome in the two groups of patients was not clearly described.

In more recent times at St Mark's the loose seton has been used with the aim of entire external sphincter preservation. Tracks and extensions outside the sphincters being widely laid open, in the past the internal sphincter was then divided to the level of the internal opening (or higher if there was a cephalad intersphincteric extension). More recently, attempts at internal sphincter conservation have been made. In the case of the high posterior trans-sphincteric track, the passage of the primary track across the sphincter complex may sometimes be accurately judged only after division of the anococcygeal ligaments, thereby dislocating the posterior sphincter attachments but allowing access to the deep postanal space.[83] The seton, passed along the primary track across the external sphincter, is then tied loosely to encircle the denuded voluntary muscle. Postoperatively, the wounds are managed by daily digitation and irrigation rather than by tight packing, with a possible repeat examination under anaesthesia at 7–10 days to ensure that all tracks have been dealt with and that healing is progressing correctly. At outpatient review, if there is evidence of good healing both of the wounds and around the seton, the latter is removed at 2–3 months. Any suspicion of ongoing sepsis requires repeat examination under anaesthesia.

A series of 34 consecutive patients with complex idiopathic trans-sphincteric fistulas treated at St Mark's Hospital between 1977 and 1984 showed that cure of the fistula without recourse to external sphincter division occurred in 44%.[96] Of those in whom the method had been successful, 83% reported full continence compared with only 32% of those in whom the external sphincter had subsequently been divided. Of the 16 patients in whom the technique failed, nine reported some degree of incontinence to formed stool; none of the patients in whom the external sphincter had been preserved reported any such disturbance of sphincter function.

A success rate of 67% was achieved in the 24 patients with similar fistulas treated in the same way between 1990 and 1991.[83] Kennedy and Zegarra[97] used a loose silk seton to treat 32 patients with high trans-sphincteric and suprasphincteric anal fistulas, and reported a success rate of 78%; the method was more successful with anterior (88%) than posterior (66%) fistulas. However, of the 25 patients successfully treated, nine had some alteration of continence.

If the technique fails and it is certain that this is not due to any missed secondary extensions (detectable by MRI), untoward aetiology, etc., there are several options available: (i) the patient may be happy living with a 'controlled' fistula with a long-term draining seton; (ii) the tight seton method may be employed; (iii) a fistulotomy may be performed and the functional results assessed postoperatively; or (iv) fistulotomy may be combined with the raising of a defunctioning colostomy, time allowed for full healing, before sphincter repair and then restoration of intestinal continuity at a final stage. The decision made must be between the individual patient and the surgeon. [Editor's note: my own personal preference is for a permanent loose seton made of No. 1 Ethibond with just one knot to avoid bulkiness and to give comfort (nylon setons tend to be sharp, silastic setons to have bulky knots) as I have lost confidence in the longer term healing of the loose seton technique described above.]

THE TIGHT SETON

The rationale of the tight or cutting seton is similar to that of the staged fistulotomy technique, in that the divided muscle is not allowed to spring apart but there is supposed to be gradual severance through the sphincter followed by fibrosis.

Misra and Kapur[98] reported the outpatient treatment of 56 anal fistulas using a braided stainless-steel tight seton, which was tightened weekly with pain being used as an indicator of tension. The two recurrences were successfully treated by rewiring. No patient reported any functional disturbances

but three patients expressed a desire for some form of anaesthesia while the wire was being tightened. However, all but eight patients had fistulas classified as simple, i.e. low trans-sphincteric, intersphincteric or superficial, but the advantages of outpatient treatment (no time off work and avoidance of a large wound) were evident.

Goldberg and Garcia-Aquilar[99] recommend the use of a tight seton whenever the fistula encircles more than 30% of the sphincter complex and when local sepsis or fibrosis precludes the raising of an advancement flap. The portion of the track outside the sphincters is laid open, although others in the USA have recommended Penrose drainage of horseshoe limbs.[100,101] The anoderm and perianal skin overlying that portion of the sphincter encircled by the seton are incised and the intersphincteric space drained by internal sphincterotomy, extended cephalad if necessary to drain any high intersphincteric (intermuscular) extension. Tightening of the seton (Goldberg uses a rubber band) does not commence until any suppuration has resolved, usually at 3 weeks postoperatively. Tightening is repeated every 2 weeks using a silk tie or Barron band until the seton has cut through.

Goldberg described the use of the cutting seton in 13 patients with trans-sphincteric fistulas between 1988 and 1992, and found that the average time for the seton to cut through was 16 weeks (range 8–36 weeks) with no recurrences at a median follow-up of 24 months (range 4–60 months). As might be expected, this cure rate was tempered by a relatively high incidence of functional morbidity: one patient suffered major incontinence, and a further seven patients (54%) complained of minor persistent loss of control to flatus or episodic loss of liquid stool.[99]

The critical aspects of management by the cutting seton must be, firstly, the elimination of acute sepsis before sphincter division[87] and, secondly, the speed with which the seton cuts through the sphincter. In a series of 24 patients with high trans-sphincteric fistulas, Christensen et al.[102] tightened the seton every second day; 62% of patients reported some degree of incontinence postoperatively, including 29% who wore a pad constantly. Published results by one of the authors of the 'snug' Silastic (elastic) seton method, aimed at cutting through the muscle much more slowly but without the need for tightening, are awaited.

THE CHEMICAL SETON

This method, enjoying a resurgence in India where it is known as *Kshara sutra*, involves the weekly reinsertion of a specially prepared thread along the fistula track. The thread is prepared in a multistage process involving multiple layers of agents derived from plants. Apart from its antibacterial and anti-inflammatory properties, the alkalinity of the thread (about pH 9.5) would appear to be the means by which the thread slowly cuts through the tissues. Indeed, the chemical nature might be the reason behind the rather slow rate of cutting, about 1 cm of track every 6 days.[103,104]

In a prospective randomised trial involving 502 patients,[105] apart from a longer healing time (8 weeks vs. 4 weeks), the results of this outpatient treatment were comparable with fistulotomy (incontinence rate 5% vs. 9%; recurrence rate at 1 year 4% vs. 11%).

A zero recurrence rate has been reported in another series using a similar technique in 80 patients from Colombo.[106] Recurrences usually occur for the same reasons as after conventional surgery, such as a missed secondary track or another internal opening,[107] but the economic advantages of such a method in a less privileged country are obvious.

For low fistulas, however, a more recent prospective randomised study from Singapore concluded that the method has no advantage over conventional fistulotomy.[108]

Advancement flaps

The use of an advancement flap was first proposed by Noble[109] for the repair of rectovaginal fistulas. Elting[110] described its use in managing anal fistula in 1912, supported by two principles: separation of the track from the communication with the bowel; and adequate closure of that communication with eradication of all diseased tissue in the anorectal wall. To Elting's principles, modern surgeons have added adequate flap vascularity and anastomosis of the flap to a site well distal to the site of the (previously excised) internal opening as important tenets. Modifications have included the use of full-thickness rectal flaps, partial-thickness flaps, curved incisions and rhomboid flaps, with or without

closure of the defect in and outside the external sphincter,[111] and distally based (anocutaneous flaps transposed upwards) flaps. Most authors agree that the flap should include part if not all of the underlying internal sphincter in order to maintain vascularity. Apart from the presence of acute sepsis, large internal openings (>2.5 cm) would be considered a contraindication as the risks of anastomotic breakdown are high;[112,113] and a heavily scarred, indurated, wooden perineum precludes adequate exposure and flap mobilisation.

Although the technique has not enjoyed much popularity because of a low success rate at St Mark's Hospital, there are several studies that have reported excellent results, with cure rates of 90–100% for idiopathic anal fistulas and little in the way of functional morbidity (**Table 13.1**). The report by Athanasiadis et al.[121] is interesting for several reasons. In the larger series of patients (N = 224), internal sphincterotomy was performed aiming to eradicate the presumed aetiological source, but this led, as might be expected, to a much higher incidence of significant postoperative continence disorders than when internal sphincterotomy had not been performed. The persistence/recurrent fistula rate was 18% for trans-sphincteric fistulas and 40% for suprasphincteric fistulas. Preservation of the internal sphincter in a subsequent group of 55 patients resulted in a much lower incidence of functional morbidity, but unfortunately fistula persistence/recurrence was not reported.

Information about fistula type has been incomplete in some reports, but the one by Kodner et al.,[113] a 10-year experience including 107 patients, is probably an accurate overall reflection of the results of the method, as well as including an excellent account of surgical management. A total of 24 patients in this series had Crohn's disease, but there was an overall initial success rate of 84% (including 27 of 31 patients with cryptoglandular fistulas), rising to 94% with revisional surgery in nine initial failures, including four patients who underwent successful repeat flap procedures. Finan[111] achieved healing in 10 of 11 patients with idiopathic infralevator trans-sphincteric fistulas and provided prospective physiological data to confirm preservation of sphincter muscle formation and anoderm sensation. A review of the technique and its results has been published.[126]

Table 13.1 • Technique and outcome of advancement flap repair of idiopathic anal fistulas. Postoperative continence is variably reported, and exact duration of follow-up difficult to determine

Reference	N	Classification	Flap thickness	Flap shape	Wound	Continence	Recurrence	Follow-up
Elting (1912)[110]	96	?	Full thickness		Pack	Incontinence	1/96	?
Oh (1983)[114]	15	'High, recurrent'	Mucosal	Tongue	Drain and pack	No change	2/15	?
Aguilar et al. (1985)[115]	189	?	Mucosal ± circular symptoms	Semilunar	Open	10% minor	3/189	12–60 months
Wedell et al. (1987)[116]	27	4 suprasphincteric 12 high trans-sphincteric 11 mid trans-sphincteric	PT circular muscle	Tongue	Open/packed	Unchanged	0/27	18–48 months
Jones et al. (1987)[117]	4	'Complex'	PT circular muscle	Tongue	Drain	?	0/4	3–67 months
Reznick & Bailey (1988)[18]	6	'High'	Mucosal (3)	Tongue	Curetted and left open	Unchanged	1/6	32 ± 36 months
Rutten & Buth (1988)[119]	3	1 suprasphincteric 2 extrasphincteric	Mucosal	Tongue	Open	Unchanged	0/3	18–24 months
Lewis & Bartolo (1990)[120]	2	High trans-sphincteric	Full thickness circular	Tongue	Curetted and drained	Unchanged	1/2	2–24 months
Kodner et al. (1993)[113]	31	?	PT circular muscle	Tongue	Curetted and drained	Unchanged	4/31	Median 7 months
Athanasiadis et al. (1994)[121]	224	189 trans-sphincteric	Mucosal (over partial internal sphincterotomy)	Tongue	Open	42/224 significant	48/224	12–96 months
Lewis et al. (1995)[122]	11	Trans-sphincteric	PT circular muscle	Tongue	Open	No change	1/11	26–30 months
Ozuner et al. (1996)[123]	19	'Complex'	PT circular muscle	Semilunar	Open	?	6/19	Median 21 months
Del Pino et al. (1996)[124]	8	Trans-sphincteric	Island flap anoplasty	Anoderm and perianal skin	Open	?	1/8	1–10 months
Jun & Choi[125]	40	35 trans-sphincteric 5 suprasphincteric	Anoderm/PT circular	Anocutaneous Tongue	Drain	Unchanged	1/40	6–24 months

PT, partial thickness.

Fibrin glue

There are several studies that have reported the successful use of fibrin glue in sealing off fistula tracks.[127–130] Autologous glues have been largely replaced by commercially available virus-inactivated fibrinogen solution from donor plasma. The glue aims to plug the tube from internal opening to external opening and promote healing through fibroblast migration and activation, and the formation of a collagen meshwork. The importance of thorough curettage to remove all granulation tissue and debris (some have used laser to destroy the chronic inflammatory lining) is stressed; the authors suspect that this, and complete plugging of the tracks, may be very difficult when dealing with serpiginous secondary tracks. Use of antibiotics is variable, but some go as far as to try to 'sterilise' the fistula track preoperatively according to the results of microbiological culture. Again, the technique is contraindicated when there is acute sepsis, this being dealt with first (and in some series always the first stage[129]) with a loose draining seton. The internal opening itself is plugged with sealant, closed simply, or an advancement flap raised. Notwithstanding these modifications, it is difficult to explain the highly variable reported success rates (14–85%). Paradoxically, treatment of short tracks appears less successful than that of longer tracks. Some reports are victims of short follow-up (most failures occur early but some occur in the long term; postoperative MRI, despite apparent healing at that time, has been shown to predict eventual outcome[131]); the reader remains ignorant about efficacy in fistulas with tortuous primary tracks or secondary extensions (strengthening the case for preoperative MRI, which would make evaluation of the technique much more comprehensive).

A randomised controlled trial has recently demonstrated no benefit in terms of healing over fistulotomy in treating low fistulas, but for those fistulas deemed unsafe to lay open, a cumulative (a second application offered in the event of initial failure) 69% success rate at 3 months[132] appears at least as good as other techniques aimed at avoiding any sphincter division.

The attractions of such a relatively simple technique are self-evident. Unfortunately, the literature fails to address those factors which are associated with success or failure, apart from those fistulas associated with specific diseases. The answers can only come from more detailed study.

Other methods

Matos et al.[133] have reported the results of a new approach to challenging high fistulas. The aims of total sphincter preservation, minimal deformity and eradication of pathology led to a technique involving eradication of intersphincteric pathology via an intersphincteric approach, combined with coring out the fistula track and anatomical closure of the cored-out tunnel. The method was used in 13 patients, of whom five had inflammatory bowel disease. Complete sphincter preservation and healing were achieved in 7 of 13, and in a further two the internal sphincter had to be divided at a second stage to achieve cure. Success was associated with good function; all failures recurred early in the postoperative period and probably represented ongoing sepsis, but the method described does not compromise more conventional treatments in the failed group, since the sphincter complex anatomy is relatively undisturbed.

Mann and Clifton[134] described a staged approach in which the extrasphincteric component of a well-established track was rerouted inwards (into the intersphincteric or submucosal planes) to a site where it could be safely laid open without puborectalis or external sphincter sacrifice. Unfortunately, only five cases were reported, but no detriment in function occurred in any of them, with complete healing and no recurrences during a follow-up period of up to 3 years.

Kupferberg et al.[135] presented a novel approach to the management of patients with recurrent high fistulas. Excision of the track was pursued as high as possible without endangering the sphincters, the proximal end of the track was closed as close to the rectal wall as possible, and gentamicin-impregnated beads were inserted into the wound before primary wound closure. After 1 week, the chains of beads were gradually withdrawn over a period of 3 weeks. At 2 years there were no recurrences in the five patients so treated.

As an adjunctive procedure in the management of complex anterior fistulas in women, the use of a labial fat pad flap (modified Martius flap) has been reported.[136] The rationale of this manoeuvre is that the space left after repair by whichever method is obliterated by a well-vascularized pedicle. Both suprasphincteric fistulas treated by this technique were eradicated.

MANAGEMENT OF THE RECURRENT FISTULA

Failure of sphincter-preserving methods and persistent symptoms may make lay open the most sensible option (although some patients may prefer to live with a long-term loose seton). After fistulotomy some patients are able to lead normal lives with the narrowest of (often fibrotic) anorectal rings, as Milligan and Morgan had stated in 1934.[82] However, some may request sphincter repair. MRI is a useful way of making sure that there is no covert pathology before embarking on repair. Over a 3-year period at St Mark's Hospital 20 patients underwent sphincteroplasty for incontinence after previous surgery for idiopathic fistulas. A good outcome (Parks' grade 1 or 2 continence score) was obtained in 13 (65%).[137]

It is important to consider the possibility of an extrasphincteric fistula when a high 'blind' track is encountered, arising from pelvic or abdominal disease or from a presacral dermoid cyst. Failure to perform imaging (fistulography, barium studies or MRI) is a major reason for delayed diagnosis of extrasphincteric fistulas. If a track is truly high and blind, this might be because the internal opening has closed, or because surgery has dealt with the primary track and recurrence is because of an overlooked secondary extension.[138] In such cases, the component of the track outside the sphincters should be laid open and curetted. As the resulting wound may be large, it is often wise to make a circular rather than a radial incision to avoid sphincter damage. Following granulation tissue with curette and probe must be done extremely carefully if false tracks and iatrogenic openings are to be avoided. If the track peters out before reaching the intersphincteric space, it is safest to stop and come back another day. If the track enters the intersphincteric space but no internal opening can be identified, it is reasonable to assume that the opening has healed or is extremely small; internal sphincterectomy of that quadrant is then justified to try to prevent recurrence.

AREAS OF FURTHER RESEARCH

Why men so often develop fistulas compared with women is unknown. It is possible that there are differences in end-organ (anal gland) sensitivity to androgens, and further research is warranted in this area (as has been done in hidradenitis suppurativa[139]), as it may lead to prospects for hormonal manipulation to ameliorate extreme cases.

Although the management of anal fistula has traditionally been purely surgical, the occasional success of fibrin glue in sealing off tracks shows that there is potential for non-surgical methods. MRI can predict failure, but we need to know what factors are associated with success. Recognition of these, and continued development of biomaterials, would represent a great leap forward.

• Key points

- A fistula has a primary track and may have secondary extensions.
- Complete eradication of both will lead to cure.
- All lay-open procedures divide some of the internal sphincter, so patients should be warned of a 1 in 20 chance of flatus incontinence and mild mucus leakage.
- Lay-open is the most certain treatment where it is possible and when the risks have been properly explained and accepted.
- Advancement flaps are intuitively attractive but practically uncertain.
- Glue is only rarely effective.
- In the balance between minor soiling with almost certain cure vs. potential recurrence with a less than certain technique, many patients allowed the choice will choose the former.
- Anterior fistulas in women are dangerous and should only rarely be laid open.
- STIR sequence MRI is the gold standard for imaging.
- A permanent, comfortable, loose seton will preserve continence and prevent much (but not all) future abscess formation, but continual discharge means all patients need continuing outpatient support and reassurance and a minority find it unacceptable in the long term.

REFERENCES

1. Marks CG, Ritchie JK, Lockhart-Mummery HE. Anal fistulas in Crohn's disease. Br J Surg 1981; 68:525–7.

2. Shukla HS, Gupta SC, Singh G, Singh PA. Tubercular fistula-in-ano. Br J Surg 1988; 75:38–9.

3. Culp CE. Chronic hidradenitis suppurativa of the anal canal: a surgical skin disease. Dis Colon Rectum 1983; 26:669–76.

4. Miles RPM. Rectal lymphogranuloma venereum. Br J Surg 1957; 45:180–8.

5. Pye G, Blundell JW. Sacrococcygeal teratoma masquerading as a fistula-in-ano. J R Soc Med 1987; 80:251–2.

6. Narashimharao KL, Patel RV, Malik AK, Mitra SK. Chronic perianal fistula: beware of rectal duplication. Postgrad Med J 1987; 63:213–14.

7. Harris GJ, Metcalf AM. Primary perianal actinomycosis. Report of a case and review of the literature. Dis Colon Rectum 1988; 31:311–12.

8. Lockhart-Mummery JP. Discussion on fistula-in-ano. Proc R Soc Med 1929; 22:1331–41.

9. Nelson RL, Prasad ML, Abcarian H. Anal carcinoma presenting as perirectal abscess or fistula. Arch Surg 1985; 120:632–5.

10. Ewerth S, Ahlberg J, Collste G, Holmstrom B. Fistula-in-ano. A six year follow up study of 143 operated patients. Acta Chir Scand 1978; 482(suppl.):53–5.

11. Sainio P. Fistula-in-ano in a defined population. Incidence and epidemiological aspects. Ann Chir Gynaecol 1984; 73:219–24.

12. Deshpande PJ, Sharma KR, Sharma SK, Singh LM. Ambulatory treatment of fistula-in-ano: results in 400 cases. Ind J Surg 1975; 37:85–9.

13. Raghavaiah NV. Anal fistula in India. Int J Surg 1976; 61:243–5.

14. Kesarwani RC. Fistula-in-ano. J Ind Med Assoc 1984; 82:113–15.

15. McColl I. The comparative anatomy and pathology of anal glands. Ann R Coll Surg Engl 1967; 40:36–67.

16. Lunniss PJ, Jenkins PJ, Besser GM, Perry LA, Phillips RKS. Gender differences in incidence of idiopathic fistula-in-ano are not explained by circulating sex hormones. Int J Colorectal Dis 1995; 10:25–8.

17. Budsberg C, Spurgeon TL, Liggitt HD. Anatomic predisposition to perianal fistulae formation in the German Shepherd Dog. Am J Vet Res 1985; 46:1468–72.

18. Vasseur PB. Results of surgical excision of perianal fistulas in dogs. J Am Vet Med Assoc 1984; 185:60–2.

19. Killingsworth CR, Walshaw R, Dunstan RW, Rosser EJ. Bacterial population and histologic changes in dogs with perianal fistula. Am J Vet Res 1988; 49:1736–41.

20. Marks CG, Ritchie JK. Anal fistulas at St Mark's Hospital. Br J Surg 1977; 64:1003–7.

21. Lilius HG. Fistula-in-ano: a clinical study of 150 patients. Acta Chir Scand 1968; 383(suppl.):3–88.

22. Sainio P. A manometric study of anorectal function after surgery for anal fistula, with special reference to incontinence. Acta Chir Scand 1985; 151: 695–700.

23. Ani AN, Solanke TF. Anal fistula: a review of 82 cases. Dis Colon Rectum 1976; 19:51–5.

24. Read DR, Abcarian H. A prospective study of 474 patients with anorectal abscess. Dis Colon Rectum 1979; 22:566–8.

25. Matt JG. Anal fistula in infants and children. Dis Colon Rectum 1960; 3:258–61.

26. Eisenhammer S. Long-tract anteroposterior intermuscular fistula. Dis Colon Rectum 1964; 7:438–40.

27. Chiari H. Uber die Analen Divertikel der Rektumschleimhaut und ihre Beziehung zu den Analfisteln. Med Jahrb Wien 1880; 8:4 419–27.

28. Herrmann G, Desfosses L. Sur la muquese de la region cloacale du rectum. C R Acad Sci (III) 1880; 90:1301–2.

29. Parks AG. The pathogenesis and treatment of fistula-in-ano. Br Med J 1961; i:463–9.

30. Fenger C, Filipe MI. Pathology of the anal glands with special reference to their mucin histochemistry. Acta Pathol Microbiol Scand 1977; 85:273–85.

31. Shafik A. A new concept of the anatomy of the anal sphincter mechanism and the physiology of defecation. X. Anorectal sinus and band: anatomic nature and surgical significance. Dis Colon Rectum 1980; 23:170–9.

32. Klosterhalfen B, Offner O, Vogel P, Kirkpatrick CJ. Anatomic nature and surgical significance of anal sinus and anal intramuscular glands. Dis Colon Rectum 1991; 34:156–60.

33. Kratzer GL, Dockerty MB. Histopathology of the anal ducts. Surg Gynecol Obstet 1947; 84:333–8.

34. Eisenhammer S. The internal anal sphincter and the anorectal abscess. Surg Gynecol Obstet 1956; 103:501–6.

   Sets the scene for Parks' 1976 classification where intersphincteric sepsis is the key.

35. Goligher JC, Ellis M, Pissides AG. A critique of anal glandular infection in the aetiology and treatment of idiopathic anorectal abscesses and fistulae. Br J Surg 1967; 54:977–83.

36. Seow-Choen F, Hay AJ, Heard S, Phillips RKS. Bacteriology of anal fistulae. Br J Surg 1992; 79:27–8.

37. Lunniss PJ, Faris B, Rees H, Heard S, Phillips RKS. Histological and microbiological assessment of the role of microorganisms in chronic anal fistulae. Br J Surg 1993; 80:1072.

38. Gordon-Watson C, Dodd H. Observations on fistula in ano in relation to perianal intermuscular glands. Br J Surg 1935; 22:703–9.

39. Lunniss PJ, Sheffield JP, Talbot IC, Thomson JPS, Phillips RKS. Persistence of anal fistula may be related to epithelialization. Br J Surg 1995; 82:32–3.

40. Thomson JPS, Parks AG. Anorectal abscesses and fistulas. Br J Hosp Med 1979; 417–24.

41. Eisenhammer S. A new approach to the anorectal fistulous abscess based on the high intermuscular lesion. Surg Gynecol Obstet 1958; 106:595–9.

42. Eisenhammer S. The final evaluation and classification of the surgical treatment of the primary anorectal, cryptoglandular intermuscular (intersphincteric) fistulous abscess and fistula. Dis Colon Rectum 1978; 21:237–54.

43. Hebjorn M, Olsen O, Haakanson T, Andersen B. A randomized trial of fistulotomy in perianal abscess. Scand J Gastroenterol 1987; 22:174–6.

44. Fucini C. One stage treatment of anal abscesses and fistulae. Int J Colorectal Dis 1991; 6:12–16.

45. Grace RH, Harper IA, Thompson RG. Anorectal sepsis: microbiology in relation to fistula-in-ano. Br J Surg 1982; 69:401–3.

The presence of gut organisms usually means a fistula; their absence excludes an underlying fistula.

46. Lunniss PJ, Phillips RKS. Surgical assessment of acute anorectal sepsis is a better predictor of fistula than microbiological analysis. Br J Surg 1994; 81:368–9.

47. Waggener HU. Immediate fistulotomy in the treatment of perianal abscess. Surg Clin North Am 1969; 49:1227–33.

48. McElwain JW, Maclean D, Alexander RM, Hoexter B, Guthrie JF. Anorectal problems: experience with primary fistulectomy for anorectal abscess. A report of 1000 cases. Dis Colon Rectum 1975; 18:646–9.

49. Schouten WR, van Vroonhoven ThJMV, van Berlo CLJ. Primary partial internal sphicterotomy in the treatment of anorectal abscess. Neth J Surg 1987; 39:43–5.

50. Schouten WR, van Vroonhoven ThJMV. Treatment of anorectal abscess with or without primary fistulectomy: results of a prospective randomized trial. Dis Colon Rectum 1991; 34:60–3.

51. Oliver I, Lacueva FJ, Perez Vicente F et al. Randomized clinical trial comparing simple drainage of anorectal abscess with and without fistula track treatment. Int J Colorectal Dis 2003; 18:107–10.

Primary fistulotomy in experienced hands is safe and effective.

52. Parks AG, Gordon PH, Hardcastle JD. A classification of fistula-in-ano. Br J Surg 1976; 63:1–12.

Landmark paper proposing the most widely used classification for anal fistula, known colloquially as the 'Parks classification'.

53. Marks CG. Classification. In: Phillips RKS, Lunniss PJ (eds) Anal fistula. Surgical evaluation and management. London: Chapman & Hall, 1996; pp. 33–46.

54. Goodsall DH, Miles WE. Diseases of the anus and rectum. London: Longmans, Green, 1890; p. 92.

55. Phillips RKS. Management of fistula-in-ano. Current medical literature. Gastroenterology 1989; 8:71–5.

56. Hawley PR. Anorectal fistula. Clin Gastroenterol 1975; 4:635–49.

57. Choen S, Burnett S, Bartram CI, Nicholls RJ. Comparison between anal endosonography and digital examination in the evaluation of anal fistulae. Br J Surg 1991; 78:445–7.

58. Fazio V. Complex anal fistulae. Gastroenterol Clin North Am 1987; 16:93–114.

59. Kuypers HC. Diagnosis and treatment of fistula-in-ano. Neth J Surg 1982; 34:147–52.

60. Gingold BS. Reducing the recurrence risk of fistula-in-ano. Surg Gynecol Obstet 1983; 156:661–2.

61. Glen DC. Use of hydrogen peroxide to identify internal opening of anal fistula and perianal abscess. Aust NZ J Surg 1986; 56:433–5.

62. Seow-Choen F, Phillips RKS. Insights gained from the management of problematical anal fistulas at St. Mark's Hospital, 1984–88. Br J Surg 1991; 78:539–41.

63. Weisman RI, Orsay CP, Pearl RK, Abcarian H. The role of fistulography in fistula-in-ano. Report of 5 cases. Dis Colon Rectum 1991; 34:181–4.

64. Pommeri F, Pittarello F, Dodi G, Pianon P, Muzzio PC. Diagnosi radiologica delle fistole anali con reperi radiopachi. Radiol Med 1988; 75:632–7.

65. Kuijpers HC, Schulpen T. Fistulography for fistula-in-ano. Dis Colon Rectum 1985; 28:103–4.

66. Tio TL, Mulder CJJ, Wijers OB, Sars PRA, Tytgat GNJ. Endosonography of perianal and pericolorectal fistula and/or abscess in Crohn's disease. Gastrointest Endosc 1990; 36:331–6.

67. Guillamin E, Jeffrey RB, Shea WJ, Asling CW, Goldberg HI. Perirectal inflammatory disease: CT findings. Radiology 1986; 161:153–7.

68. Youssem DM, Fishman EK, Jones B. Crohn's disease: perirectal and perianal findings at CT. Radiology 1988; 167:331–4.

69. Law PJ, Talbot RW, Bartram CI, Northover JMA. Anal endosonography in the evaluation of perianal sepsis and fistula-in-ano. Br J Surg 1989; 76:752–5.

70. Lunniss PJ, Barker PG, Sultan AH et al. Magnetic resonance imaging of fistula-in-ano. Dis Colon Rectum 1994; 37:708–18.

71. Lengyel AJ, Hurst NG, Williams JG. Pre-operative assessment of anal fistulas using endoanal ultrasound. Colorectal Dis 2002; 4:436–40.

72. Moscovitz I, Baig MK, Nogueras JJ et al. Accuracy of hydrogen enhanced endoanal ultra-sonography in the assessment of the internal opening. Colorectal Dis 1999; 1(suppl. 1):58.

73. Buchanan GN, Halligan S, Bartram CI, Williams AB, Cohen CRG. Anal endosonography and clinical evaluation of fistula-in-ano: prospective comparison with outcome derived gold standard. Br J Surg 2003; 90(suppl. 1):79.

74. Heiken JP, Lee JKT. MR Imaging of the pelvis. Radiology 1988; 166:11–16.

75. Koelbel G, Schmiedl U, Majer MC et al. Diagnosis of fistulae and sinus tracts in patients with Crohn disease: value of MR imaging. Am J Radiol 1989; 152:999–1003.

76. Lunniss PJ, Armstrong P, Barker PG, Reznek RH, Phillips RKS. Magnetic resonance imaging of anal fistulae. Lancet 1992; 340:394–6.

Initial demonstration of high accuracy and exquisite images of STIR images in demonstrating anal fistula tracks.

77. Beckingham IJ, Spencer JA, Ward J, Adams C, Dyke GW, Ambrose NS. Prospective evaluation of contrast enhanced magnetic resonance imaging in the evaluation of fistula *in ano*. Br J Surg 1996; 83(suppl. 1):42.

78. Buchanan GN, Halligan S, Williams AB et al. Magnetic resonance imaging for primary fistula *in ano*. Br J Surg 2003; 90:877–81.

79. Buchanan G, Halligan S, Williams A et al. Effect of MRI on clinical outcome of recurrent fistula-in-ano. Lancet 2003; 360:1661–2.

80. de Souza NM, Hau AS, Puni R et al. High resonance imaging of the anal sphincter using a dedicated endoanal coil. Comparison of magnetic resonance imaging with surgical findings. Dis Colon Rectum 1996; 92:738–41.

81. Stoker J, Fa VE, Eijkemans MJ, Schouten WR, Lameris JS. Endoanal MRI of perianal fistulas: the optimal imaging planes. Eur Radiol 1998; 8:1212–16.

82. Milligan ETC, Morgan CN. Surgical anatomy of the anal canal with special reference to anorectal fistulae. Lancet 1934; ii:1150–6, 1213–17.

The importance of the anorectal ring.

83. Lunniss PJ, Thomson JPS. The loose seton. In: Phillips RKS, Lunniss PJ (eds) Anal fistula. Surgical evaluation and management. London: Chapman & Hall, 1996; pp. 87–94.

84. Lunniss PJ, Kamm MA, Phillips RKS. Factors affecting continence after surgery for anal fistula. Br J Surg 1994; 81:1382–5.

85. Abcarian H. The 'lay open' technique. In: Phillips RKS, Lunniss PJ (eds) Anal fistula. Surgical evaluation and management. London: Chapman & Hall, 1996; pp. 73–80.

86. Friend WG. Anorectal problems: surgical incisions for complicated anal fistula. Dis Colon Rectum 1975; 18:652–6.

87. Hanley PH. Rubber band seton in the management of abscess–anal fistula. Ann Surg 1978; 187:435–7.

88. Parkash S, Lakshmiratan V, Gajendran V. Fistula-in-ano: treatment by fistulectomy, primary closure and reconstitution. Aust NZ J Surg 1985; 55:23–7.

89. Sood ID. Treatment of fistulae-in-ano and primary closure. In: Menda RK (ed.) Advances in proctology. Bombay: Indian Society for Diseases of Colon, Rectum and Anus, 1968:309–10.

90. Kronborg O. To lay open or excise a fistula-in-ano. A randomised trial. Br J Surg 1985; 72:970.

One of the few randomised trials in fistula surgery: lay open is better than fistulectomy in terms of length of time to wound healing.

91. Lewis A. Excision of fistula in ano. Int J Colorectal Dis 1986; 1:265–7.

92. Lewis A. Core out. In: Phillips RKS, Lunniss PJ (eds) Anal fistula. Surgical evaluation and management. London: Chapman & Hall, 1996; pp. 81–6.

93. Ramanujan PS, Prasad ML, Abcarian H. The role of seton in fistulotomy of the anus. Surg Gynecol Obstet 1983; 157:419–22.

94. Kuypers HC. Use of the seton in the treatment of extrasphincteric anal fistula. Dis Colon Rectum 1984; 27:109–10.

95. Parks AG, Stitz RW. The treatment of high fistula-in-ano. Dis Colon Rectum 1976; 19:487–99.

96. Thomson JPS, Ross AHMcL. Can the external sphincter be preserved in the treatment of trans-sphincteric fistula-in-ano? Int J Colorectal Dis 1989; 4:247–50.

97. Kennedy HL, Zegarra JP. Fistulotomy without external sphincter division for high anal fistula. Br J Surg 1990; 77:898–901.

98. Misra MC, Kapur BML. A new non-operative approach to fistula-in-ano. Br J Surg 1988; 75:1093–4.

99. Goldberg SM, Garcia-Aquilar J. The cutting seton. In: Phillips RKS, Lunniss PJ (eds) Anal fistula. Surgical evaluation and management. London: Chapman & Hall, 1996; pp. 95–102.

100. Held D, Khubchandani I, Sheets J, Stasik J, Rosen L, Reither R. Management of anorectal horseshoe abscess and fistula. Dis Colon Rectum 1988; 29:793–7.

101. Ustynovsky K, Rosen L, Stasik J, Reither R, Sheets J, Khubchandani IT. Horseshoe abscess fistula. Dis Colon Rectum 1990; 33:602–5.

102. Christensen A, Nilas L, Christiansen J. Treatment of trans-sphincteric anal fistulas by the seton technique. Dis Colon Rectum 1986; 29:454–5.

103. Deshpande PJ, Sharma KR. Treatment of fistula in ano by a new technique: review and follow-up of 200 cases. Am J Proctol 1973; 24:49–60.

104. Deshpande PJ, Sharma KR. Successful non-operative treatment of high rectal fistula. Am J Proctol 1976; 27:39–47.

105. Shukla NK, Narang R, Nair NG, Radha-Krishna S, Satyavati GV. Multicentric randomized controlled clinical trial of Kshaarasootra (Ayurvedic medicated thread) in the management of fistula-in-ano. Ind J Med Res 1991; 94:177–85.

Highlighted because it is a randomised controlled trial.

106. Wolffers I. Ayurvedic treatment for fistula-in-ano. Trop Doct 1986; 16:44.

107. Rangabashyam N. Management by chemical seton. In: Phillips RKS, Lunniss PJ (eds) Anal fistula. Surgical evaluation and management. London: Chapman & Hall, 1996; pp. 103–6.

108. Ho KS, Tsang C, Seoew-Choen F et al. Prospective randomized trial comparing ayurvedic cutting seton and fistulotomy for low fistula-in-ano. Tech Coloproctol 2001; 5:137–41.

Highlighted because it is a randomised controlled trial.

109. Noble GH. A new operation for complete laceration of the perineum designed for the purpose of eliminating danger of infection from the rectum. Trans Am Gynecol Soc 1902; 27:357–63.

110. Elting AW. The treatment of fistula in ano. Ann Surg 1912; 56:744–52.

111. Finan PJ. Management by advancement flap technique. In: Phillips RKS, Lunniss PJ (eds) Anal fistula. Surgical evaluation and management. London: Chapman & Hall, 1996; pp. 107–14.

112. Stone JM, Goldberg SM. The endorectal advancement flap procedure. Int J Colorectal Dis 1980; 4:188–96.

113. Kodner IJ, Mazor A, Shemesh EL, Fry RD, Fleshman JW, Birnbaum EH. Endorectal advancement flap repair of rectovaginal and other complicated anorectal fistulas. Surgery 1993; 114:682–90.

114. Oh C. Management of high recurrent anal fistula. Surgery 1983; 93:330–2.

115. Aquilar PS, Plasencia G, Hardy TG, Hartmann RF, Stewart WRC. Mucosal advancement in the treatment of anal fistula. Dis Colon Rectum 1985; 28:496–8.

116. Wedell J, Meier zu Eissen P, Banzhaf G, Kleine L. Sliding flap advancement for the treatment of high level fistulae. Br J Surg 1987; 74:390–1.

117. Jones IT, Fazio VW, Jagelman DG. The use of transanal rectal advancement flaps in the management of fistulas involving the anorectum. Dis Colon Rectum 1987; 30:919–23.

118. Reznick RK, Bailey HR. Closure of the internal opening for treatment of complex fistula-in-ano. Dis Colon Rectum 1988; 31:116–18.

119. Rutten H, Buth J. Treatment of high anorectal fistulas by anoplasty. Neth J Surg 1988; 40:93–6.

120. Lewis P, Bartolo DCC. Treatment of trans-sphincteric fistulae by full thickness anorectal advancement flaps. Br J Surg 1990; 77:1187–9.

121. Athanasiadis S, Kohler A, Nafe M. Treatment of high anal fistulae by primary occlusion of the internal ostium, drainage of the intersphincteric space, and mucosal advancement flap. Int J Colorectal Dis 1994; 9:153–7.

122. Lewis WG, Finan PJ, Holdsworth PJ. Clinical results and manometric studies after rectal flap advancement for infralevator trans-sphincteric fistula-in-ano. Int J Colorectal Dis 1995; 10:189–92.

123. Ozuner G, Hull TL, Cartmill J et al. Long-term analysis of the use of transanal rectal advancement flaps for complicated anorectal/vaginal fistulas. Dis Colon Rectum 1996; 39:10–14.

124. Del Pino A, Nelson RL, Pearl RK et al. Island flap anoplasty for treatment of transsphincteric fistula-in-ano. Dis Colon Rectum 1996; 39:224–6.

125. Jun SH, Choi GS. Anocutaneous advancement flap closure of high anal fistulas. Br J Surg 1999; 86:490–2.

126. Lunniss PJ. The role of the advancement flap technique. Semin Colon Rectal Surg 1998; 9:192–7.

127. Abel ME, Chiu YSY, Russell TR, Volpe PA. Autologous fibrin glue in the treatment of rectovaginal and complex fistulas. Dis Colon Rectum 1993; 36:447–9.

128. Cintron JR, Park JJ, Orsay CP et al. Repair of fistulas-in-ano using fibrin adhesive. Long-term follow-up. Dis Colon Rectum 2000; 43:944–50.

129. Sentovitch SM. Fibrin glue for anal fistulas. Dis Colon Rectum 2003; 46:498–502.

130. Zmora O, Mizrahi N, Rotholtz N et al. Fibrin glue sealing in the treatment of perineal fistulas. Dis Colon Rectum 2003; 46:584–9.

131. Buchanan GN, Bartram CI, Phillips RKS et al. Efficacy of fibrin sealant in the management of complex anal fistula. Dis Colon Rectum 2003; 46:1167–74.

132. Lindsey I, Smilgin-Humphreys MM, Cunningham C, Mortensen NJM, George BD. A randomized, controlled trial of fibrin glue vs. conventional treatment for anal fistula. Dis Colon Rectum 2002; 45:1608–15.

   A randomised controlled trial whose efficacy was not replicated in the St Mark's study above.

133. Matos D, Lunniss PJ, Phillips RKS. Total sphincter conservation in high fistula in ano: results of a new approach. Br J Surg 1993; 80:802–4.

134. Mann CV, Clifton MA. Re-routing of the track for the treatment of high anal and anorectal fistulae. Br J Surg 1985; 72:134–7.

135. Kupferberg A, Zer M, Rabinson S. The use of PMMA beads in recurrent high anal fistulae: a preliminary report. World J Surg 1984; 8:970–4.

136. Pinedo G, Phillips R. Labial fat pad grafts (modified Martius graft) in complex perianal fistulas. Ann R Coll Surg Engl 1998; 80:410–12.

137. Engel AF, Lunniss PJ, Kamm MA, Phillips RKS. Sphincteroplasty for incontinence after surgery for idiopathic fistula-in-ano. Int J Colorectal Dis 1997; 12:323–5.

138. Phillips RKS, Lunniss PJ. Approach to the difficult fistula. In: Phillips RKS, Lunniss PJ (eds) Anal fistula. Surgical evaluation and management. London: Chapman & Hall, 1996; pp. 177–82.

139. Harrison BJ, Read GF, Hughes LE. Endocrine basis for the clinical presentation of hidradenitis suppurativa. Br J Surg 1988; 75:472–5.

Fourteen

Minor anorectal conditions

Francis Seow-Choen and
Ming Hian Kam

HAEMORRHOIDS

The term 'haemorrhoids' is widely used but rarely fully understood. The word is derived from the Greek *haem* meaning blood and *rhoos* meaning flow. Hence, one should have bleeding in order to truly have haemorrhoids. On the other hand, the word 'piles' is derived from the Latin *pila* meaning ball or swelling. It describes the swelling that occurs when there is prolapse. However, both terms are in regular popular use, with the layman favouring 'piles'.

But what are these things we call piles or haemorrhoids? It is now widely accepted that piles are derived from anal cushions. Anal cushions are normal structures found in the anal canal, consisting of mucosa, submucosal fibroelastic connective tissues and smooth muscles on an arteriovenous channel system.[1] Anal cushions complement anal sphincter function by providing fine control over the continence of liquids and gases.[2]

Pathogenesis and aetiology

The anal cushions function normally when they are fixed in their proper sites within the anal canal by submucosal smooth muscle and elastic fibres (Treitz's muscle). These fibres may be fragmented by prolonged downward stress related to straining during defecation of hard stools. It is quite common for patients with piles to have some constipation.[3] In addition, the bleeding and pain from smaller haemorrhoids often settle with correction of bowel function alone.[4]

When the supporting submucosal fibres fragment, the anal cushions are no longer restrained from engorging excessively with blood and this results in bleeding and prolapse. Veins that traverse the anal sphincter are blocked whereas arterial flow continues, leading to increasing haemorrhoidal congestion. Defecation in the squatting position may also aggravate the tendency to prolapse.

Constipation certainly aggravates the symptoms of haemorrhoids. Interestingly, diarrhoea is also a potential risk factor and the tenesmus from diarrhoea causes straining that aggravates haemorrhoids. Other factors have been implicated, such as heredity, erect posture, absence of valves within the haemorrhoidal plexus and draining veins, as well as impedence of venous return from raised intra-abdominal pressure. Portal hypertension may lead to engorgement of the haemorrhoidal plexus. Pregnancy is associated with a higher risk of haemorrhoids and undoubtedly aggravates pre-existing disease. Per rectal bleeding or other 'haemorrhoidal' symptoms cannot be assumed to be due to haemorrhoids until proper investigations have been carried out. Patients with inflammatory bowel disease or even rectal tumours may present with similar symptoms and the diagnosis will otherwise be missed unless further tests are carried out.

Anatomy and nomenclature

External skin tags arise from the perianal skin and represent the end result of thrombosed external haemorrhoids. These usually do not require treatment unless causing discomfort to the patient, such as getting caught in clothing resulting in occasional bleeding from trauma.

External haemorrhoids comprise the dilated vascular plexuses located below the dentate line, covered by squamous epithelium.[5] They may swell and cause some discomfort. Bleeding is not usually the predominant complaint but quite severe pain can arise as a result of acute thrombosis.

Internal haemorrhoids are symptomatic arteriovenous channels sited above the dentate line and covered by transitional and columnar epithelium. They are divided into subcategories in order of severity, from first-degree to fourth-degree haemorrhoids. The definitions of each, as well as their management, are outlined in **Box 14.1**.

Management

Firstly, it must be recognised that haemorrhoids may coexist with other conditions such as rectal cancer.[6] Patients who have symptoms including blood or mucus mixed in the stools, change in bowel habit, abdominal symptoms and family history of colorectal cancer should have further evaluation of the colon and rectum.

Secondly, the anal cushions are normal functional anatomical structures. They aid in the maintenance of continence, swelling with blood at rest and being compressed at higher pressures during squeeze. They do not require treatment unless symptomatic. Therapeutic strategies then depend upon symptoms and the amount of haemorrhoidal tissue prolapsing beyond the anal verge.[7]

NON-PROLAPSING OR MILDLY PROLAPSING HAEMORRHOIDS

If the piles are not permanently prolapsed, non-operative methods should be attempted first. The

Box 14.1 • Management of internal haemorrhoids

First-degree haemorrhoids (bleeding but no prolapse)

- High-fibre diet
- Daflon (not available in the UK)

Second-degree haemorrhoids (prolapse but spontaneously reducible)

- Rubber band ligation
- Sclerotherapy
- Electrocoagulation
- (Haemorrhoidectomy)

Third-degree haemorrhoids (prolapse requiring manual reduction)

- Rubber band ligation
- Sclerotherapy
- Electrocoagulation
- (Haemorrhoidectomy)

Fourth-degree haemorrhoids (irreducible prolapse)

- Haemorrhoidectomy

primary problems of constipation and straining at stool need to be addressed. Although some patients may benefit from increased dietary fibre, many other patients may need some form of laxative to improve bowel action. A randomised controlled trial showed that a 6-week trial of fibre supplements was more effective in treating bleeding and discomfort from internal piles than placebo.

Other forms of treatment that can give more immediate symptomatic relief include rubber band ligation, injection sclerotherapy, medications such as Daflon 500 (currently not available in the UK), as well as toilet re-education. Topical applications are popular with many patients who testify to relief from bleeding and pain. There are, however, no clinical trials to demonstrate any benefit from such applications.

Rubber band ligation

In this technique, rubber bands are applied at the base of the haemorrhoidal tissue. The strangulated tissue then becomes necrotic and sloughs off in a few days, after which the wound fibroses, resulting in fixation of the mucosa.[8] The pile tissue is thus prevented from engorging and prolapsing. Up to three haemorrhoids can be banded on the same occasion. Theoretically, it is relatively painless if the bands are placed above the dentate line, but some patients have severe tenesmus and a feeling of engorgement that is only partially relieved by analgesia. Banding is usually 60–80% effective, depending on proper selection of cases.[9] There is a 2–5% risk of secondary haemorrhage, for which the patient should be warned to return for medical advice.

In a study to evaluate the long-term results of combined rubber band ligation and sclerotherapy,[10] there was a recurrence rate of 16% and the overall complication rate was 3.1% with minor bleeding being chief among them. At median follow-up of 6.5 years, there were 19% with residual symptoms of bleeding, 21% with itch and 20% with a lump; 58% were asymptomatic and only 7.7% ultimately went on to haemorrhoidectomy.

Injection sclerotherapy

Sclerosant agents used include phenol (5%) in almond oil or sodium tetradecyl sulphate. These are injected into the submucosa around the pedicle of the pile, at the level of the anorectal ring. The sclerosant is likely to cause inflammation, leading to reduced blood flow into the haemorrhoid. This technique is about 70% effective. The sclerosant also causes fibrosis, which draws minor prolapse back into the anal canal.

The correct plane is shown by elevation of the mucosa without blanching during injection. Inappropriately deep injections can cause perirectal fibrosis, infection and urethral irritation. Prostatic injection is intensely painful and the patient may develop an erection, a strong desire to void, haematuria or haemospermia. Severe sepsis is not uncommon and such patients should be admitted for antibiotics and observation until completely well.

Other methods

Daflon 500, available in Singapore but not currently available in the UK, is micronised diosmin and hesperidin, which belong to the hydroxyethylrutoside group of drugs.[11] Its pharmacological properties include noradrenaline-mediated venous contraction,[12] reduction in blood extravasation from capillaries[13]

and inhibition of prostaglandin (PGE$_2$, PGF$_2$) inflammatory response.[14]

 These properties have a proven therapeutic action in the symptomatic relief of haemorrhoidal symptoms.[15] Adverse effects have been minimal.[16,17]

These drugs are widely used in the Far East as first-line treatment for piles.[18]

Various other methods are also available. These include infrared photocoagulation, which requires additional equipment, and cryotherapy, which results in unpleasant discharge. For such reasons, these methods have not been popular. Topical preparations that may contain local anaesthetics or steroids are also available, often without prescription. To date, there is no evidence that such agents are any more effective than spontaneous remissions. Moreover, patient self-treatment may delay the diagnosis of serious diseases such as cancer and can therefore be potentially harmful.

IRREDUCIBLE PROLAPSED PILES

The majority of patients are well treated by non-surgical methods. However, when anal cushions have prolapsed or thrombosed, they no longer function effectively to maintain continence and surgery may then be needed. In fact, sensory function may be impaired and this may partially account for the complaints of minor incontinence by some patients.

Traditionally, prolapsed piles are removed by excisional haemorrhoidectomy. Although there are variations to the technique,[19–24] the main problems encountered remain similar. These are mainly postoperative pain,[20,25,26] anal incontinence[27] and haemorrhage.

 Open haemorrhoidectomy may lead to faster and more reliable wound healing where three large prolapsed irreducible piles are excised.[19]

Some authors have described post-haemorrhoidectomy pain as like passing pieces of sharp glass fragments, such that many patients would rather suffer the discomfort of large prolapsing haemorrhoids for years rather than submit to surgery.

Nonetheless, third- and fourth-degree haemorrhoids are more appropriately treated by surgery, which is conventionally performed by excision of the three primary piles. Minor variations in conventional excisional haemorrhoidectomy include whether the wounds are left to granulate or closed with sutures, whether the pedicle is ligated, or whether the piles are excised with scissors or diathermy.

Nevertheless, some patients will have more severe circumferential prolapse with massive engorgement of both external and internal haemorrhoidal plexuses. Such large haemorrhoids require extensive ablation to ensure adequate treatment in order to prevent residual or recurrent symptoms.

In the past, such haemorrhoids have been dealt with by either standard haemorrhoidectomy plus excision of the largest secondary pile with subsequent mucocutaneous reconstitution or a modification of the Whitehead or radical haemorrhoidectomy.

In a study comparing Whitehead with four-pile haemorrhoidectomy, we concluded that four-pile haemorrhoidectomy was significantly easier to perform and although residual tags and piles were left behind, the operation was preferred to radical haemorrhoidectomy.[28,29]

Currently, however, this discussion may be immaterial as stapled haemorrhoidectomy adequately addresses most circumferential prolapses.[30]

Stapled haemorrhoidectomy

Conventional surgical haemorrhoidectomy is not based on a correction of pathophysiology but on ablation of symptoms. Hence, if prolapsed piles are bleeding, painful or otherwise symptomatic, these piles are excised.

However, prolapsed haemorrhoids are not always symptomatic. Furthermore, totally asymptomatic individuals can be made to engorge their anal cushions during proctoscopy by straining or performing the Valsalva manoeuvre. This sort of engorgement is aggravated by straining in the squatting position. Once prolapse occurs, further engorgement of these vascular cushions leads to pain and an inflammatory response. Anal spasm then prevents reduction and pathological changes such as thrombosis, oedema and inflammation occur.

Chronicity is caused by a vicious cycle of prolapse and congestion of these vascular cushions. The vascular cushions hence prolapse easily and allow the anal sphincters to constrict, resulting in further congestion, oedema and pain.

Conventional haemorrhoidectomy deals with the symptoms alone without due regard to restoration of the normal physiology by fixation of the congested anal cushions. On the other hand, stapled haemorrhoidectomy tries to correct the primary pathology, resulting in resolution of haemorrhoidal symptoms.[31,32] After reduction of any prolapsed haemorrhoidal tissue, this technique then excises redundant lower rectal mucosa, fixing the prolapse back into its proper place on the wall of the anal canal. This fixation into muscle is in our opinion important to help prevent subsequent re-dislodgement and recurrence. As previously mentioned, once reduced the engorged haemorrhoidal tissue has the opportunity to decongest and shrink. We believe this theory is borne out in clinical practice. Our technique of stapled haemorrhoidectomy takes into account these pathophysiological changes and attempts to carefully correct them all.[33] Although there are concerns of long-term pain following stapled haemorrhoidectomy, this has not been seen in larger series.[34]

In a recent clinical trial by Ortiz et al.,[35] stapled haemorrhoidopexy was associated with a lower pain intensity compared with the conventional haemorrhoidectomy group. However, a total of seven patients in the stapled group re-presented within 15 months with prolapse compared with none in the conventional group. There were no significant differences in the total number of complications, the length of absence from work or control of symptoms.

However, stapled haemorrhoidectomy on its own cannot deal adequately with massive haemorrhoidal prolapse. Massive haemorrhoids are prolapsed haemorrhoids more than 3–4 cm outside the anal verge. In this situation, there is not enough space within the staple housing to contain the massive redundant tissue of the prolapsed haemorrhoids.

A modified stapled haemorrhoidectomy technique has been developed in our department to deal with massive haemorrhoidal prolapse using one circular PPH stapler, and this has been found to be safe and effective.[36] Another more expensive alternative might be to use two staplers simultaneously. In fact, stapled haemorrhoidectomy has also been used for acute thrombosed circumferentially prolapsed piles[37] and has been found to be feasible and perhaps even result in less pain, a more rapid resolution of symptoms and an earlier return to work when compared with conventional Milligan–Morgan haemorrhoidectomy.[38]

Postoperative problems

Some problems that occur after haemorrhoidectomy include severe pain, urinary retention, bleeding and faecal impaction. Studies have shown that pain is significantly diminished after stapled haemorrhoidectomy and the patient is able to go home a few hours after the operation. This has led to many advocates for stapled haemorrhoidectomy in the day-surgery setting.[39–41] Nevertheless, many surgeons perform conventional haemorrhoidectomy, both open and closed, in a day-care setting with high patient satisfaction.

Even so, whichever technique is used, pain is still an important consideration in the postoperative period. It is multifactorial, with spasm of the internal sphincter believed to play an important role.

Use of botulinum toxin has been shown to reduce pain towards the end of the first postoperative week.[42] The use of 0.2% glyceryl trinitrate (GTN) ointment is also associated with decreased postoperative pain, and contributes to more rapid healing of wounds after excisional haemorrhoidectomy by a single surgeon.[43] Others have tried lateral sphincterotomy with haemorrhoidectomy with some success,[44] but we would not advocate this because of potential permanent adverse effects.

The amount of pain after stapled haemorrhoidectomy depends on the height of mucosectomy above the anal verge. Removal of squamous epithelium results in greater intensity of postoperative pain and should be avoided.[45]

Another less frequent problem is postoperative haemorrhage. This may be primary, presenting in the immediate postoperative period and usually due to technical problems, or secondary as a result of postoperative infection. Submucosal adrenaline (epinephrine) injection[46] has been shown to be effective for addressing such bleeding and avoiding a reoperation.

Post-haemorrhoidectomy anal stricture is an uncommon occurrence seen in only 3.7% of haemorrhoidectomies.[47] The stricture usually presents at 6 weeks postoperatively and up to two-thirds may be managed conservatively with stool-bulking agents and local anaesthetic gels in the outpatient setting. The remaining one-third may require an anoplasty. Although uncommon, the key to management lies in its prevention, with the maintenance of adequate skin and mucosal bridges intraoperatively and close follow-up postoperatively to detect stricture formation early.

On the other hand, some believe that the use of an anal dilator in the course of stapled haemorrhoidectomy may be associated with a higher rate of anal sphincter damage. This has been shown to be true in a randomised trial.[48]

However, there were no differences in continence scores or anal pressures, the main difference being the persistence of internal anal sphincter fragmentation beyond 14 weeks postoperatively.

Sepsis after treatment of haemorrhoids

Sepsis after either conservative or operative treatment is uncommon, but when it occurs delay in treatment can be catastrophic. The incidence of transient bacteraemia from blood cultures after haemorrhoidectomy is 5–11%,[49] but this did not result in any cases of clinical sepsis.

In a review by Guy and Seow-Choen,[50] injection sclerotherapy has been reported to result in life-threatening retroperitoneal sepsis and rectal perforation. Urological sepsis can result from a misplaced deep anterior injection with complications such as prostatic abscess, epididymitis, chronic cystitis, seminal vesicle abscess and urinary–perineal fistula. Even with rubber band ligation, complications such as pain and haemorrhage result in 14% of patients.

It would seem that symptoms such as perineal pain, urinary retention and fever occurring at 2–7 days after treatment usually portend the onset of local sepsis and this may lead to progressive oedema and cellulitis of the perineum, thigh and abdomen. Contributory factors include immuno-deficiency and general debility. The placement of bands in a faecally loaded anorectum may theoretically result in incorporation of faeces or a local abscess. Thus administration of an enema before banding and aseptic technique, including povidone-iodine and use of sterile instruments, seems rational.

Colonisation of anal wounds occurs frequently, but the true incidence of resultant wound infection is difficult to estimate as definitions vary widely. The common colonisers include *Escherichia coli* and *Staphylococcus aureus*, followed by *Pseudomonas aeruginosa*, *Enterococcus faecalis*, *Klebsiella pneumoniae*, *Proteus vulgaris* and *Proteus mirabilis*. Culture of 'infected' haemorrhoids, on the other hand, has revealed a predominance of anaerobes like *Bacteroides fragilis* and *Peptostreptococcus*.

In a randomised trial by Carapeti et al.,[51] metronidazole was shown to reduce pain on days 5–7 after open, largely day-case haemorrhoidectomy, resulting in a shorter time to normal activity and greater patient satisfaction. It was proposed that a reduction in bacterial colonisation was an important factor.

Secondary haemorrhage, which has often been attributed to local infection, affects approximately 5% of patients undergoing haemorrhoidectomy.[25] The advocated treatment is antibiotics; the incidence does not seem to be increased after emergency haemorrhoidectomy.

Bacteraemia is also associated with haemorrhoidectomy.

A prospective randomised study of 250 patients by Maw et al.[49] showed that 11% of patients undergoing stapled haemorrhoidectomy and 5% of those undergoing diathermy haemorrhoidectomy had positive blood cultures after the operations.

These were predominantly anaerobes, commonly found in the anorectal bacterial flora. However, this transient bacteraemia did not result in serious clinical consequences such as sepsis in any of the patients.

Conclusion

Haemorrhoidal disease is a common anorectal disease. Its aetiology is likely related to inadequate dietary fibre and there is associated straining at defecation. As a result, the supports of the submucosal anal cushions weaken. Anal cushions are normal structures that line the anal canal. They contain arteriovenous channels and increase and decrease in size according to blood flow. Variation in their size has an important function in helping to seal the anal canal, thereby controlling faecal continence. When the anal cushion support is weakened, it becomes susceptible to abnormal engorgement with blood, resulting in symptomatically bleeding and prolapsing haemorrhoids.

When treating haemorrhoids, other possibly life-threatening disease such as rectal cancer has first to be excluded by adequate history, physical examination (including rectal digital examination) and, if necessary, endoscopy. Non-prolapsing and reducible prolapsing piles can usually be treated with preservation of the anal cushions. Fibre supplements alone can be effective. However, submucosal injection and rubber band ligation may accelerate symptomatic relief. Irreducible prolapsed piles may be treated either by excisional haemorrhoidectomy or, in our view preferentially, by stapled haemorrhoidectomy.

ANAL FISSURE

Anal fissures are common, representing up to 10% of new referrals to colorectal clinics. The majority of patients present with acute fissures, which respond well to local as well as oral painkillers in addition to increased dietary fibre intake. The anal pain associated with fissures classically presents during defecation and persists for a few minutes to hours afterwards. There may be associated fresh rectal bleeding and patients may have a history of an abnormal bowel habit. If there is concomitant haemorrhoidal disease, the bleeding may be more significant.

However, some patients present with chronic fissures. We define a chronic fissure as one that does not heal within 6 weeks despite adequate medical therapy.[9] If patients have signs of chronicity on examination, such as a sentinel skin tag or an intra-anal fibroepithelial polyp, then they should also be classified as having chronic fissures regardless of the duration of their symptoms, as these anatomical changes cannot have happened over a short time period.

Clinical findings

Pain may not be the predominant symptom in chronic fissures. Bleeding or the presence of a perianal skin tag may be more distressing to the patient. As always in history taking, symptoms like altered bowel habit and defecatory patterns must be elicited, and if there is a suspicion, a proximal colonic lesion must first be excluded.

Perianal and digital rectal examination usually demonstrates a skin tag (sentinel pile) overlying the external edge of a chronic anal fissure. Indeed, the fissure itself may be missed if the sentinel pile is not retracted to reveal the fissure. Although usually single and situated in the 6 o'clock position, some 2.5–10% may be sited in the 12 o'clock position.[52] If fissures are multiple or eccentrically located, inflammatory bowel disease, tuberculosis, syphilis or HIV infection must be considered.

When the pain is minimal, a gentle digital examination and proctoscopy may be done. This will show a fibrotic ulcer with white transverse internal sphincter fibres exposed. There may be a hypertrophic papilla at the internal edge of the fissure. The presence of rectal mucosal prolapse or haemorrhoids is not unusual.

Aetiology

Historically, fissures were thought to be due to the passage of a hard bolus of faeces causing a tear in the anal mucosa. A recent review by Hananel and Gordon[53] showed that only 10% of patients complained of constipation and 30% needed to strain during defecation. Another 10% developed fissures after childbirth.

Internal anal sphincter hypertonia is another hypothesis that has sparked much interest. The main determinant of resting pressure in the anal canal is the internal sphincter, which is in a continuous state of partial contraction, mediated through α-adrenergic pathways. Relaxation occurs automati-

cally in response to rectal distension due to the rectoanal inhibitory reflex.

Patients with chronic anal fissure commonly have a raised resting anal pressure from internal anal sphincter hypertonia.[54] Administration of pharmacological agents to relax the internal sphincter has been shown to lead to fissure healing, but the resting anal pressure returns to pretreatment levels once the fissure has healed and treatment ceased.[55] Internal sphincter hypertonia and anal spasm predate the onset of the fissure. This anal spasm does not seem to be a response to pain because application of topical local anaesthetics relieves pain but does not reduce the anal spasm.[56]

Over the past decade, local ischaemia has been gaining credence as a significant aetiological event in chronic fissures. There is a paucity of arterioles in the posterior commissure of 85% of cadaveric cases with reduced anodermal blood flow compared with controls.[57]

There are other hypotheses regarding aetiology. Brown et al.[58] suggested that an inflammatory process is responsible, with early myositis proceeding to fibrosis. Partial eversion of the anal canal during evacuation is inhibited anteriorly and posteriorly due to tethering, resulting in tearing of the tissue.[59] Finally, with decussation of the external sphincter muscle, there is weakness anteriorly and posteriorly, with tears occurring when hard stools are passed.[60]

Postpartum anal fissures are more commonly anterior, with the risk increasing in traumatic deliveries. Shearing forces from passage of the fetal head may be significant, compounded by the tethering of the anal mucosa to the skin. Although patients do not appear to have a raised internal anal sphincter resting pressure, they do complain of constipation, and this may contribute to fissure formation. The clinician should be wary of an underlying occult sphincter injury.

Medical treatment

Dietary modification is important. Indeed, a high-fibre diet with high water intake alone may be sufficient for acute fissures and may also contribute to healing of chronic fissures. Topical anaesthetic gels like 1% lidocaine (lignocaine) or lubricated anal dilators may be attempted for acute fissures, but results are not always satisfactory and recurrence rates are high.

The recognition of nitric oxide as a neurotransmitter mediating the relaxation of the internal sphincter[61] has led to many studies examining the use of isosorbide dinitrate and GTN to treat chronic fissures.

Different authors have tried oral, patch, sprayed and topical GTN, and 0.2% GTN topical ointment has become the standard as it achieves optimal healing in up to 70% of cases with minimal adverse effects (predominantly headaches).[62,63]

Comparisons of topical GTN with lateral sphincterotomy have also been made in recent trials.

Oettle[64] randomised 24 patients to either sphincterotomy or 0.2% GTN three times a day. All 12 patients with sphincterotomy healed whereas 2 of 12 in the GTN group did not. These two patients had no pain relief after a week and sphincterotomy led to good healing. The Canadian Colorectal Surgical Trials Group[65] randomised 82 patients to receive either sphincterotomy or 0.25% GTN three times a day. At 6 weeks, 34 (89.5%) in the sphincterotomy group had achieved healing compared with 13 (29.5%) in the GTN group. Of these 13 in the GTN group, five subsequently suffered a relapse.

Despite more favourable results from surgery, the enthusiasm for local creams has not diminished, mainly because of concerns of usually mild faecal incontinence after sphincterotomy.

Calcium channel blockers such as nifedipine and diltiazem have been shown to reduce the resting anal pressure in patients with chronic fissures.[66]

Both oral[67] and topical preparations have shown healing in up to 67% of patients. Patients who are already on these drugs for hypertension and ischaemic heart disease may be unsuitable for this form of treatment, although they are unlikely to have fissures.

The parasympathomimetic bethanecol has been shown to lower resting anal pressure and may be useful in conjunction with other topical medications. Indoramin, an α-adrenoceptor blocker, and

salbutamol, a β-adrenoceptor agonist, are further possible alternatives.

Botulinum A toxin (Botox) reduces resting anal pressure and promotes healing of anal fissures in 70–96% of patients.[68]

In a double-blind placebo-controlled trial, Maria et al.[69] showed that botulinum toxin resulted in healing of 11 of 15 anal fissures compared with only 2 of 15 in the placebo group.

The mode of action remains unclear. The toxin binds to presynaptic cholinergic nerve terminals and inhibits the release of acetylcholine at the neuromuscular junction. This should lead to relaxation of the external sphincter but should have no corresponding effect on the internal sphincter. However, Brisinda et al.[70] have shown that maximal squeeze pressures were no different from pretreatment levels at 1–2 months after injection. The site of optimal injection is still unclear and complications include transient faecal incontinence, perianal haematoma, pain and sepsis.

For all the advantages of medical treatment, there is still no answer for sentinel piles and fibrous polyps that often accompany chronic fissures. These remain distressing to the patient as there may be associated pain and bleeding from trauma to sentinel piles or persistent tenesmus or soilage due to the presence of the fibrous polyp. Surgical excision, at the time of lateral sphincterotomy, offers not only good recovery of the fissure but removes the sentinel pile and fibrous polyp at the same time.

Surgical treatment

We believe that uncontrolled anal stretch or dilatation should not be performed any longer.[71]

An uncontrolled fracturing of the internal sphincter by this method, although shown to have good rates of healing, nevertheless results in an unacceptably high incidence of incontinence with unknown long-term consequences. Posterior midline sphincterotomy is not favoured either; its results are not superior to lateral sphincterotomy and a gutter (keyhole) defect may lead to soiling.

Patients who have failed medical treatment or who have features of chronicity such as sentinel piles should be offered lateral sphincterotomy.[72,73] This may be performed by either an open or closed method, each showing similar results.[71]

A current concern is the length of optimal internal sphincter division.[74,75] Classically, sphincterotomy was done with division of the internal sphincter up to the level of the dentate line. In a tailored sphincterotomy, the sphincter is divided up to the highest point of the fissure only. In practice this is gauged by eye-balling the distance between the top of the fissure and the dentate line and performing sphincterotomy accordingly. However, it is difficult to measure the exact length of division and also to study and compare the results between the two groups. There are many variations of technique but none has been shown to be superior. Most authors have described healing rates of 85–95%.

Sphincterotomy, by virtue of its division of the internal sphincter musculature, predisposes to incontinence to flatus and faecal soilage in up to 35% of patients.[74,76] Surgical removal of the fissure (fissurectomy) with subsequent use of isosorbide dinitrate cream has been shown to be effective, with no recurrence and no internal sphincter defects on postoperative endosonography.[77] This relatively new technique is as yet unverified by a randomised controlled trial, although it presents a novel approach to an age-old problem.

Recurrent or atypical fissures

If the fissure is not in the anterior or posterior midline, then Crohn's disease or immunosuppressive conditions like AIDS must be considered. These patients should not be offered surgery at the first consultation and further intestinal and anal investigation with anal manometry and anal sphincter mapping (usually by endoanal ultrasound) should be performed. Even so, in their series Fleschner et al.[78] showed that 88% of patients with Crohn's-associated fissures healed after lateral sphincterotomy compared with only 49% on medical treatment. Furthermore, no significant increase in complications was noted in the sphincterotomy group.

Authors who believe in the ischaemic nature of chronic fissures cite this as the reason behind recurrences. Internal sphincter hypertonia leads to reduced blood flow, which in turn results in tissue hypoxia and consequent failure of healing. Hyperbaric oxygen therapy ostensibly provides increased oxygenation to hypoperfused tissue and induces neovascularisation, collagen synthesis and fibroblast replication, thus enhancing the repair process. In a study by Cundall et al.,[79] five of eight patients had healed fissures at the end of 3 months, and all showed symptomatic improvement with regard to pain and bleeding.

In patients with recurrence after lateral sphincterotomy, anal manometry and anal ultrasound are essential as they separate patients with low resting anal pressures from patients with persistently raised resting pressures and will identify those who might benefit from repeat lateral sphincterotomies in the opposite lateral quadrant.

Patients with low resting sphincter pressures may be helped by anal cutaneous advancement flaps along with fissurectomy. It is reasonable to believe that these patients will not experience improved blood flow to the fissure after sphincterotomy as sphincter hypertonia was probably not a causative factor in the first place. As such, further sphincterotomy will only increase the risk of incontinence. Nyam et al.[80] and Leong and Seow-Choen[52] have shown that an island advancement flap from the perianal skin healed most fissures.

Conclusion

Anal fissures are common and aetiology is multifactorial. There are many options for chemical sphincterotomy with good results but lateral sphincterotomy remains the gold standard for chronic anal fissures.

PRURITUS ANI

Pruritus ani is a vexing problem to both surgeons and patients. When the cause remains elusive and cure cannot be achieved, there may be intense frustration on both sides. The actual incidence is not known as many people still view this as a minor inconvenience and do not seek medical treatment in the early stages.

Aetiology and pathogenesis

Although causes of perianal itch include many anorectal and dermatological conditions (**Box 14.2**), in many instances a primary cause cannot be found. Indeed, idiopathic pruritus ani is usually associated

Box 14.2 • Secondary causes of prurutis ani

Neoplasia

- Rectal adenoma
- Rectal adenocarcinoma
- Anal squamous cell carcinoma
- Malignant melanoma
- Bowen's disease
- Extramammary Paget's disease

Benign anorectal conditions

- Haemorrhoids
- Fistula in ano
- Anal fissure
- Rectal prolapse
- Anal sphincter injury or dysfunction
- Faecal incontinence
- Radiation proctitis
- Ulcerative colitis

Infections

- Condyloma acuminatum
- Herpes simplex virus
- *Candida albicans*
- Syphilis
- Lymphogranuloma venereum

Dermatological

- Neurogenic dermatitis
- Contact dermatitis
- Lichen simplex
- Lichen planus
- Lichen atrophicus

with a minor degree of faecal incontinence. The object of history taking and examination is to find the likely cause of leakage. This may be due to local pathology permitting stool to leak to the outside, such as a fissure, fistula or prolapsing haemorrhoid, or to a high-fibre diet, leading to difficulty with anal cleaning and fragments of stool becoming trapped in the anal canal, only to seep out later and set up irritation. There may be internal sphincter dysfunction[81–83] or other contributory causes such as irritative foods (spices, alcohol and caffeine). In addition, scratching, applications of inappropriate topical creams (local anaesthetics as they are sensitive to the skin; strong steroids as they lead to dependence of the skin) and excessive cleansing of the perianal skin exacerbate this condition.

Diagnosis

The diagnosis is most often revealed by good history taking and physical examination alone, especially for causes of minor anal leakage. Important facts such as duration of symptoms, dietary habits, recent travel history and change in bowel habits should be elucidated.

Physical examination should start with a general inspection of the patient for dermatological disease elsewhere on the body. Then the perineum and underclothes should be inspected for soilage. Perianal skin changes are noted, particularly excoriation and ichthyosis, as this indicates long-standing pruritus.

Specific examination of the perineum includes a digital rectal examination for anal tone and squeeze. It may help to wipe the anus with moistened gauze; a brown stain will confirm anal leakage, a frequent cause of itching. Palpation for polyps, malignancies and fistula tracks is required and patients should also be examined while straining to exclude any prolapse. Proctoscopy should be performed. Further examination using endoscopy, radiology or laboratory tests may be required in certain cases. Skin lesions should be biopsied and examined for fungal elements.

A commonly quoted cause of pruritus ani in the young is *Enterobius* or threadworm. These may be seen on sigmoidoscopy, or 'Sellotape' may reveal the diagnosis. This involves the placement of a piece of adhesive tape to the anus. This is then removed and placed onto a glass microscopy slide. The presence of ova is indicative of infection.

Treatment

Treatment is dependent on the primary pathology. Haemorrhoids can be easily treated by rubber band ligation or haemorrhoidectomy. Perianal skin tags may be excised and fissures treated as outlined in the previous section. Threadworm infections can be treated with mebendazole or piperazine.

In primary pruritus ani, the aims of treatment are the reduction of leakage, maintenance of good personal hygiene and the prevention of further injury to the perianal skin. Leakage can be reduced by avoidance of food that produces flatulence, such as fibre, which also makes stools soft and mushy. If the stool is loose, addition of an antimotility agent such as codeine or loperamide may be beneficial until the skin has healed and dietary modification has taken effect. A somewhat mushy stool frequently gets trapped in the top of the anus at the end of defecation, whereas this does not seem to happen with a harder stool. On walking, any trapped stool tends to massage out and cause irritation. Advice to patients regarding this mechanism will help them to help themselves.

Basic hygiene should be advocated. This involves daily cleansing of the anus using water, not soap, and drying the area with a soft towel or dryer. Perfumed talcum powder should be avoided. Loose underwear made of natural fibres should be worn.

If the patient feels like scratching it is usually because of fresh leakage. Further attention to hygiene may then obviate the desire to scratch, which at times can otherwise be well nigh irresistible. Short-term use of a hydrocortisone cream may help to break the cycle but this should not last for long as the skin may atrophy or become dependent upon the steroid and itch in its absence.

In a recent study by Lysy et al.,[84] topical capsaicin has been shown to be effective in treatment of idiopathic pruritus ani; 44 patients were randomised to topical capsaicin 0.006% or placebo (menthol 1%) and crossover was carried out after 4 weeks. Of these patients, 31 experienced relief with capsaicin but not with menthol. None of the patients resistant to capsaicin were relieved with menthol.

Conclusion

Pruritus ani remains a difficult problem to manage and results of treatment of primary pruritus ani remain equivocal. Treatment is aimed at reducing leakage, whether arising from a fistula, prolapsing haemorrhoid or simply increased flatulence. Good personal hygiene remains an important aspect of treatment and prevention of further irritation to the perianal skin.

ANAL STENOSIS

Anal stenosis can be structural or functional. This section deals with structural stenosis, which is an abnormal fixed anatomical narrowing of the anal canal associated with a degree of functional obstruction at that level.[85] This is in contrast to anal canal spasm secondary to painful lesions (commonly seen in anal fissures) or to defecatory functional abnormalities but which on examination show a supple and fully compliant anus.

Aetiology

The commonest cause is post surgical,[86] usually after haemorrhoidectomy that has left only tenuous bridges, but other causes are given in **Box 14.3**. Recurrent anal fissures, perianal abscesses with repeated surgical procedures and excessive excision of perianal skin in Bowen's or Paget's disease may heal with anal canal stenosis. Chronic laxative abuse, especially those of mineral oils, over prolonged periods may lead to anal stenosis, but frequently the patient has a functional problem with anal relaxation rather than a structural one of anal stenosis.

Clinical presentation

A history of constipation, decreasing stool calibre, difficulty in voiding with the need to strain excessively and tenesmus are usually the first symptoms of anal stenosis. In severe cases, only loose stools may be passed. The clinician should be wary of some patients on laxative or enemas for their long-standing 'constipation' who may actually have a functional problem. Bleeding occurs when there is an associated anal fissure from traumatic

Box 14.3 • Aetiology of anal stenosis

Congenital

- Imperforate anus
- Anal atresia

Acquired

- Irradiation
- Lacerations
- Chronic diarrhoea
- Following surgery of anal canal/low rectum

Neoplastic

- Perianal or anal cancers
- Leukaemia
- Bowen's disease
- Paget's disease

Inflammatory

- Crohn's disease
- Tuberculosis
- Amoebiasis
- Lymphogranuloma venereum
- Actinomycosis

Spastic

- Chronic anal fissure
- Ischaemic

defecation. However, a fissure in the absence of anal spasm may be seen in patients who anally digitate and thereby traumatise the anus. These patients usually have a functional problem of obstructed defecation. The diagnosis is usual obvious on perineal inspection. Often, the passage of an index finger through the narrowing is impossible. If the finger is passed (and particularly if a proctoscope can be passed), there is usually no clinically significant stenosis. Associated surgical scars may sometimes give an indication of the cause of stenosis. A biopsy is essential if a predisposing cause for the anal stenosis is suspected. The anatomical findings may not correlate well with the magnitude of the symptoms.[87]

Treatment

The key to treatment lies firstly in its prevention. Excessive removal of the anoderm is often the cause of significant anal stenosis. Excision of the perianal skin to achieve a 'cosmetically' smooth and even skin contour does not always result in smooth anal function. Surgical judgement leaning towards only adequate excision of haemorrhoidal tissue and anoderm is often prudent. Eversion of any haemorrhoidal mass and excision may often lead to excessive removal of the anoderm. In particular, the Whitehead procedure for circumferential haemorrhoids may put the anal canal at risk of developing anal stenosis[88] and associated mucosal ectropion as the scar contracts towards the perineum. In a review of 704 patients who had undergone excisional haemorrhoidectomy (500 elective and 204 emergency cases) over a 2-year period, 3.8% developed clinical evidence of anal stenosis.[89] No difference was seen between either elective or emergency cases.

ANAL DILATATION

Treatment of anal stenosis depends on the severity and level of stenosis within the anal canal, as well as when it has arisen if in relation to a precipitating anal operation. Mild or moderate stenosis (tight anal canal but permitting the passage of the index finger on pressure or forceful dilatation) may be treated with bulk laxatives, which will increase the stool calibre and provide a dilatory effect.

This may be supplemented with regular stretching, the patient using either his or her own finger or an appropriately sized anal dilator (e.g. St Mark's anal dilator or size 18 Hagar dilator). Initial dilatation may need to be performed under anaesthesia. The patient should understand how to use the dilator before hospital discharge. This may be performed in the left lateral position or with the patient squatting and bearing down onto a well-lubricated (4% lidocaine jelly) finger or anal dilator. The patient should be guided to pass the dilator beyond the anal stricture twice daily for 2 weeks. Good functional results may be achieved in this manner, particularly if a postsurgical stenosis is caught early. The additional use of topical steroids has no documented benefits.

Severe anal stenosis, with inability to pass the index finger through the stenosis, will always require at least some initial form of surgical intervention, if only examination under anaesthesia with graded Hagar's dilatation. The principles of surgical treatment are outlined in **Box 14.4**.

Four-finger manual dilatation performed under anaesthesia should be discouraged and is anyway unnecessary. It may lead to excessive damage of the anal sphincters with resultant incontinence, especially in the hands of a novice. Jensen et al.[90] and MacDonald et al.[91] both reported a high rate of faecal incontinence after dilatation (39% and 24% respectively), especially in the female patients who already have a pre-existing anatomically shorter anal canal. However, a very scarred and stenotic anus, or one associated with Crohn's disease, may be self-maintained using Hagar's dilators after initial Hagar's graded dilatation under general anaesthesia.

SPHINCTEROTOMY

If the 'stenosis' is due to a hypertrophied internal anal sphincter, then lateral anal sphincterotomy will be indicated. Localised scars in the anal canal are not likely to cause stenosis. Circumferential mucosal scarring will usually require some form of relining of the anal canal, usually by an anoplasty. However, we believe that there is a role for sphincterotomy in a circumferentially scarred anus. It is simple to perform and if a single sphincterotomy is insufficient to open up the stenosis, multiple sphincterotomies may be done at different positions. Open sphincterotomy has the advantage of allowing the ingrowth of anoderm to maintain the increase in diameter of the anal canal. Sphincterotomy will provide immediate relief of any pain and apprehension associated with bowel opening in these patients. Associated complications are infrequent and minor and include inadvertent nicking of the haemorrhoidal vessels (0.3–0.8%), failed healing (2–6%) and abscess formation when the anoderm is accidentally breached in closed haemorrhoidectomy (0–2%). Impaired faecal continence has been reported to vary from 11 to 25%, while late faecal incontinence of some degree varies from 4 to 35%.[92,93] If there is circumferential mucosal or cutaneous scarring, restenosis is likely.

FLAP PROCEDURES

Mucosal advancement flap

This involves the advancement of anal mucosa into the stenotic area by way of a vertical incision made in the stenotic area perpendicular to the dentate line in the lateral position. An anal sphincterotomy and excision of the scar tissue allows widening of the stenosis. The incision is then undermined for about 2 cm and closed in a transverse manner with vicryl 3/0, stitching the mucosal edge down onto the skin edge of the anoderm. This creates a minor mucosal ectropion, which will keep the stenosis open.

Y-V advancement flap

Originally described by Penn in 1948, a Y incision is made, with the vertical limb of the Y in the anal canal above the proximal level of the stenosis. The 'V' of the Y is drawn on the lateral perianal skin. The skin is incised and a V-shaped flap is raised; the length to breadth ratio must be less than 3. After excision of the underlying scar tissue in the anal canal with or without an additional lateral sphincterotomy, the flap can be mobilised into the anal canal and stitched into place. This may be done bilaterally with good results[94,95] and provides relief in 85–92% of cases. Tip necrosis occurs in 10–25% of cases and stenosis may then recur.

V-Y advancement flap

Unlike the Y-V advancement flap, the V-Y flap has the advantage of bringing a wider piece of skin into the stenosis to keep it open. The V is drawn with the wide base parallel to the dentate line about 2 cm long. A similar length-to-base ratio as in the

---

Box 14.4 • Principles of surgical treatment for anal stenosis

- Stool bulking
- Increase anal outlet dimensions
- Examination under anaesthesia with graded Hagar's dilatation followed by postoperative self-maintenance
- Sphincter narrowing: internal sphincterotomy
- Removal of cutaneous scarring
- Maintain correction
- Skin advancement (inwards)
- Mucosal advancement (outwards)
- Colostomy

Y-V flap should be maintained. The scar tissue is excised. Marking out of the skin flap is followed by its mobilisation such that it may move without tension into the anal canal. Sufficient subcutaneous tissue must be mobilised with the flap, which derives its blood supply from the perforating vessels arising within the fat. The skin is then closed behind the flap to produce the limb of the Y. A treatment success rate of 96% has been reported with this flap.

Island advancement flap

First described in 1986 by Caplin and Kodner,[96] the island flap may be constructed in various shapes (e.g. diamond, house or U-shaped). The flap is mobilised from its lateral margins together with the subcutaneous fat after the scar tissue in the stenotic area has been excised. A lateral sphincterotomy may or may not be performed. A broad skin flap (up to 50% of the circumference) may be brought into the entire length of the anal canal and simultaneously allow for closure of the donor site. Improvement of symptoms may be as high as 91% at 3 years of follow-up;[97,98] 18–50% suffer minor wound separation.

S-anoplasty

This procedure mobilises bilateral gluteal skin into the entire anal canal after excision of the scar tissue up to the dentate line. The incision is designed in an S shape, hence the name of the flap. The breadth-to-length ratio must be more than 1, with the base of the S being about 7–10 cm. The skin is rotated to line the anal canal in a tension-free manner. This extensive procedure is rarely used. Prior full bowel preparation and perioperative antibiotic cover is advocated.

Conclusion

Most of the above treatments and surgical procedures will adequately deal with postsurgical anal canal stenosis, which usually involves the lower anal canal. Occasionally, a higher stenosis (above the dentate line) is encountered. In this instance, we believe a lateral sphincterotomy or division of the fibrotic band may be sufficient as the anal canal is more distensible at this level. However, in perianal Crohn's disease-related anal stenosis, we usually try to provide symptomatic relief with anal dilators, sometimes after prior examination under anaesthesia, in the hope of avoiding surgical wound problems.

• **Key points**

- Haemorrhoidal disease is common but other life-threatening diseases must first be excluded. Treatment by fibre supplements, submucosal injection, rubber band ligation or micronised flavonoids allow for symptomatic relief but consideration should be given to stapled in favour of excisional haemorrhoidectomy for prolapsing piles.
- Anal fissures are common and their aetiologies multifactorial. Although chemical sphincterotomies have been performed with good results, lateral sphincterotomy remains the gold standard for chronic anal fissures.
- Pruritis ani may result from many anorectal or dermatological conditions and remains a difficult problem to manage and treat. Reduction of anal leakage and good personal hygiene remain important aspects of treatment.
- Anal stenosis has many aetiologies but the commonest is a result of anal surgery. Treatments range from anal dilatation to flap procedures, and sphincterotomies may provide immediate symptomatic relief.

REFERENCES

1. Haas PA, Fox TA, Haas GP. The pathogenesis of haemorrhoids. Dis Colon Rectum 1984; 27:442–50.

2. Jorge JM, Wexner SD. Anorectal manometry: techniques and clinical applications. South Med J 1993; 86:924–31.

3. Johanson JF, Sonnenberg A. Constipation is not a risk factor for haemorrhoids: a case–control study of potential etiological agents. Am J Gastroenterol 1994; 89:1981–6.

4. Moesgaard F, Nielsen ML, Hansen JB, Knudsen JT. High fibre diet reduces bleeding and pain in patients with haemorrhoids. Dis Colon Rectum 1992; 25:454–6.

5. Gordon PH, Santhat Nivatvongs (eds) Haemorrhoids. Principles and practice of surgery for the colon, rectum and anus. 2nd edn. Marcel Dekker, 1999.

6. Ho YH, Goh HS. Current value of anorectal physiology and biofeedback in clinical practice. Asian J Surg 1995; 18:244–56.

7. Ho YH. Management of haemorrhoidal disease: a review. Phlebology 1997; 15:3–6.

8. Nicholls J, Glass R. Coloproctology. Diagnosis and outpatient management. Berlin: Springer-Verlag, 1985.

9. Keighley MRB, Williams NS. Surgery of the anus, rectum and colon. London: WB Saunders, 1993.

10. Chew SS, Marshall L, Kalish L et al. Short-term and long-term results of combined sclerotherapy and rubber band ligation of haemorrhoids and mucosal prolapse. Dis Colon Rectum 2003; 46:1232–7.

11. Wadworth AN, Faulds D. Hydroxyethylrutosides. A review of its pharmacology and therapeutic efficacy in venous insufficiency and related disorders. Drugs 1992; 44:1013–32.

12. Duhalt J. Mecanism d'action de Daflon 500mg sur le tonus veineux noradrenergique. Arteres Veines 1992; 11:217–18.

13. Galley P. A double-blind, placebo-controlled trial of a new venoactive flavonoid fraction (S5682) in the treatment of symptomatic fragility. Int Angiol 1993; 12:69–71.

14. Damon M. Effect of chronic treatment with purified flavonoid fraction on inflammatory granuloma in the rat. Study of prostaglandin E2 and F2 and thromboxane B2 release and histological changes. Arzneimittelforschung 1987; 37:1149–53.

15. Cospite M. Double-blind versus placebo evaluation of clinical activity and safety of Daflon 500 mg in the treatment of acute haemorrhoids. Angiology 1994; 6:566–73.

Inflammation, congestion, oedema and prolapse were more markedly improved in the Daflon 500 group, giving quicker and more pronounced symptomatic relief.

16. Ho YH, Foo CL, Seow-Choen F, Goh HS. Prospective randomized controlled trial of micronized flavonidic fraction to reduce bleeding after haemorrhoidectomy. Br J Surg 1995; 82:1034–5.

Postoperative Daflon reduced the risk of secondary haemorrhage without any adverse effects.

17. Ho YH, Goh HS. Unilateral anal electrosensation: modified technique to improve quantifications of anal sensory loss. Dis Colon Rectum 1995; 38:239–44.

18. Ho YH, Tan M, Seow-Choen F. Micronized purified flavonidic fraction compared favourably with rubber band ligation and fiber alone in the management of bleeding haemorrhoids. Dis Colon Rectum 2000; 43:66–9.

19. Ho YH, Seow-Choen F, Tan M, Leong APFK. Randomised trial of open and closed haemorrhoidectomy. Br J Surg 1997; 84:1729–30.

Open haemorrhoidectomy leads to faster and more reliable wound healing.

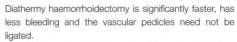

20. Seow-Choen F, Ho YH, Ang HG, Goh HS. Prospective, randomized trial comparing pain and clinical function after conventional scissor excision/ligation vs. diathermy excision without ligation of symptomatic prolapsed haemorrhoids. Dis Colon Rectum 1992; 35:1165–9.

Diathermy haemorrhoidectomy is significantly faster, has less bleeding and the vascular pedicles need not be ligated.

21. Ho YH, Seow-Choen F, Goh HS. Haemorrhoidectomy and disordered rectal and anal physiology in patients with prolapsed haemorrhoids. Br J Surg 1995; 82:596–8.

22. Ho YH, Seow-Choen F, Low JY, Tan M, Leong APKF. Effect of trimebutine (anal sphincter relaxant) on post haemorrhoidectomy pain tested in a controlled prospective randomized trial. Br J Surg 1997; 84:377–9.

Although Proctolog reduced mean resting anal pressure at 4 hours after application, this did not affect pain after haemorrhoidectomy.

23. Ho KS, Eu KW, Heah SM, Seow-Choen F, Chan YW. Randomized clinical trial of haemorrhoidectomy under a mixture of local anaesthesia versus general anaesthesia. Br J Surg 2000 Apr; 87(4): 410–3.

(Topical anaesthetics and local anaesthesia can provide an effective alternative to general anaesthesia for patients undergoing haemorrhoidectomy.)

24. Jane Tan JY, Seow-Choen F. Prospective randomised trial comparing diathermy and harmonic scalpel haemorrhoidectomy. Dis Colon Rectum 2001; 44:677–9.

25. Eu KW, Seow-Choen F, Goh HS. Comparison of emergency and elective haemorrhoidectomy. Br J Surg 1994; 81:308–10.

26. Ibrahim S, Tsang C, Lee YL, Eu KW, Seow-Choen F. Prospective, randomized trial comparing pain and complications between diathermy and scissors for closed hemorrhoidectomy. Dis Colon Rectum 1998; 41:1418–20.

Diathermy closed haemorrhoidectomy required less postoperative medication than scissors except in the first 24 hours.

27. Ho YH, Tan M. Ambulatory anorectal manometric findings in patients before and after haemorrhoidectomy. Int J Colorectal Dis. 1997; 12(5): 296–7.

28. Seow-Choen F, Low HC. Prospective randomized study of radical versus four piles haemorrhoidectomy for symptomatic large circumferential prolapsed piles. Br J Surg 82:188–9.

Patient satisfaction was greater in four-pile haemorrhoidectomy although there was a higher incidence of anal skin tags and symptomatic residual piles. There were five cases of wound dehiscence after radical haemorrhoidectomy and the stricture rate was almost equal.

29. Kraemer M, Seow-Choen F. Whitehead haemorrhoidectomy in older patients. Tech Coloproct 2000; 4:79–82.

30. Seow-Choen F. Stapled haemorrhoidectomy: pain or gain. Br J Surg 2000; 88:1–3.

31. Seow-Choen F. Surgery for haemorrhoids: ablation or correction. Asian J Surg 2002; 25:265–6.

32. Corman ML, Gravie JF, Hager T, Loudon MA, Mascagni D, Nystrom PO, Seow-Choen F, Abcarian H, Marcello P, Weiss E, Longo A. Stapled haemorrhoidopexy: a consensus position paper by an international working party - indications, contra-indications and technique. Colorectal Dis. 2003 Jul; 5(4): 304–10. Review.

33. Lloyd D, Ho KS, Seow-Choen F. Modified Longo's haemorrhoidectomy. Dis Colon Rectum 2002; 45:416–17.

34. Cheetham MJ, Mortensen NJ, Nystrom PO, Kamm MA, Phillips RK. Persistent pain and faecal urgency after stapled haemorrhoidectomy. Lancet 2000; 356:730–3.

35. Ortiz H, Marzo J, Armendariz P. Randomized clinical trial of stapled haemorrhoidopexy versus conventional diathermy haemorrhoidectomy. Br J Surg 2002; 89:1376–81.

Although stapled haemorrhoidectomy had significantly less pain, the rate of recurrent prolapse was also higher.

36. Jayne D, Seow-Choen F. Modified stapled haemorrhoidectomy for treatment of massive circumferentially prolapsing piles. Tech Coloproctol 2002; 6:191–3.

37. Brown SR, Ballan K, Ho E, Ho YH, Seow-Choen F. Stapled mucosectomy for acute thrombosed circumferentially prolapsed piles: a prospective randomized comparison with conventional haemorrhoidectomy. Colorectal Dis 2001; 3:175–8.

Stapled mucosectomy is feasible for thrombosed piles and results in less pain, more rapid symptom resolution and earlier return to work.

38. Milligan ETC, Morgan CN, Jones LE, Officer R. Surgical anatomy of the anal canal and the operative treatment of haemorrhoids. Lancet 1937; ii:1119–24.

39. Ho YH, Lee J, Salleh I, Leong A, Eu KW, Seow-Choen F. Randomized controlled trial comparing same-day discharge with hospital stay following haemorrhoidectomy. Aust NZ J Surg 1998; 68:334–6.

Same-day discharge reduced the total hospitalisation stay and in turn reduced cost without affecting pain scores, analgesia requirements, postoperative complications, patient satisfaction and time off work.

40. Guy RJ, Ng CE, Eu KW. Stapled anoplasty for haemorrhoids: a comparison of ambulatory vs. in-patient procedures. Colorectal Dis 2003; 5:29–32.

41. Ho YH, Cheong WK, Tsang C et al. Stapled hemorrhoidectomy: cost and effectiveness. Randomized, controlled trial including incontinence scoring, anorectal manometry, and endoanal ultrasound assessments at up to three months. Dis Colon Rectum 2000; 43:1666–75.

Stapled hemorrhoidectomy is a safe and effective option in treating irreducible prolapsed piles. It is more expensive but less painful, with less time needed off work. Total complications, anorectal manometry and endoanal ultrasound showed no differences when compared with conventional surgery.

42. Davies J, Duffy D, Boyt N, Aghahoseini A, Alexander D, Leveson S. Botulinum toxin (Botox) reduces pain after haemorrhoidectomy: results of a double-blind, randomized study. Dis Colon Rectum 2003; 46:1097–102.

Using a visual analogue scale, it was shown that although there was no significant difference in morphine usage within 24 hours postoperatively, there was significantly less pain towards the end of the first week. This was presumed to be due to a reduction in internal sphincter spasm.

43. Hwang do Y, Toon SG, Kim HS, LeeJK, Kim KY. Effect of 0.2 percent glyceryl trinitrate ointment on wound healing after a haemorrhoidectomy: results of a randomized, prospective, double-blind, placebo-controlled trial. Dis Colon Rectum 2003; 46:950–4.

This study shows more rapid healing with glyceryl trinitrate ointment at 3 weeks of 74.5% vs. 42% using placebo. There was no difference in consumed amounts of analgesics.

44. Mathai V, Ong BC, Ho YH. Randomized controlled trial of lateral internal sphincterotomy with haemorrhoidectomy. Br J Surg 1996; 83:380–2.

The addition of lateral sphincterotomy to conventional haemorrhoidectomy did not provide any benefit and carries the risk of incontinence.

45. Correa-Rovelo JM, Tellez O, Obregon L et al. Prospective study of factors affecting postoperative pain and symptom persistence after stapled rectal mucosectomy for haemorrhoids: a need for preservation of squamous epithelium. Dis Colon Rectum 2003; 46:955–62.

46. Nyam DCNK, Seow-Choen F, Ho YH. Submucosal adrenaline injection for post-haemorrhoidectomy haemorrhage. Dis Colon Rectum 1995; 38:776–7.

47. Eu KW, Teoh TA, Seow-Choen F, Goh HS. Anal stricture following haemorrhoidectomy: early diagnosis and treatment. Aust NZ J Surg 1995; 65:101–3.

48. Ho YH, Seow-Choen F, Tsang C, Eu KW. Randomized trial assessing anal sphincter injuries after stapled haemorrhoidectomy. Br J Surg 2001; 88:1449–55.

Internal anal sphincter fragmentation persisting to 14 weeks was found in four patients after stapled haemorrhoidectomy using the anal dilator but there was no difference in continence scores and anal pressures. This may become problematic with ageing.

49. Maw A, Concepcion R, Eu KW et al. Prospective randomized study of bacteremia in diathermy and stapled haemorrhoidectomy. Br J Surg 2003; 90:222–6.

50. Guy RJ, Seow-Choen F. Septic complications after treatment of haemorrhoids. Br J Surg 2003; 90:147–56.

51. Carapeti EA, Kamm MA, McDonald PJ, Phillips RKS. Double-blind randomized controlled trial of effect of metronidazole on pain after day-case haemorrhoidectomy. Lancet 1998; 351:169–72.

Prophylactic metronidazole afforded better pain relief at 5–7 days postoperatively and allowed for earlier return to work.

52. Leong AFPK, Seow-Choen F. Lateral sphincterotomy compared with anal advancement flap for chronic anal fissure. Dis Colon Rectum 1995; 38:69–71.

53. Hananel N, Gordon PH. Re-examination of clinical manifestations and response to treatment of fissure-in-ano. Dis Colon Rectum 1997; 40:229.

54. Keck JO, Staniunas RJ, Coller JA, Barrett RC, Oster ME. Computer-generated profiles of the anal canal in patients with anal fissure. Dis Colon Rectum 1995:38; 72–9.

55. Lund JN, Parsons JL, Scholefield JH. Spasm of the internal anal sphincter in anal fissure: cause or effect? Gastroenterology 1996; 110:A711.

56. Minguez M, Tomas-Ridocci M, Garcia A, Benages A. Pressure of the anal canal in patients with haemorrhoids or anal fissure: effect of the topical application of an anaesthetic gel. Rev Esp Enfirm Dig 1992; 81:103–7.

57. Klosterhalfen B, Vogel P, Rixen H, Mittermayer C. Topography of the inferior rectal artery: a possible cause of chronic, primary anal fissure. Dis Colon Rectum 1989; 32:43–52.

58. Brown AC, Sumfest JM, Rozwadowski JV. Histopathology of the internal anal sphincter in chronic anal fissure. Dis Colon Rectum 1989; 32:680.

59. Schouten WR, Briel JW, Auwerda JJ, De-Graaf EJ. Ischaemic nature of anal fissure. Br J Surg 1996; 83:63–5.

60. Smith LE. Anal fissure. Neth J Med 1990; 37:S33.

61. Chakder S, Rattan S. Release of nitric oxide by activation of noradrenergic noncholinergic neurons of internal anal sphincter. Am J Physiol 1993; 264:G7.

62. Lund JN, Scholefield JH. A randomized, prospective, double-blind, placebo-controlled trial of glycerin trinitrate ointment in the treatment of anal fissure. Lancet 1997; 349:11–14.

Sustained relief of pain in patients with anal fissure was demonstrated. Over two-thirds of patients treated with topical GTN avoided surgery.

63. Carapeti EA, Kamm MA, McDonald PJ, Chadwick SJ, Melville D, Phillips RK. Randomized controlled trial shows that glyceryl trinitrate heals anal fissures, higher doses are not more effective, and there is a high recurrence rate. Gut 1999; 44:727–30.

Two-thirds of patients had resolution of fissures with topical GTN and one-third of those healed suffered a recurrence. Headaches were reported in 72% of patients on GTN.

64. Oettle GJ. Glyceryl trinitate versus sphincterotomy for treatment of chronic fissure-in-ano: a randomized controlled trial. Dis Colon Rectum 1997; 40:1318–20.

Local GTN healed 80% of fissures while sphincterotomy healed 100%.

65. Richard CS, Gregorie R, Plewes EA et al. Internal sphincterotomy is superior to topical nitroglycerin in the treatment of chronic anal fissure: results of a randomized trial by the Canadian Colorectal Surgical Trials Group. Dis Colon Rectum 2000; 43:1048–57.

66. Jonas M, Neal KR, Abercrombie JF, Scholefield JH. A randomized trial of oral vs topical diltiazem for chronic anal fissure. Dis Colon Rectum 2001; 44:1074–8.

Topical diltiazem was shown to be more effective than the oral form.

67. Cook TA, Humphreys MMS, McC Mortensen NJ. Oral nifedipine reduces resting anal pressure and heals chronic anal fissure. Br J Surg 1999; 86:1269–73.

68. Maria G, Sganga G, Civello IM, Brisinda G. Botulinum neurotoxin and other treatments for fissure-in-ano and pelvic floor disorders. Br J Surg 2002; 89:950–61.

69. Maria G, Cassetta E, Gui D, Brisinda G, Bentivoglio AR, Albanese A. A comparison of botulinum toxin and saline for the treatment of chronic anal fissure. N Engl J Med 1998; 338:217–20.

70. Brisinda G, Maria G, Bentivoglio AR, Cassetta E, Gui D, Albanese A. A comparison of injections of botulinum toxin and topical nitroglycerin ointment

for the treatment of chronic anal fissures. N Engl J Med 1999; 341:65–9.

71. Nelson R. Operative procedures for fissure in ano (meta-analysis). Cochrane Library, vol. 3, 2003.

Botulinum toxin was effective in treatment of anal fissure, with a healing rate of 73%.

72. Griffith J. Anal fissure: Aetiology and current management choices. Proceedings: Fourth Singapore General Hospital Colorectal Week 1998.

73. Lund JN, Scholefield JH. Aetiology and treatment of anal fissure. (Review) Br J Surg 1996 Oct; 83(10): 1335–44.

74. Khubchandani IT, Reed JF. Sequelae of internal sphincterotomy for chronic fissure-in-ano. Br J Surg 1989; 76:431.

75. Littlejohn DR, Newstead GL. Tailored lateral sphincterotomy for anal fissure. Dis Colon Rectum 1997; 40:1439–42.

76. Garcia-Aguilar J, Belmonte C, Wong WD, Lowry AC, Madoff RD. Open vs closed sphincterotomy for chronic anal fissure: long-term results. Dis Colon Rectum 1996; 39:440–3.

77. Engel AF, Eijsbouts QAJ, Balk AG. Fissurectomy and isosorbide dinitrate for chronic fissure-in-ano not responding to conservative treatment. Br J Surg 2002; 89:79–83.

78. Fleschner PR, Schoetz DJ Jr, Roberts PL, Murray JJ, Coller JA, Veidenheimer MC. Anal fissure in Crohn's disease: a plea for aggressive management. Dis Colon Rectum 1995; 38:1137–43.

79. Cundall JD, Gardiner A, Laden G, Grout P, Duthie GS. Use of hyperbaric oxygen to treat chronic anal fissure. Br J Surg 2003; 90:452–3.

80. Nyam DCNK, Wilson RG, Stewart KJ, Farouk R, Bartolo DC. Island advancement flaps in the management of anal fissures. Br J Surg 1995; 82:326–8.

81. Eyers AA, Thomson JP. Pruritis ani: is anal sphincter dysfunction important in aetiology? Br Med J 1979; 2:1549–51.

82. Allan A, Ambrose NS, Silverman S, Keighley MR. Physiological study of pruritis ani. Br J Surg 1987; 74:576–9.

83. Farouk R, Duthie GS, Pryde A, Bartolo DC. Abnormal transient internal sphincter relaxation in idiopathic pruritis ani: physiological evidence from ambulatory monitoring. Br J Surg 1994; 81:603–6.

84. Lysy J, Sistiery-Ittah M, Israelit Y et al. Topical capsaicin: a novel and effective treatment for idiopathic intractable pruritus ani. A randomised, placebo controlled, crossover study. Gut 2003; 52:1323–6.

Capsaicin was effective in treatment of pruritis ani in 31 of 44 patients.

85. Luchtefeld MA, Mazier WP. Anal stenosis. In: Fazio VW (ed.) Current therapy in colon and rectal surgery. Philadelphia: BC Decker, 1990; pp. 46–59.

86. Khubchandani IT. Anal stenosis. Surg Clin North Am 1994; 74:1353–60.

87. Tang CL. Anal stenosis. Proceedings: Fourth Singapore General Hospital Colorectal Week, 1998; 20–22.

88. Rosen L. Anoplasty. Surg Clin North Am 1988; 68:1441–6.

89. Eu KW, Teoh TA, Seow-Choen F, Goh HS. Anal stricture following haemorrhoidectomy: early diagnosis and treatment. Aust NZ J Surg 1995; 65:101–3.

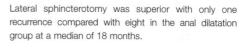

90. Jensen SL, Llund F, Nielsen OV, Tange G. Lateral subcutaneous sphincterotomy versus anal dilatation in the treatment of fissure-in-ano in outpatients: a prospective randomised study. Br Med J 1984; 289:528–30.

Lateral sphincterotomy was superior with only one recurrence compared with eight in the anal dilatation group at a median of 18 months.

91. MacDonald A, Smith A, McNeill AD, Finlay IG. Manual dilatation of the anus. Br J Surg 1992; 79:1381–2.

92. Senogore AJ. Surgery for chronic anal fissure and stenosis. In: Hicks TC, Bek DE, Opelka FG, Timmcke AE (eds) Complications of colon and rectal surgery. Baltimore: Williams and Wilkins, 1996; pp. 193–202.

93. Prager E. Common ailments of the anorectal region: anal stenosis. In: Block GE, Moossa AR (eds) Operative colorectal surgery. Philadelphia: WB Saunders, 1994; pp. 413–14.

94. Angelchik PD, Harms BA, Stanley JR. Repair of anal stricture and mucosal ectropion with YV or pedicle flap anoplasty. Am J Surg 1993; 166:55–9.

95. Ramanujam PS, Venkatesh KS, Cohen M. YV anoplasty for severe anal stenosis. Contemp Surg 1998; 3:62–8.

96. Caplin DA, Kodner IJ. Repair of anal stricture and mucosal ectropion by single flap procedures. Dis Colon Rectum 1986; 29:92.

97. Pidala MJ, Slezak FA, Porter JA. Island advancement anoplasty for anal canal stenosis and mucosal ectropion. Am Surg 1994; 60:194–6.

98. Sentovich SM, Falk PM, Christensen MA, Thorson AG, Blatchford GJ, Pitsch RM. Operative results of house advancement anoplasty. Br J Surg 1996; 83:1242–4.

Fifteen

Sexually transmitted diseases and the anorectum

Charles B. Whitlow and
David E. Beck

INTRODUCTION

Sexually transmitted diseases (STDs) are important to colorectal surgeons as many of them cause gastro-intestinal symptoms and produce lesions in the perineum, anus and rectum. An explosive growth in their prevalence and variety has occurred in the past two decades, which can be traced to increases in promiscuity, homosexuality and the use of the anorectum for sexual gratification. Anogenital, oro-anal and other anal-based erotic practices have increased, with approximately 2–2.5 million British citizens regularly using the anorectum for sexual fulfilment.[1,2] Similarly, 4–13% of the adult male population of the USA are predominantly homo-sexual or bisexual for at least a significant portion of their lives.[3] Promiscuity also plays a major role in the transmission of the vast majority of these diseases. It has been estimated that the average homosexual has about 1000 sexual partners during his lifetime,[3,4] while other studies suggest that even a 'moderately active' homosexual man will have sexual relations with 100 men a year.[5,6]

STDs of the anorectum also affect females who participate in anal intercourse. Review of surveys of sexual practices suggests that heterosexual anal intercourse is far more common than generally realised, more than 10% of American women and their male consorts engaging in the act with some regularity.[7]

The frequent occurrence of STDs (estimated at over 15 million cases a year in the USA) and the gastrointestinal symptoms associated with these infections mandate a high index of suspicion in order to make an accurate diagnosis. Providers must remember that these patients commonly have more than one disease.[8,9] The diseases presented in **Table 15.1** are categorised by aetiological agent. Medications and dosages are suggested, but clinicians are reminded to consult the full prescribing information before using any medication mentioned in this chapter.

VIRAL

Cytomegalovirus

Cytomegalovirus (CMV) is a ubiquitous DNA virus. Positive cultures or serology are very common in immunosuppressed patients. More than 90% of patients with acquired immunodeficiency syndrome (AIDS) develop an active CMV infection and it is the most commonly identified pathogen in culture-negative diarrhoea in AIDS patients.[10,11] CMV can cause inflammation, haemorrhage, ulceration or perforation of the gastrointestinal tract. Ileocolitis

Table 15.1 • Sexually transmitted and infectious organisms that cause anorectal pathology

Organism	Symptoms	Anoscopy and proctoscopy	Laboratory test	Treatment
Viral				
Cytomegalovirus	Rectal bleeding	Multiple small white ulcers	Biopsy, viral culture, antigen assay of ulcers	Intravenous ganciclovir, foscarnet
Herpes simplex	Anorectal pain, pruritus	Perianal erythema, vesicles, ulcers, diffusely inflamed, friable rectal mucosa	Cytological examination of scrapings or viral culture of vesicular fluid	Symptomatic: aciclovir, famciclovir, valaciclovir (see text)
Human immunodeficiency virus (AIDS)	See text	See text	Western blot	Nucleoside analogues, non-nucleoside reverse transcriptase inhibitors, protease inhibitors
Human papillomavirus (condylomata acuminatum)	Pruritus, bleeding, discharge, pain	Perianal warts	Excisional biopsy with viral analysis	Destruction, imiquimod (see text)
Molluscum contagiosum	Painless dermal lesions	Flattened round umbilicated lesions	Excisional biopsy	Excision, cryotherapy
Bacterial				
Campylobacter jejuni	Diarrhoea, cramps, bloating	Erythema, oedema, greyish-white ulcerations of rectal mucosa	Culture stool using selective media	Oral erythromycin 500 mg q.i.d. for 7 days
Chlamydia	Tenesmus	Friable, often ulcerated rectal mucosa ± rectal mass	Serological antibody titre, biopsy for culture	Oral doxycycline 100 mg b.i.d. or oral erythromycin 500 mg q.i.d. for 7 days, oral azithromycin 1 g single dose
Lymphogranuloma venereum	Enlarged inguinal nodes, fever, malaise, anorexia	Friable, often ulcerated rectal mucosa	Serological antibody titre, complement fixation test	Oral doxycycline 100 mg b.i.d. or oral erythromycin 500 mg q.i.d. for 21 days
Haemophilus ducreyi (chancroid)	Anal pain	Anorectal abscesses and ulcers	Culture	Oral erythromycin 500 mg q.i.d. for 7 days, oral ciprofloxacin 500 mg b.i.d. for 3 days, single-dose ceftriaxone 250 mg i.m., single-dose oral azithromycin 1 g

Table 15.1 • (*Cont'd*) Sexually transmitted and infectious organisms that cause anorectal pathology

Organism	Symptoms	Anoscopy and proctoscopy	Laboratory test	Treatment
Bacterial				
Neisseria gonorrhoeae (gonorrhoea)	Rectal discharge	Proctitis, mucopurulent discharge	Thayer–Martin culture of discharge	Ceftriaxone 125 mg i.m. single dose plus oral doxycycline 100 mg b.i.d. for 7 days
Calymmatobacterium granulomatis (granuloma inguinale)	Perianal mass	Hard, shiny perianal masses	Biopsy of mass	Oral doxycycline 100 mg b.i.d., oral trimethoprim–sulfamethoxazole (double strength) one tablet b.i.d., oral ciprofloxacin 750 mg b.i.d., oral erythromycin 500 mg q.i.d. for 21 days (see text)
Mycobacterium avium-intracellulare	Watery diarrhoea	Normal	Acid-fast stain of stool, ileal biopsy	Oral clarithromycin 500 mg b.i.d. or oral azithromycin 250 mg q.d. plus oral ethambutol 15 mg/kg daily and oral rifabutin 300 mg q.d.
Treponema pallidum (syphillis)	Rectal pain	Painful anal ulcer	Dark-field examination of fresh scrapings	Benzathine benzylpenicillin 2.4 million units i.m.
Parasitic				
Entamoeba histolytica (amoebiasis)	Bloody diarrhoea	Friable rectal mucosa; shallow ulcers with yellowish exudate and ring of erythema	Fresh stool examination (microscopy)	Oral metronidazole 750 mg t.i.d. for 10 days, then oral iodoquinol 650 mg t.i.d. for 20 days
Cryptosporidium	Bloody, mucoid diarrhoea, dehydration	Normal	Rectal biopsy (oocysts)	Hydration
Isospora	Vomiting, fever, abdominal pain	Normal	Acid-fast stain of stool, endoscopic biopsy	Oral trimethoprim–sulfamethoxazole (double strength) b.i.d. for 7 days

secondary to CMV is the most common intestinal manifestation of AIDS. Symptomatic CMV proctitis presents with tenesmus, diarrhoea, weight loss, melaena or haematochezia. Endoscopic findings vary from submucosal haemorrhage and erythematous patches to multiple, wide, deep ulcers. The differential diagnosis includes *Clostridium difficile*, ulcerative colitis and Crohn's colitis. Biopsy helps to confirm the diagnosis. Microscopic findings on biopsy demonstrate vasculitis, neutrophilic infiltration and large basophilic intranuclear cytomegalic viral inclusions. Viral cultures of biopsy specimens may also reveal CMV.

Medical treatment of CMV requires either ganciclovir or foscarnet.[12] Ganciclovir has a similar formula to aciclovir but is 50 times more effective against CMV.[13] Both ganciclovir and foscarnet are virostatic and must be given intravenously. Relapse of clinical symptoms is common after the drugs are discontinued and thus lifelong oral maintenance therapy may be necessary. Surgery is required for refractory haemorrhage or perforation. Pathology due to CMV has been an infrequent indication for emergency laparotomy in AIDS patients. The most successful results are obtained after subtotal colectomy with end ileostomy. However, these are high-risk procedures in very sick patients and 30-day mortality exceeds 50%.[10,14]

Herpes simplex

Herpes simplex virus (HSV) is a DNA virus that is endemic in the USA population. Two serotypes cause clinical problems. Type 1 (HSV-1) is usually associated with oral lesions; however, it has been estimated that 2–15% of all HSV-1-seropositive patients have genital involvement by HSV-1.[15] Type 2 (HSV-2) is typically associated with genital infections.[8] Up to 95% of homosexual males have positive serological tests confirming infection with HSV-2 and 6–30% of homosexual patients with rectal symptomatology have positive rectal cultures for HSV.[16–18] In 1987, the Centers for Disease Control (CDC) revised the diagnostic criteria for AIDS to include chronic mucocutaneous HSV infection. This infection is also included in the more recent 1993 diagnostic criteria.[19,20] Ulcerative perianal HSV-2 (among other varieties) present for

at least 1 month in a patient with no other identifiable cause of immunodeficiency or with laboratory evidence of human immunodeficiency virus (HIV) infection is diagnostic of AIDS.

The virus is transmitted by direct contact to the skin or mucosa and causes symptoms more commonly than most other anorectal infections. After a latent period (4–21 days), multiple 1–2 mm vesicular lesions form in infected skin or rectal mucosa (proctitis).[17,21] During the acute phase, the anorectum will usually be exquisitely tender, and an accurate examination may be impossible without topical anaesthesia. Acute cutaneous lesions range from small (1–2 mm) vesicles with red aureoles, to larger ruptured vesicles (**Fig. 15.1**) to aphthous coalesced ulcers. These lesions are usually painful, contain clear fluid and occur on the perianal skin, in the anal canal or, less frequently, in the rectum. Shallow perianal ulcers may coalesce and extend to the sacrococcygeal area in a butterfly distribution.

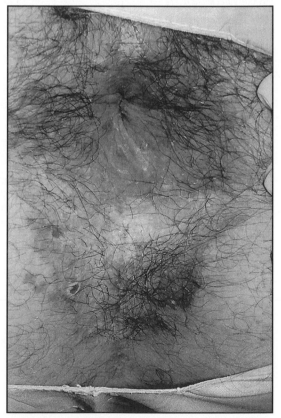

Figure 15.1 • Perianal herpes simplex virus. The vesicles have already ruptured.

The lesions usually resolve in 1–2 weeks, but initially may recur. The disease is highly contagious, from the first appearance of the vesicles until perianal re-epithelialisation is complete. Rarely, HSV is transmitted even after complete healing.

The pain associated with proctitis is exacerbated by enemas, intercourse and bowel movements. Other findings include mucoid or bloody bowel movements, tenesmus, psychogenic constipation and, less commonly, the systemic manifestations of fever, chills and malaise.[17] Bilateral tender inguinal lymphadenopathy is reported occasionally.[22]

Some patients also develop a constellation of symptoms associated with lumbosacral radiculopathy (urinary dysfunction, sacral paraesthesia, impotence and pain in the lower abdomen, thighs and buttocks). This syndrome is found in up to 50% of HSV-infected men.[23] The symptoms of the radiculopathy and a deep-seated severe pelvic pain often outlive the active clinical infection.[24]

The sigmoidoscopic findings of HSV proctitis typically include friable mucosa, diffuse ulcerations and occasional intact vesicles and pustules. These changes are almost always limited to the distal 10 cm of the rectum. Ulcerations in the anal canal may become secondarily infected and appear as greyish crypts with erythematous borders. Crusting of the lesions is followed by healing in approximately 2 weeks. A chronic relapsing course is common, with recurrence rates of 40%.[25] In some patients, an inciting factor such as trauma, exposure to sunlight, cold or heat stress, concurrent infection and menstruation may be related to the recurrence. Lesions usually recur in the same dermatome distribution as the initial infection. Sacral paraesthesiae and severe perianal and buttock pain often precede the recurrence of vesicles by several days. Cytological scrapings or biopsies taken from the bed of an ulcer will reveal the typical intranuclear inclusion bodies or multinucleated giant cells (**Fig. 15.2**) diagnostic of the virus.[26] Crypt abscesses and lamina propria neutrophils occur in about half of all specimens. Although routine stains are usually sufficient for recognising typical cytological alterations, intranuclear inclusion bodies can be selectively stained with anti-HSV-2 antiserum using special techniques. Viral culture and direct immunofluorescent staining of the vesicular fluid are also diagnostic.[27]

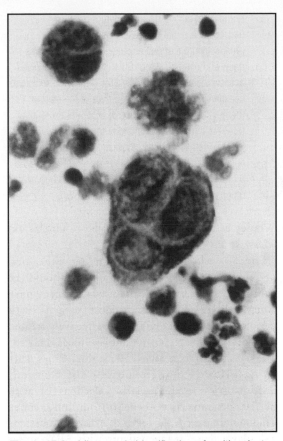

Figure 15.2 • Microscopic identification of multinucleate giant cells from the cytological scraping of a perianal ulcer.

Treatment is directed at two areas. First is to provide symptomatic relief of the skin and mucosal lesions. Helpful measures include analgesics, cool compresses, lidocaine (lignocaine) ointment, sitz baths, etc. Hygiene is important to prevent bacterial superinfection. The second concern is direct treatment of severe active infections or of patients with frequent reinfections (more than six per year). Therapy with aciclovir, a synthetic guanine analogue, reduces the duration and severity of symptoms but does not eradicate HSV or cure the disease.[28,29] Oral and topical aciclovir has been effective in reducing the length of the asymptomatic period, promoting healing of lesions and reducing the period of viral shedding.[29] Oral aciclovir may suppress the frequency of recurrence, provided the drug is taken for life.[30–32] Similar benefits and effects have also been shown for therapy with oral famciclovir and valaciclovir.[33]

Rompalo et al.[34] enrolled 29 homosexual men with first-episode rectal HSV-2 in a double-blind prospective trial of oral aciclovir (400 mg five times daily) and placebo. About 80% of those who received aciclovir compared with only 25% of placebo recipients ceased viral shedding within 3 days of the start of therapy. The median duration of both viral excretion from the herpetic lesions and of the presence of the lesions themselves was significantly shorter in the aciclovir-treated group. This latter group also reported a more rapid resolution of rectal pain, discharge and other subjective symptoms of proctitis.

Whitley et al.[35] reported very similar results, as did Mertz et al.[36]

Topical aciclovir is less effective than either oral or intravenous therapy.[37] Treatment should be continued until all mucocutaneous surfaces have completely re-epithelialised. Most patients with perianal herpes infections can be effectively treated with oral aciclovir 200–400 mg five times daily for 10 days. Oral famciclovir 250 mg three times daily or valaciclovir 1 g twice daily may also be used.[38] Patients with severe perianal infections or with herpes proctitis may benefit from intravenous aciclovir at a dose of 5 mg/kg every 8 hours for 5–7 days. Since many patients with AIDS suffer from frequent recurrences, suppressive therapy is possible. CDC recommends the following regimens for daily suppressive therapy: oral aciclovir 400 mg twice daily; oral famciclovir 250 mg twice daily; or oral valaciclovir 500 mg once daily (for patients with fewer than ten recurrences per year). Oral valaciclovir 1 g once daily is recommended for patients with ten or more recurrences per year.[38] However, treatment during an episode does not affect the rate or severity of recurrences. AIDS patients with HSV perianal ulcerations resistant to aciclovir may be candidates for either foscarnet or vidarabine.[39–41]

Stamm et al.[42] and Holmberg et al.[43] have independently reported a statistically significant association between HSV-2 infection and subsequent HIV infection. Thus HSV-2 must be recognised not only as an ulcerative pathogen but as a harbinger of HIV infection. All patients with anorectal herpes infections should be counselled regarding HIV testing. Manifestations at primary infection frequently include fever, malaise and lymphadenopathy. Recurrences are often different from the primary infection and appear to be due to reactivation of latent HSV. In some patients, an inciting factor (e.g. trauma, exposure to sunlight) may be related to the recurrence. Recurrent lesions usually develop in the same dermatome distribution as the initial infection.

Human immunodeficiency virus

HIV is an RNA retrovirus that infects human T lymphocytes.[10] The virus is spread by contaminated body fluids and after a variable latent period of up to 2 years, it produces diminished immunological function.[44,45] The incidence of infection with HIV is increasing. CDC reported more than 807 000 cases of AIDS as of 2001, with 57% having died.[46] Cases have been reported in all states of the USA, and it is estimated that 1–1.5 million American patients have been exposed to the virus. While the incidence of HIV infection has apparently levelled in the USA, the numbers of new AIDS cases and deaths from AIDS have decreased. This is in large part due to highly active antiretroviral therapy (HAART): combinations of potent anti-HIV drugs that act as nucleoside analogues, non-nucleoside reverse transcriptase inhibitors and protease inhibitors. Proctological conditions are common in HIV patients, and in the absence of routine screening these complaints may be the primary reason for seeking medical help.[47,48] A systematic approach allows appropriate management of these patients.

The initial evaluation should include a complete history, physical examination, laboratory studies (complete blood count, biochemical profile, serological tests for common STDs) and invasive diagnostic procedures (spinal tap). An adequate history is essential in order to obtain the correct diagnosis for any proctological complaint. The presenting symptoms should be explored, with particular attention given to bowel activity, sexual history and overall health. A patient's risk for HIV infection or AIDS should be explored with specific questions about sexual preference, intravenous drug usage and exposure to blood products or to HIV-positive individuals. Alterations in body functions or symptoms may direct the investigations towards specific diseases. In known HIV-positive patients, several symptoms have been proposed in order to classify the disease stage. These include the Walter Reed classification system and that of the CDC (Box 15.1).[49,50] An essential feature of each system is that early-stage patients (e.g. CDC Clinical Category A) have minimal alterations in their gross immunological or healing ability. Patients with later disease stages (CDC Clinical Category C) have significant immunological dysfunction, resulting in accentuated morbidity and mortality. Some authors have attempted to use the CD4+ count to predict healing while others have not found this helpful.[8,51–53] This discrepancy may be explained by the use of newer medications in the treatment of HIV infection, which may improve a patient's ability to heal despite a low CD4+ count.

In HIV-positive patients with gastrointestinal symptoms, it is essential to evaluate the stool for pathogens by cultures and stains.[10,54] In addition, any abnormal lesion of the perirectal area or rectal

Box 15.1 • Centers for Disease Control (CDC) classification system for HIV

CD4+ T-lymphocyte category
• Category 1: >500 cells/μL
• Category 2: 200–499 cells/μL
• Category 3: <200 cells/μL

Clinical category
Category A
• Asymptomatic HIV infection
Category B
• Symptomatic infection: conditions that are not listed in Category C and (i) are attributed to HIV infection or indicate a defect in cell-mediated immunity or (ii) conditions which are considered to have a clinical course or require management that is complicated by HIV infection
Category C
• Contitions listed in the 1993 AIDS surveillance case definition

Adapted from Centers for Disease Control 1993 revised classification system for HIV infection and expanded surveillance case definition for AIDS among adolescents and adults. MMWR 1992; 41(RR-17).

mucosa should be biopsied to complete the evaluation. Since HIV is transmitted sexually and via contaminated needles, infected body fluids and perhaps tissue, infection control measures are very important. Examiners should observe universal precautions, and any activity with the potential for body fluid contact requires eye and skin protection, including use of gloves, goggles, mask and barrier gowns.[10] Most patients require only a proctoscopic or anoscopic examination for adequate evaluation; for convenience, we use disposable instruments. Traditional sterilisation measures are used if nondisposable instruments are required.

The diseases identified in HIV-infected patients can be grouped into three categories. The first group includes the common proctological conditions (e.g. haemorrhoids, fissures, pruritus) routinely discovered in the general population.[55] Second are diseases associated with high-risk groups. Diseases associated with homosexuality in males include candidiasis, cryptosporidiosis, cytomegalic inclusion disease, pneumonia (*Pneumocystis carinii*), herpes simplex and herpes zoster, whereas intravenous drug use is associated with hepatitis (hepatitis B virus). The third group includes those illnesses associated with HIV infections, such as unusual opportunistic infections, Kaposi's sarcoma and lymphoma.

The exact incidence of these conditions is not accurately known due to the absence of routine screening and selection biases in the published series. The experience reported by Beck et al.[55] in 1990 included 677 HIV-positive patients. The majority of these patients were early-stage disease (78% Walter Reed stage I or II) and male (95%). Non-sexually related anorectal conditions were found in 6% of these patients, and more than 60% had at least one other STD. *Chlamydia* and hepatitis were the most common conditions, serology proving positive in 51% and 31% respectively, followed by anal condylomas (18%). Combining patients with non-sexually related anorectal diseases and those with anal condylomas, 24% had treatable anorectal conditions. A more recent report of 1117 HIV-positive patients treated at the University of Amsterdam[56] found 7.4% with anorectal disease that required a surgical consultation. Many of these 83 patients had more than one problem, including perianal sepsis (55%), condylomata acuminatum (34%), anorectal ulcers (33%), haemorrhoids

(17%), invasive anorectal carcinoma (17%) and polyps (11%). Finally, in 1998 Barrett et al.[57] reported their experience with 260 consecutive HIV-positive patients with perianal disease between 1989 and 1996. The most common disorders were condyloma (42%), fistula (34%), fissure (32%) and abscess (25%). Neoplasms were present in 7% of patients; 66% of patients had more than one disorder.

The management of these anorectal conditions in the HIV-positive patient deserves additional comment. Unlike in other patients, the primary therapeutic goal in HIV-positive patients is to eliminate or reduce symptoms. A secondary goal is resolution of the condition and healing of the wound.

Abscesses with pus usually present with pain and require drainage. Efforts are directed towards keeping the wounds small. Drainage with a latex Pezzer catheter is very effective.[58] Symptomatic fistulas are treated with a standard fistulotomy in early-stage patients and can be expected to heal.[56] Late-stage patients are treated in order to minimise symptoms. This usually entails establishing adequate drainage. Extensive procedures to resolve the fistula are contraindicated as healing is rare and the result is often larger non-healing wounds.

Anal ulcers (**Fig. 15.3**) can be caused by a number of infectious agents described in this chapter. The ulcers caused by HIV are deep and chronic, with overhanging edges. They are often eccentric or multiple, cavitating and oedematous with a bluish-purple hue. It is important to differentiate these HIV anal ulcers from benign anal fissures and neoplasms. Routine anal fissures are either posterior or anterior, accompanied by skin tags and readily visible on buttock retraction. Anal ulcers usually cause pain when there is 'pocketing' or inadequate drainage of the associated ulcer cavity. Any HIV-positive patient with anal pain should receive an examination under anaesthesia to exclude undrained pus. If a deep cavitating ulcer is identified, it should be unroofed to establish drainage. This usually resolves the pain. Gottesman[59] has also recommended injection of a long-acting steroid into the base of the ulcer to relieve symptoms. Prior to the widespread use of HAART, AIDS anal ulcers were an increasing problem. The absence of recent literature on this topic correlates with our personal experience that

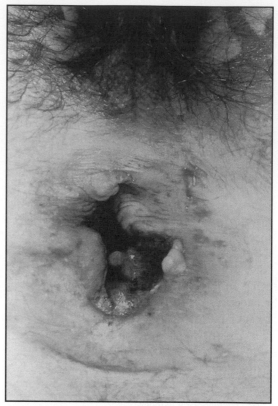

Figure 15.3 • HIV anal ulcer.

this condition is much less common in the era of HAART.

HIV-infected patients are afflicted with a variety of neoplastic disorders related to their immuno-compromised state.[60] Kaposi's sarcoma, non-Hodgkin's lymphoma and epidermoid anal carcinoma all present as anal masses or ulcers. Incisional biopsies confirm the diagnosis. Unfortunately, the associated immunodeficiency limits therapeutic options and the prognosis remains poor.

Limited information is available on the treatment of HIV infection. Early studies of HIV-infected patients with perianal disease noted poor healing and high morbidity rates. Recent changes in the systemic treatment of HIV infection and newer drug regimens that include combinations of protease inhibitors and nucleoside analogues have greatly improved the prognosis for HIV-infected patients.[57] Certain measures directed at control of infectious organisms have been shown to be of benefit. Localised infections (e.g. abscesses) require drainage.

However, previous reports grouped all HIV patients (asymptomatic, seropositive, AIDS and AIDS-related complex) together. Previously cited data reflect findings of markedly altered immunological function associated with advanced disease. These patients had very significant morbidity and mortality, and the results of operative therapy were dismal. We have not performed aggressive surgical procedures on late-stage patients. Conservative proctological procedures in early-stage patients have resulted in a good initial outcome, and on follow-up these patients have continued to do well.[55,56] Treatment of the identified anorectal conditions included stool bulking agents for haemorrhoidal disease and fissures. Abscesses were drained and condylomas, fistulas or pilonidal disease were treated according to the patient's HIV disease status. Late-stage patients were managed conservatively, whereas early-stage patients were offered standard operative procedures as described elsewhere in this book. There were no significant operative complications, and the result of this therapy was similar to that in patients who were not HIV positive.

Human papilloma virus

PATHOPHYSIOLOGY

Anal condylomas, or condylomata acuminatum, are the most common STD seen by colorectal surgeons and result from infection with human papilloma virus (HPV). There are over 80 subtypes of HPV but subtypes 6 and 11 are most commonly responsible for HPV infection. Subtypes 16 and 18 behave more aggressively and have been more frequently associated with dysplasia and malignant transformation.[61,62] The incidence of condyloma has been rising steadily over the past three decades.[63] It is estimated that 30–50% of sexually active adults are infected with HPV and it has been found in 40–70% of homosexual men.[64] HIV-positive homosexual males have an HPV infection rate of 93%. While data on incidence are difficult to obtain, there are approximately 5.5 million new cases of HPV infection every year in the USA.[65] The highest rates of infection are found in women aged 19–22 years and in men aged 22–26 years. Only 1–2% of the infected population have clinically apparent warts of the anogenital region.[63] Scholefield et al.[66] used magnification, colposcopy and HPV typing to deter-mine the incidence of HPV in perianal tissue that was not grossly condylomatous. Palmer et al.[67] have reported similar findings.

Nash et al.[68] reported 20 cases of histologically atypical and mucosal lesions, ranging from atypical condylomas to carcinoma in situ. About 92% of the patients were male and 75% of these were known homosexuals. Croxson et al.[69] reported seven homosexual men in whom condylomas revealed carcinoma in situ. Other authors have noted homosexual men to be at increased risk for the development of invasive anal carcinoma.[70–72] Gal et al.[73] have used immunohistochemical techniques to implicate HPV in anal squamous cell carcinoma in homosexual men.

Associated genital condylomas are common in 80% of women (on the external genitalia, vagina or cervix) and in 16% of men (on the penis).[10] Urethral warts have also been reported, and warts may occur in the anal canal. Symptoms are related to the location of the lesions and patients without visible anogenital warts may be asymptomatic. As many as 50–75% of asymptomatic homosexual men will harbour anal canal condylomas,[74] leading to important epidemiological implications. Sohn and Robilotti[74] reported that in only 6% of symptomatic homosexual males were the condylomas confined to the perianal area, whereas in 84% both perianal and intra-anal lesions were noted. Furthermore, 10% of the symptomatic patients had only intra-anal condylomas. This highlights the importance of anoscopy performed with adequate sphincter relaxation, good direct lighting, and possible colposcopy, acetic acid staining or loupe magnification (H.R. Bailey, personal communication).[67]

Symptoms include pruritis ani, bleeding, discharge, persistent perianal wetness and pain.[37] Very few patients complain of a lump or mass. The lesions can be single, pinkish-white, cauliflower-like pinhead lesions or multiple vast clusters that appear to form a confluent sheet that may obliterate the anus from view (**Fig. 15.4**). This latter pattern is typically seen in the AIDS patient.[75] The differential diagnosis of these lesions includes condylomata latum, molluscum contagiosum and hypertrophied anal papillae. Condylomata latum (secondary syphilitic sores) are smoother, flatter and moister than condylomata acuminatum and demonstrate spirochaetes on dark-field examination. Molluscum

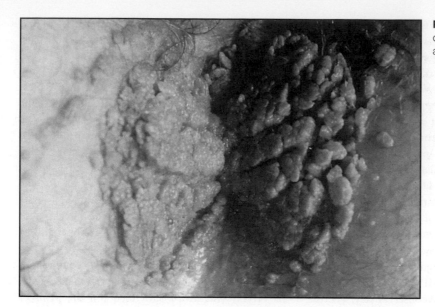

Figure 15.4 • Anal condylomas (condylomata acuminatum).

contagiosum comprises small, raised and centrally umbilicated pinkish-white lesions, while hypertrophied anal papillae are usually not as friable as condylomas.

Microscopically, condylomata acuminatum show marked acanthosis of the epidermis with hyperplasia of the prickle cells, parakeratosis and an underlying chronic inflammatory cell infiltration.[76] Vacuolisation of the upper prickle layer (koilocytosis) may also be present and orthokeratosis is often seen.

Successful therapy requires accurate diagnosis and eradication of all warts. Therefore, all patients should undergo anoscopy, proctosigmoidoscopy and either a vaginal or penile examination. In addition, other coexisting alimentary or sexually transmitted pathogens (as described in this chapter) should be identified and treated.

The significance of the potential premalignant type of HPV in perianal condylomas in clinically occult HPV infection cannot be overemphasised. Grossly or microscopically infected areas may undergo malignant transformation and develop into either squamous intraepithelial lesions (high or low grade) or invasive carcinoma. This relationship between HPV and the development of anal squamous intraepithelial lesions and anal canal cancer is believed to be similar to the well-established role of HPV in cervical dysplasia and cervical cancer because the anal canal is a transitional zone from columnar to squamous epithelium, analogous to the squamocolumnar junction of the cervix.[77]

THERAPY

Multiple types of therapy have been utilised to manage anal condylomas. Options include observation, excision, destruction (by a variety of methods such as chemicals, fulguration, freezing, laser) and immunotherapy with intralesional injection of d-interferon and other substances.[78–80] Evaluation of each method has been complicated by occasional spontaneous regression of the warts, uncertainty as to whether the warts identified after treatment are true recurrences or reinfection, and the lack of prospective controlled clinical trials. Results of therapy have varied, with reported recurrence rates averaging 10–75%.[8] The method used to eliminate the warts appears to be less important than limiting the damage to the surrounding normal skin. Each method has advantages and disadvantages, which are presented below.

Excision

Excision of condylomas can be performed either in the general practitioner's surgery under local anaesthesia or in the outpatient operating room using a regional block. Excision allows precise removal of the condylomas and complete histopathological microscopic examination. This is especially important in view of the rising incidence of malignant transformation of condylomas.[71]

Our excisional technique involves giving the patient two disposable phosphate enemas 30–60 minutes before the procedure. The patient is positioned in the prone jack-knife position with the buttocks taped apart. A solution of 0.5% Xylocaine with 0.25% bupivacaine and 1 in 200 000 adrenaline (epinephrine) is used to obtain a perianal field block. If regional or general anaesthesia is used, a 1 in 200 000 adrenaline solution is still used as it acts to reduce blood loss and elevates and separates the warts, improving the operator's ability to excise individual warts accurately and with minimal damage to intervening skin. Before wart excision, anoscopy and proctoscopy should be undertaken if they have not been already. The warts are then individually excised with a fine iris or fistula scissors. Preservation of anoderm and especially anal canal mucosa is of paramount importance in order to minimise perioperative discomfort, complications and healing time. The vast majority of patients can have all their condylomas excised in a single session. The most frequent complication is postoperative bleeding (2–3%);[78] electrocautery applied to the base of each wart helps prevent early postoperative bleeding, although it increases tissue destruction and delayed bleeding after the eschar sloughs is still possible. The rate of recurrence is less than 10%.[81]

Podophyllin/podophyllotoxin

Podophyllin is the resin of podophyllum, an agent that is cytoxic to condylomas and very irritating to normal skin. It is generally applied in either liquid paraffin or tincture of benzoin, the latter adhering best to the warts. Although concentrations of 5–50% have been used, a 25% suspension is readily available and seems optimal. The mixture is carefully applied directly to the condylomas, ensuring that the intervening normal skin bridges are not treated. A sharpened wooden dowel is a good vehicle for delivery. After application, talcum powder is applied to the skin. After 6–8 hours, the patient should wash the entire area thoroughly to prevent skin damage.

Because of autoinoculation, multiple treatments are often required to eradicate all warty tissue. Furthermore, because podophyllin is toxic to skin

or mucosa, it cannot be applied to anal canal warts. Local complications include skin necrosis, fistula in ano, dermatitis and anal stenosis. In addition, large doses may result in systemic effects, including hepatic, renal, gastrointestinal, respiratory and neurological problems.[82,83] Particularly disturbing is the fact that podophyllin causes histological changes in the treated warts that are difficult to distinguish from carcinoma in situ.[76] These histological changes, including dispersion of chromatin, paranuclear vacuolisation and nuclear changes, reverse within 4 weeks of the last podophyllin application.[84]

Jensen[85] reported a prospective randomised trial in which 25% podophyllin application was compared with surgical excision in 60 patients with first-episode condylomas. The podophyllin was applied on a weekly basis for up to 6 weeks. Although 77% of patients treated with podophyllin had resolution of their warts, 65% had recurrence at 12 months. This compared with 93% resolution and 29% recurrence after surgical excision. Thus excision produced more rapid initial clearance and a lower incidence of recurrence than did podophyllin.

A purified form of the active component of podophyllin is available. Podophyllotoxin is applied to a total surface area of less than 10 cm² (as a 0.5% topical gel or solution) by the patient, twice a day for 3 days followed by 4 days without treatment. This cycle can be repeated for up to 2 months. Local adverse effects are rarely significant enough to warrant cessation of treatment but include erythema, pruritis, burning sensation and tenderness. Clearance rates of 70–80% and recurrence rates of 10–20% have been reported.[86,87]

Bichloroacetic acid/trichloroacetic acid

Bichloroacetic acid (BCAA) and trichloroacetic acid (TCAA) can be applied to warts in a similar way to podophyllin. The major differences are that BCAA and TCAA can be applied to anal canal warts, do not have systemic toxicity and do not cause histological changes that mimic carcinoma in situ. There are few clinical trials assessing effectiveness despite fairly widespread use but reported resolution rates range from 20 to 70%. The recurrence rate is approximately 25% after a mean of five treatments, and up to 13 treatments are necessary to achieve resolution of the condylomas.[79] Treatments can be performed at weekly intervals. BCAA has become extremely difficult to find commercially in the USA.

Electrocoagulation

Electrocoagulation requires the use of local or regional anaesthesia. The aim is to produce a white coagulum, which is the equivalent of a superficial second-degree burn. The procedure is best effected with a high current setting. Patients are prepared and positioned as described for excision. The cautery tip is placed near, but not into, the wart and a spark gap is created.[76] A white coagulum is produced which can then be wiped away. If any black eschar appears, a deep second- or third-degree burn has been created. This is a major drawback to this procedure, especially in the anal canal. The procedure may also cause intense pain and sphincter spasm, both during and after the procedure. For this reason general anaesthesia may be necessary when a large number of condylomas are present. Furthermore, an ample quantity of oral analgesics should be given to the patient on discharge home. Obviously, anal stenosis is a potential complication. Recurrence rates range from 10 to 25%.

Cryotherapy

Advocates of cryotherapy report that anaesthesia is unnecessary, but this has not been the overall experience. The procedure is inexact as the depth of destruction cannot be accurately gauged intraoperatively. Typically, wide deep wounds are created that are associated with delayed painful tissue sloughing. Moreover, a foul-smelling discharge accompanies the sloughing ulcer. A cotton-tipped applicator may be used to carefully treat individual warts. However, since liquid nitrogen is cumbersome to store and has a limited shelf-life, cryotherapy has little if any value.[88]

Laser

A laser can also be used to destroy warts. Although advocates claim that this modality is followed by less pain and results in fewer recurrences than other therapies, randomised studies have not yet confirmed this.

Billingham and Lewis[89] treated 38 patients with extensive warts with a carbon dioxide laser on the right half of the anus and with electrocautery on the left. The patients were blinded as to which half was treated with which modality. Laser treatment was accompanied by more pain and by a more rapid recurrence of condylomas.

An additional risk of using the laser is the problem of aerosolised active viral particles in the laser plume (smoke). Viable viral particles have been recovered from this plume,[90,91] and cases of medical providers developing condylomas in their respiratory tract after using a laser to treat condylomas have been reported.[92] To reduce this possibility, special filter masks and devices to evacuate the smoke are recommended whenever a laser is used.[93] Transmission of viral particles appears to be less of a problem with the larger particle smoke from electrocautery.[91] Finally, the laser is vastly more expensive than cautery and requires special training by both the physician and the ancillary staff. For these reasons many colorectal surgeons have been reluctant to abandon the less expensive and equally effective cautery for the laser.

During any operative or therapeutic procedure, several condylomas should be biopsied for pathological review. This confirms the clinical diagnosis and excludes the presence of an invasive squamous cell cancer (Buschke–Lowenstein tumour) that may mimic condylomas.

Immunotherapy

Immunotherapy has been described by Abcarian and Sharon.[94,95] At least 5 g of condylomas are used for preparation of an autologous vaccine. Intramuscular injections of 0.5 mL of the vaccine are given every week for 6 weeks. No adverse sequelae of the injections have been reported. Of the 200 patients treated by Abcarian, 84% experienced disappearance of the warts and all remained free of disease during the 46-month follow-up.[95] An additional 11% had significant reductions in the volume of condylomas that permitted complete eradication after a single session of local excision. Only 5% of patients did not benefit from the vaccine, and half of those responded to a second course of immunotherapy. Others have subsequently reported similar results.[96] There are a variety of logistical problems limiting the widespread use of immunotherapy: the vaccine must be prepared locally and stored properly, and patients must commit to 6 weeks of injections.

Interferon

Several studies have reported the use of interferon alpha-2b, injected either intramuscularly or intralesionally.

> Schonfeld et al.[97] treated 22 patients in a double-blind trial with either 2 million units of intramuscular interferon or placebo. Complete remission was reported in 82% of the former group and 18% of the latter.

Gall et al.[98] used 5 million units of intralesional interferon on a daily basis for 1 month and noted complete responses in 69% of patients and partial responses in 25%. Eron et al.[99] used 1 million units intralesionally thrice weekly for 3 weeks. One week after the conclusion of therapy there was a 62% decrease in the area of the warts compared with a 1% increase in the placebo group. Twelve weeks later the interferon group still showed a 40% reduction, whereas the placebo group displayed a 46% increase. Friedman-Kien et al.[100] reported a double-blind randomised trial in which 62% of interferon-treated patients had complete elimination or improvement of warts compared with only 21% of placebo-treated patients. The adverse effects of interferon include fever, chills, myalgia, headache, fatigue and leucopenia. Because of this adverse effect profile and the availability of equally effective but safer agents, the use of interferon is not indicated. Topical interferon, like intralesional interferon, has had mixed results, with wart clearance in 30–60%. In their 1998 study, Gross et al.[101] showed a recurrence of 54–62% when topical interferon gel was used as an adjunct to ablative therapy compared with a 75% recurrence in the placebo group. These results, combined with the cost and the adverse effects (including local skin irritation, burning and flu-like symptoms), limit the utility of topical interferon.

Imiquimod

Imiquimod is a more recently available drug that has an immunomodulatory effect. This treatment is unique among all recommended therapies for condylomas in that it does not rely on physical destruction of the lesions but is directed at eradication of the causative agent, HPV. Through immune mechanisms, imiquimod enhances cell-mediated cytolytic activity against HPV. It should be applied topically at bedtime, three times a week, for a maximum of 16 weeks. On the morning after application (6–10 hours later), the treated area should be cleansed with soap and water. Warts may clear in 8–10 weeks, or earlier. Treatment may take up to 16 weeks. A randomised controlled study has shown that 5% imiquimod achieved a 50% complete response rate with a recurrence rate of 11%.[102] Currently, imiquimod is not approved for use in the anal canal due to the possibility of significant ulceration and bleeding. However, a number of investigators are working on a formula to be delivered intra-anally, with encouraging results.[103] Imiquimod currently can be used as monotherapy or as an adjunct to surgery, either preoperatively to debulk large lesions or postoperatively after healing to treat residual disease. Local skin reactions, including erythema, erosion, excoriation and flaking, are common and are usually mild to moderate in severity. Systemic reactions have not been reported. Imiquimod has not been studied for use during pregnancy, although it is not a teratogen.[63]

MANAGEMENT OF CONDYLOMAS IN HIV-POSITIVE PATIENTS

A recent clinical problem of increasing importance has been the management of condylomas in HIV-positive patients. Beck et al.[104] reported on 119 HIV-positive patients with anal condylomas who comprised 18% of the authors' overall HIV patients and had demographics and risk factors similar to those of the other HIV-positive patients. About 60% of the patients also had at least one other STD. Based on their experience, Beck et al. recommended that asymptomatic and late-stage HIV-positive patients with anal condylomas be observed. Symptomatic patients with warts limited to the anal margin are treated with one to two applications of BCAA, and patients with anal canal lesions are offered excision and fulguration utilising general or regional anaesthesia. In the series of HIV-positive patients reported by Beck et al., 23% had excision and fulguration under general or regional anaesthesia. All had biopsy-proven condylomata acuminatum, with no significant perioperative complications and good wound healing. In follow-up, averaging more than 1 year, the recurrence rate for condylomas in the treated patients was 26% after local treatment with podophyllin and 4% after fulguration and excision. However, these HIV-positive patients with condylomas were a select group of military personnel who were young, healthy and identified on asymptomatic screening. Other HIV-positive patients may not have the same good results.

The diagnosis and management of patients with squamous intraepithelial lesions associated with HPV is not clear-cut. Screening of HIV-positive homosexual males without gross evidence of HPV has been recommended using cytology specimens collected with Dacron swabs. The time interval for this screening is unclear, although every 2–3 years is one recommended schedule. Once squamous intra-epithelial lesions are identified, either on screening or at time of excision of gross lesions, a mapping technique using acetic acid, Lugol's solution and an operating microscope is used to identify further areas for destruction.[77]

Molluscum contagiosum

Molluscum contagiosum is caused by a virus of the pox group and is transmitted by direct body contact. After an incubation period of 3–6 weeks, the patient develops painless, 3-mm, flattened, round, umbilicated lesions. Biopsy with viral analysis confirms the diagnosis. Although the disease is benign and self-limiting, treatment is used to prevent spread and for cosmetic purposes. Therapy based on physical removal of the lesions has been considered most effective.[63] Options include local destruction with phenol, surgical removal and cryotherapy.[8] Antiviral and immuno-modulatory therapies include topical imiquimod and cidofovir.[63]

BACTERIAL

Campylobacter jejuni

Campylobacter jejuni has recently been recognised as a common cause of enterocolitis or infectious diarrhoea. This curved, motile, non-spore-forming, Gram-negative rod can be transmitted by ingestion of infected milk or meat. There is a male pre-dominance, perhaps related to homosexual activity, but sexual transmission is uncertain.[105] The organism infects the small and large bowel and produces endotoxins similar to Vibrio cholerae.[106] After an incubation period of 1–5 days, the patient develops crampy diarrhoea containing some blood, associated with abdominal pain. Additional symptoms have included chills, fever, weight loss, skin rash, arthritis, pericarditis and paralysis.[13] These infections are usually self-limiting and resolve without sequelae within 1 week. The diagnosis is confirmed by stool culture. If symptoms persist for more than 1 week or if recurrent attacks occur, the patient can be treated with oral erythromycin 500 mg q.i.d. for 7 days.

Chlamydia

Chlamydia are small intracellular organisms related to bacteria, and have been implicated in a number of clinical syndromes including cervicitis, non-gonococcal urethritis and proctitis.[8] It is currently the most common STD, with over 3 million estimated cases in the USA. Symptoms result from inflammation of the infected mucosa. Of the 15 known immunotypes of Chlamydia trachomatis, serotypes D to K are responsible for proctitis.

Symptoms of rectal infection generally include fever, malaise, anorexia, headache, joint pain, tenesmus, rectal pain and a mucoid or bloody rectal discharge. Sigmoidoscopic findings generally include severe non-specific granular proctitis with mucosal erythema, friability and ulceration. Late findings may include an intraluminal stricture or mass, although this is more common in women. Biopsy of the rectal mucosa will reveal findings consistent with infectious proctitis; these microscopic features include crypt abscesses, infectious granulomas and giant cells.[107,108] Because Chlamydia is an obligate intracellular pathogen, rectal culture is usually unrewarding and the complement fixation test may not be positive.[109] The microimmunofluorescent antibody titre is the most sensitive serotyping test and is becoming more readily available.[110] In its absence, the diagnosis can be confirmed by culture of a biopsy of the inflamed rectal mucosa obtained under direct visualisation and transported in sucrose phosphate media on ice for immediate tissue culture inoculation. Antichlamydial antibody titres, as determined by the complement fixation test, are 1:80 or greater.[108] Titre elevation generally occurs 1 month or more after infection. However, low-level antibody response should not form the cornerstone of diagnostic reliability: either micro-immunofluorescent or tissue culture testing must be positive for confirmation.

Infections with *C. trachomatis* generally respond to oral doxycycline 100 mg b.i.d. for 7 days or oral erythromycin base 500 mg q.i.d. for 7 days, or oral azithromycin 1 g as a single dose.[38] For severe proctitis a 6-month course of vibramycin, two capsules daily, has been suggested.[111] Routine follow-up cultures are not needed, but all sexual partners should be simultaneously treated.

Residual rectal strictures have been reported as a late complication of these infections.[112] Symptomatic strictures are treated with a 3-week course of erythromycin, tetracycline or doxycycline. If this does not relieve symptoms, sphincter-saving excisional surgery may be the only curative alternative.

Lymphogranuloma venereum is caused by L1–3 serotypes of *C. trachomatis*. After an incubation period of 1–4 weeks, a small vesicular lesion develops. This lesion resolves quickly and the inguinal lymph nodes enlarge, progressing to an indurated mass with erythema of the overlying skin. This may be associated with malaise, anorexia, fever, headache and joint pain. Chronic inflammation of the lymph nodes may result in lymphoedema and rectal strictures may occur as a late complication.[1,112] The diagnosis is confirmed by complement fixation test or the more sensitive microimmunofluorescent antibody titre.[1] Treatment includes oral doxycycline 100 mg b.i.d. for 21 days or oral erythromycin base 500 mg q.i.d. for 21 days.[33]

Chancroid

Chancroid is caused by *Haemophilus ducreyi*, a small Gram-negative, non-motile, non-spore-forming, aerobic bacillus. The infection is characterised by adenopathy, multiple perineal abscesses and ulcers.[8] The diagnosis is confirmed by culture. Treatment is accomplished with four equally effective antibiotic regimens: a single dose of ceftriaxone 250 mg i.m.; a single dose of oral azithromycin 1 g; oral erythromycin base 500 mg q.i.d. for 7 days; or oral ciprofloxacin 500 mg b.i.d. for 3 days. Ciprofloxacin is contraindicated in persons younger than 18 years and in pregnant or lactating women.[33] Antibiotic susceptibility of this organism varies. If clinical improvement does not occur after the initial course of therapy, antibiotics should be changed. Resolution of the adenopathy will lag behind resolution of the ulcers.[113]

Gonorrhoea

Gonorrhoea is a common disease that has a decreasing annual incidence, most recently estimated at 650 000.[65] The causative organism, *Neisseria gonorrhoeae* (a Gram-negative intracellular diplococcus that occurs in pairs or clusters), can infect the mucous lining of all body orifices. Up to 55% of homosexual men seen in screening clinics harbour gonorrhoea.[114]

The rectum is the only site infected in 40–50% of these patients, and the majority are asymptomatic.[115] Transmission is by anal intercourse and is followed by an incubation period of 2–5 days, after which proctitis and/or cryptitis results.[22] In women, gonorrhoea can result from anal-receptive intercourse; however, the vast majority of cases are caused by autoinoculation of vaginal gonorrhoea into the lower rectum. Stansfield[116] reported that only 6% of women have rectal gonorrhoea in the absence of cervical or urethral involvement.

After an incubation period of 2–5 days, the organism produces an inflammatory response of varying degree. Up to half of anorectal infections may be asymptomatic. When symptoms do occur they include pruritis ani, bloody or mucoid rectal discharge, or tenesmus. In advanced cases, disseminated disease can occur, including perihepatitis, meningitis, endocarditis, pericarditis and gonococcal arthritis. The latter manifestation is probably the most common of the disseminated group and tends to be a unilateral migratory purulent arthritis of large joints.

A mucopurulent discharge is the most suggestive diagnostic clue, especially when seen in combination with proctitis. This discharge appears as a

298

Chapter Fifteen • Sexually transmitted diseases and the anorectum

thick, viscid, yellow exudate. Symptoms are non-specific and include pruritus ani, tenesmus and haematochezia.[117] Lubrication of the anoscope with anything other than water is not advisable since many lubricants and creams contain antibacterial agents. On endoscopic evaluation, the anal canal is classically uninvolved, whereas the rectum displays oedema, friability, erythema, ulceration and mucus. One classic finding is the ability to express the mucopus from the anal crypts. This is done by applying gentle external pressure while the anoscope is in place.

Diagnosis should be made by immediate culture on Thayer–Martin or Stuart's (anaerobic) medium. One can blindly swab the anal canal by inserting a pledget 2–2.5 cm into the anal canal and then rotating it from side to side for several seconds. However, swabbing the mucopus under direct anoscopic visualisation raises the positive yield on Gram stain from 34 to 79%.[118–120] Rarely are the Gram-negative intracellular diplococci seen, although positive identification facilitates immediate therapy. However, many non-diagnostic Gram stains are subsequently revealed to be false negatives. For this reason, a high index of suspicion warrants empirical treatment pending final culture results. Conversely, positive identification of N. gonorrhoeae does not provide irrefutable proof of its responsibility for the patient's symptoms. Many homosexual male patients have coexistent STDs. Neisseria meningitidis may also be cultured from the rectum of homosexual male patients.[121]

Treatment must include screening for repeat gonorrhoeal infection in 3 months, as failure of initial treatment occurs in up to 35% of cases.[122] The current preferred treatment for uncomplicated gonorrhoea is a single dose of ceftriaxone 125 mg i.m. plus oral doxycycline 100 mg b.i.d. for 7 days. Other recommended treatment regimens include ceftriaxone and azithromycin, cefixime plus azithromycin or doxycycline, and ciprofloxacin plus azithromycin or doxycycline.[38]

As with other STDs, all sexual contacts must be treated to prevent recurrence. The importance of close follow-up examination with culture to assess disease eradication cannot be overemphasised. With careful follow-up and treatment of all sexual partners, a 95% cure rate is a reasonable expectation.[8]

Granuloma inguinale

Granuloma inguinale, or donovanosis, is caused by Calymmatobacterium granulomatis, a Gram-negative bacillus. It produces chronic granulomatous infections that present as hard and shining masses in the perianal area. The diagnosis is confirmed by biopsy. Treatment is oral doxycycline 100 mg b.i.d. or trimethroprim–sulfamethoxazole, one double-strength tablet b.i.d. Alternative regimens include oral ciprofloxacin 750 mg b.i.d. or oral erythromycin 500 mg q.i.d. All of the regimens are administered for a minimum of 3 weeks and should be continued until all lesions have thoroughly healed.[33]

Syphilis

Syphilis is one of the oldest infectious diseases and remains common. Primary anal syphilis is largely a disease of homosexual men.[8,123] The causative agent, Treponema pallidum, is a motile spirochaete that produces a primary chancre 2–5 weeks after infection at the site of contact.[8] The chancre is a raised, 1–2 cm, circular, indurated lesion which may occur at the anal margin or canal (**Fig. 15.5**). The lesions are eccentrically located, multiple or irregular, and two ulcers may be opposite each other in a 'mirror image' or 'kissing' configuration. The ulcers are usually painful and associated with a discharge and inguinal adenopathy. Chancres heal spontaneously in 2–4 weeks.[112] Proctitis has been reported in the absence of anogenital lesions and is accompanied by tenesmus, mucoid discharge and rectal pain.[8]

The second stage of syphilis appears several weeks later and presents as fever, malaise, lymphadenopathy, arthropathy and disseminated cutaneous eruptions that mimic many other skin diseases. In addition, the patient develops multiple, raised, flat lesions (condylomata latum) around the anus that produce an exudate rich in Treponema. If syphilis is untreated for several years, the tertiary stage develops with involvement of the nervous and vascular system and formation of gummas.

The clinical disease can be confirmed in several ways. Dark-field microscopic examination of the exudate from the primary chancre or condylomata latum will demonstrate T. pallidum. Additional with a single dose of benzathine benzylpenicillin (penicillin G) 2.4 million units i.m. Patients with disease present for more than 1 year or those with tertiary syphilis require one weekly dose of benzathine benzylpenicillin 2.4 million units i.m. for three successive weeks. Patients who are allergic to pencillin may be given alternative treatments, such as doxycycline, tetracycline or erythromycin, or they may undergo desensitisation to penicillin.[124] Patients with neural involvement require cerebrospinal fluid examination. If the cerebrospinal fluid is involved, additional therapy is indicated.

PARASITIC

Amoebiasis

Entamoeba histolytica is a protozoan that commonly infects humans. Transmission is related to sanitation measures, and this organism is endemic in several parts of the world (Mexico, Russia, rural America, etc.). After amoebic cysts contaminating food and drink are ingested, the amoeba invades the gut mucosa and submucosa, producing ulcers that may become secondarily infected by bacteria. The amoeba may also penetrate the bowel wall and pass via the portal venous system to the liver where they may produce amoebic abscesses.

After an incubation period of 7–10 days, the disease may take several forms, the most common being an acute infection that produces diarrhoea; this may be severe enough to result in dehydration. The attack is usually self-limited and resolves after several days. A more severe colonic infection may progress to toxic colonic dilatation, which is often fatal. Some patients develop recurrent intermittent attacks of diarrhoea or amoebic dysentery. A final pattern is an asymptomatic carrier state that may or may not have been associated with one of the acute presentations. In all forms, amoebic cysts are passed intermittently in the stool.[22] The diagnosis can be confirmed by identification of amoeba or cysts in stool, pus or mucosal biopsy. Amoebic blood titres may also be useful. Therapy includes oral metronidazole 750 mg t.i.d. plus a luminal amoebicide such as oral iodoquinol 650 mg t.i.d. for 20 days. Large liver abscesses will usually require drainage and intravenous metronidazole.

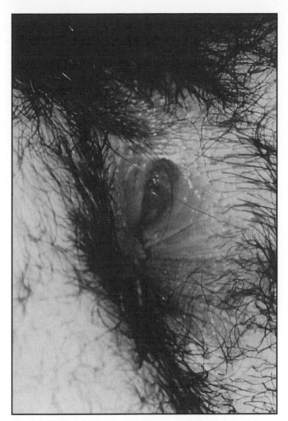

Figure 15.5 • Anal chancre (from syphilis).

confirmation is provided by serological tests. The rapid plasma reagin (RPR) and the Venereal Disease Research Laboratory (VDRL) slide test are non-specific screening tests. The RPR can be automated and is used in mass screening of serum. The VDRL also uses serum and has greater specificity. Both tests become positive within 1–2 weeks of infection and may remain positive for long periods even after treatment. The fluorescent treponemal antibody absorption test is a serum test that uses an indirect immunofluorescence method. It also becomes positive 2 weeks after infection but converts to a negative range after treatment. It is specific and sensitive but more expensive.[8] As multiple infections are common with STDs, each patient should be completely evaluated. This includes swabs of the genitourinary tract, oral cavity and rectum.

Treatment for syphilis is guided by the stage of disease. Patients with primary, secondary or latent disease of less than 1 year's existence can be treated

Cryptosporidium

Cryptosporidia are tiny protozoans that inhabit intestinal microvilli.[8] They can cause life-threatening colitis in immunocompromised patients, characterised by profuse, bloody, mucoid diarrhoea. Endoscopically, a mucoid proctocolitis is frequently observed. Demonstration of characteristic oocysts with an acid-fast stain of stool or endoscopic biopsy establishes the diagnosis. Treatment is supportive, with intravenous hydration and nutrition. Antiparasitic agents have failed to be helpful.

Isospora

Isospora belli is an opportunistic protozoan with a lower incidence than that of *Cryptosporidium* but with similar symptoms (diarrhoea, vomiting, fever and abdominal pain), although the quantity of diarrhoea is usually less. Diagnosis is made by a modified acid-fast stain of fresh stool or endoscopic biopsy. Fortunately, this organism is well controlled by trimethoprim and sulfamethoxazole.[8]

> ### • Key points
>
> - Sexually transmitted diseases are common and increasing.
> - A high index of suspicion and knowledge of lesions is required.
> - Patients and their partners must be treated.
> - Aciclovir will shorten the course of herpes infection and has a role in suppression.
> - HAART is effective in HIV-positive patients.
> - Excision has produced the best results for anal condylomas.
> - Review of current treatment recommendations is suggested for managing uncommon lesions.

REFERENCES

1. Felman YM, Morrison JM. Examining the homosexual male for sexually transmitted diseases. JAMA 1977; 238:2046–7.
2. Wilcox RR. The rectum as viewed by the venereologist. Br J Venereal Dis 1981; 57:1–6.
3. Kinsey AC, Pomeroy WB, Martin LE. Sexual behavior in the human male. Philadelphia: WB Saunders, 1948; pp. 650–1.
4. Darrow WW, Barrett D, Jay K et al. The gay report on sexually transmitted diseases. Am J Public Health 1981; 71:1004–11.
5. Gebhard PH. The exposure factor. The venereal disease crisis. Report of International Venereal Disease Symposium. St Louis: Pfizer Laboratories, 1978 (entire issue).
6. William DC. The sexual transmission of parasitic infections by gay men. J Homosex 1980; 5:291–4.
7. Voeller B. AIDS and heterosexual anal intercourse. Arch Sex Behav 1991; 20:233–76.
8. Wexner SD, Beck DE. Sexually transmitted and infectious diseases. In: Beck DE, Wexner SD (eds) Fundamentals of anorectal surgery. New York: McGraw-Hill, 1992; pp. 402–22.
9. Kazal HL, Sohn N, Carrasco JI et al. The gay bowel syndrome: clinico-pathologic correlation in 260 cases. Ann Clin Lab Sci 1976; 6:184–92.
10. Wexner SD, Beck DE. Acquired immunodeficiency syndrome. In: Beck DE, Wexner SD (eds) Fundamentals of anorectal surgery. New York: McGraw-Hill, 1992; pp. 423–39.
11. Goodgame RW. Viral causes of diarrhea. Gastroenterol Clin North Am 2001; 30:779–95.
12. Whitley RJ, Jacobson MA, Friedberg DN et al. Guidelines for the treatment of cytomegalovirus diseases in patients with AIDS in the era of potent antiretroviral therapy. Recommendations of an international panel. Arch Intern Med 1998; 158:957–69.
13. Smith LE. Sexually transmitted diseases. In: Gordon PH, Nivatvongs S (eds) Principles and practice of surgery for the colon, rectum, and anus. St Louis: Quality Medical Publishing, 1992; pp. 317–36.
14. Wexner SD, Smithy WB, Trillo C et al. Emergency colectomy for cytomegalovirus ileocolitis in patients with the acquired immune deficiency syndrome. Dis Colon Rectum 1988; 31:755–61.
15. Schomogyi M, Wald A, Corey L. Herpes simplex virus-2 infection: an emerging disease? Infect Dis Clin North Am 1998; 12:47–61.
16. Goldmeier D. Proctitis and herpes simplex virus in homosexual men. Br J Venereal Dis 1980; 56:111–14.
17. Goodell SE, Quinn TC, Mkritchian EE et al. Herpes simplex virus: an important cause of acute proctitis in homosexual men (abstract). Gastroenterology 1981; 80:1159.
18. Nerurkar L, Goedert J, Wallen W et al. Study of antiviral antibodies in sera of homosexual men. Fed Proc 1983; 42:6109.

19. Revision of the CDC surveillance case definition for acquired immunodeficiency syndrome. MMWR 1987; 36(suppl. 1):1s–15s.

20. Centers for Disease Control. 1993 revised classification system for HIV infection and expanded surveillance case definition for AIDS among adolescents and adults. MMWR 1992; 41(RR-17).

21. Jacobs E. Anal infections caused by herpes simplex virus. Dis Colon Rectum 1976; 19:151–7.

22. Buls JB. Sexually transmitted diseases of the anorectum. In: Goldberg SM, Gordon PH, Nivatvongs S (eds) Essentials of anorectal surgery. Philadelphia: JB Lippincott, 1980; pp. 150–2.

23. Samarasinghe PL, Oates JK, MacLennan IPB. Herpetic proctitis and sacral radiomyelopathy: a hazard for homosexual men. Br Med J 1979; 2:365–6.

24. Baringer JR. Recovery of herpes simplex virus from human sacral ganglions. N Engl J Med 1974; 291:828–30.

25. Goldmeier D. Herpetic proctitis and sacral radiculomyelopathy in homosexual men (letter). Br Med J 1979; 2:549.

26. Goodell SE, Quinn TC, Mkrtichian EE et al. Herpes simplex virus proctitis in homosexual men: clinical, sigmoidoscopic, and histopathologic features. N Engl J Med 1983; 308:868–71.

27. Rotterdam H, Sommers SC. Alimentary tract biopsy lesions in the acquired immune deficiency syndrome. Pathology 1985; 17:181–92.

28. Quinn TC, Corey L, Chaffee RG et al. The etiology of anorectal infections in homosexual men. Am J Med 1981; 71:395–406.

29. Bryson YJ, Dillon M, Lovett M et al. Treatment of first episodes of genital herpes simplex virus infection with oral acyclovir: a randomized double-blind controlled trial in normal subjects. N Engl J Med 1983; 308:916–21.

30. Reichman RC, Badger GJ, Merttz GJ et al. Treatment of recurrent genital herpes simplex infections with oral acyclovir. A controlled trial. JAMA 1984; 251:2103–7.

31. Douglas JM, Critchlow C, Benedetti J et al. A double-blind study of oral acyclovir for suppression of recurrences of genital herpes simplex virus infection. N Engl J Med 1984; 310:1551–6.

32. Straus SE, Takiff HE, Seidlin M et al. Suppression of frequently recurring genital herpes: a placebo-controlled double-blind trial of oral acyclovir. N Engl J Med 1984; 310:1545–50.

33. Brown TJ, Angela YM, Tyring SK. An overview of sexually transmitted diseases. Part I. J Am Acad Dermatol 1999; 41:661–77.

34. Rompalo AM, Mertz GJ, Davis LG et al. Oral acyclovir for treatment of first-episode herpes simplex virus proctitis. JAMA 1988; 259:2879–81.

A prospective controlled trial of homosexual men with rectal herpes simplex infection which demonstrated that treatment with aciclovir reduced viral shedding and symptoms.

35. Whitley RJ, Levin M, Barton N et al. Infections caused by herpes simplex virus in the immuno-compromised host: natural history and topical acyclovir therapy. J Infect Dis 1984; 150:323–9.

36. Mertz GJ, Jones CC, Mills J et al. Long-term acyclovir suppression of frequently recurring genital herpes simplex virus infection. A multicenter double-blind trial. JAMA 1988; 260:201–6.

37. Wexner SD. Sexually transmitted diseases of the colon, rectum, and anus. The challenge of the nineties. Dis Colon Rectum 1990; 33:1048–62.

38. Centers for Disease Control and Prevention. Sexually transmitted diseases treatment guidelines 2002. MMWR 2002; 51(RR-6):12–17.

39. Erlich KS, Mills J, Chatis P et al. Acyclovir-resistant herpes simplex virus infections in patients with the acquired immunodeficiency syndrome. N Engl J Med 1989; 320:293–6.

40. Chatis PA, Miller CH, Schrager LE et al. Successful treatment with foscarnet of an acyclovir-resistant mucocutaneous infection with herpes simplex virus in a patient with acquired immunodeficiency syndrome. N Engl J Med 1989; 320:297–300.

41. Wexner SD. Treatment of AIDS patients with herpes simplex virus infections resistant to acyclovir. Colon Rectal Surg Outlook 1989; 2:1–2.

42. Stamm WE, Handsfield HH, Rompalo AM et al. The association between genital ulcer disease and acquisition of HIV infection in homosexual men. JAMA 1988; 260:1429–33.

43. Holmberg SD, Stewart JA, Gerber AR et al. Prior herpes simplex virus type 2 infection as a risk factor for HIV infection. JAMA 1988; 259:1048–50.

44. Ranki A, Valle S-L, Krohn M et al. Long latency precedes overt seroconversion in sexually trans-mitted human-immunodeficiency-virus infection. Lancet 1987; ii:589–93.

45. Lifson AR, Rutherford GW, Jaffe HW. The natural history of human immunodeficiency virus infection. J Infect Dis 1988; 158:1360–7.

46. Centers for Disease Control and Prevention. CDC HIV/AIDS Surveillance Report 2001; 135–6.

47. Dworkin B, Wormser GP, Rosenthal WS et al. Gastrointestinal manifestations of the acquired immunodeficiency syndrome: a review of 22 cases. Am J Gastroenterol 1985; 80:774–8.

48. Gelb A, Miller S. AIDS and gastroenterology. Am J Gastroenterol 1986; 81:619–22.

49. Redfield RR, Wright DC, Tramont EC. The Walter Reed staging classification for HTLV-III/LAV infection. N Engl J Med 1986; 314:131–2.

50. Centers for Disease Control. Classification system for human T-lymphotropic virus type III/lymphadenopathy-associated virus infections. MMWR 1986; 35:334–9.

51. Morandi E, Merlini D, Salvaggio A et al. Prospective study of healing time after hemorrhoidectomy. Influence of HIV infection, acquired immunodeficiency syndrome, and anal wound infection. Dis Colon Rectum 1999; 42:1140–4.

52. Lord RVN. Anorectal surgery in patients infected with human immunodeficiency virus. Factors associated with delayed wound healing. Dis Colon Rectum 1998; 41:177–9.

53. Nadal SR, Manzione CR, Galvao VD et al. Healing after fistulotomy. Comparative study between HIV-positive and HIV-negative patients. Dis Colon Rectum 1994; 37:439–43.

54. Goldberg GS, Orkin BA, Smith LE. Microbiology of human immunodeficiency virus anorectal disease. Dis Colon Rectum 1994; 37:439–43.

55. Beck DE, Jaso RG, Zajac RA. Proctologic management of the HIV-positive patient. South Med J 1990; 83:900–3.

56. Consten ECJ, Slors FJM, Noten HJ, Oosting H, Danner SA, van Lanschot JJ. Anorectal surgery in human immunodeficiency virus-infected patients. Dis Colon Rectum 1995; 38:1169–75.

57. Barrett WL, Callahan TD, Orkin BA. Perianal manifestations of human immunodeficiency virus infection: experience with 260 patients. Dis Colon Rectum 1998; 41:606–11.

58. Beck DE, Fazio VW, Lavery IC, Jagelman DG, Weakley FL. Catheter drainage of ischiorectal abscesses. South Med J 1988; 81:444–6.

59. Gottesman L. Treatment of anorectal ulcers in HIV positive patients. Perspect Colon Rectal Surg 1991; 4:19–33.

60. Soler ME, Gottesman L. Anal and rectal ulceration. In: Allen-Mersh TG, Gottesman L (eds) Anorectal disease in AIDS. London: Hodder & Stoughton, 1991; pp. 121–2.

61. Gissmann L, Schwarz E. Persistence and expression of human papillomavirus DNA in genital cancer. Ciba Found Symp 1986; 120:90–7.

62. Syrjanen SM, von Krogh G, Syrjanen KJ. Detection of human papillomavirus DNA in anogenital condylomata in men using in-situ DNA hybridisation applied to paraffin sections. Genitourin Med 1987; 63:32–9.

63. Brown TJ, Angela YM, Tyring SK. An overview of sexually transmitted diseases. Part II. J Am Acad Dermatol 1999; 41:661–77.

64. Carr G, William DC. Anal warts in a population of gay men in New York City. Sex Transm Dis 1977; 4:56–7.

65. Centers for Disease Control and Prevention. Tracking the hidden epidemics. Trends in STDs in the United States. 2000:1–26.

66. Scholefield JH, Sonnex C, Talbot IC et al. Anal and cervical intraepithelial neoplasia: possible parallel. Lancet 1989; ii:765–9.

67. Palmer JG, Scholefield JH, Coates PJ et al. Anal cancer and human papillomaviruses. Dis Colon Rectum 1989; 32:1016–22.

68. Nash G, Allen W, Nash S. Atypical lesions of the anal mucosa in homosexual men. JAMA 1986; 256:873–6.

69. Croxson T, Chabon AB, Rorat E, Barash IM. Intraepithelial carcinoma of the anus in homosexual men. Dis Colon Rectum 1984; 27:325–30.

70. Cooper HS, Patchefsky AS, Marks G. Cloacogenic carcinoma of the anorectum in homosexual men: an observation of four cases. Dis Colon Rectum 1979; 22:557–8.

71. Wexner SD, Milsom JW, Dailey TH. The demographics of anal cancers are changing: identification of a high-risk population. Dis Colon Rectum 1987; 30:942–6.

72. Peters RK, Mack TM. Patterns of anal carcinoma by gender and marital status in Los Angeles county. Br J Cancer 1983; 48:629–36.

73. Gal AA, Meyer PR, Taylor CR. Papillomavirus antigens in anorectal condyloma and carcinoma in homosexual men. JAMA 1987; 257:337–40.

74. Sohn N, Robilotti JG Jr. The gay bowel syndrome: a review of colonic and rectal conditions in 200 male homosexuals. Am J Gastroenterol 1977; 67:478–84.

75. Wexner SD, Smithy WB, Milson JW, Dailey TH. The surgical management of anorectal diseases in AIDS and pre-AIDS patients. Dis Colon Rectum 1986; 29:719–23.

76. Connors RC, Ackerman AB. Histologic pseudo-malignancies of the skin. Arch Dermatol 1976; 112:1767–80.

77. Zbar AP, Fenger C, Efron J et al. The pathology and molecular biology of anal intraepithelial neoplasia: comparisons with cervical and vulvar intraepithelial carcinoma. Int J Colorectal Dis 2002; 17:203–15.

78. Thomson JPS, Grace RH. The treatment of perianal and anal condylomata acuminata: a new operative technique. J R Soc Med 1978; 71:180–5.

79. Swerdlow DB, Salvati EP. Condyloma acuminatum. Dis Colon Rectum 1971; 14:226–31.

80. Abcarian H, Smith D, Sharon N. The immunotherapy of anal condylomata acuminatum. Dis Colon Rectum 1976; 19:237–44.

81. Gollock JM, Slatford K, Hunter JM. Scissor excision of anorectal warts. Br J Venereal Dis 1982; 58:400–1.

82. Moher LM, Maurer SA. Podophyllum toxicity: case report and literature review. J Fam Pract 1979; 9:237–40.

83. Montaldi DH, Giambrone JP, Courey NG, Taefi P. Podophyllum poisoning associated with the treatment of condyloma acuminatum: a case report. Am J Obstet Gynecol 1974; 119:1130–1.

84. Prasad ML, Abcarian H. Malignant potential of perianal condyloma acuminatum. Dis Colon Rectum 1980; 23:191–7.

85. Jensen SL. Comparison of podophyllin application with simple surgical excision in clearance and recurrence of perianal condyloma acuminata. Lancet 1985; ii:1146–8.

   A prospective randomised trial comparing surgical excision and topical podophyllin for anal condylomas. Excision produced more rapid clearance and a lower incidence of recurrence.

86. von Krogh G, Lacey CJN, Gross G et al. European course on HPV associated pathology: guidelines for primary care physicians for the diagnosis and management of anogenital warts. Sex Transm Infect 2000; 76:162–8.

87. Tyring S, Edwards L, Cherry LK et al. Safety and efficacy of 0.5% Podofilox gel in the treatment of anogenital warts. Arch Dermatol 1998; 134:33–8.

88. Corman ML. Colon and rectal surgery, 2nd edn. Philadelphia: JB Lippincott, 1989.

89. Billingham RP, Lewis FG. Laser versus electrical cautery in the treatment of condylomata acuminata of the anus. Surg Gynecol Obstet 1982; 155:865–7.

   A prospective trial comparing wart destruction with electrocautery and laser. The laser was associated with more pain and a higher recurrence rate.

90. Garden JM, O'Banion MK, Shelnitz LS et al. Papillomavirus in vapor of carbon dioxide laser-treated verrucae. JAMA 1988; 259:1199–1202.

91. Sawchuk WS, Weber PJ, Lowy DR, Dzubow LM. Infectious papillomavirus in the vapor of warts treated with carbon dioxide laser or electrocoagulation: detection and protection. J Am Acad Dermatol 1989; 21:41–9.

92. Voien D. Intact viruses in CO_2 laser plumes spur safety concern. Clin Laser Monthly 1987; 5:101–3.

93. Sawchuk WS, Felten RP. Infectious potential of aerosolized particles. Arch Dermatol 1989; 125:1689–92.

94. Abcarian H, Sharon N. Long-term effectiveness of the immunotherapy of anal condyloma acuminatum. Dis Colon Rectum 1982; 25:648–51.

95. Abcarian H, Sharon N. The effectiveness of immunotherapy in the treatment of anal condylomata acuminatum. J Surg Res 1977; 22:231–6.

96. Eftaiha MS, Amshel AL, Shonberg IL, Batshon B. Giant and recurrent condyloma acuminatum: appraisal of immunotherapy. Dis Colon Rectum 1982; 25:136–8.

97. Schonfeld A, Nitke S, Schattner A et al. Intramuscular human interferon-B injections in treatment of condylomata acuminata. Lancet 1984; i:1038–42.

   A prospective controlled trial of intramuscular interferon to treat condylomas. Treatment produced a higher remission rate than placebo.

98. Gall SA, Hughes CE, Whisnant J, Weck P. Interferon for the therapy of condyloma acuminatum. Am J Gynecol 1985; 153:156–63.

99. Eron LJ, Judson F, Tucker S et al. Interferon therapy for condyloma acuminata. N Engl J Med 1986; 315:1059–64.

100. Friedman-Kien AE, Eron LJ, Conant M et al. Natural interferon alpha for treatment of condylomata acuminata. JAMA 1988; 259:533–8.

101. Gross G, Rogozinski T, Schofer H et al. Recombinant interferon beta gel as an adjuvant in the treatment of recurrent genital warts: results of a placebo-controlled double-blind study in 120 patients. Dermatology 1998; 196:330–4.

102. Edwards L, Ferenczy A, Eron L et al. Self-administered topical 5% imiquimod cream for external anogenital warts. Arch Dermatol 1998; 134:25–30.

103. Kaspari M, Gutzmer R, Kaspari T et al. Application of imiquimod by suppositories (anal tampons) efficiently prevents recurrences after ablation of anal canal condyloma. Br J Dermatol 2002; 147:757–9.

104. Beck DE, Jaso RG, Zajac RA. Surgical management of anal condylomata in the HIV-positive patient. Dis Colon Rectum 1990; 33:180–3.

105. Blaser MJ. Campylobacter enteritis in the United States. A multicenter study. Ann Intern Med 1983; 98:360–5.

106. Whelan RL. Other proctitides. In: Beck DE, Wexner SD (eds) Fundamentals of anorectal surgery. New York: McGraw-Hill, 1992; pp. 477–500.

107. Quinn TC, Goodell SE, Mkrtichian E et al. Chlamydia trachomatis proctitis. N Engl J Med 1981; 305:195–200.

108. Levine JS, Smith PD, Brugge WR. Chronic proctitis in male homosexuals due to lymphogranuloma venereum. Gastroenterology 1980; 79:563–5.

109. Goodell SE, Quinn TC, Mkrtichian EE et al. The infectious etiology and histopathology of proctitis and enteritis in homosexual men (abstract). Gastroenterology 1981; 80:1159.

110. Wang SP, Grayston JT, Alexander ER, Holmes KK. A simplified microimmunofluorescence test with trachoma–lymphogranuloma venereum (*Chlamydia trachomatis*) antigens for use as a screening test for antibody. J Clin Microbiol 1975; 1:250–5.

111. Rodier B, Catalan F, Harboun A. Severe proctitis due to chlamydia of serotype D. Coloproctology 1987; 9:341–4.

112. Goligher JC. Sexually transmitted diseases. In: Goligher JC (ed.) Diseases of the anus, rectum, and colon, 5th edn. London: Baillière Tindall, 1985; pp. 1033–45.

113. Baker DA. Clinical management of sexually transmitted diseases, vol. 2. Treatment and management of STDs. Charlotte, NC: Burroughs Welcome, 1989.

114. Schwarcz SK, Zenilman JM, Schnell D et al. National surveillance of antimicrobial resistance in *Neisseria gonorrhoeae*. The Gonococcal Isolate Surveillance Project. JAMA 1990; 264:1413–17.

115. Baker RW, Peppercorn MA. Gastrointestinal ailments of homosexual men. Medicine 1982; 61:390–405.

116. Stansfield VA. Diagnosis and management of anorectal gonorrhea in women. Br J Venereal Dis 1980; 56:319–21.

117. Fluker JL, Deherogada P, Flatt DJ et al. Rectal gonorrhea in male homosexuals: presentation and therapy. Br J Venereal Dis 1980; 56:397–9.

118. Deherogada P. Diagnosis of rectal gonorrhea by blind anorectal swabs taken via proctoscope. Br J Venereal Dis 1977; 53:311–13.

119. Danielsson D, Johannisson G. Culture diagnosis of gonorrhoea: a comparison of the yield with selective and non-selective gonococcal culture media inoculated in the clinic after transport of specimens. Acta Derm Venereol (Stockh) 1973; 53:75–80.

120. William DC, Felman YM, Riccardi NB. The utility of anoscopy in the rapid diagnosis of symptomatic anorectal gonorrhea in men. Sex Transm Dis 1981; 8:16–17.

121. Janda WM, Bohnhoff M, Morello JA, Lerner SA. Prevalence and site-pathogen studies of *Neisseria meningitidis* and *N. gonorrhoeae* in homosexual men. JAMA 1980; 244:2060–4.

122. Klein EJ, Fisher LS, Chow AW, Guze LB. Anorectal gonococcal infection: a clinical review. Ann Intern Med 1977; 86:340–6.

123. Catterall RD. Sexually transmitted diseases of the anus and rectum. Clin Gastroenterol 1975; 4:659–69.

124. Centers for Disease Control. Sexually transmitted diseases treatment guidelines. MMWR 1993; 42(RR-14):1–97.

CHAPTER
Sixteen
Minimally invasive colorectal surgery

Jared Torkington and
Ara Darzi

INTRODUCTION

This chapter covers a spectrum of related surgical techniques rather than a single condition. It is important to make this distinction early, as minimally invasive surgery is a method of administering treatment rather than a treatment in its own right. The same operation, for example colectomy, is performed whether it is carried out by laparoscopic or open surgery. However, in some circumstances the application of minimally invasive techniques may dramatically alter the procedure performed. An example of this would be the local excision of an early rectal cancer by transanal endoscopic microsurgery as opposed to radical abdominoperineal resection. Minimally invasive colorectal surgery refers to a combination of innovation and the latest technology in an attempt to minimise the surgical trauma caused to the patient in the treatment of a variety of common colorectal conditions.

In this chapter we discuss some of the reasons why minimally invasive colorectal surgery has not achieved the uptake in the UK that was predicted during the surgical equivalent of the Californian gold rush, with the explosion of interest in laparoscopic techniques in the early 1990s. Bearing in mind this initial surge in interest and publications and subsequent developments and modifications in

technique, we have tried to keep the references as recent as possible without overlooking the major papers from the first decade of minimally invasive surgery. We cover the arguments for and against minimally invasive colorectal surgery while looking at the two main types of procedure that this somewhat generic term covers, namely laparoscopic colorectal surgery and transanal endoscopic microsurgery (TEMS).

MINIMISING THE TRAUMA OF ACCESS

There has been, and remains, confusion over nomenclature in this field of surgery.[1] Many reports use different terms, such as 'minimal invasive', 'minimal access', 'laparoscopic' and 'laparoscopic-assisted', to describe what may or may not be the same procedure. Further techniques and terminology, such as 'hand-assisted laparoscopic surgery', have heightened this effect. The terms 'minimally invasive' and 'minimal access' have been used interchangeably and refer to the ability to perform surgical procedures via the smallest possible incisions. They also imply the use of laparoscopy. All colorectal procedures that involve resection or excision require a means for removal of the specimen. Morcellating the specimen within a bag and retrieving it through a port site is not feasible since an intact specimen is required for pathological examination. Therefore, the only operation that might be described as a true laparoscopic resection is the laparoscopic abdominoperineal resection as the specimen can be retrieved through the perineal wound. Anterior resection specimens and colectomy specimens require an incision, albeit a small one, and these procedures may be better described as 'laparoscopically assisted'.

Colorectal surgery requires access to the diseased organ in order to facilitate its resection or bypass. The easiest and traditional method of doing this is through a midline laparotomy incision. When performing procedures such as anterior resection, which requires not only pelvic dissection but also usually mobilisation of the splenic flexure and a proportion of the transverse colon, a long midline wound is required simply in order to access the various quadrants of the abdomen where the surgery is to be performed. This incision of access causes pain and a decrease in mobility (with its associated risks), may increase the incidence of wound infection and incisional hernia, and leads to issues of cosmesis for the patient. A number of studies have pointed to the significance of the midline wound as a cause of the major trauma associated with abdominal surgery by measuring inflammatory and acute-phase proteins. It has been shown that these physiological markers are not as dramatically raised in procedures carried out laparoscopically. Leung et al.[2] studied 34 patients in a randomised controlled trial and demonstrated reduced levels of the cytokines interleukin 1, interleukin 6 and C-reactive protein in laparoscopic anterior resection compared with open surgery.

 Similar changes were seen in a randomised study of open vs. laparoscopic colectomy in 97 patients; no significant changes were seen in cortisol or prolactin levels.[3]

However, Tang et al.[4] found no significant demonstrable difference in systemic immune response between laparoscopic and conventional open surgery in a randomised trial of 236 patients. Overall the evidence seems to support the hypothesis that despite the same intra-abdominal operation being performed, it is the trauma of access that has been diminished. This is the physiological underpinning

of the argument in favour of laparoscopic or minimally invasive treatment. Minimise the trauma of access and the surgeon can minimise the overall physiological trauma experienced by the patient.

OTHER EFFECTS OF MINIMALLY INVASIVE SURGERY (Box 16.1)

The pneumoperitoneum of surgery induces a number of potential and real physiological changes related to increased intra-abdominal pressure and is exacerbated by the sometimes prolonged Trendelenburg position of the patient. This is considered further in the discussion of anaesthesia below.

Measuring postoperative pain is difficult: a variety of psychosocial as well as physiological and pathological processes play a part in the individual experience and expression of pain. However, a number of studies have shown that patients who

Box 16.1 • Advantages and disadvantages of laparoscopy vs. open colorectal surgery

Advantages

- Decreased acute-phase response
- Less pain
- Earlier resolution of ileus
- Earlier return to normal activity
- Better cosmesis
- Better oncological outcome???

Disadvantages

- Longer procedure
- Pathophysiology of pneumoperitoneum
- Technically difficult
  - Interpreting two-dimensional image in performing a three-dimensional task
  - Use of long instruments
  - Loss of tactile feedback
- Training issues
- Expense of capital equipment
- Worse oncological outcome???

have a laparoscopic colorectal resection suffer less postoperative pain than patients undergoing an open resection.

 Braga et al.[5] in a randomised study of 79 patients showed that laparoscopic colorectal surgery induced a reduced acute-phase response and reduced postoperative pain.

One measure used in many studies is the length of postoperative stay. This is influenced by a number of different factors, such as patient and surgeon motivation, domestic and social circumstances and the facility for out-of-hospital home care. Nevertheless, many studies use this as a measure to demonstrate the benefits of laparoscopic surgery.[6] The same factors make measurement of return to work or normal activity difficult to measure. One of the major determinants in the time taken for patients to return to normal and resume work is whether they are self-employed. However, once again the same studies and others demonstrate earlier return to normal activity.

Traditionally, surgeons have paid great attention to the ileus suffered by the bowel following major abdominal surgery. This led to early postoperative confinement of the bowel followed by introduction of sips of water, then 30–60 mL hourly, and thus stepwise back to full diet depending on the presence of bowel sounds and the passage of flatus. The minimally invasive era has led to a rewriting of the rule book on this subject. Perhaps compelled to demonstrate the dramatic effect of this new technique, laparoscopic surgeons encouraged their patients to eat and drink much earlier in the postoperative period. In addition, novel ideas such as chewing gum in the immediate postoperative period have been found to be useful in reducing the duration of ileus but not the length of stay.[7] This philosophy of early feeding was soon adopted by surgeons caring for patients operated on conventionally, and is now the norm in most surgical units after elective colorectal surgery. This is one way in which minimally invasive surgery has contributed to the development of conventional surgery.

By incorporating a number of these techniques that speed up recovery following colorectal surgery, many surgeons operating conventionally have reproduced the improvements in physical and psycho-logical function in the immediate postoperative period and have achieved earlier discharge from hospital.[8] However, laparoscopy is useful as one of a range of techniques in the so-called 'multimodal rehabilitation' of patients following surgery.[9–11] Thus early reports heralding the dramatically positive effects of laparoscopic surgery must now be considered with regard to the wholesale changes in the way that patients undergoing conventional open surgery are managed. This is reflected in most modern reports, where the gap between laparoscopic and open surgery is closing when considering outcome measures such as resolution of ileus, mobilisation, analgesic requirements and discharge from hospital.

Finally, and perhaps most indisputably, the development of minimally invasive techniques has had a dramatic effect on attitudes towards cosmesis. Recall some elderly patients operated on in their youth, when an appendicectomy was performed through a large grid-iron incision that was not closed with an eye on cosmesis and the resultant disfiguring scar. No surgeon now would perform appendicectomy in such a manner, and while curing the disease remains paramount, few surgeons and fewer patients would dispute that cosmesis is a welcome addition to the successful outcome of any operation. Hopefully the only reminder of the procedure that patients carry with them always is their scar, so why not make it neat and cosmetically acceptable? How much the effect of cosmesis contributes to the overall quality of life experienced by patients is difficult to measure. Many studies have examined quality of life as a secondary outcome measure.

 The so-called COST (Clinical Outcomes of Surgical Therapy) study from the USA showed advantages in quality of life but only assessed this in the short term.[12]

Whether better cosmesis enhances quality of life in the longer term remains to be seen.

TECHNICAL CONSIDERATIONS

Minimally invasive surgery requires different skills from those normally a prerequisite in open surgery. These skills focus mainly on the ability to manipulate long unwieldy instruments, cope with diminished tactile feedback and reinterpret a three-dimensional real-time image from a two-dimensional image projected on a screen. Using this two-dimensional image the surgeon is required to perform a number of complex three-dimensional fine motor movements, often in more than one quadrant of the abdomen, which are frequently associated with paradoxical movements of the hands in relation to the tips of the instruments. Ergonomic studies have demonstrated unique physical stresses in the laparoscopic surgeon compared with the open surgeon.[13,14] Furthermore, a study of heart rate variability in operating surgeons suggests that despite the decrease in stress response in the patients, there may be an increase in stress for the surgeon.[15] The ability to deal with these issues was a major constraint for many surgeons in the early days of minimally invasive colorectal surgery as no open surgical task really trains these techniques. However, today's trainees have grown up in an era where laparoscopic cholecystectomy is a standard procedure performed almost as commonly as inguinal hernia repair. It is likely that these basic skills, learnt early on in surgical training, will be of major benefit to the next generation of surgeons starting in the more complex field of minimally invasive colorectal surgery.

GETTING STARTED

Laparoscopic cholecystectomy was first performed in 1987,[16] and has now become the gold standard operation for the treatment of cholelithiasis, with the consequence that most surgeons upon completion of training will have performed many more laparoscopic than open cholecystectomies. This trend has not been reflected in laparoscopic colorectal surgery (first described in 1991[17]), which is the first-line approach to colorectal disease in very few UK centres. Therefore the reverse occurs in terms of experience, with plentiful exposure to open colectomy but little if any exposure to laparoscopic colorectal procedures. This creates difficulties for surgeons who wish to offer this service within their practice.

Getting started requires forethought and planning. Ideally, identifying suitable training posts at home or abroad within specialist registrar training, attending the wide variety of available courses and seeking helpful preceptors when attempting the first few cases is essential. One major determinant in beginning minimal colorectal surgery is finding the time to ensure that anaesthetists, theatre staff, an assistant and indeed the surgeon are fully conversant with the new technique. A dedicated list for performing colorectal surgery should be available in order to relieve the pressure inevitably placed on the normal operation list by the length of initial laparoscopic procedures. Keeping the same anaesthetist and camera and theatre staff is immensely helpful as the whole team learns together.

Minimally invasive colorectal surgery cannot be performed without all the necessary equipment. This comprises the laparoscopic stack with monitor, light source, camera and insufflator, laparoscopes, trocars and suitable laparoscopic instrumentation. The laparoscopes used may be either 0 or 30° telescopes, the former giving a straight-ahead view, the latter an angled illumination and view that some surgeons find helpful when operating in the pelvis. A number of specific instruments are required, such as non-traumatic bowel graspers (5 mm diameter) and endoscopic stapling devices that allow intracorporeal stapling and division of bowel under direct vision, in much the same manner as open surgery. Careful consideration must be given to the different types of dissection technology. Much dissection can be performed with conventional laparoscopic scissors or hook with attached unipolar diathermy. Many surgeons now consider technologies such as the Harmonic Scalpel (Ethicon, USA) or the non-disposable equivalent Sonosurg (Olympus, UK) to be essential for the majority of the dissection. Both of these instruments use ultrasonic technology, where the high-frequency oscillation of an active blade causes vaporisation of the tissue, producing a safe and haemostatic dissecting tool.[18]

TRAINING

The conclusions of the report of the Working Party chaired by Professor Sir Alfred Cuschieri and published in March 1993 highlighted the differences between open and minimally invasive surgery.[19] The report suggested that the introduction of minimally invasive surgery had been largely industry driven and that there was a clear need for training guidelines to be established by the Royal Colleges and specialty associations. In particular the report recommended that dedicated regional skills centres be established that should 'provide intensive, practical experience of the component skills necessary for safe laparoscopic surgery' and 'be involved in the development of objective assessments of skills and technical competence'.

There is evidence that training junior surgeons only on real patients is expensive due to the increased operating time required for training. One report from the USA which examined 62 different types of operation categories involving 14 452 cases found that resident operating times were longer than faculty times in 46 categories. The authors extrapolated their findings to estimate that the training of 1014 general surgery residents would cost $53 million annually.[20]

The consequence of these factors, not to mention political and patient expectations, means that an increasing amount of surgical skills training must take place outside theatre, away from 'real' patients, in a simulated environment on simulated patients or tissues. The Royal Surgical Colleges in the UK have begun to address this issue by setting up and franchising recognised courses, such as the Basic Surgical Skills Course, which gives an early introduction to minimal access surgery. The use of simulators may allow trainees to perform an operation on a patient for the first time, having already progressed some way along the learning curve.[21,22] Simulation may also provide an opportunity to replicate unwanted intraoperative scenarios, such as significant haemorrhage, and practise managing them. Theoretically, it should be possible to provide surgeons with a comprehensive experience in dealing with all manner of complications. Illustrating this point, Sackier,[23] both a surgeon and a keen private pilot, states that 'the first time that a resident deals with crisis management should not be a situation of true crisis.'

In summary, training in laparoscopic colorectal surgery should ideally commence with a solid grounding in basic laparoscopic skills gained in the classroom and from experience of laparoscopic cholecystectomy, all allied to a comprehensive sub-specialty training in coloproctology.

INDICATIONS AND CONTRAINDICATIONS

The indications for laparoscopic surgery are the same as those for open surgery in both benign and malignant disease. If the patient requires the operation, the use of minimally invasive techniques may be used to facilitate this. Specific contraindications that would dictate an open approach rather than laparoscopy include gross peritonitis, toxic megacolon and obstructing carcinoma. Relative contraindications include morbid obesity, extensive previous abdominal surgery and severe cardiorespiratory disease.

PREOPERATIVE MANAGEMENT

It is imperative that the correct diagnosis has been made preoperatively, in particular that there has been accurate location of the lesion to be resected. Because of limited tactile feedback during laparoscopy, resection of the wrong segment of bowel, missing the lesion altogether or overlooking a synchronous lesion is entirely possible. In this regard it may be considered wise to have performed contrast imaging rather than endoscopy alone, which is notorious for deceiving the endoscopist as to the true position of a lesion. A small lesion can be marked at endoscopy preoperatively using India ink.

In all other respects, preoperative preparation for the patient undergoing laparoscopic colorectal surgery is the same as for the open procedure, with bowel preparation, antibiotic and thromboembolic prophylaxis and stoma site marking. (While acknowledging that all the published evidence points to bowel preparation having little effect on patient outcome, it is particularly useful in laparoscopic surgery should on-table colonoscopy be required to locate a lesion.)

Finally, consenting the patient should include the specific risks of laparoscopic surgery and the risk of conversion. Ideally, this should be based on local experience and audit but a risk of conversion of 20–30% seems reasonable based on literature rates that vary from 0 to 48%. The conversion rate is highly dependent on not only surgeon experience but also case selection. Reasons for conversion are numerous and range from equipment failure, dense adhesions, uncertain anatomy to tumour fixity. Additionally, and importantly, there comes a point in any procedure when the length of time the surgery is taking negates the benefit to the patient of having the operation performed laparoscopically, and consideration should be given to conversion.

ANAESTHETIC CONSIDERATIONS

Laparoscopic colorectal surgery exerts a number of physiological changes due in part to the pneumo-peritoneum and to the adoption of the extreme Trendelenburg position required to facilitate a good laparoscopic view of the pelvis. Both of these factors can cause splinting of the diaphragm and respiratory compromise. These potential consequences have not always been borne out in clinical practice; a randomised study of laparoscopic or conventional colorectal resection of 60 patients showed that pulmonary function was less affected by the minimally invasive technique.[24] Cardiovascular effects may also occur, such as variation in venous return due to pneumoperitoneum or the Trendelenburg position. Prolonged surgery can result in excess absorption of carbon dioxide and systemic acidosis. A good working relationship with the anaesthetist is therefore required, and a willingness to deflate the pneumoperitoneum quickly if requested.

SPECIFIC CONDITIONS

While almost all colorectal procedures have been performed laparoscopically, some conditions seem particular suited to the technique.

Crohn's disease

Crohn's disease is not cured by surgery. Surgery cures the current symptomatology that the patient is experiencing due to the inflammation, fistulisation or stenosis of the segment to be resected. Consequently, many patients undergo many surgical procedures over the course of a lifetime. Therefore the benefits of laparoscopic surgery, such as cosmesis, earlier return to normal activity and potential for fewer adhesions, are particularly suited to this pre-

dominantly young group of patients.[25] The benefits can be offset against the difficulties encountered in Crohn's disease: thickened mesenteries and friable bowel in often malnourished immunosuppressed patients. The commonest site of Crohn's is the terminal ileum and the operation of ileocaecectomy in a fit thin Crohn's patient is one of the more straightforward laparoscopic operations when embarking on this type of surgery. It is important to inspect the rest of the bowel by hand-over-hand movement with bowel-grasping forceps to identify other areas of disease and estimate the remaining length of bowel. Finally, consideration should be given to the site of incision for specimen extraction. Bearing in mind that these patients may ultimately go on to have ileostomy formation at some point, avoiding a right iliac fossa incision seems sensible. When the right colon is fully mobilised, it is simple to remove it through a 3–4 cm incision in the mid-line (partly hidden in the umbilicus), exteriorise the bowel and perform an extracorporeal stapled or hand-sewn anastomosis.

The only randomised trial published of 60 patients undergoing either open or laparoscopic ileocolic resection for Crohn's disease showed a significant benefit for laparoscopy in recovery of pulmonary function but a longer operating time and no significant difference in time to discharge (5 days for laparoscopy vs. 6 days for open resection).[26]

Laparoscopic surgery in cases of recurrent Crohn's disease and previous surgery has been described with good results but a higher conversion rate.[27,28]

Cancer

The National Institute for Clinical Excellence (NICE) published its guidelines on the use of laparoscopic surgery for colorectal cancer in December 2000.[29] This stated that:

1. for colorectal cancer, open rather than laparoscopic resection should be the preferred surgical procedure;
2. laparoscopic surgery should be undertaken for colorectal cancer as part of a randomised controlled clinical trial.

These guidelines were based on evidence from literature review, submissions by the Association of Endoscopic Surgeons of Great Britain and Ireland, manufacturers, professional groups, patient groups and external expert and patient advocates. The NICE guidelines were to be reviewed in August 2003.

The NICE guidelines reflected to a certain extent the grave concerns about the reports of port-site metastases, a potential consequence of laparoscopic surgery. The safety of the laparoscopic approach for the resection of cancer is a contentious issue. Colonic cancer is the second commonest cancer in the Western world, and surgery offers a potential cure in 50% of patients. Therefore, it has been essential to ensure that the laparoscopic procedure is at least as effective a cure as the open procedure. On the technical front there are worries that the loss of tactile feedback may result in greater manipulation of, or inadvertent incision into, the tumour. One of the greatest concerns is whether resection margins and nodal sampling are compromised during laparoscopic resection. Circumferential resection margins are particularly important in rectal cancer as inadequate clearance of the mesorectum or margin is the principal cause of local recurrence.

The MRC-funded CLASICC (Conventional versus Laparoscopic-Assisted Surgery in Colorectal Cancer) trial was set up in 1996 specifically to help answer these questions. The trial has now stopped recruiting and although no data have yet been published, the demographic data of the 794 patients have been presented at a number of meetings. These initial data from the CLASICC trial appear to confirm findings of randomised studies from other countries, namely that laparoscopic surgery can achieve similar results to open surgery in terms of lymph node harvest and resection margin clearance. However, it is important to acknowledge that long-term data will not be available for some time.

The debate over port-site metastases merits some discussion in its own right as it has been the major argument against the performance of laparoscopic resection of malignancy. The early reports of this phenomenon were enough for Berends et al.,[30] when reporting three cases in a series of 14 resections (20%), to suggest that 'laparoscopic resection of colorectal cancer should be abandoned'. The concern regarding port-site metastases generated much research into all possible mechanisms, such as the

so-called chimney effect of laparoscopic smoke through port sites, where aerosolised tumour cells implant at the wound as the gas rushes out during deflation of the pneumoperitoneum, or factors related to the use of humidified carbon dioxide as an insufflating gas. Many precautions have been suggested for preventing port-site metastases, such as the use of wound protectors at the time of specimen extraction. The cause has not been truly elucidated but concern has diminished for two main reasons. Firstly, when looking at open surgery in greater depth it is clear that wound recurrence is a phenomenon of all surgery and not an issue peculiar to laparoscopy at all. Secondly, the early reports of high incidences of port-site metastases have not been borne out by the many case series and randomised studies published recently and in the latter part of the last decade (Table 16.1). The general consensus among surgeons now is that port-site metastases are

Table 16.1 • Port-site metastases (series greater than 100 patients)

Reference	Number of port-site metastases/ total patients	Percentage
Lumley et al. (1996)[31]	1/103	1.0
Kwok et al. (1996)[32]	1/83	1.2
Fleshman et al. (1996)[33]	4/372	1.1
Franklin et al. (1996)[34]	0/180	0
Vukasin et al. (1996)[35]	5/480	1.1
Huscher et al. (1996)[36]	0/146	0
Lacy et al. (1997)[37]	0/106	0
Fielding et al. (1997)[38]	2/149	1.3
Larach et al. (1997)[39]	0/108	0
Croce et al. (1997)[40]	1/134	0.9
Leung et al. (1999)[41]	1/217	0.65
Poulin et al. (1999)[42]	0/172	0
Schiedeck et al. (2000)[43]	1/399	0.25
Total	**16/2649**	**0.6**

After Chung C, Tsang W, Kwok S, Li M. Laparoscopy and its current role in the management of colorectal disease. Colorectal Dis 2003; 5:528–43, with permission from Blackwell Publishing Ltd.

not an integral risk of laparoscopic colon resection for malignancy but that the high incidence in the early days of the procedure was an unfortunate consequence of the learning curve of surgeons undertaking a procedure in evolution. In this respect there is an analogy with the high incidence of bile duct injury at the inception of laparoscopic cholecystectomy.

The most explosive paper that has been published to date on the subject of laparoscopic surgery for colorectal cancer comes from Barcelona.[44] In this well-conducted randomised controlled trial of 219 patients with colon cancer, laparoscopic surgery not only gave significant benefits in terms of morbidity, recovery and postoperative stay but multifactorial analysis also demonstrated improved cancer-related survival in patients with stage III disease.

Recent evidence such as this, and the facts that concerns about port-site metastases have largely been allayed and that the major UK trial for laparoscopic treatment of colorectal cancer (CLASICC trial) has closed, suggests that an urgent revisit of the NICE guidelines is required.

Rectal prolapse

There is a multitude of operative procedures described for the treatment of rectal prolapse (see Chapter 10). These can be divided into perineal and abdominal procedures. Broadly speaking, the perineal procedures have a higher risk of recurrence but avoid the risks and discomfort of abdominal surgery. Laparoscopic surgery might very well be less painful than abdominal procedures but more effective than perineal procedures. The commonest procedures to be performed laparoscopically are sutured or stapled rectopexy and resection rectopexy. A randomised trial of 40 patients with full-thickness rectal prolapse that compared laparoscopic and abdominal rectopexy showed significantly less pain and earlier mobility for the laparoscopic group, although operating time was longer.[45] In addition, a number of case series have been published. Results from 48 patients undergoing stapled rectopexy at St Mary's Hospital showed a median time to discharge of 5 days, with one conversion and two recurrences at 18 months' follow-up.[46] Larger series

are starting to be published[47–49] but in general follow-up has been short and more substantial follow-up times are required.

Overall, published results indicate that laparoscopic repair of rectal prolapse is as good as the open procedure in terms of functional outcome and recurrence, with the added benefit of improved short-term benefits such as postoperative pain and cosmesis. The benign nature of the condition obviates the need for a resected specimen with adequate margins, and the full benefits of a laparoscopic procedure can be realised. The population that commonly presents with rectal prolapse is post-retirement age and therefore less able to tolerate major abdominal surgery. Although perineal procedures have been advocated for this group of patients, the functional outcome is arguably not as good. Laparoscopic repair extends the spectrum of patients to whom an abdominal procedure can be offered.

Diverticular disease

The use of laparoscopic surgery in diverticular disease has the advantage that none of the oncological concerns apply, although there is the disadvantage that the disease can present some of the most challenging situations for the abdominal surgeon. Fistulising disease, abscess formation and severe inflammation can all accompany diverticular disease. A multicentre study of over 300 patients undergoing laparoscopic resection of the sigmoid colon for diverticular disease had an overall conversion rate of 7.2%.[50] The less severe cases, for example those with stenosis or recurrent attacks of inflammation, had a conversion rate of 4.8% compared with 18.2% in complicated diverticular disease. Complications were also higher in this latter group (31.8% vs. 14.8%). Another study of 170 patients has been reported with a lower conversion rate of 4% and good functional outcomes.[51] Overall, the published data[52,53] point to a role for laparoscopy in the treatment of diverticular disease.

Other conditions

A wide range of other conditions, such as functional bowel disease with colonic inertia, endometriosis, volvulus and segmental resection for colonic polyps, have all been performed laparoscopically. Furthermore, there may be a role for laparoscopy, specifically the use of laparoscopic ultrasound, in the staging of colorectal cancer in order to characterise equivocal liver lesions found on computed tomography or conventional ultrasound.

SPECIFIC PROCEDURES

Although the aim of this chapter is not to provide a comprehensive guide to operative technique, it may be helpful to consider a few aspects of individual procedures and how they apply to individual conditions.

Laparoscopic colorectal surgery

RIGHT HEMICOLECTOMY

Right hemicolectomy, or ileocaecetomy, is a good operation for the surgeon early in their laparoscopic experience. It uses many of the necessary dissecting skills and while the dissection is performed intracorporeally, vascular division can be performed laparoscopically or via a small incision if needed. The resection and anastomosis are performed extracorporeally before closure of the incision, which can be made in a number of positions. We have found the best position to be within the umbilicus and extended for 3 cm in the midline (**Fig. 16.1**). This allows minimal tension on the transverse colon and gives an incision that is largely hidden within the umbilicus.

SIGMOID COLECTOMY/ANTERIOR RESECTION

In general, a left-sided resection requires four to five ports situated as shown in **Fig. 16.2**. The mobilisation is performed intracorporeally. There are essentially two methods of doing this: a conventional mobilisation along the white line of Toldt, or a medial to lateral approach where the inferior mesenteric vessels can be identified and divided early. Mobilisation of the left colon and sigmoid is carried out in the Trendelenburg position and the position reversed for mobilisation of the splenic flexure. The rectum can be mobilised down to the

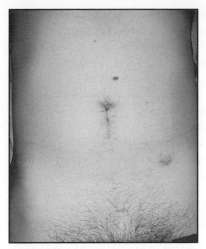

Figure 16.1 • Postoperative picture of a patient with Crohn's disease who had undergone ileocaecal resection showing the incision for specimen extraction partly hidden within the umbilicus.

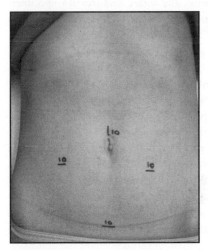

Figure 16.2 • One possible configuration of port placement for laparoscopic sigmoid resection.

pelvic floor if necessary in the 'holy plane' of total mesorectal excision, with the added benefit that the magnification in laparoscopic surgery can aid in the performance of a nerve-sparing dissection. The rectum can then be divided at the selected height using an endoscopic gastrointestinal anastomosis (GIA) stapler. When the division point is low in the rectum, it is beneficial to use a GIA stapler that allows rotation of the head in order to minimise the angle of division. A small incision is made either in the left iliac fossa, extending a port site, or suprapubically as a Pfannenstiel incision. The latter has the advantage that it can be extended to provide relatively easy access to the pelvis if required and is cosmetically better placed. The proximal colon and specimen are removed through this incision, with or without a wound protector, and the proximal resection margin selected. Once divided and the specimen removed, the anvil of a circular stapling gun is placed with a pursestring suture and dropped back into the abdomen. The small wound is closed and pneumoperitoneum established. The anastomosis is then completed intracorporeally by grasping the anvil and connecting it to the gun passed up through the rectal stump.

ABDOMINOPERINEAL RESECTION

Abdominoperineal resection and non-resection rectopexy are perhaps the only truly laparoscopic procedures. No abdominal incision is required for either procedure: the latter requires no specimen removal, while in the former the specimen is removed via the perineal incision as in the conventional procedure. The abdominal part of the operation is carried out in the same way as for anterior resection described above. However, the key to the operation is that the abdominal dissection stops circumferentially at the level of the coccyx and the rest of the procedure is completed by the perineal operator ensuring good oncological clearance. One technical point is that the proximal colon division should be performed before the perineal dissection begins, as attempting to do this when the pneumoperitoneum has been lost is difficult and potentially hazardous.

RECTOPEXY

Laparoscopic rectopexy involves mobilising the rectum to the pelvic floor without division of the lateral ligaments because this may reduce the incidence of postoperative constipation. The rectum can then be sutured or stapled to the sacral promontory. Interestingly, this is the only laparoscopic colorectal operation where suturing is regularly required, although proficiency in this skill can be useful in unexpected circumstances in any procedure. If a resection is to be carried out, this is performed in the same way as for an anterior resection, with a small left iliac fossa incision to remove the specimen and insertion of the anvil of the stapling gun.

REVERSAL OF HARTMANN'S PROCEDURE

Many patients who undergo an emergency Hartmann's procedure, with resection of a diseased segment (usually sigmoid or upper rectum) and the formation of a colostomy, never have their stoma reversed. The reasons for this are multifactorial: the disease process or comorbidity may make reversal inadvisable; the patient (and surgeon) may not wish to undergo more major surgery; and these patients often do not get priority in the already hard-pressed practice of many colorectal surgeons. A minimally invasive approach to these patients can make a difference to some but not all of these factors. Laparoscopy will avoid reopening a long midline wound, with the attendant increased risk of wound infection associated with reversal of stoma. In addition, the potential for less pain and quicker recovery may make the operation a more attractive proposition for patients. The initial part of the operation is mobilisation of the stoma in the conventional manner until completely free. The head of a stapling gun can then be introduced with a pursestring suture and the bowel dropped back into the abdomen. By passing a finger through this wound it is possible to aid safe insertion of the first port at the umbilicus. On closing the wound and establishing pneumoperitoneum, dissection of the rectal stump can then be performed. This is greatly facilitated if there has been little or no pelvic dissection at the initial operation. The use of a rectal probe can facilitate identification of the stump. End-to-end anastomosis can then be performed in the usual way. The greatest obstacle and the cause of most conversions in this group of patients is the presence of dense pelvic adhesions. There have been no randomised controlled trials in this group of patients but several small series attest to its effectiveness.[54,55]

HAND-ASSISTED LAPAROSCOPIC SURGERY

Hand-assisted laparoscopic surgery is a newer technique. The argument for its use in resectional surgery is that if an incision is likely to be needed in order to remove the specimen, then why not make it at the beginning of the procedure and put a hand through it. It involves the intra-abdominal placement of a hand through a mini-laparotomy incision while pneumoperitoneum is maintained by one of a number of commercially available sleeves or ports. In this way the hand can be used as in an open procedure to palpate organs or tumours, retract atraumatically, identify vessels and dissect bluntly along a tissue plane, and also to provide finger pressure to bleeding points while proximal control is achieved. Additionally, it might be argued that this approach is more economical than a totally laparoscopic approach, reducing both the number of laparoscopic ports and the number of instruments required. Some advocates of the technique claim that it is also easier to learn and perform than totally laparoscopic approaches. Certainly, it might act as a halfway house in the process of learning laparoscopic surgery and may also be a useful step when conversion is being contemplated during laparoscopic surgery.

SUMMARY

Laparoscopic surgery is regularly described as a new technique. In fact, laparoscopic colorectal surgery has been around for over a decade. Despite this, it has not become absorbed into the everyday practice of colorectal surgery in the same way that laparoscopic cholecystectomy has become the gold standard operation for cholelithiasis. This is because of the complexity of the surgery and a result of early concerns about its efficacy and oncological safety. The balanced view would seem to be an acceptance that laparoscopic surgery offers benefits to some patients. As a specialty we readily accept the small benefit given to certain groups of patients by adjuvant chemotherapy and we should therefore support the adoption of laparoscopic surgery in providing the benefits of less pain, quicker recovery and better cosmesis that are so tangible to the patient. Ultimately, with a much more informed public, the demand for laparoscopic colorectal surgery may find itself becoming a very patient-driven subspecialty for the colorectal surgeon.

Transanal endoscopic microsurgery

The development of new technologies often rekindles interest in old ideas. The concept of local excision of rectal lesions is not a new one. Parks'

peranal excision is well established and two other sphincter-cutting techniques, namely those of Kraske[56] and York Mason,[57] held popularity for a brief period. The advent of TEMS, as developed by Buess et al. in 1984,[58] has heralded an increase in the number of patients undergoing local excision and also an apparent widening of the indications for such surgery. Combining the concepts of local excision with the technology of minimally invasive surgery, a greater area of the rectum became accessible to surgeons attempting to remove tumours peranally.

There is no debate about the usefulness of local excision by TEMS or peranal excision as described by Parks in the circumstances of benign disease, a patient unfit for a lengthy abdominal procedure or for palliation of the symptoms caused by a rectal tumour in a patient with incurable disease. However, there is controversy surrounding the use of local excision in the situation of a potentially curable rectal tumour. Traditional surgical treatment has involved wide segmental excision of such a tumour along with its lymphovascular pedicle. The excision is part curative by removing any residual or metastatic disease and part prognostic by allowing accurate staging of the disease. Therefore, local excision of the tumour alone prevents the potential therapeutic and prognostic information provided by a radical abdominal procedure.

The argument for local excision is that some tumours have such a low probability of lymph node metastases that this small risk is more than offset by avoidance of the morbidity and mortality associated with major resectional surgery. Thus, the crux of the matter is the ability to predict the likelihood of lymph node metastases using conventional preoperative staging techniques.

Radiological preoperative staging of rectal cancer uses two main techniques, magnetic resonance imaging (MRI) and endorectal ultrasound (EUS). With regard to assessment of the crucial circumferential resection margin in advanced rectal tumours, the evidence appears to fall heavily in favour of MRI. However, when trying to distinguish between T1 stage (confined to the submucosa) and T2 stage (breaching the submucosa), the greater spatial resolution of EUS has the edge. However, while good for T stage, various studies of the ability of EUS to predict nodal status (N stage) of a rectal tumour have not shown much improvement from the early work of Beynon et al., which demonstrated an accuracy of 78% for the detection of positive and negative nodes.[59] The importance of accurate staging of a rectal tumour becomes important when considering the seminal work of Hermanek and Gall[60] who on examining the complete radical resection specimens of 1588 rectal cancers were able to identify low-risk and high-risk cancers for lymph node metastases (3% and 12% respectively) (**Table 16.2**).

This corresponded with the assertion of Lockhart-Mummery and Dukes in 1952 that the three factors that affected local recurrence following local excision were depth of invasion, grade of malignancy and adequate margin of tissue around the tumour.[61] Bearing this in mind, reasonable selection criteria for tumours to be treated via TEMS include those less than 5 cm in size and well-differentiated or moderately differentiated tumours that appear to be T1 stage on EUS.

TECHNIQUE

All patients should be warned of the possibility of conversion to a laparotomy if a complication arises or if the lesion is found to be extensive but still resectable. Bowel preparation and antibiotic and antithrombotic therapy should be used as for any bowel surgery.

Apart from anterior tumours in the upper third of the rectum that have to be considered with care as full-thickness excision here will enter the peritoneal

cavity, the whole of the rectum is accessible using TEMS. The patient is generally positioned such that the lesion to be excised lies inferiorly; this requires care with an anterior tumour as the patient is often balanced on the table with the hips and knees fully flexed in a praying position. The 4-cm diameter operating sigmoidoscope has four airtight ports through which can be passed instruments for grasping, cutting, coagulation and suction. The view within the rectum is maintained by steady insufflation of carbon dioxide, and the image is unusual for minimally invasive surgery because the use of a sophisticated binocular viewing system allows a three-dimensional (as opposed to the usual two-dimensional) image to be displayed for the operating surgeon. Use of a simple attachment allows this to be projected onto a television monitor so that the assistant and scrub nurse can follow the procedure. This is also vital for training purposes.

Surgeons are split on the subject of full- or partial-thickness excision of the lesion. The advantage of full-thickness excision is that it gives a greater chance of complete excision and is quicker and easier to learn. The resultant defect can be sutured or left open provided it does not enter the peritoneal cavity. The disadvantage of full-thickness excision is that if histology were to dictate radical resection, then the plane of dissection has been disturbed, making further surgery potentially more difficult.

CLINICAL RESULTS

Results from several studies of TEMS demonstrate favourable levels of morbidity (0–14%). Complications of bleeding, perforation, suture disruption, rectovaginal fistula, incontinence, rectal stricture and urinary problems have all been reported. There have been concerns expressed about possible functional impairment following the introduction of such a large instrument through the sphincters; however, these concerns have not been borne out in large physiological studies. Mortality is extremely rare. The crucial measure of the success of TEMS is local recurrence. Winde et al.[62] performed a randomised controlled study of 50 patients with T1 rectal cancers undergoing either TEMS ($N = 24$) or radical resection ($N = 26$). There was one case of local recurrence in the TEMS group and one case of distant metastases in the radical resection group, leading to 96% 5-year survival in both groups.

Table 16.2 • Characteristics of T1 tumours that predict the risk of lymph node metastases

	Low risk*	High risk†
Tumour diameter (cm)	<3	>3
Differentiation	Well/moderate	Poor/signet
Lymphatic invasion	No	Yes
Vascular invasion	No	Yes

*3% risk of lymph node metastases.
†12% risk of lymph node metastases.
From Hermanek P, Gall F. Early (microinvasive) colorectal cancer. Pathology, diagnosis, surgical treatment. Int J Colorectal Dis 1986; 1:79–84, with permission from Springer–Verlag ©.

The most extensive analysis of TEMS is provided by the originators of the technique.[63] Since 1983 they have analysed the data from 326 patients, 274 of whom have been included in a prospective clinical trial. Both operative time and complication rate were higher in the group with carcinomatous lesions, attributable to the larger extent of the resection. Another series from Cologne showed successful therapeutic excision of lesions in 84% of 286 patients.[64] Radical surgery was performed in 7.6% of patients where histology of the lesion showed poorly differentiated or advanced tumours.

Despite these successful results, there are some practical drawbacks to the technique. Equipment is costly and training is difficult as the procedure is predominantly a one-operator technique.

SUMMARY

Local excision has all the advantages of a minimally invasive therapy. Major resections, with their concurrent mortality, colostomy rate and loss of sphincters, can be avoided. Nevertheless, completeness of local excision of lesions is essential to avoid recurrence. Published results are encouraging, although it is unlikely that this is a skill that will need to be acquired by all colorectal surgeons or indeed every hospital as the number of cases that are suitable constitute a small percentage of the colorectal workload. Ultimately, TEMS is a technique for performing local excision. Whether local excision should be performed in a particular case boils down to a statistical argument regarding competing risks allied to the patient's understanding of what it all means. Some patients terrified by cancer may consider local excision unacceptable, even for low-risk tumours. Others, properly informed, will accept its potential benefits.

Key points

- Laparoscopy has proven benefits in reducing the acute-phase response to the trauma of surgery.
- The extent of the benefit of laparoscopic colorectal surgery over open surgery has been narrowed by the introduction of more aggressive preoperative, perioperative and postoperative multimodal therapies.
- Laparoscopic surgery is particularly useful in Crohn's disease where patients can expect a number of surgical interventions over a lifetime.
- Modern results indicate at least equivalence for the oncological safety of laparoscopic surgery for cancer, although long-term data from the major randomised trials are not yet available.
- Use of TEMS technology extends the area of the rectum accessible to local excision of early rectal cancer.
- There are tried and tested criteria in predicting rectal cancers with a low risk of lymph node metastases according to preoperative staging.
- Extending these criteria necessitates the use of adjuvant therapies and ideally should be performed within a trial setting.

REFERENCES

1. Mathur P, Seow-Choen F. The difference between laparoscopic and keyhole surgery. Br J Surg 2003; 90:1029–30.

2. Leung KL, Lai PB, Ho RL et al. Systemic cytokine response after laparoscopic-assisted resection of rectosigmoid carcinoma: a prospective randomized trial. Ann Surg 2000; 231:506–11.

3. Delgado S, Lacy A, Filella X et al. Acute phase response in laparoscopic and open colectomy in colon cancer. Dis Colon Rectum 2001; 44:638–46.

   A good example of the studies looking at the acute-phase response in laparoscopic surgery.

4. Tang CL, Eu KW, Tai BC, Soh JG, MacHin D, Seow-Choen F. Randomized clinical trial of the effect of open versus laparoscopically assisted colectomy on systemic immunity in patients with colorectal cancer. Br J Surg 2001; 88:801–7.

5. Braga M, Vignali A, Zuliani W et al. Metabolic and functional results after laparoscopic colorectal surgery: a randomized, controlled trial. Dis Colon Rectum 2002; 45:1070–7.

   Another good example of the work on the patho-physiology of laparoscopy.

6. Braga M, Vignali A, Gianotti L et al. Laparoscopic versus open colorectal surgery: a randomized trial on short-term outcome. Ann Surg 2002; 236:759–66; disscussion 767.

7. Asao T, Kuwano H, Nakamura J, Morinaga N, Hirayama I, Ide M. Gum chewing enhances recovery from postoperative ileus after laparoscopic colectomy. J Am Coll Surg 2002; 195:30–2.

8. Anderson A, McNaught C, MacFie J, Tring I, Barker P, Mitchell C. Randomised clinical trial of multimodal optimisation and standard perioperative surgical care. Br J Surg 2003; 90:1497–504.

9. Senagore A, Duepree H, Delaney C, Brady K, Fazio V. Results of a standardised technique and postoperative care plan for laparoscopic sigmoid colectomy: a 30-month experience. Dis Colon Rectum 2003; 46:503–9.

10. Kehlet H, Wilmore D. Multimodal strategies to improve surgical outcome. Am J Surg 2002; 183:630–41.

11. Wilmore D, Kehlet H. Management of patients in fast track surgery. Br Med J 2001; 322:473–6.

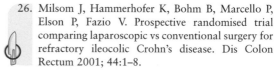
12. Weeks J, Nelson H, Gelber S, Sargent D, Schroeder G. Short-term quality-of-life outcomes following laparoscopic-assisted colectomy vs. open colectomy for colon cancer: a randomised trial. JAMA 2002; 287:321–8.

13. Gillette J, Quick N, Adrales G, Shapiro R, Park A. Changes in postural mechanics associated with different types of minimally invasive surgical training exercises. Surg Endosc 2003; 17:259–63.

14. Berguer R. Surgical technology and the ergonomics of laparoscopic instruments. Surg Endosc 1998; 12:458–62.

15. Bohm B, Rotting N, Schwenk W, Grebe S, Mansmann U. A prosepctive randomised trial on heart rate variability of the surgical team during laparoscopic and conventional sigmoid resection. Arch Surg 2001; 136:305.

16. Dubois E, Icard P, Berthelot G, Levard H. Coelioscopic cholecystectomy: preliminary report of 36 cases. Ann Surg 1990; 211:60–2.

17. Jacobs M, Verdeja J, Goldstein H. Minimally invasive colon resection (laparoscopic colectomy). Surg Laparosc Endosc 1991; 1:144–50.

18. Gossot D, Buess G, Cuschieri A et al. Ultrasonic dissection for endoscopic surgery. The EAES Technology Group. Surg Endosc 1999; 13:412–17.

19. Cuschieri A. Minimal access surgery: implications for the NHS. London: Department of Health and the Scottish Office Home and Health Department, 1993.

20. Bridges M, Diamond D. The financial impact of teaching surgical residents in the operating room. Am J Surg 1999; 177:28–32.

21. Hunter J. The learning curve in laparoscopic cholecystectomy. Minim Invasive Ther Allied Technol 1997; 6:24–5.

22. Lirici M. New techniques, new technologies and educational implications. Minim Invasive Ther Allied Technol 1997; 6:102–4.

23. Sackier J. Evaluation of technical surgical skills: lessons from minimal access surgery. Surg Endosc 1998; 12:1109–10.

24. Schwenk W, Bohm B, Witt C, Junghans T, Grundel K, Muller JM. Pulmonary function following laparoscopic or conventional colorectal resection: a randomized controlled evaluation. Arch Surg 1999; 134:6–12; discussion 13.

25. Dunker M, Stiggelbout A, Van Hogezand R, Ringers J, Griffioen G, Bemelman W. Cosmesis and body image after laparoscopic-assisted and open ileocolic resection for Crohns disease. Surg Endosc 1998; 12:1334–40.

26. Milsom J, Hammerhofer K, Bohm B, Marcello P, Elson P, Fazio V. Prospective randomised trial comparing laparoscopic vs conventional surgery for refractory ileocolic Crohn's disease. Dis Colon Rectum 2001; 44:1–8.

   One of the few randomised studies looking at the clinical effects of laparoscopic surgery in Crohn's disease.

27. Schmidt C, Talamini M, Kaufman H, Lilliemoe K, Learn P, Bayless T. Laparoscopic surgery for

Crohn's disease: reasons for conversion. Ann Surg 2001; 233:733–9.

28. Evans J, Poritz L, Macrae H. Influence of experience on laparoscopic ileocolic resection for Crohn's disease. Dis Colon Rectum 2002; 45:1595–600.

29. National Institute for Clinical Excellence. Guidance on the use of laparoscopic surgery for colorectal cancer. Technology Appraisal Guidance No. 17. London: NICE, 2000.

30. Berends F, Kazemier G, Bonjer H, Lange J. Subcutaneous metastases after laparoscopic colectomy. Lancet 1994; 344:58.

31. Lumley JW, Fielding GA, Rhodes M, Nathanson LK, Siu S, Stitz RW. Laparoscopic-assisted colorectal surgery. Lessons learned from 240 consecutive patients. Dis Colon Rectum 1996; 39:155–9.

32. Kwok SP, Lau WY, Carey PD, Kelly SB, Leung KL, Li AK. Prospective evaluation of laparoscopic-assisted large bowel excision for cancer. Ann Surg 1996; 223:170–6.

33. Fleshman JW, Nelson H, Peters WR et al. Early results of laparoscopic surgery for colorectal cancer. Retrospective analysis of 372 patients treated by Clinical Outcomes of Surgical Therapy (COST) Study Group. Dis Colon Rectum 1996; 39(10 suppl.):S53–S58.

34. Franklin M, Rosenthal D, Abrego-Medina D. Prospective comparison of open vs laparoscopic colon surgery for carcinoma: five year results. Dis Colon Rectum 1996; 39:s35–s46.

35. Vukasin P, Ortega AE, Greene FL et al. Wound recurrence following laparoscopic colon cancer resection. Results of the American Society of Colon and Rectal Surgeons Laparoscopic Registry. Dis Colon Rectum 1996; 39(10 suppl.):S20–S23.

36. Huscher C, Silecchia G, Croce E et al. Laparoscopic colorectal resection. A multicenter Italian study. Surg Endosc 1996; 10:875–9.

37. Lacy AM, Garcia-Valdecasas JC, Delgado S et al. Postoperative complications of laparoscopic-assisted colectomy. Surg Endosc 1997; 11:119–22.

38. Fielding GA, Lumley J, Nathanson L, Hewitt P, Rhodes M, Stitz R. Laparoscopic colectomy. Surg Endosc 1997; 11:745–9.

39. Larach SW, Patankar SK, Ferrara A, Williamson PR, Perozo SE, Lord AS. Complications of laparoscopic colorectal surgery. Analysis and comparison of early vs. later experience. Dis Colon Rectum 1997; 40:592–6.

40. Croce E, Azzola M, Russo R, Golia M, Olmi S. Laparoscopic colectomy: the absolute need for a standard operative technique. JSLS 1997; 1:217–24.

41. Leung KL, Yiu RY, Lai PB, Lee JF, Thung KH, Lau WY. Laparoscopic-assisted resection of colorectal carcinoma: five-year audit. Dis Colon Rectum 1999; 42:327–32; discussion 332–3.

42. Poulin EC, Mamazza J, Schlachta CM, Gregoire R, Roy N. Laparoscopic resection does not adversely affect early survival curves in patients undergoing surgery for colorectal adenocarcinoma. Ann Surg 1999; 229:487–92.

43. Schiedeck TH, Schwandner O, Baca I et al. Laparoscopic surgery for the cure of colorectal cancer: results of a German five-center study. Dis Colon Rectum 2000; 43:1–8.

44. Lacy A, Garcia-Valdecasas J, Delgado S, Castelis A, Taura P, Pique J. Laparoscopy-assisted colectomy versus open colectomy for treatment of non-metastatic colon cancer: a randomised trial. Lancet 2002; 359:2224–9.

Perhaps the most important recent paper regarding laparoscopic surgery in malignancy, showing a survival benefit in stage III disease.

45. Solomon MJ, Young CJ, Eyers AA, Roberts RA. Randomized clinical trial of laparoscopic versus open abdominal rectopexy for rectal prolapse. Br J Surg 2002; 89:35–9.

46. Cheshire N, Scott H, Nduka C, Darzi A. Stapled laparoscopic rectopexy for rectal prolapse. Br J Surg 1996; 83(suppl. 1):2.

47. Kessler H, Jerby BL, Milsom JW. Successful treatment of rectal prolapse by laparoscopic suture rectopexy. Surg Endosc 1999; 13:858–61.

48. Heah S, Hartley J, Hurley J, Duthie G, Monson J. Laparoscopic suture rectopexy without resection is effective treatment for full thickness rectal prolapse. Dis Colon Rectum 2000; 43:638–43.

49. Xynos Chrynos E, Tsiaoussis J, Epanomeritakis E, Vassilakis J. Resection rectopexy for rectal prolapse. The laparoscopic approach. Surg Endosc 1999; 13:862–4.

50. Kockerling F, Schneider C, Reymond MA et al. Laparoscopic resection of sigmoid diverticulitis. Results of a multicenter study. Laparoscopic Colorectal Surgery Study Group. Surg Endosc 1999; 13:567–71.

51. Trebuchet G, Lechaux D, Lecalve J. Laparoscopic left colon resection for diverticular disease. Surg Endosc 2002; 16:18–21.

52. Schlachta CM, Mamazza J, Poulin EC. Laparoscopic sigmoid resection for acute and chronic diverticulitis. An outcomes comparison with laparoscopic resection for nondiverticular disease. Surg Endosc 1999; 13:649–53.

53. Eijsbouts QA, Cuesta MA, de Brauw LM, Sietses C. Elective laparoscopic-assisted sigmoid resection for diverticular disease. Surg Endosc 1997; 11:750–3.

54. Lucarini L, Galleano R, Lombezzi R, Ippoliti M, Ajraldi G. Laparoscopic-assisted Hartmann's

reversal with the Dexterity Pneumo Sleeve. Dis Colon Rectum 2000; 43:1164–7.

55. Regadas F, Siebra J, Rodrigues L, Nicodemo A, Reis Neto J. Laparoscopically assisted colorectal anastomosis post-Hartmann's procedure. Surg Laparosc Endosc 1996; 6:1–4.

56. Kraske P. Zur exstirpation hochsitzender mastdarmkrebse. Verhdt Chir 1885; 14:464.

57. Mason A. Trans-sphincteric exposure for low rectal anastomosis. Proc R Soc Med 1972; 65:974.

58. Buess G, Hutterer F, Theiss J et al. Das system fur die transanale rektum operation. Chirurg 1984; 55:677–80.

59. Beynon J, Mortensen N, Foy D, Channer J, Rigby H, Virjee J. Preoperative assessment of mesorectal lymph node involvement in rectal cancer. Br J Surg 1989; 76:276–9.

60. Hermaneck P, Gall F. Early (microinvasive) colorectal cancer. Pathology, diagnosis, surgical treatment. Int J Colorectal Dis 1986; 1:79–84.

61. Lockhart-Mummery H, Dukes C. The surgical treatment of malignant rectal polyps. Lancet 1952; ii:751–5.

62. Winde G, Nottberg H, Keller R, Schmid K, Bunte H. Surgical cure for early rectal carcinomas (T1). Transanal endoscopic microsurgery vs anterior resection. Dis Colon Rectum 1998; 41:526–7.

63. Buess G, Mentges B, Manncke K et al. Technique and results of TEM in early rectal cancer. Am J Surg 1992; 163:63–70.

64. Said S, Huber P, Pichlmaier H. Technique and results of endorectal surgery. Surgery 1993; 113:65–75.

Seventeen
Intestinal failure

Alexander G. Heriot and
Alastair C.J. Windsor

DEFINITION

Intestinal failure is defined as the inability to maintain adequate nutritional, fluid and electrolyte status without supportive therapy. This is the result of loss of functioning gut mass to below that required for absorption of nutrients, fluid and electrolytes.[1] The pathophysiology was first described experimentally by Senn in 1888,[2] and clinically by Flint in 1912 and Hammond in 1935.[3,4] The vast majority of cases of intestinal failure are transient, without significant gut pathology, and are routinely managed in district general hospitals. These cases are generally of short duration (<3 weeks), have straightforward management and frequently occur secondary to postoperative ileus. However, there is a group of cases distinguished by loss of functional gut that results in prolonged intestinal failure lasting from months to years, some patients requiring permanent parenteral nutrition. Management of these cases may be complex, prolonged and expensive, in terms of both financial cost and clinical input. Care may be optimised by involvement of a multidisciplinary unit devoted to the management of intestinal failure. This unit will include a nutrition support team with the capacity to facilitate the transition of the patient's care from a hospital environment to a home environment.

EPIDEMIOLOGY

It is unclear precisely how many individuals suffer from intestinal failure, but consideration of patients requiring home parenteral nutrition (HPN) indicates an incidence around 2 per million.[5] However, a more recent European study of HPN reported a higher incidence of 3 per million, with a prevalence of 4 per million.[6] Both these figures are likely to underestimate the true incidence of some degree of intestinal failure, as 50–70% of patients who initially require total parenteral nutrition (TPN) can be weaned off it, particularly children, and some patients never require TPN at all during their management.

Around half the patients on HPN may be suitable for small bowel transplantation. Estimates from Switzerland[7] and Finland[8] put the figure for those patients suitable for small bowel transplantation at 0.5–1.5 per million per year. At St Mark's Hospital there are 85 patients being maintained on HPN out of approximately 300 in the country.

CAUSES

The underlying causes of chronic intestinal failure differ between adults and children and are summarised in **Box 17.1**.

Box 17.1 • Aetiology of short bowel syndrome

Adults

- Mesenteric thrombus
- Crohn's disease
- Midgut volvulus
- Trauma
- Mesenteric desmoid
- Pseudo-obstruction
- Radiation enteritis

Children

- Midgut volvulus
- Necrotising enterocolitis
- Congenital atresia
- Gastroschisis
- Hirschsprung's disease
- Pseudo-obstruction

Surgery

RESECTION

Surgical resection of bowel may result in short bowel syndrome (SBS) where the amount of remaining bowel is inadequate. This may be the result of multiple resections for recurrent Crohn's disease or due to an isolated massive enterectomy that may be necessary following a vascular catastrophe, such as mesenteric arterial thrombosis or embolism, venous thrombosis, volvulus, trauma or, in the case of children, necrotising enterocolitis or gastroschisis.

The amount of bowel removed that results in SBS is variable and is influenced by the age of the patient, the site of resection and the presence or absence of colon. The normal small bowel is around 600 cm in length but may range between 300 and 800 cm. The important figure is not how much small bowel is removed but how much remains. An approximate figure of less than 100 cm in the presence of an ileostomy or less than 50 cm with colon present is likely to result in dependence on TPN at 3 months. Children may function with less bowel as small bowel adaptation (see below) may be very dramatic. The function of the remaining bowel may also be influenced by the presence of active Crohn's disease

as well as the aforementioned presence or absence of colon since this may have a significant absorptive function.

FUNCTIONALLY SHORT BOWEL

Fistulous disease may bypass otherwise normal functional small intestine. This is usually the result of an enterocutaneous fistula, but hidden internal fistula may also be responsible. The majority of fistulas occur in postoperative patients[9,10] and are most commonly the consequence of breakdown of anastomoses. Risks for anastomotic breakdown include the age of the patient, the state of the bowel undergoing anastomosis, preoperative nutritional status and the site of anastomosis.[9] When associated with malignancy, factors including tumour fixity, presence of obstruction, previous radiotherapy, associated abscess and surgical technique all increase the risk.

The other common causes of fistulas are Crohn's disease, colorectal cancer and diverticular disease. Rarer conditions include congenital fistulas, such as a patent vitello-intestinal tract. Traumatic wounding or inadvertent unrecognised iatrogenic damage may occur during surgery. Tuberculosis may fistulate as a complication of an ileal mass, and actinomycosis is an alternative possibility. Ulcerative colitis may fistulate, but this is more commonly postoperational, and occasionally the diagnosis needs reviewing as to the possibility of Crohn's disease. Radiation damage due to small bowel being caught in the pelvic field may occur, the resulting fistulas usually being complex and entero-enteric and carrying a high mortality. Frequently, there is an associated surgical procedure contributing to the cause.

Decreased intestinal absorptive capacity

Inflammatory conditions of the small bowel, which result in non-functioning of the enterocytes, may reduce the absorptive capacity of the small bowel. These include sprue, scleroderma, amyloid, coeliac disease and radiation enteritis.

Decreased functional ability

Dysmotility conditions of the small bowel may inhibit function. This may be acute, as seen in postoperative ileus, or chronic, such as in pseudo-obstruction, visceral myopathy or autonomic neuropathy.

The detailed management of decreased intestinal absorptive capacity and decreased functional ability will not be covered, but the principles of nutritional support as described later still apply.

THE THREE STAGES OF INTESTINAL FAILURE

Three stages of intestinal failure can be recognised following the initiating event.

Stage I: hypersecretory phase
This may last 1–2 months and is characterised by copious diarrhoea and/or high stoma or fistula outputs, resulting in fluid and electrolyte depletion. The high output is contributed to by gastric hypersecretion, and all these factors result in malnutrition. Treatment is focused on fluid and electrolyte replacement. TPN is usually required to maintain nutrition.

Stage II: adaptation phase
This lasts 3–12 months, during which intestinal adaptation occurs. The amount of adaptation varies with patient age, underlying disease, extent, and site of resection. Having controlled fluid and electrolyte balance, there is a gradual introduction of enteral feeding, with the patient requiring a variable combination of enteral feeding, subcutaneous or intravenous fluids, and parenteral nutrition.

Stage III: stabilisation phase
Maximum intestinal adaptation may take up to 1–2 years and the extent and route of nutritional support will vary. The overall goal for the patient is to achieve as normal a lifestyle as possible, which means achieving stability at home.

PATHOPHYSIOLOGY

In order to manage the fluid and nutritional sequelae of intestinal failure, an appreciation of the pathophysiology of small bowel function is vital.

Fluid and electrolytes

Every day approximately 6 L of fluid enter the duodenum from gastric, pancreatic and biliary sources;

in addition, the small intestine itself secretes another litre daily. Of this, 6 L are reabsorbed proximal to the ileocaecal valve and 800 mL are reabsorbed in the colon, leaving just 200 mL of water in the faeces.

Sodium absorption in the small bowel is actively linked to the absorption of glucose and certain amino acids. Water absorption is passive and follows the sodium. The jejunum is freely permeable to water, so the contents remain isotonic.

Movement of sodium into the lumen occurs if sodium concentration is low, but absorption of sodium, and hence water, occurs only when the concentration is greater than 100 mmol/L.[11]

Normally, sodium is reabsorbed in the ileum and colon (**Fig. 17.1**). If the ileum and colon are absent, the absence of reabsorptive capacity results in dilute luminal contents with a sodium loss of around 100 mmol/L. If there is a high fistula or jejunostomy, there will be a net loss of sodium and therefore a net loss of water from the body, often amounting to 3–4 L of water and 300–400 mmol of sodium per day (**Fig. 17.2**). With increasing low sodium fluid intake, namely water, more sodium will diffuse into the jejunal lumen, followed passively by water, increasing sodium and water loss. Enteral intake will also increase sodium and water losses. Conversely, a drink containing a high concentration of sodium (>90 mmol/L) and glucose promotes sodium and water absorption by the small bowel.[11] The sodium concentration that is absorbable is limited by palatability.[12]

The colon has a significant absorptive capacity, amounting to 6–7 L of water, up to 700 mmol of sodium and 40 mmol of potassium per day, even against a steep electrochemical gradient.[13] Connection of colon in continuity with the residual small bowel will significantly reduce water and sodium losses.

Potassium absorption is usually adequate unless there is less than 60 cm of small bowel.[14] In this scenario, standard daily intravenous requirements of 60–100 mmol of potassium are required. Magnesium is usually absorbed in the distal jejunum and ileum. Loss of these will result in significant magnesium loss and deficiency. Magnesium deficiency may precipitate calcium deficiency because hypomagnesaemia impairs the release of parathyroid hormone.

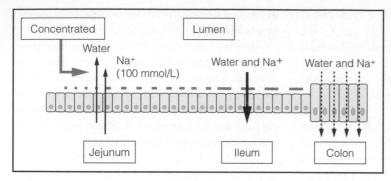

Figure 17.1 • Sodium is secreted into the jejunum and is passively followed by water. The jejunum is freely permeable to water, so the contents remain isotonic. Sodium is actively reabsorbed in the ileum and colon and is passively followed by water.

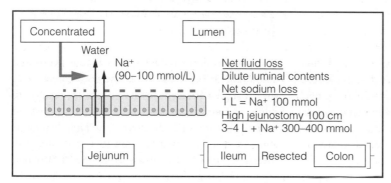

Figure 17.2 • Absence of the ileum and colon and their reabsorptive capacity results in dilute luminal contents, with a sodium loss of around 100 mmol/L. With increasing low-sodium fluid intake, namely water, more sodium will diffuse into the jejunal lumen, followed passively by water, increasing sodium and water loss. Enteral intake will also increase sodium and water losses. Conversely, a drink containing a high concentration of sodium (>90 mmol/L) and glucose promotes sodium and water absorption by the small bowel.

Nutrients

CARBOHYDRATES, PROTEINS AND WATER-SOLUBLE VITAMINS

The upper 200 cm of jejunum absorbs most carbohydrates, protein and water-soluble vitamins. Nitrogen is the macronutrient least affected by a decrease in the absorptive surface and utilisation of peptide-based diets rather than protein-based ones has demonstrated no benefit.[15] Water-soluble vitamin deficiencies are rare in patients with SBS, although thiamine deficiency has been reported.[16]

FAT, BILE SALTS AND FAT-SOLUBLE VITAMINS

Fat and the fat-soluble vitamins (A, D, E and K) are absorbed over the length of the small intestine.[17] Hence loss of ileum will impair absorption. Bile salts are also reabsorbed in the ileum and bile salt deficiency will contribute to reduced fat absorption. However, bile salt supplements such as cholestyramine have shown no benefit and may worsen steatorrhoea due to binding of dietary lipid[18] and may also worsen fat-soluble vitamin deficiency.

In view of multifactorial metabolic bone disease, vitamin D_2 supplements are often given empirically along with calcium supplements. Vitamin A and E deficiencies have been reported, but usually an awareness that visual or neurological symptoms may indicate deficiency combined with infrequent monitoring of serum levels are all that is necessary. If the patient is wholly dependent on TPN, then replacement along with vitamin K injections is required. Most patients have lost their terminal ileum and so require vitamin B_{12} replacement. Trace elements appear not to be a problem, with normal levels being found in patients on long-term TPN.

Loss of bowel results in not only decreased absorptive capacity but also rapid transit. Reduced time for absorption will exacerbate nutritional deficiencies.

Colon and colonic complications of SBS

The colon has significant absorptive capacity, not only for fluid and electrolytes as described above but also for short-chain fatty acids.[18,19] These are an energy substrate and in the region of 500 kcal may be derived in this way. It is estimated that having a colon is the equivalent of approximately 50 cm of small bowel for energy purposes.[20] The colon will also slow intestinal transit, particularly if the ileocaecal valve is present, which will improve absorption.

Having overcome the immediate problems of fluid balance and nutritional replacement, a frequent problem for those patients who still have their large bowel in continuity is diarrhoea. Excessive carbohydrate entry into the colon may result in osmotic diarrhoea.[21,22] Alternatively, choleric diarrhoea may be brought on by failure to reabsorb bile salts completely. Colonic bacteria deconjugate and dehydroxylate these into bile acids, which stimulate water and electrolyte secretion. In the more extreme cases of SBS, bile salt depletion may occur that will then give rise to steatorrhoea from incompletely digested long-chain fatty acids. Bile salts increase colonic permeability to oxalate. As the undigested fatty acids bind calcium in preference to oxalate, there is a resultant increase in enteric oxalate uptake and hence increased renal stone formation.[23]

 There is also an increased frequency of mixed gallstones, possibly because of interruption of the enterohepatic circulation.[24]

Lastly, D-lactate acidosis[25] is a rare syndrome that comprises headache, drowsiness, stupor, confusion, behavioural disturbance, ataxia, blurred vision, ophthalmoplegia and/or nystagmus. The exact mechanism is unknown. It may be provoked by a carbohydrate load and is relieved by antibiotics. Whether it is a direct result of D-lactate or whether this is a marker for some other substance is unclear. There is anecdotal evidence that neomycin or vancomycin has led to improvements.

Adaptation

Following massive small bowel resection there are changes in the mucosal surface of the remaining small intestine. Most experimental work has been in small animals such as rats. It appears that adaptation will occur only if there is enteral feeding. Patients who are wholly dependent on TPN have mucosal atrophy, which is reversed on refeeding enterally. The mechanism for this is at present unknown, but various trophic factors have been proposed. Current theory is that increased crypt cell proliferation leads to lengthening of villi and deepening of crypts, so resulting in increased surface area. Because the ileum has shorter villi it is able to adapt further, but is unfortunately more frequently resected. The stimulation to adapt appears to be threefold: (i) direct absorption of enteral nutrients leading to local mucosal hyperplasia; (ii) enteral nutrition resulting in the release of trophic hormones and a paracrine effect; and (iii) increased fluid and protein secretion with subsequent resorption, leading to increased enterocyte workload and adaptation.[26]

Another form of adaptation occurs in neonates, infants and young children, where continued developmental growth of the small intestine may make the difference between dependence on TPN and managing with an enteral diet.[27]

SURGICAL CATASTROPHE AND MANAGEMENT

Patients often develop intestinal failure in the setting of some form of surgical catastrophe. This may follow an acute event, such as a mesenteric embolus necessitating massive enterectomy, or occur as a complication following elective surgery, such as an anastomotic leak. In the latter scenario, though early surgical reintervention in the first week may be beneficial (e.g. by creating a defunctioning stoma), intervention after this and before 3 months is often fraught with danger, as the surgical environment of the abdomen becomes very hazardous secondary to adhesions. This scenario – of reoperation resulting in multiple enterotomies, closures then leaking, the patient developing enterocutaneous fistulas, and finally laparostomy – is not unusual. Prevention of this is the aim, with judicious timing of reoperation important, particularly avoidance of repeat surgery if more than 10 days after an initial laparotomy if at all possible. However, in the presence of generalised peritonitis, repeat surgery is obviously unavoidable, along with its potential complications. In the case of enterocutaneous fistulas, Chapman et al.[28] commented 'when the fistula appears there is a tendency to do nothing at first, see how bad it is going to be and by the time the full impact of catastrophe has struck, the patient is septic, anaemic, nutritionally depleted, often severely dehydrated with extensive breakdown of the skin'.

It is important to have a management strategy that can be applied to patients with intestinal failure. Certain aspects are more applicable to patients with intestinal failure associated with enterocutaneous fistulas, but the general principles are applicable to all patients developing intestinal failure. Management can be summarised in terms of the four Rs, representing resuscitation, restitution, reconstruction and rehabilitation.

Resuscitation

As discussed above, the scenarios in which patients usually develop intestinal failure are often acute catastrophes, and the very nature of intestinal failure is such that patients are often severely fluid and electrolyte depleted. In the light of this, urgent fluid and electrolyte replacement is vital. This will often have been undertaken when the patient was first admitted to hospital, prior to transfer to a specialist intestinal failure centre.

Restitution

The key components of restitution may be summarised by the acronym SNAPP, representing sepsis, nutrition, anatomy, protection of skin and planned surgery. Each is considered in turn.

SEPSIS

Sepsis is often present in patients who have developed intestinal failure and adversely influences outcome.

In a study of patients with enterocutaneous fistulas, Reber et al.[9] reported an overall mortality of 11%, with 65% of these associated with sepsis. In patients who had their sepsis controlled within 1 month the mortality was 8%, with spontaneous closure of the fistula in 48%. In those where sepsis remained uncontrolled the mortality was 85%, with a spontaneous closure rate of 6%.

Awareness of the high probability of associated sepsis is vital, and if the suspicion arises patients should be thoroughly investigated. This may include plain radiology, ultrasound or computed tomography to identify collections. Management includes appropriate antibiotics and drainage of sepsis. This is often possible radiologically, but if not it must be undertaken surgically. This may involve local surgical drainage, but can extend to formation of a laparostomy in the situation of multiple inter-loop abscesses. It cannot be stressed too strongly that sepsis must be eliminated in order for the patient to have a more favourable outcome.

NUTRITION

Not only are patients fluid and electrolyte depleted on presentation but many patients who suffer from inflammatory bowel disease are already in a state of malnutrition prior to surgery. Associated peritonitis and sepsis in a subgroup of patients increase the metabolic challenge, with the patient often developing a catabolic state, thereby worsening their nutritional status. Replacement of fluid and electolytes and nutrients, including carbohydrate, protein, fat and vitamins, is vital. Hiram Studley in 1936 commented that 'Weight loss is a basic indicator of surgical risk' and this still remains true today.

Fluid and electrolytes

Following resuscitation, fluid and electrolyte requirements will depend on the patient's losses. As described above, the first stage of intestinal failure is a hypersecretory phase, with high outputs and gastric hypersecretion. Fluid and electrolyte replacement should be by the intravenous route, with the following requirements:

Water: losses + 1 L
Na^+: losses (100 mmol/L effluent) + 80 mmol
K^+: 80 mmol/day
Mg^{2+}: 10 mmol/day

Nutritional support

Initial nutritional support should be via the parenteral route, and should be introduced only when the patient is haemodynamically stable and fluid and electrolyte replacement complete. Overall energy requirements depend on the size and weight of the patient, activity levels and metabolic status, with sepsis increasing demand. The rule of thumb is that males require 25–30 kcal/day and females 20–25 kcal/day of non-protein energy. For research purposes, more exact estimates can be made using the Harris–Benedict equation:

Male energy expenditure
$$= [66 + (13.7 + W) + (5 + H) - (6.8 + A)] + SF$$

Female energy expenditure
$$= [665 + (9.6 + W) + (1.7 + H) - (4.7 + A)] + SF$$

where W represents weight (kg), H height (cm), A age (years) and SF stress factor. However, the Harris–Benedict equation is inconvenient for daily use. Replacement should also include 1.0–1.5 kg/day of protein.

Daily requirements from the American Gastroenterological Association[29] for patients with SBS are recorded in **Box 17.2**.

Parenteral nutrition will provide calories (carbohydrate and fat), protein (amino acids), vitamins and trace elements. The volume should also be considered as part of the daily fluid requirement, with additional fluid requirements given as normal saline.

Reduction of output

Losses from stomas, fistulas or per anus may be very substantial, making replacement and simple management difficult. A number of strategies should be introduced to reduce these losses. Patients should be restricted to around 500 mL of water orally per day, as hypotonic drinks will increase output in patients with SBS as described above. They should instead be cautioned against consumption of plain

water and be given electrolyte solution, which will reduce intestinal fluid and electrolyte losses. There are several comercially available formulas. St Mark's electrolyte solution is made from 1 L of water to which is added 20 g of glucose (six tablespoons), 3.5 g of sodium chloride (one level 5-mL teaspoon) and 2.5 g of sodium bicarbonate (one heaped 2.5-mL teaspoon). This provides 100 mmol of sodium per litre. The problem is palatability, although this may be improved by the addition of orange squash or similar flavourings. The World Health Organization recommendations are similar but also contain 20 mmol of potassium chloride.[30]

Medication is also given to reduce gastric hypersecretion. H_2 receptors can reduce gastric hypersecretion,[31] as can proton pump inhibitors, but not always enough to obviate the need for parenteral fluid supplements.[32,33]

Patients are routinely started on omeprazole to reduce gastric output. Octreotide produces a similar action but is more expensive and is usually of benefit only to patients with net fluid secretion.[34] Medication to slow intestinal transit or gastric emptying should in theory improve absorption,[35] so both codeine phosphate and loperamide[36,37] are used on an empirical basis. They are given before meals and often at higher doses than normal. However, codeine runs the risk of addiction and clinical trials are equivocal as to the benefit of both,[38] so monitoring the effluent and weighing patients daily are essential for individual assessment. Bulking agents have shown no benefit in reducing stomal effluent.

Box 17.2 • Dietary macronutrient recommendations for short bowel syndrome

	Colon present	Colon absent
Carbohydrate	Complex carbohydrate, 30–35 kcal/kg daily Soluble fibre	Variable, 30–35 kcal/kg daily
Fat	MCT/LCT, 20–30% of caloric intake, with or without low fat/high fat	LCT, 20–30% of caloric intake, with or without low fat/high fat
Protein	Intact protein, 1.0–1.5 g/kg daily, with or without peptide-based formula	Intact protein, 1.0–1.5 g/kg daily, with or without peptide-based formula

LCT, long-chain triglyceride; MCT, medium-chain triglyceride.
From AGA technical review on short bowel syndrome and intestinal transplantation. Gastroenterology 2003; 124:1111–34, with permission.

Cholestyramine may be used to treat hyperoxaluria, but it has no place in those with a jejunostomy, and in those with a colon in continuity it may reduce jejunal bile salt concentration to a level below the minimal micellar concentration for absorption of fat, resulting in steatorrhoea. A review of long-term medication is always useful, paying particular heed to site of uptake. Enteric-coated tablets are unlikely to be useful.

Dietary modification

Though feeding should initially be parenteral, the enteral route is preferable. Oral feeding should be introduced gradually with additions made one at a time and assessed. Patients should remain fluid restricted and continue on oral rehydration solution, gastric antisecretory drugs and antidiarrhoeal medication, the latter taken 30–60 minutes before meals. Drinking should be avoided during meals as this increases losses. It is important to continue intravenous maintenance therapy during this time as this will reduce the pressure on the patient to drink. In the early part of the second clinical stage it may be necessary to feed the patient wholly using TPN, as gastric hypersecretion in response to even the smallest volume of enteral feeding can prejudice newly stabilised fluid balance.

 A change of eating pattern to one of 'grazing' or 'little and often' increases the absorption window for the small intestine. Alternatively, overnight nasogastric tube or percutaneous endoscopic gastrostomy feeding can utilise otherwise unproductive absorption time.[39]

If intestinal losses remain high, octreotide may be started at a dose of 50–100 µg s.c. three times daily. Oral magnesium oxide capsules, 12–16 mmol daily, are started and intravenous therapy is gradually withdrawn. Magnesium replacement may need to remain intravenous, albeit intermittent.

The precise balance between oral and parenteral requirements will vary between patients. As a rule of thumb, daily stoma/fistula losses below 1500 mL may be managed with oral replacement alone; losses between 1500 and 2000 mL require sodium and water replacement, usually as subcutaneous or intravenous fluids, but no parenteral nutrition; and losses of more than 2000 ml per day require parenteral nutrition. Requirements will change over time as adaptation occurs; this can continue for up to 2 years and in the case of children can be very dramatic.

Outcome aims and monitoring

Clinically, the aim is for the patient to have no thirst or signs of dehydration, with acceptable strength, energy and appearance. Biochemical targets should include the following:

Gut loss: <2 L/day
Urine: >1 L/day
Urine Na^+: >20 mmol/L
Serum Mg^{2+}: >0.7 mmol/L
Body weight within 10% of normal

The mainstays of monitoring in the first stage are those used in the normal postoperative patient (temperature, pulse, blood pressure, postural hypotension, urinary output, and daily urea and electrolytes), combined with random estimations of urinary sodium osmolality. If urinary sodium content falls below 20 mmol/L, then deficiency is likely. As the patient stabilises, fluid balance is monitored with daily weight estimation and the acute observations are reduced in frequency. A meticulous watch is kept on the input/output volumes, with specifically designed charts for ease and clarity of recording. With the fluid balance under control and the eradication of any associated septic foci, reassessment of the underlying trend of the patient's nutritional status is performed. This is done by calculating body mass indices, skinfold thickness and serum albumin, and by making an estimate of likely return to normal activities. As the patient moves into the third stage of maximum adaptation, the common nutrient deficiencies are assessed (**Table 17.1**) and the rarer complications are clinically looked for (**Box 17.3**).

Total parenteral nutrition

TPN is used either as a temporary measure to maintain fluid and energy intake while the remaining small bowel undergoes adaptation or as definitive treatment in itself. It may also be used as non-total parenteral nutrition in the third clinical stage. The advantages of maintaining some enteral nutrition, even if unable to be totally sufficient in terms of energy needs, include maintenance of normal gut

Table 17.1 • Supplementation required in patients with intestinal failure depending on whether the patient needs partly enteral or wholly parenteral feeding

Nutrient	Parenteral	Partly enteral	Route
Potassium	Yes	If <60 cm and a jejunostomy	In TPN or oral supplement
Magnesium	Common with a jejunostomy Uncommon with a colon		Magnesium oxide 12–24 mmol daily
Calcium	Uncertain	Vitamin D_2 400–900 IU daily	
Vitamin D	Uncertain		
Vitamin A	Uncommon		Watch for visual and neurological symptoms and monitor levels 3-yearly
Vitamin E	Uncommon		
Vitamin K	Yes	Normal	Monthly injections
Vitamin B complex	Yes	Normal	In TPN
Vitamin C	Yes	Normal	In TPN
Vitamin B_{12}	If terminal ileum lost (most patients)	Bimonthly hydroxycobalamin 1000 μg	
Iron	Yes	Normal	In TPN
Zinc	Yes	Normal	In TPN
Copper	Yes	Normal	In TPN

TPN, total parenteral nutrition.

flora, increased gastrointestinal adaptation and prevention of biliary sludge accumulation. With better understanding has come a willingness to maintain patients at home on TPN. This is a great advantage for those who are dependent on TPN and who have not otherwise responded to medical therapy. The benefits of the home environment cannot be overestimated in terms of morale and psychological well-being in an otherwise chronically hospitalised patient.[40] Home TPN depends upon a stable physiological condition, other medical pathology, a suitable social set-up and good patient education, coupled with a dedicated TPN team providing technical support and advice. Even then, it is not without complications, the chief among them being catheter sepsis.[41,42] Meticulous aseptic technique on the part of the team and patient is essential if this is to be avoided. It takes about 3 weeks as an inpatient for the nursing staff to teach sufficiently rigorous self-care of the feeding line. Other complications, such as catheter occlusion, hepatic dysfunction, gallstones and bone disease, may occur.[43] Guidelines to its use are well established.[44]

ANATOMY

Defining the anatomy of the clinical scenario is important in terms of both planned management and prediction of long-term outcome. This may vary from determining how much small bowel remains, which may give an indication of the likely necessity of permanent parenteral nutrition, to defining the anatomy of enterocutaneous fistulas that will enable planned surgery later. The key facts to identify therefore are small bowel anatomy, site of origin of a fistula (if present) and the anatomy of fistulous tracts.

Radiological contrast studies are the investigations of choice and may include small bowel follow-throughs or enemas, and fistulograms. Active discussion between the intestinal failure team and the radiologists is essential as each case is unique and poses different questions.

PROTECTION OF SKIN

Protection of the skin is an essential component of management of patients with intestinal failure. It is critically important and may require urgent surgery for control, thereby affecting subsequent surgical

Box 17.3 • Complications of intestinal failure

Early

- Dehydration
- Hyponatraemia
- Shock
- Hypokalaemia

Intermediate

- Morale
- Weight loss
- Immune compromise
- Peptic ulcers
- Gastro-oesophageal reflux disease
- Proximal small bowel inflammation
- Diarrhoea
- Bacterial overgrowth
- Peristomal excoriation

Late

- Vitamin deficiency syndromes
- Growth retardation in children
- Depression
- TPN-induced liver disease
- Recurrent sepsis
- Intravenous line-related complications
- Cholelithiasis
- D-Lactic acidosis
- Urolithiasis

TPN, total parenteral nutrition.

approaches. Small bowel output is caustic and excoriation of skin around a stoma or fistula is a painful, demoralising and highly visible immediate complication. The extent of the problem will vary, ranging from a standard end ileostomy, through patients with an enterocutaneous fistula, to those with a laparostomy wound and multiple open loops of small bowel visible in the wound. This requires specialist stoma care from highly skilled nurses who will use a wide variety of shaped appliances, wide-necked bags and protective dressings and pastes to protect the skin and contain the small bowel

contents. In some situations, emergency surgery is indicated to either refashion a stoma or construct a controlled proximal stoma in the presence of a more distal enterocutaneous fistula.

The resolution of wounds over time may be very significant. This is usually a factor of time, nutrition and skin protection. In the case of patients with laparostomies, there is usually significant reduction in the diameter of the wound and bowel loops become indistinguishable following growth of granulation tissue over them.

PLANNED SURGERY

Surgical intervention should be planned and frequently delayed. In the case of intestinal failure associated with enterocutaneous fistulas, early operative intervention to close the fistula is contraindicated by the associated high mortality due to sepsis, malnutrition and difficulties with fluid balance.[28] Indications for early surgery include the following:[45]

1. drainage of pus;
2. excision of ischaemic bowel;
3. laying open of abscess cavities in the abdominal wall;
4. construction of a controlled proximal stoma;
5. catastrophic anastomotic failure, by exteriorisation of proximal and distal bowel ends.

These are usually the most septic patients and there is an associated high mortality with these procedures. Only in life-threatening situations should surgery be undertaken early in these patients and the decision should not be taken lightly as early surgery can result directly in multiple complications.

Reconstruction

When considering reconstructive surgery, the aim is to have a well patient, with no signs of dehydration or evidence of sepsis and with a good nutritional status. The aim of the management described above is to produce this scenario, such that surgery can be undertaken as safely as possible. The decisions then concern when to operate and what to do.

The decision about when to operate is vital. In the 1960s, Edmunds et al. proposed that early intervention using a conservative approach was associated with 80% mortality compared with 6% mortality for an operative approach. Supportive care has changed significantly since that time, however, particularly the use of TPN. In 1978, Reber et al.[9] proposed planned intervention following eradication of sepsis. In the case of enterocutaneous fistulas, they reported a proportion of spontaneous closures, of which 90% occurred within 1 month, 10% within the next 2 months and none thereafter.

As discussed above, early surgery is made extremely difficult by the severity of the adhesions. It is important to delay surgery until these adhesions have softened, thereby reducing the risk of iatrogenic complications.

This will often necessitate a delay of 5–6 months following the patient's previous surgical intervention. Clinically, this may be indicated by the identification of prolapse of stomas or fistulas, and by the impression, on examination, that the abdominal wall is moving separately to the underlying bowel.

The second decision is what definitive reconstruction to undertake and this must be individualised. It may range from connecting an end ileostomy to the remaining colon, with the aim of bringing the colon into continuity, to specialist surgery to increase nutrient and fluid absorption by either slowing intestinal transit or increasing intestinal surface area. This is usually only considered at a stage when maximal adaptation has occurred.

Reversed small bowel segments,[46–48] colonic interposition, and tapering with small bowel lengthening[49–51] are the surgical procedures that have found clinical application. The first two attempt to slow the transit of luminal contents by antiperistaltic activity or interposition of colonic tissue. They have achieved some clinical success but run the risk of further sacrifice of small bowel, obstruction or anastomotic leakage. Tapering with small bowel lengthening has been applied in children with some success.[52] It involves dividing the dilated adapted bowel in two longitudinally, while maintaining mesenteric blood supply via careful dissection in the axis of the mesentery, allocating vessels to either segment. The bowel is then tubularised and joined sequentially.[53–55] However, no new mucosa is formed and there are risks of multiple adhesions and stenosis from the long anastomotic line.

Artificial valves, recirculation loops, electrical pacing,[56–58] tapering and plication, growth of neomucosa and mechanical tissue expansion[59] are all experimental techniques that are either untried in clinical practice or limited to case reports only.

ENTEROCUTANEOUS FISTULA

High-output proximal small bowel fistulas are associated with intestinal failure by producing functionally short bowel, and are often associated with significant problems with sepsis, malnutrition and difficulties with fluid balance.[28] Initial management is as described above.

Natural resolution of the fistula depends on the underlying pathology. Postoperative fistulas heal in around 70% of cases,[60] usually within the first 6 weeks of starting TPN. Factors preventing healing may be specific to the fistula itself, as indicated in **Box 17.4**, or general, including ongoing sepsis, nutritional deficiency, and infiltration of the tract by underlying disease such as malignancy, Crohn's or tuberculosis.

Surgical intervention tends to be somewhat 'freestyle' as, despite detailed investigations, findings

Box 17.4 • Factors influencing spontaneous fistula closure

	Unfavourable	Favourable
Anatomy	Jejunum Short and wide fistula Mucocutaneous continuity Discontinuity of the bowel	Ileum Long and narrow fistula Mucocutaneous discontinuity Continuity of the bowel
Small bowel	Active disease Distal obstruction	No active disease No distal obstruction
Enteral feeding	???	???

at surgery may be unexpected. General principles are well described.[61] The abdominal cavity is entered and the small bowel mobilised carefully as the adhesions are usually considerable. The fistula-bearing segment(s) of bowel is resected en bloc and the remaining ends of bowel reanastomosed. This includes resection of any cutaneous abdominal wall component of the fistulous tract. If an anastomosis is likely to be in an area of residual sepsis, a stoma may be used. Abdominal wall closure may be problematic and may necessitate use of Vicryl mesh in order to obtain fascial closure due to tissue loss from the abdominal wall.

Rehabilitation

The goal of therapy is for the patient to resume work and a normal lifestyle, or as normal a one as possible. This can be a considerable undertaking as the patient will generally have spent a prolonged period of time in hospital, often up to 6 months. Rehabilitation must be multidisciplinary, involving stoma care, physiotherapy, dietetics and occupational health. There needs to be detailed stoma care for patients with high-output stomas and referral to community continence service for patients with intestinal continuity and incontinence due to liquid stools. Referral to a medical social worker for assistance with social security benefits is important. A proportion of patients will need to remain on intravenous therapy, either saline or TPN. Patients must be taught how to manage their tunnelled feeding lines appropriately in order to allow them to move from a hospital environment to home.

Considerable psychological support may be required and patients should be put in contact with supporting organisations. Long-term sequelae must also be considered. This may involve long-term HPN or recurrence of the underlying disease. Long-term care will include regular monitoring and review of therapy, vitamin B_{12} replacement if more than 1 m of terminal ileum has been resected, and review of other nutrients such as zinc, iron and folic acid and fat-soluble vitamins.

SUPPORTING ORGANISATIONS

Like most chronic conditions, a supporting structure has evolved to assist in overall management.

The patient support group is Patients on Intravenous and Nasogastric Nutrition Therapy (PINNT, 258 Wennington Road, Rainham, Essex RM13 9UU). The paediatric version is called half-PINNT. Apart from the functions of providing advice and understanding from patients in a similar condition, the association also enables the borrowing of portable equipment to allow holidays away from home.

The professional supporting body is the British Association of Parenteral and Enteral Nutrition (BAPEN, PO Box 922, Maidenhead, Berkshire SL6 4SH). Keeping an overall view of intestinal failure is the British Artificial Nutritional Survey (BANS, 4 Low Moor Road, Lincoln LN 3JY), which maintains a census of patients on long-term nutritional support. Most importantly, the pharmaceutical firms that supply the various nutritional mixtures are also involved in providing and delivering the bags to patients at home; this also includes maintenance contracts that ensure continued functioning of the necessary fridges and emergency back-up in case of failure.

MULTIDISCIPLINARY TEAM

A fundamental principle of the care of patients with intestinal failure is the multidisciplinary approach of the team involved. The care of patients with intestinal failure is prolonged and involves specialist gastroenterological, surgical and nursing input. The nursing staff on the ward and in clinic, specialist nutrition nurses and the HPN team are the backbone of delivery of care to these patients and their families. The different functions of each of these groups and their separate physical locations make it imperative that all are coordinated in their approach to each patient. Failure to achieve this results in confusion and demoralisation of this psychologically vulnerable group of patients, who have been faced with prolonged hospital admission, a debilitating illness, the prospect of no longer being able to eat normally or at all and the likelihood of less than fully functional recovery. Those who do survive find it difficult to accept the major limitations to their opportunities in life, especially in the case of young adults who constitute a significant proportion of these patients. For the adolescent, a period of teenage rebellion against the strictures of medical care is potentially life-threatening. A high level of technical training in the carers is required, which necessitates a specialist centre to maintain the technical base to these skills. In addition, congenial working conditions will help prevent high staff turnover and consequent loss of skills. Coordination is achieved by a sense of team purpose and familiarity, consultant-led weekly multidisciplinary rounds, and a consensus approach to patient management that is explicitly stated in a protocol, but which allows flexibility for medical and social demands.

OUTCOME OF SBS PATIENTS AND SMALL BOWEL TRANSPLANTATION

Around two patients per million commence HPN and 50% are suitable for consideration of small bowel transplantation. In the UK, this results in a possible 50 cases per year (50% children). A study of 124 consecutive adult SBS patients with non-malignant disease at two centres in France reported survival of 86% at 2 years and 75% at 5 years.[62] Dependence on TPN was 49% at 2 years and 45% at 5 years. A review of 225 patients on HPN from the Mayo Clinic reported similar findings.[63] Small bowel transplantation remains an experimental procedure. At the last update of the international registry, 474 intestinal transplants had been performed on 446 patients in 46 different centres in 16 different countries. This included intestine-only transplants (216, 45%), combined intestine/liver transplants (186, 40%) and multivisceral transplants (72, 15%). The majority have been performed in patients under the age of 16 years (62%).[64] The most recent evaluation has reported a 1-year patient and graft survival of 79% and 64% respectively for intestine-only transplants, and 50% and 49% respectively for intestine/liver transplants. Long-term patient and graft survival for intestine-only transplants is 62% and 49% repectively at 3 years, and 50% and 38% at 5 years.[65] Because survival is poorer than that of patients on HPN, the indication for transplantation is SBS not maintainable on dietary supplements, and in whom TPN is no longer possible due to severe complications. These usually include lack of access sites because of central venous occlusion, or cholestatic liver disease progressing to fibrosis and cirrhosis. The possibility of gut-lengthening operations must be considered first. The portal vein must be patent and should be

checked by Doppler studies, as should the other great veins, in a search for vascular access for the perioperative period.

Complications are chiefly due to graft rejection and immunosuppression. Rejection leads to bacterial translocation and sepsis in an immunosuppressed patient who is often already malnourished. Current immunosuppressives such as tacrolimus have adverse effects of neurotoxicity, nephrotoxicity and glucose intolerance. The antiproliferative agents may cause bone marrow suppression. The consequences of chronic steroid use are osteoporosis, cataracts and diabetes, and growth retardation in children. Opportunistic infections are a major problem, particularly cytomegalovirus.[66]

Recently, a report of an experimental procedure in beagles described the transplantation of ileal mucosa to the colonic lumen. This raises the possibility of autogenic allotropic small bowel mucosa transplantation. As progress is made in the understanding of immunosuppression and new agents come on line, transplantation will be a more realistic option for those who are not otherwise at risk of imminent death. However, at present TPN is the best treatment for those with severe SBS.

INTESTINAL FAILURE: CRITERIA FOR REFERRAL

The following criteria[67] are an indication of the type of cases that warrant referral to a nationally designated intestinal failure unit.

1. Persistence of intestinal failure beyond 6 weeks, without any evidence of resolution and/or complicated by venous access problems.
2. Multiple intestinal fistulation in a totally dehisced abdominal wound.
3. An intestinal fistula outside the expertise of the referring unit (e.g. recurrent in a non-specialist unit) or second and third recurrences in a colorectal centre.
4. Total or near-total small bowel enterectomy, resulting in less than 30 cm of residual small bowel.
5. Recurrent venous access problems in patients needing sustained parenteral nutrition. This definition includes recurrent severe infections and recurrent venous thrombosis where all

upper limb and cervical venous access routes have become obliterated.

6. Persistent intra-abdominal sepsis, complicated by severe metabolic derangement (characterised by hypoalbuminaemia), that is not responding to radiological/surgical drainage of sepsis and provision of nutritional support.

7. Metabolic complications relating to high-output fistulas and stomas and to prolonged intravenous feeding, not responsive to medication and adjustment of the feeding regimen. Disorders of hepatic and renal function associated with intravenous nutrition that are resistant to metabolic and nutritional supplementation.

8. Chronic intestinal failure (from whatever cause) in a hospital without adequate experience/expertise to manage the medical/surgical and nutritional requirements of such patients.

SUMMARY

Intestinal failure is a developing field. Recent developments, including HPN and a greater understanding of the pathophysiology of massive intestinal resection, have allowed clinicians to treat and maintain such patients, resulting in long-term survival. These patients are complex medical and surgical cases whose management is prolonged and multidisciplinary (**Box 17.5**). To facilitate this, the Government have set up and funded two supraregional units in England through the National Specialist Commissioning Advisory Body. One is at St Mark's Hospital in London (Northwick Park, Watford Road, Harrow, Middlesex HA1 3UJ); the other is at Hope Hospital in Salford (Hope Hospital, Stott Lane, Salford, Manchester M6 8HD). It is hoped that by concentrating expertise, progress in the care of these clinically challenging patients will be maintained.

• Key points

- There are three stages in patients with intestinal failure: hypersecretory phase, characterised by diarrhoea/high stoma outputs and fluid and electrolyte depletion; adaptation phase, during which intestinal adaptation occurs; and stabilisation phase, aiming to achieve as normal a lifestyle as possible, which will involve achieving stability at home.
- A clear understanding of normal intestinal physiology with respect to fluid and electrolyte and nutritional transport is vital to understanding the pathophysiology of intestinal failure.
- The management of intestinal failure can be summarised as resuscitation, restitution, reconstruction and rehabilitation.
- The key components of restitution may be summarised by the acronym SNAPP, representing sepsis, nutrition, anatomy, protection of skin and planned surgery.
- A fundamental principle of the care of patients with intestinal failure is the multidisciplinary approach involving specialist gastroenterological, surgical and nursing input. Referral to a specialist intestinal failure unit should be considered.

Box 17.5 • St Mark's intestinal failure protocol

Stage 1: Establish stability

1. Restrict oral fluids to 500 mL daily

Achieve and maintain reliable venous access

1. Administer intravenous sodium chloride 0.9% until the concentration of sodium in the urine is greater than 20 mmol/L

Maintain equilibrium by infusing:

1. Fluid: calculated from the previous day's losses and daily body weight records

2. Sodium: 100 mmol/L for every litre of previous days' intestinal loss plus 80 mmol (more if the intestinal loss is excessive)

3. Potassium: 60–80 mmol daily

4. Magnesium: 8–14 mmol daily

5. Calories, protein, vitamins, trace elements: only if enteral absorption is inadequate

Stage 2: Transfer to oral intake

1. Continue intravenous maintenance therapy

2. Start low-fibre meals

3. Start antidiarrhoeal medication 30–60 minutes before meals

4. Start gastric antisecretory drugs

5. Start oral rehydration solution. Discourage drinking around meal times

6. Restrict the intake of non-electrolyte drinks to 1 L daily

7. Encourage snacks and supplementary nourishing drinks, within above limits

Consider the need for enteral tube feeding

1. Start oral magnesium oxide capsules 12–16 mmol daily

2. If intestinal losses remain high, start octreotide 50–100 mg s.c. t.d.s.

3. Gradually withdraw intravenous therapy

Stage 3: Rehabilitation

1. The patient and family should by now understand the physiological changes that have occurred and the rationale for treatment

2. There needs to be detailed stoma care for patients with high-output stomas

3. Referral to community continence service for patients with intestinal continuity and incontinence due to liquid stools

4. Referral to medical social worker for assistance with social security benefits

5. If intravenous therapy cannot be withdrawn because of continuing intestinal losses (>2 L/day), teach the patient/family to perform intravenous therapy at home

Stage 4: Long-term care

1. Regular monitoring and review of therapy

2. Vitamin B_{12} replacement if more than 1 m of terminal ileum resected

3. Review other nutrients such as zinc, iron and folic acid and also fat-soluble vitamins

REFERENCES

1. Ladefoged K, Christensen KC, Hegnhoj J, Jarnum S. Effect of a long acting somatostatin analogue SMS 201-995 on jejunostomy effluents in patients with severe short bowel syndrome. Gut 1989; 30:943–9.

2. Senn N. An experimental contribution to intestinal surgery with special reference to the treatment of intestinal obstruction. II. Enterectomy. Ann Surg 1888; 7:99–115.

3. Flint JM. The extent of extensive resection of the small intestine. Bull Johns Hopkins Hosp 1912; 127–44.

4. Hammond HE. Massive resection of the small intestine. Surg Gynecol Obstet 1935; 61:693–705.

5. Mughal M, Irving M. Home parenteral nutrition in the United Kingdom and Ireland. Lancet 1986; ii:383–6.

6. Van Gossum A, Bakker H, Bozetti F et al. Home parenteral nutrition in adults: a European multicentre study in 1997. Clin Nutr 1999; 18:135–40.

7. Barri YM, Graves GS, Knochel JP. Calciphylaxis in a patient with Crohn's disease in the absence of end-stage renal disease. Am J Kidney Dis 1997; 29:773–6.

8. Pakarinen M, Halttunen J, Rintala R, Kuusanmaki P. Gut failure in pediatric and adult patients. Candidates for small-bowel transplantation in southern Finland. Scand J Gastroenterol 1995; 30:764–70.

9. Reber HA, Roberts C, Way LW, Dunphy JE. Management of external gastrointestinal fistulas. Ann Surg 1978; 188:460–7.

   Classic paper describing principles of management of enterocutaneous fistulas that remains very current.

10. McIntyre PB, Ritchie JK, Hawley PR, Bartram CI, Lennard-Jones JE. Management of enterocutaneous fistulas: a review of 132 cases. Br J Surg 1984; 71:293–6.

11. Spiller RC, Jones BJM, Silk DBA. Jejunal water and electrolyte absorption from two proprietary enteral feeds in man: importance of sodium content. Gut 1987; 28:671.

   Role of sodium and water metabolism in the small bowel critically assessed.

12. Lennard-Jones JE. Oral rehydration solutions in short bowel syndrome. Clin Ther 1990; 12(suppl. A): 129–37.

13. Fordtran JS, Rector FC Jr, Carter NW. The mechanism of sodium absorption in the human small intestine. J Clin Invest 1968; 47:884–900.

14. Nightingale JM, Lennard-Jones JE, Walker ER, Farthing MJ. Jejunal efflux in short bowel syndrome. Lancet 1990; 336:765–8.

15. McIntyre PB, Fitchew M, Lennard-Jones JE. Patients with a high jejunostomy do not need a special diet. Gastroenterology 1986; 91:25–33.

16. Alloju M, Ehrinpreis MN. Shortage of intravenous multivitamin solution in the United States. N Engl J Med 1997; 337:54–5.

17. Borgstrom B, Dahlqvist A, Lundh G, Sjoval J. Studies of intestinal digestion and absorption in the human. J Clin Invest 1957; 36:1521–36.

18. Hoffman AF, Poley R. Role of bile acid malabsorption in pathogenesis of diarrhoea and steatorrhea in patients with ileal resection. Gastroenterology 1972; 62:918–34.

19. Gouttebel MC, Saint-Aubert B, Astre C, Joyeux H. Total parenteral nutrition needs in different types of short bowel syndrome. Dig Dis Sci 1986; 31:718–23.

20. Jeppesen PB, Mortensen PB. Significance of a preserved colon for parenteral energy requirements in patients receiving home parenteral nutrition. Scand J Gastroenterol 1998; 33:1175–9.

21. Spiller RC, Brown ML, Phillips PJ. Decreased fluid tolerance, accelerated transit, and abnormal motility of the human colon induced by oleic acid. Gastroenterology 1986; 91:100–7.

22. Ammon HV, Phillips SF. Inhibition of colonic water and electrolyte absorption by fatty acids in man. Gastroenterology 1973; 65:744–9.

23. Dobbins JW, Binder HJ. Importance of colon in enteric hyperoxaluria. N Engl J Med 1977; 296:298–301.

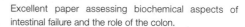
24. Nightingale JM, Lennard-Jones JE, Gertner DJ, Wood SR, Bartram CI. Colonic preservation reduces need for parenteral therapy, increases incidence of renal stones, but does not change high prevalence of gall stones in patients with a short bowel. Gut 1992; 33:1493–7.

   Excellent paper assessing biochemical aspects of intestinal failure and the role of the colon.

25. Oh MS, Phelps KR, Traube M, Barbosa-Saldivar JL, Boxhill C, Carroll HJ. D-Lactic acidosis in a man with the short bowel syndrome. N Engl J Med 1979; 301:249–52.

26. Vanderhoof JA, Langnas AN. Short-bowel syndrome in children and adults. Gastroenterology 1997; 113:1767–78.

27. Kurkchubasche AG, Rowe MI, Smith SD. Adaptation in short-bowel syndrome: reassessing old limits. J Pediatr Surg 1993; 28:1069–71.

28. Chapman R, Foran R, Dunphrey JE. Management of intestinal fistulas. Am J Surg 1964; 108:157–64.

29. AGA technical review on short bowel syndrome and intestinal transplantation. Gastroenterology 2003; 124:1111–34.

   Evidence-based guidelines from the American Gastroenterological Association on SBS and intestinal transplantation.

30. Treatment and prevention of dehydration in diarrhea diseases: a guide for use at the primary level. Geneva: World Health Organization, 1976.

31. Thompson JS, Edgar J. Poth Memorial Lecture. Surgical aspects of the short-bowel syndrome. Am J Surg 1995; 170:532–6.

    Excellent evidence-based assessment of surgical approaches to short bowel syndrome.

32. Goldman CD, Rudloff MA, Ternberg JL. Cimetidine and neonatal small bowel adaptation: an experimental study. J Pediatr Surg 1987; 22:484–7.

33. Jacobsen O, Ladefoged K, Stage JG, Jarnum S. Effects of cimetidine on jejunostomy effluents in patients with severe short-bowel syndrome. Scand J Gastroenterol 1986; 21:824–8.

34. Aigrain Y, Cornet D, Cezard JP, Boureau M. Longitudinal division of small intestine: a surgical possibility for children with the very short bowel syndrome. Z Kinderchir 1985; 40:233–6.

35. Nightingale JM, Kamm MA, van der Sijp JR et al. Disturbed gastric emptying in the short bowel syndrome. Evidence for a 'colonic brake'. Gut 1993; 34:1171–6.

36. Schlemminger R, Lottermoser S, Sostmann H, Kohler H, Nustede R, Schafmayer A. Metabolic parameters and neurotensin liberation after resection of the small intestine, syngeneic and allogeneic segment transplantation in the rat. Langenbecks Archiv Chir 1993; 378:265–72.

37. Farthing MJ. Octreotide in dumping and short bowel syndromes. Digestion 1993; 54(suppl. 1): 47–52.

38. Rodrigues CA, Lennard-Jones JE, Thompson DG, Farthing MJ. The effects of octreotide, soy polysaccharide, codeine and loperamide on nutrient, fluid and electrolyte absorption in the short-bowel syndrome. Aliment Pharmacol Ther 1989; 3:159–69.

39. McIntyre PB, Wood SR, Powell-Tuck J, Lennard-Jones JE. Nocturnal nasogastric tube feeding at home. Postgrad Med J 1983; 59:767–9.

    Value of utilisation of 'wasted' nocturnal time for feeding.

40. Gulledge AD, Gipson WT, Steiger E, Hooley R, Srp F. Home parenteral nutrition for the short bowel syndrome. Psychological issues. Gen Hosp Psychiatry 1980; 2:271–81.

41. Kurkchubasche AG, Smith SD, Rowe MI. Catheter sepsis in short-bowel syndrome. Arch Surg 1992; 127:21–4.

42. Lake AM, Kleinman RE, Walker WA. Enteric alimentation in specialized gastrointestinal problems: an alternative to total parenteral nutrition. Adv Pediatr 1981; 28:319–39.

43. Foldes J, Rimon B, Muggia-Sullam M et al. Progressive bone loss during long-term home total parenteral nutrition. J Parenter Enteral Nutr 1990; 14:139–42.

44. Anonymous. Guidelines in the use of total parenteral nutrition in hospital patients. J Parenter Enteral Nutr 1987; 10:441–5.

45. Keighley MRB. Intestinal fistula. In: Keighley MRB, Williams NS (eds) Surgery of the anus, rectum and colon. London: WB Saunders, 1993; pp. 2014–43.

46. Pigot F, Messing B, Chaussade S, Pfeiffer A, Pouliquen X, Jian R. Severe short bowel syndrome with a surgically reversed small bowel segment. Dig Dis Sci 1990; 35:137–44.

47. Panis Y, Messing B, Rivet P et al. Segmental reversal of the small bowel as an alternative to intestinal transplantation in patients with short bowel syndrome. Ann Surg 1997; 225:401–7.

48. Hennessy K. Nutritional support and gastrointestinal disease. Nurs Clin North Am 1989; 24:373–82.

49. Thompson JS, Pinch LW, Murray N, Vanderhoof JA, Schultz LR. Experience with intestinal lengthening for the short-bowel syndrome. J Pediatr Surg 1991; 26:721–4.

50. Thompson JS, Vanderhoof JA, Antonson DL. Intestinal tapering and lengthening for short bowel syndrome. J Pediatr Gastroenterol Nutr 1985; 4:495–7.

51. Weinberg GD, Matalon TA, Brunner MC, Patel SK, Sandler R. Bleeding stomal varices: treatment with a transjugular intrahepatic portosystemic shunt in two pediatric patients. J Vasc Intervent Radiol 1995; 6:233–6.

52. Bianchi A. Longitudinal intestinal lengthening and tailoring: results in 20 children. J R Soc Med 1997; 90:429–32.

53. Pokorny WJ, Fowler CL. Isoperistaltic intestinal lengthening for short bowel syndrome. Surg Gynecol Obstet 1991; 172:39–43.

54. Boeckman CR, Traylor R. Bowel lengthening for short gut syndrome. J Pediatr Surg 1981; 16:996–7.

55. Dionigi P, Spada M, Alessiani M et al. Potential small bowel transplant recipients in Italy. Italian National Register of Home Parenteral Nutrition. Transplant Proc 1994; 26:1444–5.

56. Cullen JJ, Kelly KA. The future of intestinal pacing. Gastroenterol Clin North Am 1994; 23:391–402.

57. Gladen HE, Kelly KA. Electrical pacing for short bowel syndrome. Surg Gynecol Obstet 1981; 153:697–700.

58. Brousse N, Canioni D, Rambaud C et al. Small bowel transplant cyclosporine-related lymphoproliferative disorder: report of a case. Transplant Proc 1994; 26:1424–5.

59. Stark GB, Dorer A, Walgenbach KJ, Grunwald F, Jaeger K. The creation of a small bowel pouch by

tissue expansion: an experimental study in pigs. Langenbecks Archiv Chir 1990; 375:145–50.

60. Levy E, Frileux P, Sandrucci S et al. Continuous enteral nutrition during the early adaptive stage of the short bowel syndrome. Br J Surg 1988; 75:549–53.

   Paper reporting the importance of enteral nutrition in small bowel adaptation.

61. Fazio VW. Intestinal fistulas. In: Keighley MRB, Pemberton JH, Fazio VW, Parc R (eds) Atlas of colorectal surgery. New York: Churchill Livingstone, 1996; pp. 363–71.

62. Carbonnel F, Cosnes J, Chevret L et al. The role of anatomic factors in nutritional autonomy after extensive small bowel resection. J Parenter Enteral Nutr 1996; 20:275–80.

63. Scolapio JS, Fleming CR, Kelly DG et al. Survival of home parenteral nutrition-treated patients: 20 years of experience at the Mayo Clinic. Mayo Clin Proc 1999; 74:217–22.

64. Grant D. Intestinal transplantation: 1997 report of the international registry. Transplantation 2000; 69:555–9.

65. US Scientific Registry of Transplant Recipients and the Organ Procurement and Transplantation Network. 2000 Annual Report. Transplant data 1990–1999. Rockville, MD and United Network of Organ Sharing, Richmond, VA: US Department of Health and Human Services, Health Resources and Services Administration, Office of Special Programs, Division of Transplantation.

66. Pirenne J. Short-bowel syndrome. Medical aspects and prospects of intestinal transplantation. Acta Chir Belg 1996; 96:150–4.

67. Anonymous. Intestinal failure: criteria for referral. London: St Marks Hospital, 1999 (internal).

Index

diverticular disease (*cont.*)
    antibiotics, 114, 122–123, 124
    conservative, 121–122, 122–123, 125
    considerations, 111
    controversies, 120, 124–125
    dietary, 114
    follow-up, 120
    surgical *see surgical management (below)*
  misdiagnosis, 121
  mortality, 111, 122f
  pathology, 112–114
    diverticulum formation, 112, 112f
    sites, 112
  presentation, 114–116
  recurrence rates, 125
  right-sided, 111
  surgical management
    elective surgery, 114, 120, 125
    emergency *see emergency surgery (above)*
    evidence base, 112, 112f
    laparoscopic, 121, 125, 126t, 312
    operative strategies, 123–124
    recommendations, 122–124
DNA repair, HNPCC and, 26
double-Z-plasty, 215–216, 216f
doxycycline
  Chlamydia infections, 297
  gonorrhoeal infections, 298
  granuloma inguinale, 298
drug-induced disorders, constipation, 233–234
Duhamel procedure, 235
Dukes' C classification of rectal tumours, 70
Dukes' D classification of colonic tumours, 51, 59, 59t
duodenum
  fistulas, Crohn's disease, 177
  polyps, in FAP, 33, 33t
  strictureplasty, Crohn's disease, 177
Dutch Colorectal Cancer Study Group, radiotherapy in rectal cancer trial, 78, 79, 91
dysentery, amoebiasis, 299

economic issues, surgery training, 309
Eisenhammer proctoscope, 248
Ekehorn's rectopexy, 203
elderly patients, rectal prolapse treatment, 203
elective surgery *see specific conditions*
electrical sensation, measurement, 5, 6
electrical stimulation, gracilis neosphincter, 218–220, 220f
electrocautery, condylomata acuminatum, 294
electrocoagulation, condylomata acuminatum, 294
electrolytes, intestinal failure and, 323, 324f, 326
  output reduction, 327–328
electromyography (EMG), 8

incontinence investigation, 214
electrophysiology, 7–10
  electromyography, 8, 214
  pudendal nerve terminal motor latency, 8–10, 9f
  rectal prolapse, 202
  somatosensory evoked potentials, 10
  spinal motor latency, 10
  see also specific techniques
endocoil receiver MRI, 11–12, 12f, 14
endorectal ultrasound (EUS), 11
  rectal cancer, 12, 79, 315
    MRI *vs.*, 13
    prostate involvement, 69f
    role, 67
endoscopy
  biopsy, 135–136, 170
  complications, 136
  Crohn's disease, 169–170
  gonorrhoeal infections, 298
  Peutz–Jeghers syndrome, 35
  transanal microsurgery, 315–317
  ulcerative colitis, 135–136
  see also specific techniques
endotoxins, diarrhoea, 296
enemas, constipation treatment, 235
energy balance/requirements, 326–327
  male *vs.* female, 327
  short bowel syndrome, 325
Entamoeba histolytica (amoebiasis), 135, 285t, 299
enteral nutrition, Crohn's disease, 173
Enterobius infections, 274–275
enterocutaneous fistulas
  Crohn's disease, 178–179
  intestinal failure, 331–332
  spontaneous closure, 331, 331t
enteropathy, ulcerative colitis, 132
enteroperineal fistula, Crohn's disease, 182, 182f
environmental factors
  Crohn's disease, 164
  ulcerative colitis, 130
EORTC 22921 trial, 89
episcleritis, ulcerative colitis and, 134
epithelium, 1, 131
erectile dysfunction, following rectal excision, 77
erythema nodosum, ulcerative colitis and, 134
erythrocyte sedimentation rate (ESR), Crohn's disease, 168
erythromycin
  granuloma inguinale, 298
  Haemophilus ducreyi (chancroid), 297
Escherichia coli, colon cancer and, 44
ethnic variations, Crohn's disease, 163
evacuation proctography, 10, 15
exercise, colon cancer and, 44
exophytic adenomas, 42
extended abdominal rectopexy, 197
extended pelvic lymphadenectomy
  anal cancer, 103
  rectal cancer, 70–71

external anal sphincter
  anatomy, 1–2
  conservation in fistulotomy, 254
  continence role, 250
  electromyography, 8
  obstetric injury, 216
  physiology, 218
  resting tone, 218
  sepsis, 243
  two-part model, 2
extrasphincteric fistulas, 246, 247f
eye(s), ulcerative colitis and, 134

faecal continence
  anatomy and physiology, 2–3, 250
  failure *see* faecal incontinence
  preservation in rectal surgery, 74–77
faecal impaction
  anal fissures, 271
  post-haemorrhoidectomy, 269
  see also constipation
faecal incontinence, 211–230
  aetiologies, 211–213, 211t
    congenital abnormalities, 211t, 213
    constipation treatment, 236
    iatrogenic, 106, 212, 272
    neurogenic, 212, 217
    rectal prolapse, 193–194, 202
    trauma, 211t, 212
    ulcerative colitis, 132
  biofeedback treatment, 214–215
  Cleveland Clinic scoring system, 213t
  conservative treatment, 214–223
  epidemiology, 211
  examination, 213–214
  history-taking, 213
  investigations, 214
    imaging studies, 13–14, 214
    vector volume manometry, 5, 214
  medical treatment, 214, 223
  presentation, 213–214
  psychosocial issues, 211
  surgical treatment, 215–223
    artificial sphincters, 221–223, 225
    choice, 215
    failure, 224, 225–226
    plication procedures, 218
    preoperative preparation, 215
    results, 223–226
    sacral nerve stimulation, 223, 223f, 226
    Silastic implants, 221
    sphincter augmentation, 218–221, 219f, 220f, 221f, 225, 226
    sphincter repair, 215–218, 216f, 217f, 223–225, 224t
    stoma formation, 223
    total pelvic floor repair, 217–218, 225
  see also specific techniques
faecal occult blood (FOB), colon cancer screening, 47, 61
famciclovir, herpes simplex infection, 287